# THE MYELODYSPLASTIC SYNDROMES
## Pathobiology and Clinical Management

edited by
## John M. Bennett

*James P. Wilmot Cancer Center and
University of Rochester Medical Center
Rochester, New York*

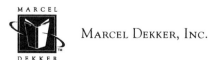

MARCEL DEKKER, INC.　　　　　　　　NEW YORK • BASEL

**ISBN: 0-8247-0782-6**
This book is printed on acid-free paper.

**Headquarters**
Marcel Dekker, Inc.
270 Madison Avenue, New York, NY 10016
tel: 212-696-9000; fax: 212-685-4540

**Eastern Hemisphere Distribution**
Marcel Dekker AG
Hutgasse 4, Postfach 812, CH-4001 Basel, Switzerland
tel: 41-61-261-8482; fax: 41-61-261-8896

**World Wide Web**
http://www.dekker.com

The publisher offers discounts on this book when ordered in bulk quantities. For more information, write to Special Sales/Professional Marketing at the headquarters address above.

Current printing (last digit):
10 9 8 7 6 5 4 3 2 1

**PRINTED IN THE UNITED STATES OF AMERICA**

To my wife, Carol, and my children, Robert, Elizabeth, and Douglas,
without whose support and encouragement over the years
my career in academic medicine and the study of hematological malignancies
would never have occurred.

To Patricia Foley,
for outstanding technical support for my cytomorphology investigations.

To the thousands of patients with MDS,
who have taught me more about life and disease
than could be found in the medical literature.

# Series Introduction

The current volume, *The Myelodysplastic Syndromes: Pathobiology and Clinical Management*, is the twenty-seventh in the Basic and Clinical Oncology series. Many of the advances in oncology have resulted from close interaction between the basic scientist and the clinical researcher. The current volume illustrates the success of this relationship as demonstrated by new insights into clinical drug resistance and means of circumventing this potential obstacle to effective cancer treatment.

As editor of the series, my goal is to recruit volume editors who not only have established reputations based on their outstanding contributions to oncology, but who also have an appreciation for the dynamic interface between the laboratory and the clinic. To date, the series has consisted of monographs on topics that are of a high level of current interest. *The Myelodysplastic Syndromes* certainly fits into this category and is a most important addition to the series.

*Bruce D. Cheson*

# Preface

The myelodysplastic syndromes (MDS) are a group of potentially acute myeloid leukemic disorders that have attracted considerable interest over the past two decades. A delicate balance exists between accelerated program cell death (apoptosis) and proliferation of the leukemic hematopoietic stem cell that permits many patients to survive for years, but when the balance shifts toward proliferation of the leukemic clone, acute myeloid leukemia (AML) develops, with a poor outcome for most but not all patients. Best estimates indicate that the incidence of MDS is at least twice as common as AML. With the vast majority of cases occurring over the age of 70 years, therapeutic options that have been available for "de novo" AML are often not utilized.

As the median age of our population increases, more cases will be recognized. In addition, the successful application of combination chemotherapy and radiation therapy has resulted in long-term remissions and cure of an increasing number of neoplasms. Unfortunately, a small percentage of these patients (varying from 1% to as high as 15%) will develop MDS/AML as a result of the therapy. This could contribute an additional 10% to the overall incidence.

Progress in understanding the pathobiology of MDS has evolved rapidly, as have an increasing number of myeloablative and supportive care strategies. In this book I have solicited chapters from many of the world's leading authorities to provide current and timely information for those involved with the diagnosis and management of patients with MDS.

The book contains 18 chapters that cover the entire range of MDS, including the recent changes in classification by the World Health Organization; a review of the incidence and prevalence of MDS; insights into possible exogenous factors that could contribute to the causation of MDS; cytogenetics and molecular genetics; the relationship between hypocellular MDS, AML, and aplastic anemia; and the critical importance of the role of apoptosis. The mid-section encompasses prognostic factors and response criteria, mechanisms of drug resistance, and a most provocative chapter on pediatric MDS patients. The final chapters discuss the importance of recognizing patients who would benefit from supportive care programs including erythropoietin, growth factors and immune modulation as well as new approaches, including anti-antigenic agents, anti-cytosine agents and new agents that appear to interfere with important biological pathways such as farnesyl transferase inhibitors. The book concludes with detailed discussions of intensive chemotherapy, auto- and allo-bone marrow transplantation, and a summary chapter on overall approaches to patient care management.

This volume provides a wealth of information by many of the world's leading authorities on the pathogenesis, staging, and management strategies on the most common neoplastic hematological disorder recognized today. It should be of considerable interest to hematopathologists, hematologists, and clinicians who are involved in the diagnosis and care of patients with MDS. In addition, scientists engaged in developing new agents for hematological neoplasms will find the chapters of considerable value in understanding the rationale for the urgent need for novel pharmaceuticals to improve the survival and quality of life for our patients.

*John M. Bennett*

# Contents

# Contributors

**Jeanne E. Anderson**   Department of Medicine, University of Washington, Seattle, Washington

**Carlo Aul**   Department of Hematology, Oncology, and Clinical Immunology, St. Johannes Hospital, Duisburg, Germany

**A. John Barrett**   Hematology Branch, National Heart, Lung, and Blood Institute, National Institutes of Health, Bethesda, Maryland

**John M. Bennett**   Professor Emeritus of Medicine, Laboratory Medicine, and Pathology, Hematology-Medical Oncology Division, James P. Wilmot Cancer Center and University of Rochester Medical Center, Rochester, New York

**David T. Bowen**   Department of Molecular and Cellular Pathology, University of Dundee and Ninewells Hospital, Dundee, Scotland

**Bruce D. Cheson**   Cancer Therapy Evaluation Program, National Cancer Institute, Bethesda, Maryland

**Theo M. de Witte**   Department of Hematology, University Medical Center, Nijmegen, The Netherlands

**Guillermo Garcia-Manero**   Department of Leukemia, University of Texas M.D. Anderson Cancer Center, Houston, Texas

**Robert B. Geller**   Bone Marrow Transplant Program, Arizona Cancer Center, University of Arizona College of Medicine, Tucson, Arizona

**Ulrich Germing**   Department of Hematology, Oncology, and Clinical Immunology, Heinrich-Heine-Universität, Düsseldorf, Germany

**Aristoteles Giagounidis**   Department of Hematology, Oncology, and Clinical Immunology, St. Johannes Hospital, Duisburg, Germany

**Lucy A. Godley**   Section of Hematology/Oncology, Department of Medicine, The University of Chicago, Chicago, Illinois

**Terry J. Hamblin**   Department of Haematology, South Hampton University and Royal Bournemouth Hospital, Bournemouth, England

**Henrik Hasle**   Department of Pediatrics, Skejby Hospital and Aarhus University, Aarhus, Denmark

**Eva Hellström-Lindberg**   Karolinska Institute and Huddinge University Hospital, Stockholm, Sweden

**Hagop M. Kantarjian**   Department of Leukemia, University of Texas M.D. Anderson Cancer Center, Houston, Texas

**Peter A. Kouides**   Hematology Unit, Rochester General Hospital and University of Rochester School of Medicine, Rochester, New York

**Richard A. Larson**   Section of Hematology/Oncology, Department of Medicine, The University of Chicago, Chicago, Illinois

**Michelle M. Le Beau**   Section of Hematology/Oncology, Department of Medicine, The University of Chicago, Chicago, Illinois

**Martha S. Linet**   Radiation Epidemiology Branch, National Cancer Institute, Rockville, Maryland

**Alan F. List**   Bone Marrow Transplant Program, Arizona Cancer Center, University of Arizona College of Medicine, Tucson, Arizona

**Dragana Milojković**   Department of Haematological Medicine, Guy's, King's, and St Thomas' School of Medicine, and King's College Hospital, London, England

**Gareth J. Morgan** Academic Unit of Hematology and Oncology, School of Medicine, University of Leeds, Leeds, England

**Ghulam J. Mufti** Department of Haematological Medicine, Guy's, King's, and St Thomas' School of Medicine and King's College Hospital, London, England

**Kazuhiro Nagai** Molecular Medicine Unit, Department of Hematology, Atomic Bomb Disease Institute, Nagasaki University School of Medicine, Nagasaki City, Japan

**Charlotte Niemeyer** Department of Pediatric Hematology/Oncology, Universitats-Kinderklinik, Freiburg, Germany

**Harold J. Olney** Hematology-Blood Bank, Department of Medicine, Centre Hospitalier de l'Université de Montreal, Montreal, Quebec, Canada

**Margriet Oosterveld** Department of Hematology, University Medical Center, Nijmegen, The Netherlands

**John T. Phelan II** Hematology and Medical Oncology Units, Rochester General Hospital and University of Rochester School of Medicine, Rochester, New York

**Martyn T. Smith** School of Public Health, University of California, Berkeley, California

**Masao Tomonaga** Molecular Medicine Unit, Department of Hematology, Atomic Bomb Disease Institute, Nagasaki University School of Medicine, Nagasaki, Japan

**Yataro Yoshida** Division of Hematology, Department of Medicine, Takeda General Hospital, Kyoto, Japan

**Neal S. Young** Hematology Branch, National Heart, Lung, and Blood Institute, National Institutes of Health, Bethesda, Maryland

# THE MYELODYSPLASTIC SYNDROMES

# 1
# Myelodysplastic Syndromes: Historical Aspects and Classification

**John T. Phelan II and Peter A. Kouides**
*Rochester General Hospital and University of Rochester School of Medicine, Rochester, New York*

**John M. Bennett**
*James P. Wilmot Cancer Center and University of Rochester Medical Center, Rochester, New York*

## I. INTRODUCTION

The first published reports (1–7), dating back to at least 1913, of what is now designated the myelodysplastic syndromes (MDS) were individual case reports and single-institution case series of refractory anemia. The reports usually contained detailed case information describing characteristic presenting symptoms, physical examination findings, peripheral blood film findings, bone marrow morphology as determined through biopsy, and clinical outcome. Typically, individuals were reported as presenting with fatigue and pallor and were found to have anemia that did not respond to "hematinic" treatment. Peripheral blood films typically showed red cell anisocytosis. Bone marrow biopsies showed unexpected erythroid lineage hypercellularity. When long-term follow-up was reported, progression to trilineage peripheral blood dysplasia was described. Final outcome in the early case reports was usually death from progressive anemia, hemorrhage, infection, or acute leukemia.

Saarni and Linman, in 1973, published the first literature review of "preleukemic anemia" (8); preleukemic anemia along with "pseudoaplastic anemia," "leukanemia," "refractory normoblastic anemia," "DiGuglielmo's syndrome," "preleukemia," "panmyelosis," and "acute smoldering leukemia" (7,9) were early terms used to describe MDS. Saarni and Linman excluded reports involving individuals with Down syndrome or having certain immunological-deficiency states, reports of identical twin siblings where one sibling had acute leukemia, and reports of individuals exposed to high levels of ionizing radiation. Ultimately, they reviewed 143 cases of "preleukemia."

Fatigue, pallor, and mucosal hemorrhage were the most frequently reported presenting features and physical examination findings documented in the review. Anisocytosis, poikilocytosis, macrocytosis (Fig. 1), normochromia, and nucleated red blood cells were the most frequently described peripheral red blood cell findings. The most frequently reported leukocyte abnormalities were immature appearing granulocytes (Fig. 1), monocytosis, and pseudo Pelger-Huet cells. Thrombocytopenia was reported in two-thirds of the cases reviewed. The most commonly reported bone marrow findings were marrow hypercellularity, erythroid hyperplasia (Fig. 2), left-shifted granulocytic maturation, and multilineage megaloblastic changes. Qualitative morphological abnormalities specifically relating to the megakaryocytic lineage were rarely discussed. Finally, in cases where outcome was reported, patients typically succumbed to refractory anemia, hemorrhage, infection, or acute leukemia.

Based on their review, Saarni and Linman proposed that these patients suffered from a primary marrow disorder that is distinct from acute leukemia and is characterized by inexorably progressive peripheral blood cytopenias, marrow hypercellularity, disordered precursor maturation, and ultimate progression to acute myelogenous leukemia (AML). The retrospective data suggested a seem-

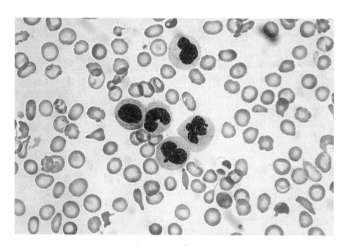

**Fig. 1** Peripheral blood: dimorphic red blood cells with hypochromia and macrocytosis. Granulocytes are hypogranular to agranular with excessive condensation of the nuclear chromatin. MGG stain. (Courtesy of J.E. Goasguen, Laboratoire d'Hematologie, Hospital SUD, Rennes Cedex, France.)

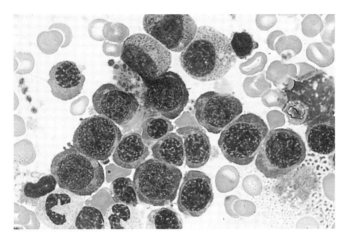

**Fig. 2**   Bone marrow: marked megaloblastoid hyperplasia. MGG stain. (Courtesy of J.E. Goasguen, Laboratoire d'Hematologie, Hospital SUD, Rennes Cedex, France.)

ingly uniform clinical picture (peripheral blood cytopenias, marrow hypercellularity, progression to AML), which would be better clarified by prospective clinical investigation and more firm diagnostic criteria.

## II.  DIAGNOSTIC CRITERIA: THE FAB SYSTEM

The development of diagnostic criteria was first addressed in 1974–1975. At that time, seven prominent hematologists [J.M. Bennett, D. Catovsky, M.T. Daniel, G. Flandrin, D.A.G. Galton, H.R. Gralnick, and the late C.S. Sultan—the French-American-British (FAB) Cooperative Group] had worked to refine the nomenclature and classification of acute leukemias. The FAB Cooperative Group identified two broad categories of "dysmyelopoietic syndrome"; one category was designated "refractory anemia with excess of blasts" (Fig. 3) and the other was designated "chronic myelomonocytic leukemia" (Fig. 4). The FAB Cooperative Group, in its original report (1976), characterized refractory anemia with excess blasts by erythropoietic hyperplasia and dyserythropoietic marrow changes, with or without the presence of ringed sideroblasts, as well as by neutropenia, the appearance of hypogranular/agranular granulocytes, and hypercellular marrow with 10–30% blasts and promyelocytes. Chronic myelomonocytic leukemia was characterized by peripheral blood monocytosis ($>1000/\mu l$), marrow hypercellularity with 10–30% blasts and promyelocytes, increased promonocytes/monocytes, and elevated serum lysozyme concentrations. In addition, the FAB Coop-

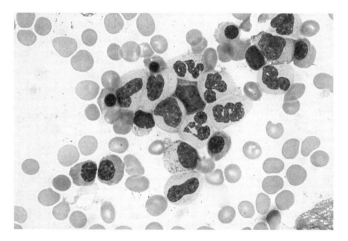

**Fig. 3** Bone marrow: megaloblastoid erythroid precursors; hypogranular myelocytes and metamyelocytes, rare myeloblasts. (RAEB). MGG stain. (Courtesy of J.E. Goasguen, Laboratoire d'Hematologie, Hospital SUD, Rennes Cedex, France.)

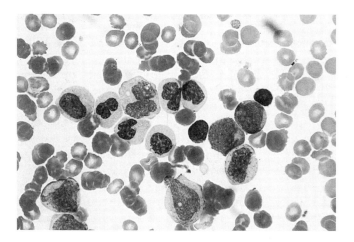

**Fig. 4** Bone marrow: hypogranular myelocytes and metamyelocytes, monocytes, myeloblasts (one with a single Auer rod) (CMML in transformation). MGG stain. (Courtesy of J.E. Goasguen, Laboratoire d'Hematologie, Hospital SUD, Rennes Cedex, France.)

erative Group identified "a range of conditions for which an immediate recommendation to start therapy cannot be made or may not be indicated. These are disorders associated with bone-marrow hypercellularity in which confusion with acute myeloid leukaemia is possible" (10).

By 1982, the FAB Cooperative Group acknowledged that "it has become clear that the range of morphologic appearances in the PB [peripheral blood] and BM [bone marrow] consistent with a diagnosis of MDS [not dysmyelopoietic syndrome as first reported in 1976] is very wide, that there is a great variation in the risk of transformation to a blastic phase, and that the risk appears to be correlated with the morphologic features" (11). In addition, the two broad categories defined in 1976 (refractory anemia with excess blasts and chronic myelomonocytic leukemia) did not incorporate well-defined features for predicting progression to AML. Because of these issues, the FAB Cooperative Group examined more cases of MDS (as defined by their 1976 criteria) to determine whether morphological features could be used to differentiate subtypes according to the likelihood of the MDS transforming to AML. This process, conducted from 1980 to 1982, resulted in definition of the five FAB subtypes of MDS in use today: refractory anemia (RA), refractory anemia with ringed sideroblasts (RARS), refractory anemia with excess blasts (RAEB), refractory anemia with excess blasts in transformation (RAEB-t), and chronic myelomonocytic leukemia (CMML) (11). The 1982 revisions:

1.  Changed the definition of RAEB to >5–20% blasts in the marrow and <5% blasts in the peripheral blood.
2.  Added the RAEB-t category to define patients who, in the FAB Cooperative Group's experience, were at greater risk than those with RAEB for developing AML. RAEB-t was defined as ≥5% blasts in the peripheral blood, ≥20–30% blasts in the bone marrow, or Auer rods in the peripheral blood or bone marrow granulocytic precursors.
3.  Redefined AML as >30% marrow blasts.
4.  Added RARS, a category for patients with a slightly poorer prognosis than those with RA, and defined RARS as <1% peripheral blood blasts, <5% marrow blasts, and >15% ringed sideroblasts in the marrow (Fig. 5).
5.  Included specific cytological and histochemical features to record when analyzing MDS cases, such as:

Marrow and peripheral blood blasts (%)
Dyserythropoietic features:
  ringed sideroblasts (%)
  nucleated red cells
  multinuclearity
  nuclear fragments

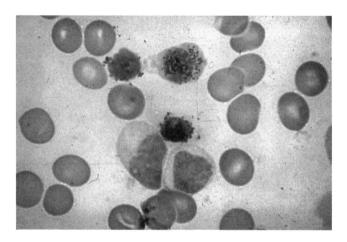

**Fig. 5**  Bone marrow: ringed sideroblasts. Prussian Blue stain.

      nucleocytoplasmic abnormalities
      erythroblasts (%)
Dysmegakaryocytopoietic features:
      micromegakaryocytes (Fig. 6)
      large mononuclear forms
      multiple small nuclei
      reduced numbers
Dysgranulopoietic features:
      nuclear abnormalities
      hypogranular cytoplasm
      Auer rods
Monocytosis
Hyper/hypocellularity

    The FAB classification system proved to be a milestone in the study of myelodysplastic syndromes. This system laid the conceptual groundwork for further study of the biology of MDS. Furthermore, worldwide clinical experience with the FAB classification system since its 1982 publication has validated the original reported findings of risk for AML correlating with marrow and peripheral blood morphology (11–13).

    Despite these advances, the FAB classification system is not all-encompassing. Hypoplastic MDS, childhood MDS, treatment-related MDS, and difficult-to-categorize transitional forms are not readily incorporated or addressed by

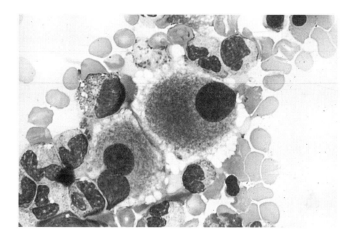

**Fig. 6** Bone marrow: micromegakaryocytes. MGG stain. (Courtesy of J.E. Goasguen, Laboratoire d'Hematologie, Hospital SUD, Rennes Cedex, France.)

the FAB classification system; these entities, however, comprise a small portion of reported MDS cases. In addition, within-class variability for survival was large, with some patients living many years with minimal or no treatment. Therefore, additional objective prognostic criteria were needed to risk-stratify patients.

## III. OTHER SCORING SYSTEMS

To address this need, studies (14–20) were carried out between 1982 and 1996 to facilitate development of scoring systems that better predict survival of MDS patients. These studies demonstrated that:

1. FAB subtype, age (relative to 60 years) at diagnosis, amount of marrow blasts ($<$ or $\geq 5\%$), and peripheral blood cytopenias (particularly a platelet count of $\leq 100,000/\mu l$) significantly correlated with survival in multivariate regression analysis.
2. Survival for patients having RA and RARS was significantly better than for those having RAEB and RAEB-t.
3. Occurrence of abnormal localization of immature myeloid precursors significantly correlated with survival, FAB subtype, AML evolution, and presence/absence of marrow blasts.
4. RA showed an increased frequency of evolution to AML relative to that of RARS.

Also throughout the late 1980s and into the 1990s, the prognostic significance of cytogenetic analysis in predicting MDS clinical outcome became more
widely appreciated (21,22). However, there were few multi-institutional studies
(23,24) in which well-defined clinical and cytogenetic parameters were evaluated
as predictors of clinical outcomes for MDS patients. For this reason, Greenberg et
al. (25) analyzed multiple clinical, demographic, hematological, and cytogenetic
variables in 816 primary MDS patients from centers in Japan, the United States,
United Kingdom, and Europe. Univariate analysis showed that the major variables predictive of survival were: FAB classification, percentage of bone marrow
blasts, number of cytopenias, cytogenetic pattern, age, and gender. Variables predictive of AML evolution were: FAB classification, percentage of marrow blasts,
cytogenetic pattern, and number of cytopenias. Specifically, poor outcome was
noted for patients with RAEB (greater than 10% marrow blasts) or RAEB-t, two
to three peripheral blood cytopenias, or "poor" cytogenetics, defined as complex
cytogenetic abnormalities ($\geq$3 chromosomal anomalies) or chromosome 7 anomalies. However, relatively "good" outcome was noted for individuals with normal cytogenetics or with del(5q) only, del(20q) only, and $-$Y only. All other
cytogenetic patterns were designated "intermediate."

Multivariate analysis showed that the most significant independent variables for determining outcome were percentage of marrow blasts, number of
cytopenias, cytogenetic subgroup (good, intermediate, poor), and gender. Marrow
blast percentage, number of cytopenias, and cytogenetic subgroup were then chosen as the final set of variables for a prognostic model; these variables were
chosen on both clinical and statistical grounds in that they were significant for
both survival and AML evolution. Risk scores were generated for each significant
variable and a scoring system, the International Prognostic Scoring System
(IPSS), was developed. Patients could then be stratified into four well-defined
risk groups regarding survival and AML evolution: low risk, 0; Int-1 (intermediate risk-1), 0.5–1.0; Int-2 (intermediate risk-2), 1.5–2.0; and high risk, $\geq$2.5.

When the same patients were analyzed for outcomes based upon their disease classification according to previously published prognostic systems [FAB
(Bennett, 11), Spanish (Sanz, 17), and Lille (Morel, 20)], the IPSS showed greater
discrimination between good- and poor-prognosis patients (smaller probability,
*p*, of error). This was in spite of more stringent entry criteria (i.e., previously
treated patients excluded) in the IPSS study. (The sole exception to greater discrimination by IPSS was in regard to CMML, as patients diagnosed with CMML
were present in all four IPSS risk groups.) The IPSS also better clarifies the role
of age as a prognostic factor in MDS; younger patients (groupings of $\leq$60 years
vs. $\leq$70 years) in the Int-1 or low-risk groups had a greater probability of survival
than older patients or than any patient in the Int-2 or high-risk groups. This discrepancy (i.e., age effect in Int-1 and low-risk groups only) may be due to the
greater propensity of the Int-2 and high-risk IPSS group patients to develop poor-

prognosis AML, an adverse clinical outcome regardless of age. Within the low and Int-1 risk group, older patients may be more likely to die from the progressive effects of prolonged marrow failure (hemorrhage, infection, anemia, transfusion refractoriness).

Overall, the IPSS is the most comprehensive prognostic scoring system developed for MDS. This can be attributed to the broad geographic distribution of the enrolled patients, stringent entry criteria, and central review of cytogenetics by the Workshop Cytogenetics Committee of the Myelodysplastic Syndromes Foundation, which, all together, results in improved prognostic evaluation. The IPSS clarifies the prognostic significance of age and cytogenetic abnormalities in MDS. Further, it may improve prediction of MDS clinical outcome and may provide a useful framework for future study of various molecular determinants (i.e., oncogenes, cytokines, cell surface molecules) in the etiology of MDS and its evolution to AML.

The prognostic scoring systems for MDS published to date rely on the 1982 revision of the FAB classification system for morphological classification and risk stratification. However, worldwide experience with the FAB system has shown that the categories (RA, RARS, RAEB, RAEB-t, CMML) have considerable overlap and heterogeneity with regard to outcome (i.e., progression to AML, survival, and morbidity). For example, several investigators have shown that individuals with RA or RARS can differ widely with respect to AML progression, morbidity, and mortality (26,27). The RAEB category (marrow blasts ≥5–20%), like that of RA and RARS, also incorporates individuals with markedly heterogeneous outcomes (28–30). Other investigators have questioned the inclusion of CMML as a myelodysplastic syndrome; compelling observations and data have shown that many (but not all) cases of CMML have clinical and hematological features more characteristic of a myeloproliferative disorder (31–33). In addition, clinical experience over the last 18 years has shown that it is very difficult to morphologically distinguish RAEB-t from AML with trilineage dysplasia and that the outcome for individuals with >20% marrow blasts and for individuals with >30% marrow blasts (defined as AML, according to the FAB criteria) is essentially identical (29,30). Because RAEB-t is virtually indistinguishable from AML, some investigators have questioned the clinical relevance of the RAEB-t category. Finally, individuals manifesting hypoplastic MDS (as many as 10% of the cases in some registries) (34), or MDS with myelofibrosis (as seen in individuals with HIV), or treatment-related MDS are very difficult to classify according to the 1982 revised FAB system.

To better incorporate newly defined clinical entities and produce more homogeneous, clinically relevant categories, prominent hematologists and hematopathologists have collaborated under the auspices of the World Health Organization (WHO) to produce a revised MDS classification system (Table 1) (35). The salient features of the WHO system include elimination of the RAEB-t category,

**Table 1**  Myelodysplastic Syndrome Classification 2000

| Category | Peripheral blood | Bone marrow |
|---|---|---|
| 1a. RA without dysplasia | Blasts < 1%; monocytes < 1000/mm³ | Blasts < 5%; ringed sideroblasts < 15% |
| 1b. RA with dysplasia | Same + dysgranulocytes and/or giant platelets | Same + dysgranulocytes and/or dysmegakaryocytes |
| 2a. RARS without dysplasia | Blasts < 1%; monocytes < 1000/mm³ | Blasts < 5%; > 15% ringed sideroblasts |
| 2b. RARS with dyplasia | Same + dysgranulocytes and/or giant platelets | Same + dysgranulocytes and/or dysmegakaryocytes |
| 3a. RAEB-I | Blasts 1–5%; monocytes < 1000/mm³ | Blasts 5–10% |
| 3b. RAEB-II | Blasts 6–20%; monocytes < 1000/mm³ | Blasts 11–20% |
| 4. CMML[a] | Blasts < 1–20%; monocytes > 1000/mm³ | Blasts 0–20% |

RA indicates refractory anemia; RARS, refractory anemia with ringed sideroblasts; RAEB, refractory anemia with excess blasts; CMML, chronic myelomonocytic leukemia.
[a] List under other French-American-British subtypes when white blood cell count <13,000/mm³; otherwise list under myeloproliferative disorders (chronic myeloid leukemias).
*Source*: Ref. 35.

redefinition of AML as 20% marrow or peripheral blood myeloblasts, recognition that multilineage dysplasia in individuals previously classified as RA or RARS significantly impacts on prognosis, and inclusion of CMML as a myelodysplastic syndrome only if the total white blood cell count is <13,000/µl. Although discrete categories for hypoplastic MDS, MDS with myelofibrosis, and treatment-related MDS were not created, it is likely that these entities will be more readily and uniformly categorized in the WHO system than in the revised FAB system.

Germing et al. have evaluated and validated the WHO classification system for MDS (36). They retrospectively applied the WHO classification system to the data contained in the Dusseldorf MDS registry; this registry is maintained by the Department of Hematology at the Heinrich Heine University in Dusseldorf and includes data on 1600 patients diagnosed with primary MDS at the University between 1970 and 1999. All of these MDS cases had been classified according to the FAB system; 26% (418) were RA, 20% (328) were RARS, 22% (344) were RAEB, 17% (273) were RAEB-t, and 15% (237) were CMML. After reclassification by the WHO criteria, 80% (217) of the RAEB-t cases and 49% (116) of the CMML cases were excluded; this represented 21% of all cases in the registry. The 56 remaining RAEB-t cases were reclassified as RAEB-I (5–10% marrow blasts) or RAEB-II (11–20% marrow blasts). The RAEB-t patients with a marrow blast count >20% had a median survival time of 5 months, whereas those with RAEB-t, with or without Auer rods, and a marrow blast count of <20% had a median survival time of 11 months ($p = 0.05$), which was comparable to the prognosis of RAEB patients in this registry. The 121 remaining CMML patients (myelodysplastic CMML) were reclassified as follows: 22 (18%) as either RA or RARS with dysplasia, 78 (65%) as RAEB-I, and 21 (17%) as RAEB-II. The patients originally designated as having RAEB were reclassified as well, such that the final distribution was 52% RAEB-I and 48% RAEB-II.

Of the 418 original RA patients, 18 were placed in a separate 5q- category and 9 were not further considered because megakaryopoiesis could not be evaluated. Of the remaining 391 RA cases, 107 (27%) were reclassified as pure RA (refractory anemia without granulocytic or megakaryocytic dysplasia) and 284 (73%) were reclassified as refractory anemia with granulocytic and/or megakaryocytic dysplasia (refractory cytopenia with multilineage dysplasia) as put forth by the WHO criteria. Similarly for the RARS patients, seven were placed in a separate 5q- category. Of the remaining 321 RARS cases, 138 (43%) were reclassified as RARS without granulocytic or megakaryocytic dysplasia and 183 (57%) were reclassified as refractory anemia with granulocytic and/or megakaryocytic dysplasia.

Data from the newly reclassified cases were then applied to four validated scoring systems, IPSS (25), Dusseldorf (19), Bournemouth (16), and Spanish (17). As a result, risk groups were defined using these scoring systems and the new WHO criteria. Graphic plots of the risk for AML transformation for these registry patients showed that the risk was minimal in the RA/RARS-without-dysplasia groups but significantly higher in the RA/RARS-with-dysplasia groups as well as with the RAEB-I and RAEB-II groups. Median survival in the RA/RARS-without-dysplasia groups was 69 months, whereas the median survival in the RA/RARS-with-dysplasia groups was 33 and 32 months, respectively. There was no significant difference in survival by age (relative to 60 years) in the different WHO subgroups.

These retrospective data drawn from a large, well-maintained MDS registry readily demonstrate the capacity of the WHO classification system to identify relatively poor-prognosis patients (i.e., those having RA/RARS-with-dysplasia and RAEB-II) who would have been grouped with better-prognosis patients in the revised FAB system. Also, the RA/RARS-with-dysplasia categories may allow for inclusion of MDS patients who were previously unclassifiable by the revised FAB system. In addition, at least in this registry, the CMML group was eliminated and these patients were reclassified as having either a myeloproliferative or a myelodysplastic disorder and the myelodysplastic CMML patients were redistributed to other (mostly poorer prognosis) WHO categories of MDS. Overall, it would appear that when applied retrospectively, the WHO MDS criteria reduce the number of unclassifiable cases, provide more homogeneity within MDS categories, and, thus, provide more uniform and accurate prognostic data. Prospective studies are needed, however, to ensure validation of the WHO criteria as presented by Germing et al. and to provide data for future revision of these criteria.

## REFERENCES

1.  Nageli O. Handb d.Spez.Pathol u.Therop. 8. 2d ed. Vienna, 1913.
2.  Gunewardine TH. Br J Child Dis 1920; 17:9.
3.  Parkes-Weber F. Polycythaemia, Erythrocytosis, and Erythraemia (Vaquez-Osler Disease). London, 1921.
4.  Sinek F, Kohn E. Folia Haematol 1930; 42:241.
5.  Elman C, Marshall S. Lancet 1936; 2:1094.
6.  Hamilton-Patterson JL. Preleukemic anaemia. Acta Haematol 1949; 2:309–316.
7.  Dacie JV, Smith MD, White JC, Mollin DL. Refractory normoblastic anaemia: a clinical and haematological study of seven cases. Br J Haematol 1959; 5:56–82.
8.  Saarni MI, Linman JW. Preleukemia. The hematologic syndrome preceding acute leukemia. Am J Med 1973; 55:38–48.
9.  Block M, Jacobson LO, Berthard WF. Preleukemic acute human leukemia. JAMA 1953; 152:1018–1023.
10. Bennett JM, Catovsky D, Daniel MT, Flandrin G, Galton DAG, Gralnick HR, Sultan C. French-American-British (FAB) co-operative group. Proposals for the classification of the acute leukaemias. Br J Haematol 1976; 33:451–458.
11. Bennett JM, Catovsky D, Daniel MT, Flandrin G, Galton DAG, Gralnick HR, Sultan C. The French-American-British (FAB) Co-operative Group. Proposals for the classification of the myelodysplastic syndromes. Br J Haematol 1982; 51:189–199.
12. Delacretaz F, Schmidt PM, Piguet D, Bachmann F, Costa J. Histopathology of myelodysplastic syndromes. The FAB classification (proposals) applied to bone marrow biopsy. Am J Clin Pathol 1987; 87:180–186.
13. Kerkhofs H, Hermans J, Haak HL, Leeksma CH. Utility of the FAB classification for myelodysplastic syndromes: investigation of prognostic factors in 237 cases. Br J Haematol 1987; 65:73–81.
14. Coiffier B, Adeleine P, Gentilhomme O, Felman P, Treille-Ritouet D, Bryon PA. Myelodysplastic syndromes. A multiparametric study of prognostic factors in 336 patients. Cancer 1987; 60:3029–3032.
15. Foucar K, Langdon RM, Armitage JO, Olson DB, Carroll TJ. Myelodysplastic syndromes. A clinical and pathologic analysis of 109 cases. Cancer 1985; 56:553–561.
16. Mufti GJ, Stevens JR, Oscier DG, Hamblin TJ, Machin D. Myelodysplastic syndromes: a scoring system with prognostic significance. Br J Haematol 1985; 59: 425–433.

17. Sanz GF, Sanz MA, Vallespi T, Canizo MC, Torrabadella M, Garcia S, Irriguible D, San Miguel JF. Two regression models and a scoring system for predicting survival and planning treatment in myelodysplastic syndromes: a multivariate analysis of prognostic factors in 370 patients. Blood 1989; 74:395–408.
18. Tricot G, Vlietinck R, Boogaerts MA, Hendrickx B, De Wolf-Peeters C, Van den Berghe H, Verwilghen RL. Prognostic factors in the myelodysplastic syndromes: importance of initial data on peripheral blood counts, bone marrow cytology, trephine biopsy, and chromosomal analysis. Br J Haematol 1985; 60:19–32.
19. Aul C, Gattermann N, Heyll A, Germing U, Derigs G, Schneider W. Primary myelodysplastic syndromes: analysis of prognostic factors in 235 patients and proposals for an improved scoring system. Leukemia 1992; 6:52–59.
20. Morel P, Declercq C, Hebbar M, Bauters F, Fenaus P. Prognostic factors in myelodysplastic syndromes: critical analysis of the impact of age and gender and failure to identify a very-low-risk group using standard mortality ratio techniques. Br J Haematol 1996; 94:116–119.
21. Mufti GJ. Chromosomal deletions in the myelodysplastic syndrome (review). Leuk Res 1992; 16:35–41.
22. Seo IS, Li CY, Yam LT. Myelodysplastic syndrome: diagnostic implications of cytochemical and immunocytochemical studies. Mayo Clin Proc 1993; 68:47–53.
23. Guerci AP, Feldmann L, Humbert JC, Guerci O. Refractory anemia with excess of blasts: a multivariate analysis of prognostic factors in 91 patients and a simplified scoring system for predicting survival. Eur J Haematol 1995; 54:241–244.
24. Parlier V, van Melle G, Beris P, Schmidt PM, Tobler A, Haller E, Bellomo MJ. Prediction of 18-month survival in patients with primary myelodysplastic syndrome. A regression model and scoring system based on the combination of chromosome findings and the Bournemouth score. Cancer Genet Cytogenet 1995; 81:158–165.
25. Greenberg P, Cox C, Le Beau MM, Fenaux P, Morel P, Sanz G, Sanz M, Vallespi T, Hamblin T, Oscier D, Ohyashiki K, Toyama K, Aul C, Mufti G, Bennett J. International scoring system for evaluating prognosis in myelodysplastic syndromes. Blood 1997; 89:2079–2088.
26. Matsuda A, Jinnai I, Yagasaki F, Kusumoto S, Minamihisamatsu M, Honda S, Murohashi I, Bessho M, Hirashima K. Refractory anemia with severe dysplasia: clinical significance of morphological features in refractory anemia (see comments). Leukemia 1998; 12:482–485.
27. Rosati S, Mick R, Xu F, Stonys E, LeBeau MM, Larson R, Vardiman JW. Refractory cytopenia with multilineage dysplasia: further characterization of an "unclassifiable" myelodysplastic syndrome. Leukemia 1996; 10:20–26.
28. Aul C, Gattermann N, Germing U, Runde V, Heyll A, Schneider W. Risk assessment in primary myelodysplastic syndromes: validation of the Dusseldorf score. Leukemia 1994; 8:1906–1913.
29. Germing U, Strupp C, Giagounidis AS, Meckenstock G, Aul C. RAEB-T: a heterogeneous entity? Leuk Res 1999; 23(suppl 1):A169.
30. Seymour JF, Estey EH. The prognostic significance of auer rods in myelodysplasia (see comments). Br J Haematol 1993; 85:67–76.
31. Bennett JM, Catovsky D, Daniel MT, G Flandrin, Galton DA, Gralnick H, Sultan C, Cox C. The chronic myeloid leukaemias: guidelines for distinguishing chronic

granulocytic, atypical chronic myeloid, and chronic myelomonocytic leukaemia. Proposals by the French-American-British Cooperative Leukaemia Group (see comments). Br J Haematol 1994; 87:746–754.

32. Germing U, Gattermann N, Minning H, Heyll A, Aul C. Problems in the classification of CMML—dysplastic versus proliferative type (see comments). Leuk Res 1998; 22:871–878.

33. Michaux JL, Martiat P. Chronic myelomonocytic leukaemia (CMML)—a myelodysplastic or myeloproliferative syndrome? (review). Leuk Lymphoma 1993; 9:35–41.

34. Tuzuner N, Cox C, Rowe JM, Watrous D, Bennett JM. Hypocellular myelodysplastic syndromes (MDS): new proposals (see comments). Br J Haematol 1995; 91:612–617.

35. Bennett JM. World Health Organization classification of the acute leukemias and myelodysplastic syndrome. Int. J Hematol 2000; 72:131–133.

36. Germing U, Gattermann N, Strupp C, Aivado M, Aul C. Validation of the WHO proposals for a new classification of primary myelodysplastic syndromes: a retrospective analysis of 1600 patients. Leuk Res 2000; 24:983–992.

# 2
# Epidemiology of the Myelodysplastic Syndromes

**Terry J. Hamblin**
*South Hampton University and Royal Bournemouth Hospital, Bournemouth, England*

## I. INCIDENCE

### A. Difficulties in Establishing the True Incidence

The true incidence of the myelodysplastic syndromes (MDS) is not known. Because these syndromes have been recognized only recently, the *International Classification of Diseases* (ICD), 9th edition (1) did not identify them as nosological entities and therefore they tended to get lost under a disparate variety of headings. Chronic myelomonocytic leukemia (CMML), for example, was included in ICD-9, but only as a type of chronic myeloid leukemia. Furthermore, the term "myelodysplasia" in the ICD-9 manual refers to congenital defects of the spinal canal. The more specialized diagnostic manual, the *International Classification of Disease for Oncology*, suffers from the same defect, and thus it is that cancer registries, death certification, and hospital discharge data are of little value in establishing the prevalence of myelodysplastic syndromes. Indeed, the nonuniform classification scheme for MDS is exemplified by a Swedish study that found myelodysplastic syndromes recorded in Cancer Registries under five different diagnoses (2).

In addition to classification inconsistencies, another problem in establishing the true incidence of MDS is the difficulty in making the diagnosis. Especially in refractory anemia (RA), the diagnostic features may be extremely subtle. And for the new category of single-lineage RA, recently introduced by the World Health Organization (WHO) (3), this is even more so. Such diagnostic subtleties are highlighted by a study by Fernández-Ferrero and Ramos (4) demonstrating that dysplastic features occur in the bone marrow of healthy subjects, most frequently in the elderly and among smokers. These investigators found dyserythropoiesis in 0.4–7.6% of cells in subjects under 50 years of age compared with 4.0–28% of cells in subjects older than 50. Similarly, dysgranulopoiesis was found in 3.0–12.5% of cells and 6.0–29% of cells in the two age groups, respectively. A history of smoking raised the percentage of cells affected by an average of 3.7%.

The problem of establishing the true incidence of MDS is further complicated by the suggestion that some patients might have "biological MDS" without any morphological features. In 1990, Allan Jacobs coined the terms "not quite MDS" and "not yet MDS" to describe this phenomenon (5). He initiated a study to look for clonal hematopoiesis in patients who survived for a long time after having received chemotherapy for lymphoma. Although the assays have proved insensitive since skewed lyonization occurs relatively frequently in healthy women as they age (6), individual case reports suggest that "not yet MDS" is a true entity (7).

In the United States, the authoritative database of cancer incidence, mortality, and survival—the Surveillance, Epidemiology, and End Results (SEER) Program of the National Cancer Institute—does not yet require registration of MDS, and therefore reliable American incidence data are lacking. An early estimate of the incidence of MDS by Linman and Bagby (8) in 1978 suggested 1500 new cases per year in the United States, but this was limited to cases with fewer than 5% blasts in the marrow and this figure is clearly a marked underestimate.

## B. European Population Studies

In the mid-1980s, the Leukaemia Research Fund (LRF) in the United Kingdom conducted a study in 26 counties in England and Wales surveying about 16 million people (9), which is just over a quarter of the population of Great Britain. Hospital hematologists retrospectively reported cases diagnosed in their laboratories to a central registry. This method of data collection has several flaws because many patients with mild MDS are diagnosed on incidental blood tests that may not result in further investigation or hospital admission. In addition, permanent records are likely to be kept only if a bone marrow examination has been performed and older patients especially may decline this investigation. Importantly, patients aged 80 and older were not included in this study.

Nevertheless, the LRF found a much higher incidence than had been expected. A total of 1806 cases were reported during a 5-year period for an overall incidence of 3.6 per 100,000. This incidence rate, however, disguises a fourfold variation between counties, with centers that had a hematologist interested in the syndrome recording the highest incidence. More than 90% of cases consisted of individuals >55 years of age at diagnosis. The male-to-female ratio was 1.4, but owing to the greater number of women alive at older ages, the standardized, gender-specific incidence rates were even more biased toward males: 4.69 and 2.51 per 100,000, respectively. In the age group 75–79, the incidence rates were 34 per 100,000 for males and 17 per 100,000 for females.

A subsequent LRF publication (10) explored the incidence in individuals older than 80 years of age and extended the data collection period from 5 to 10 years. During the 10-year period, 1919 cases were reported among those >80 years of age compared with 3641 cases among those aged <79. In other words, 34.5% of cases occurred in an age group that comprises only 3.9% of the British population (i.e., persons older than 80 years of age). The standardized incidence rates for the >80 age group were 61.72 per 100,000 for males, 28.37 for females, and 38.85 overall. Even this is probably an underestimate as the rate peaks in the 85–89 age group at 41.7 per 100,000 and decreases in the >90 age group. There is no logical reason for the reported decline in the >90 age group other than a reluctance on the physician's part to investigate the very old.

A second major investigation to determine the incidence of MDS was undertaken by the Düsseldorf group (11). The study, a retrospective reanalysis of bone marrow aspirates, covered a 16-year period from 1975 to 1990. The catchment population studied was 1.2 million, which generated 18,416 bone marrow evaluations during the period. Of these, 584 cases of MDS could be recognized from the diagnostic reports. Prior to 1983, before the French-American-British (FAB) Cooperative Group classification scheme for myelodysplastic and myeloproliferative disorders was in use, the following diagnoses were surveyed for examples: panmyelopathy with hypercellular marrow, sideroblastic anemia, CMML, and smoldering leukemia.

In this investigation, the most reliable incidence data came from a substudy of the 547,000 people of the town of Düsseldorf itself where more accurate estimates of the denominator could be obtained. For the period 1986–1990, the incidence, at 4.1 per 100,000, was very similar to that found by the LRF (i.e., 3.6 per 100,000; see Ref. 9). The increasing incidence with age was also confirmed: in the <50 age group, MDS incidence was 0.22 per 100,000; in the 50–69 age group, the incidence was 4.88 per 100,000; and in the >70 age group, 22.8 per 100,000.

Following the publication of these seminal observations, several groups have estimated the incidence of MDS in their own communities. A Swedish study found an incidence of 3.6 per 100,000 (12) and a French study reported an incidence of 3.2 per 100,000 (13). A small study from the Basque country in France (14) found an incidence of 7.7 per 100,000 in contrast to a Japanese study (15) that found an incidence of only 1 per 100,000. Additionally, two of the counties

**Table 1**   Annual Incidence Rates of MDS as Determined by Individual Studies

| Country or community studied | Years studied | Annual incidence rate (per 100,000) | Ref. |
|---|---|---|---|
| England and Wales (LRF study) | 1984–1988 | 3.6 | 9 |
| England and Wales (LRF study) | 1984–1993 | 38.85 (for persons >80 years) | 10 |
| Düsseldorf, Germany | 1975–1990 | 4.1 | 11 |
| Sweden | 1978–1992 | 3.6 | 12 |
| France | 1980–1990 | 3.2 | 13 |
| French Basque country | 1993–1996 | 7.7 | 14 |
| Japan | 1991 | 1 | 15 |
| Bournemouth, UK | 1981–1990 | 12.6 | 16 |
| Somerset County, UK | 1985–1993 | 9.3 | 17 |

LRF: Leukaemia Research Fund.

with the highest incidence rates in the LRF study have reported their data separately: Bournemouth had an incidence rate of 12.6 per 100,000 (16) and Somerset, a rate of 9.3 per 100,000 (17). All studies, except the German one, have shown male predominance and all have shown increasing incidence with age. Table 1 summarizes the annual incidence rates for various regions as calculated in the studies discussed above.

## C.   Is Incidence Increasing?

In 1991, Reizenstein and Dabrowski conducted an opinion poll among a group of hematologists recognized internationally for their interest in MDS (2). Of the 41 surveyed, 91% felt that the incidence of these disorders had increased by at least 100% in the past 10–20 years. More than 80% felt that the rise was real and not due to improved diagnosis. They reported that the most likely cause was increased exposure to leukemogenic agents in the workplace or during medical treatment. Atomic bombs, nuclear power station accidents, automobile exhausts, and pesticides were likely culprits.

From the LRF study (9), there is clear evidence of an increasing incidence in MDS. In 1984, the standardized incidence rate was 75% of the mean, and in 1988 it was 125%. This trend was confirmed by the subsequent publication from the same group covering the next 5 years (10). In the 10-year period, the standardized incidence rate had risen from 2.38 per 100,000 in 1984 to 4.59 per 100,000 in 1993. The Düsseldorf group reported a very similar increase: an annual incidence of 1.3 per 100,000 for the years 1976–1980 increased to 4.1 per 100,000 for 1986–1990 (11). Interestingly, in those counties with highest incidence in the LRF study, no increase has been observed during the period 1980–2000 (16,17) and this has been our observation in Bournemouth as well (unreported observation).

The Düsseldorf group (18) considered whether there was evidence for increased exposure to medical or environmental leukemogens during the observation period, but felt that this explanation was not convincing. Only 31 cases were secondary to treatment with ionizing radiation or cytotoxic drugs, and in all but an additional 12 cases, exposure to significant levels of organic solvents could be ruled out. The Düsseldorf group felt that the most likely explanation for the apparent increase in incidence was a greater willingness to perform bone marrow investigations on older subjects. In 1975, patients older than 60 years of age comprised 42% of those having bone marrow aspirates compared with 54% in 1990. During the same period, the percentage of patients >80 years of age climbed from 2.5% to 9%.

The possibility that there is a large group of asymptomatic and undiagnosed patients with MDS was investigated by the Bournemouth group (16). This group had already claimed the highest annual incidence of MDS (12.6 per 100,000) of any group in the world, and had found an incidence of 89 per 100,000 in the >80 age group. From among 10,200 individuals registered with a single family-practitioner group practice of six partners located close to the hospital, the Bournemouth group identified a cohort of 2926 older than age 55. These individuals were invited to give a blood sample, either by attending the outpatient phlebotomy service or by a home visit. A total of 1388 agreed and blood samples were drawn and analyzed. Five years later, it was established that 785 of the 1388 were still alive and living in the area; these individuals were invited to give a second sample. On this occasion, 657 samples were analyzed. In the first survey, three previously unknown and asymptomatic cases of sideroblastic anemia were discovered, and in the second survey two new cases of CMML were discovered. Both of the latter patients had had normal blood counts 5 years previously.

Over the 10-year period that encompassed these surveys, an additional 10 patients from the same family practice had been diagnosed as having MDS following conventional investigation of symptomatic or unrelated disease. Of these 10, three had been too young to be included in the initial cohort study [one with 5q-syndrome, one with refractory anemia with excess blasts (RAEB), and one with refractory anemia with excess blasts in transformation (RAEB-t)]; four (two with CMML and one each with RA and RAEB) had declined the invitation to come for a blood test, while two [with RA and refractory anemia with ringed sideroblasts (RARS)] had had a normal blood count on the first occasion. Two other patients with MDS joined the practice from other parts of the country during the 10-year period.

Although the small numbers make it difficult to have great confidence in the precision of the reported annual incidence of 14.7 per 100,000 for this practice, the rate is of the same order of magnitude as that reported for the Bournemouth group overall (i.e., 12.6 per 100,000). The finding suggests that for every case of MDS known to hematologists there are perhaps two other asymptomatic cases waiting to be discovered by intensive screening.

The high prevalence of asymptomatic MDS in the elderly was confirmed by Beloosesky et al. (19), who studied 3275 patients admitted to a geriatric department for the "cognitively different" in Israel. Over a 4-year period, 245 were found to have unexplained cytopenia, macrocytosis, or monocytosis. Of these, 37 were diagnosed as having MDS.

## D.  Incidence of MDS in Relation to Other Hematological Malignancies

According to the LRF study (9,10), MDS is by far the most common hematological malignancy in the very old, three times as common as acute myeloid leukemia (AML), twice as common as chronic lymphocytic leukemia (CLL) and myeloma, and more common than all non-Hodgkin's lymphomas put together. MDS becomes more common than AML when age increases above 65 years; MDS and AML are equally common among those 60–64 years of age; and AML is more common among those younger than age 60. The Düsseldorf group found MDS to be twice as common as AML for the general population, and three times as common for the >70 age group (11). In Sweden (12), the two conditions were thought to be equally common whereas in Bournemouth county, MDS was believed to be six times as common as AML (16).

In the new WHO classification (4), most AML in the elderly is included as AML/MDS and is considered to be part of the same disease process as MDS. Thus, the distinction between the two disorders will simply reflect how assiduously asymptomatic cases are sought.

## E.  MDS Incidence in Childhood

Childhood MDS will be considered in detail in Chapter 12, but a brief reference to its epidemiology is appropriate here. In the LRF study (9,10), childhood MDS was found to be very rare with only 21 cases reported in the <20 age group for the entire 10-year period. This is probably an underestimate owing to diagnostic confusion as the classification of childhood MDS is still developing.

Although cases of MDS similar to adult MDS are seen in children, two other MDS-like syndromes are more common: juvenile myelomonocytic leukemia (JMML) and transient myeloproliferative syndrome. JMML is quite unlike

CMML (20) and is almost always seen in patients under 5 years of age, with a strong male predominance. Transient myeloproliferative syndrome is seen in perhaps 10% of newborns with Down syndrome (21). Although some authors also segregate a specific monosomy 7 syndrome, it seems to this author to be insufficiently distinct to sustain a separate classification.

## II. PREDISPOSING CAUSES

Most cases of MDS are idiopathic. In a few cases, a preexisting hematological disease, such as aplastic anemia (22) or paroxysmal nocturnal hemoglobinuria (23), can be identified and therapy-related MDS following treatment for other cancers is well recognized. However, an exploration of the genetic and environmental predisposing factors for primary MDS provides clues to its etiology.

## A. Genetic Factors

Childhood MDS is commonly preceded by predisposing genetic disorders, including Down syndrome and transient myeloproliferative disorder, as mentioned above. Several other syndromes associated with obscure eponyms have also been associated with MDS. Both Shwachman-Diamond syndrome and Noonan syndrome may predispose to MDS. Shwachman-Diamond syndrome (24) is an autosomal recessive disorder characterized by pancreatic insufficiency, metaphyseal dysostosis, and bone marrow dysfunction. Noonan syndrome (25) is a major dysmorphic syndrome with craniofacial abnormalities, cardiac abnormalities, hypertelorism, webbed neck, and fetal pads on fingers and toes. Note that some confusion may arise with a syndrome that goes by the same acronym as MDS and that is also associated with a cytogenetic abnormality involving the short arm of chromosome 17. The Miller-Dieker syndrome (26) consists of lissencephaly, abnormal facies, and growth retardation. Whereas MDS and the Miller-Dieker syndrome are both associated with 17p chromosomal abnormalities, the latter is not a bone marrow disorder.

Neurofibromatosis is another genetic disorder that predisposes to MDS. Type 1 neurofibromatosis is a common autosomal dominant disorder with an incidence of 1 in 3500 (20). About 15% of patients with JMML have the clinical features of neurofibromatosis, and a further 15% have mutations of the neurofibromatosis gene *NF1* (27). Of course, JMML develops only very rarely in patients with neurofibromatosis.

Fanconi syndrome was first described in 1927 as pancytopenia with physical abnormalities (28). It is defined by characteristic chromosomal breaks after clastogenic stress. The most common physical abnormalities are skin pigmentation, hypoplastic thumbs and radii, undeveloped genitalia, and abnormalities of head and neck. About a quarter of those with Fanconi syndrome have renal abnormalities. Aplastic anemia occurs in two-thirds of all individuals with Fanconi syndrome, and MDS occurs in 2–3% of such individuals.

Dyskeratosis congenita is an inherited disease characterized by the triad of abnormal skin pigmentation, nail dystrophy, and mucosal leukoplakia (29). Most cases have an X-linked recessive form of inheritance, with an abnormal gene, *DKC1*, mapped to Xq28. Around two-thirds of the deaths among individuals with dyskeratosis congenita are due to bone marrow failure and approximately 1–2% of individuals with dyskeratosis congenita develop MDS.

Kostmann's syndrome (30) describes severe congenital neutropenia that responds to treatment with granulocyte colony-stimulating factor (G-CSF). MDS and acute leukemia are rare complications.

In general, about a third of cases of childhood MDS have an associated predisposing condition including platelet storage pool disorder, Pierre Robin syndrome, Xanthogranulomata, various constitutional chromosomal abnormalities including trisomy 8 mosaicism and abnormalities of chromosomes 5 and 7, immunodeficiencies, and congenital autoimmune syndromes (31–35).

Onset of MDS in adulthood may also have a familial or genetic basis, as demonstrated by Lucas et al. (36), who identified 5 of 193 individuals with first-degree relatives who also had MDS. Sometimes the same constitutional abnormalities on chromosomes 5 and 7 are implicated (37–39), but often no linkage is found (40–42). Occasionally, MDS may supervene in familial Pelger-Hüet anomaly (43).

An underlying genetic disorder is also suggested for those cases that seem to have been caused by environmental toxins. One example is the enzyme glutathione S-transferase, which is involved in the detoxification of carcinogens. It has been postulated that deficiency of this enzyme might be associated with a greater risk of MDS. Davies et al. (44) calculated an odds ratio of 2.0 [95% confidence interval (CI): 1.3–3.1] for the *GSTM1* null genotype in patients with AML/MDS compared with controls. Chen et al. (45) found an odds ratio of 4.3 (95% CI: 2.5–7.4) for the *GSTT1* null genotype.

Alternatively, enzyme systems required to produce leukemogenic metabolites from potential environmental toxins may also be important. Some phase I cytochrome P450 enzymes are encoded by polymorphic genes and have been associated with an enhanced risk for several cancers, presumably by this mechanism, although the increased frequency of the CYP2D5-PM allele in AML may be related to poor detoxification of carcinogens (46).

Although MDS is characterized by chromosomal deletions, it is not completely understood why such chromosome breaks occur. Nevertheless, it appears that some individuals may have an increased propensity for the induction of fragile sites by pesticides (47).

## B.  Environmental Factors

Anemic episodes preceding the development of acute leukemia after exposure to ionizing radiation were reported anecdotally in the early literature (48–50). Survivors of the atom bomb attacks in Japan exhibited features in their blood that today would be termed as MDS (51).

It is now well established that secondary MDS occurs following bone marrow injury by alkylating agents and ionizing radiation used in cancer chemotherapy regimens. (This topic is dealt with in detail in Chapter 7.) The chromosomal abnormalities found in therapy-related MDS, mainly involving chromosomes 5 and 7, are those most frequently found in primary MDS, implying that similar, though unknown, chemicals are responsible for marrow injury in such cases.

The earliest reports of an environmental toxin causing preleukemia relate to benzene (52–54). Few of us encounter raw benzene these days and a number of case-control studies have explored the possibility that exposure to common chemicals or other environmental factors might have a role in the pathogenesis of MDS.

A pilot study, evaluating a methodology previously used to establish a link between environmental exposure and solid tumors, implicated petrol and diesel liquid and vapor as well as ammonia (55). A larger, definitive study by the same group identified exposure to ionizing radiation, metals, halogenated organics, and petroleum products as significant risk factors (56). An American study found an increased exposure to pesticides and solvents among MDS cases compared with controls (57) and this was subsequently confirmed by an Italian study (58). A Japanese study found drinking alcohol to be the only significant risk factor (59), but a larger study by the same group found the risk to be confined to former rather than current drinkers, and also implicated the use of hair dyes (60). Most recently, a French study has found that agricultural workers, textile operators, health professionals, and machine operators all have a significantly greater risk of developing MDS than members of other occupations. The high risk also applies to those living near industrial plants, smokers, and those exposed to mineral oil (61).

## III.  CONCLUDING REMARKS

The interpretation of MDS incidence and prevalence data is intertwined with the etiology of MDS. Consideration of predisposing genetic and environmental factors contributes to our understanding of the epidemiology of MDS. However, as noted above, most cases of MDS are idiopathic. Thus, inconsistencies in disease classification and diagnosis constitute the most significant challenge of characterizing the epidemiology of MDS today. With the acceptance of worldwide definitions and diagnostic criteria, it is hoped that accurate incidence, demographic, and other epidemiological data can be collected.


## REFERENCES

1. International Classification of Diseases. Manual of the International Statistical Classification of Diseases, Injuries and Causes of Death. 9th ed. Geneva: World Health Organization, 1977.
2. Reizenstein P, Dabrowski L. Increasing prevalence of the myelodysplastic syndrome. An international Delphi study. Anticancer Res 1991; 11:1069–1070.
3. Harris NL, Jaffe ES, Diebold J, Flandrin G, Muller-Hermelink HK, Vardiman J, Lister TA, Bloomfield CD. World Health Organization classification of neoplastic diseases of the hematopoietic and lymphoid tissues: report of the Clinical Advisory Committee meeting, Airlie House, Virginia, November 1997. Histopathology 2000; 36:69–86.
4. Fernandez-Ferrero S, Ramos F. Dyshaemopoietic bone marrow features in healthy subjects are related to age. Leuk Res 2001; 25:187–189.
5. Jacobs A. Leukaemia Research Fund annual guest lecture 1990. Genetics lesions in preleukaemia. Leukemia 1991; 5:277–282.
6. Busque L, Mio R, Mattioli J, Brais E, Blais N, Lalonde Y, Maragh M, Gilliland DG. Nonrandom X-inactivation patterns in normal females: lyonization ratios vary with age. Blood 1996; 88:59–65.
7. Cachia PG, Taylor C, Thompson PW, Tennant GB, Masters G, Pettersson T, Whittaker JA, Burnett AK, Jacobs A, Padua RA. Non-dysplastic myelodysplasia. Leukemia 1994; 8:677–681.
8. Linman JW, Bagby GC, Jr. The preleukemic syndrome (hemopoietic dysplasia) (review). Cancer 1978; 42(suppl 2):854–864.
9. Cartwright RA, Alexander FE, McKinney PA, Ricketts TJ. Leukaemias and Lymphoma: an atlas of distribution within areas of England and Wales 1984–1988. London: Leukaemia Research Fund, 1990:32–40.
10. Cartwright RA, McNally RJQ, Rowland DJ, Thomas J. The Descriptive Epidemiology of Leukaemia and Related Conditions in Parts of the United Kingdom 1984–1993. London: Leukaemia Research Fund, 1997:9–100.
11. Aul C, Gattermann N, Schneider W. Age-related incidence and other epidemiological aspects of myelodysplastic syndromes. Br J Haematol 1992; 82:358–367.
12. Radlund A, Thiede T, Hansen S, Carlsson M, Engquist L. incidence of myelodysplastic syndromes in a Swedish population. Eur J Haematol 1995; 54:153–156.
13. Mayanadie M, Verret C, Moskovtchenko P, Mugneret F, Petrella T, Caillot D, Carli PM. Epidemiological characteristics of myelodysplastic syndrome in a well-defined French population. Br J Cancer 1996; 74:288–290.
14. Bauduer F, Ducout L, Dastugue N, Capdupuy C, Renoux M. Epidemiology of myelodysplastic syndromes in a French general hospital of the Basque country. Leuk Res 1998; 22:205–208.

15. Shimizu H, Matsushita Y, Aoki K, Nomura T, Yoshida Y, Mizogushi H. Prevalence of myelodysplastic syndromes in Japan. Int J Hematol 1995; 61:17–22.

16. Williamson PJ, Kruger AR, Reynolds PJ, Hamblin TJ, Oscier DG. Establishing the incidence of myelodysplastic syndrome. Br J Haematol 1994; 87:743–745.

17. Phillips MJ, Cull GM, Ewings M. Establishing the incidence of myelodysplastic syndrome. Br J Haematol 1994; 88:896–897.

18. Aul C, Germing U, Gattermann N, Minning H. Increasing incidence of myelodysplastic syndromes: real or fictitious? Leuk Res 1998; 22:93–100.

19. Beloosesky Y, Cohen AM, Grosman B, Grinblat J. Prevalence and survival in myelodysplastic syndrome of the refractory anemia type in hospitalized cognitively different geriatric patients. Gerontology 2000; 46:323–327.

20. Emanuel PD. Myelodysplasia and myeloproliferative disorders in childhood: an update. Br J Haematol 1999; 105:852–863.

21. Lange BJ, Kobrinsky N, Barnard DR, Arthur DC, Buckley JD, Howells WB, Gold S, Sanders J, Neudorf S, Smith FO, Woods WG. Distinctive demography, biology and outcome of acute myeloid leukemia and myelodysplastic syndrome in children with Down syndrome: Children's Cancer Group Studies 2681 and 2891. Blood 1998; 91:608–615.

22. de Planque MM, Kluin-Nelemans HC, van Krieken HJ, Kluin PM, Brand A, Beverstock GC, Willemze R, van Rood JJ. Evolution of acquired severe aplastic anaemia to myelodysplasia and subsequent leukaemia in adults. Br J Haematol 1988; 70:55–62.

23. Ishihara S, Nakakuma H, Kawaguchi T, Nagakura S, Horikawa K, Hidaka M, Asou N, Mitsuya H. Two cases showing clonal progression with full evolution from aplastic anemia-paroxysmal nocturnal hemoglobinuria syndrome to myelodysplastic syndromes and leukemia. Int J Hematol 2000; 72:206–209.

24. Faber J, Lauener R, Wick F, Betts D, Filgueira L, Seger RA, Gungor T. Shwachman-Diamond syndrome: early bone marrow transplantation in a high risk patient and new clues to pathogenesis (review). Eur J Pediatr 1999; 158:995–1000.

25. Bertola DR, Sugayama SM, Albano LM, Kim CA, Gonzalez CH. Noonan syndrome: a clinical and genetic study of 31 patients. Rev Hosp Clin Fac Med Sao Paulo 1999; 54:147–150.

26. Stratton RF, Dobyns WB, Airhart SD, Ledbetter DH. New chromosomal syndrome: Miller-Dieker syndrome and monosomy 17p13. Hum Genet 1984; 67:193–200.

27. Side LE, Emanuel PD, Taylor B, Franklin J, Thompson P, Castleberry RP, Shannon KM. Mutations of the NF1 gene in children with juvenile myelomonocytic leukemia without clinical evidence of neurofibromatosis, type 1. Blood 1998; 92:267–272.

28. Alter BP. Inherited bone marrow failure syndromes. In: Handin RI, Lux SE, Stossel TP, eds. Blood: Principles and Practice of Hematology. Philadelphia: JB Lippincott Company, 1995:227–291.

29. Dokal I. Dyskeratosis congenita in all its forms (review). Br J Haematol 2000; 110:768–779.

30. Kostmann R. Infantile genetic agranulocytosis: a new recessive lethal disease in man. Acta Paediatr Scand 1956; 45:1–12.

31. Passmore SJ, Hann IM, Stilier CA, Ramani P, Swansbury GJ, Gibbons B, Reeves

BR, Chessels JM. Pediatric myelodysplasia: a study of 68 children and a new prognostic scoring system. Blood 1995; 85:1742–1750.

32. Grimwade DJ, Stephenson J, De Silva C, Dalton RG, Mufti GJ. Familial MDS with 5q-abnormality. Br J Haematol 1993; 84:536–538.

33. Kardos G, Veerman AJ, de Waal FC, van Oudheusden LJ, Slater R. Familial sideroblastic anemia with emergence of monosomy 5 and myelodysplastic syndrome. Med Pediatr Oncol 1996; 26:54–56.

34. Luna-Fineman S, Shannon KM, Atwater SK, Davis J, Masterson M, Ortega J, Sanders J, Steinherz P, Wienberg V, Lange BJ. Myelodysplastic and myeloproliferative disorders of childhood: a study of 167 patients. Blood 1999; 93:459–466.

35. Hasle H, Kerndrup G, Jacobsen BB. Childhood myelodysplastic syndrome in Denmark: incidence and predisposing conditions. Leukemia 1995; 9:1569–1572.

36. Lucas GS, West RR, Jacobs A. Familial myelodysplasia. Br Med J 1989; 299:551.

37. Olopade OI, Roulston D, Baker T, Narvid S, Le Beau MM, Freireich EJ, Larson RA, Golomb HM. Familial myeloid leukemia associated with the loss of the long arm of chromosome 5. Leukemia 1996; 10:669–674.

38. Wakita A, Komatsu H, Banno S, Ando M, Nitta M, Takada K, Mitimo Y, Ueda R. Myelodysplastic syndrome developed in a mother and her son whose bone marrow karyotype showed monosomy 7. Rinsho Ketsueki 1996; 37:311–316 [Japanese].

39. Kardos G, Veerman AJ, de Waal FC, van Oudheusden LJ, Slater R. Familial sideroblastic anemia with emergence of monosomy 5 and myelodysplastic syndrome. Med Pediatr Oncol 1996; 26:54–56.

40. Gao Q, Horwitz M, Roulston D, Hagos F, Zhao N, Freireich EJ, Golomb HM, Olopade OI. Susceptibility gene for familial acute myeloid leukaemia associated with loss of 5q and/or 7q is not localized on the commonly deleted portion of 5q. Genes Chromosomes Cancer 2000; 28:264–272.

41. Kumar T, Mandla SG, Greer WL. Familial myelodysplastic syndrome with early age of onset. Am J Hematol 2000; 64:53–58.

42. Mandla SG, Goobie S, Kumar RT, Hayne O, Zayed E, Guernsey DL, Greer WL. Genetic analysis of familial myelodysplastic syndrome: absence of linkage to chromosomes 5q31 and 7q22. Cancer Genet Cytogenet 1998; 106:113–118.

43. Hiraga H, Yabe H, Nagai K, Nakayama S. Myelodysplastic syndrome in a patient with familial Pelger-Huet anomaly. Rinsho Ketsueki 1991; 32:1453–1457 [Japanese].

44. Davies SM, Robison LL, Buckley JD, Radloff GA, Ross JA, Perentesis JP. Glutathione S-transferase polymorphisms in children with myeloid leukemia: a Children's Cancer Group study. Cancer Epidemiol Biomarkers Prev 2000; 9:563–566.

45. Chen H, Sandler DP, Taylor JA, Shore DL, Liu E, Bloomfield CD, Bell DA. Increased risk for myelodysplastic syndrome in individuals with glutathione transferase theta 1 (GSTT1) gene defect. Lancet 1996; 347:295–297.

46. Shpilberg O, Dorman JS, Shahar A, Kuller LH. Molecular epidemiology of hematological neoplasms—present status and future directions (review). Leuk Res 1997; 21:265–284.

47. Sbrana I, Musio A. Enhanced expression of common fragile site with occupational exposure to pesticides. Cancer Genet Cytogenet 1995; 82:123–127.

48. Moreland HS. The occurrence of malignancy in radioactive persons. Am J Cancer 1931; 15:2435–2516.
49. Hamilton-Paterson JL. Pre-leukaemic anaemia. Acta Haematol 1949; 2:307–316.
50. Evans RD. The effects of skeletally deposited alpha-ray emitters in man. Br J Radiol 1966; 39:881–895.
51. Finch SC, Hoshino T, Lamphere JP, Ishimaru T. Peripheral blood changes preceding the development of leukemia in atom bomb survivors in Hiroshima and Nagasaki. In: Seno S, Takaku F, Irino S, eds. Topics in Haematology, 16th International Congress of Haematology. Amsterdam: Exerpta Medica, 1977:97–98.
52. Browning E. Toxicity and Metabolism of Industrial Solvents. Amsterdam: Elsevier, 1965:3–65.
53. Aksoy M, Erdem S, Dincol G. Types of leukemia in chronic benzene poisoning. A study in thirty-four patients. Acta Haematol 1976; 55:65–72.
54. Aksoy M. Malignancies due to occupational exposure to benzene. Am J Indust Med 1985; 7:395–402.
55. Farrow A, Jacobs A, West RR. Myelodysplasia, chemical exposure and other environmental factors. Leukemia 1989; 3:33–35.
56. West RR, Stafford DA, Farrow A, Jacobs A. Occupational and environmental exposures and myelodysplasia: a case control exposure. Leuk Res 1995; 19:127–139.
57. Goldberg H, Lusk E, Moore J, Nowell PC, Besa EC. Survey of exposure to genotoxic agents in primary myelodysplastic syndrome: correlation with chromosomal patterns and data on patients without hematological disease. Cancer Res 1990; 50:6876–6881.
58. Rigolin GM, Cuneo A, Roberti MG, Bardi A, Bigoni R, Piva N, Minotto C, Agostini P, De Angeli C, Del Senno L, Spanedda R, Castoldi G. Exposure to myelotoxic agents and myelodysplasia: case-control study and correlation with clinicobiological findings. Br J Haematol 1998; 103:189–197.
59. Ido M, Nagata C, Kawakami N, Shimizu H, Yoshida Y, Nomura T, Mizoguchi H. A case-control study of myelodysplastic syndromes among Japanese men and women. Leuk Res 1996; 20:727–731.
60. Nagata C, Shimizu H, Hirashima K, Kakishita E, Fujimura K, Niho Y, Karasawa M, Oguma S, Yoshida Y, Mizoguchi H. Hair dye use and occupational exposure to organic solvents as risk factors for myelodysplastic syndrome. Leuk Res 1999; 23:57–62.
61. Nisse C, Haguenoer JM, Grandbastien B, Preudhomme C, Fontaine B, Brillet JM, Lejeune R, Fenaux P. Occupational and environmental risk factors of the myelodysplastic syndromes in the north of France. Br J Haematol 2001; 112:927–935.

# 3

# Causative Agents in the Etiology of Myelodysplastic Syndromes and the Acute Myeloid Leukemias

**Martyn T. Smith**
*School of Public Health, University of California, Berkeley, California*

**Martha S. Linet**
*National Cancer Institute, Rockville, Maryland*

**Gareth J. Morgan**
*University of Leeds, Leeds, England*

## I. INTRODUCTION

Myeloid malignancies and related disorders originate in pluripotential precursor cells that normally give rise to red blood cells, polymorphonuclear neutrophils, monocytes, and platelets. Disruptions of the normal hierarchy of myeloid maturation result in hematological disorders characterized by either excesses or deficiencies of the mature effector cells (1). The disorders of myeloid origin include acute myeloid leukemia (AML), myelodysplastic syndromes (MDS), and myeloproliferative disorders such as chronic myeloid leukemia (CML).

The interrelationship of myeloid disorders becomes clearer when the stem cell origin of these conditions is considered. When myeloid stem cell maturation is blocked by genetic changes, the result is transformation to AML. By contrast, MDS and CML are the clinical consequences of disordered, but relatively complete, maturation (1). Although stem cells in MDS and CML vary in their capacity to differentiate toward functional cells, both conditions may transform to AML.

From the epidemiological perspective, it is important to recognize the variable antecedent history of AML. AML may arise de novo or following a myelodysplastic or myeloproliferative state, with de novo AML and secondary AML being morphologically similar in appearance. The antecedent history of AML is taken into account in the World Health Organization (WHO) classification with the designations of secondary AML (sAML), which arises following a prior MDS phase, and therapy-related AML (tAML), which arises following treatment with leukemogenic agents. Therapy-related MDS (tMDS) and tAML are part of the same disease spectrum, although the specific cytogenetic and molecular characteristics of chemotherapy-related tAML may differ according to the form of chemotherapy used (2).

## II. CHARACTERISTICS AND PATHOGENESIS OF AML AND MDS

AML is characterized by the accumulation of blasts in the bone marrow. Experimental data suggest that an early precursor or stem cell is the transformed cell in AML (3). An accumulation of blast cells (which grow rapidly and fail to differentiate) leads to substantially diminished production of normal erythrocytes, granulocytes, and platelets, and the corresponding clinical manifestations of anemia, infection, and hemorrhage. It is the extent of differentiation that determines the morphological appearance of the AML subtypes. The French-American-British (FAB) Cooperative Group classification scheme defines AML as leukemia characterized by at least 30% blasts, and recognizes eight morphologically distinct subtypes (4–6). These include M0, defined as minimally differentiated AML; M1 and M2, representing further differentiation; M3 as promyelocytic; M4 and M5 as monocytic; M6 as erythroid; and M7 as megakaryocytic in lineage.

In contrast to AML, myelodysplastic syndromes are characterized by bone marrow hyperplasia and peripheral cytopenias, and morphologically recognizable abnormal differentiation in all three blood cell lines. For certain subtypes of MDS, excess blast cells are present. (The classification of MDS is considered in detail in Chapter 1.) The FAB classification recognizes five distinct categories of MDS in adults: refractory anemia (RA, comprised of less than 5% blasts), refractory anemia with ringed sideroblasts (RARS), refractory anemia with excess blasts (RAEB, comprised of more than 5% but less than 20% blasts), refractory anemia with excess blasts in transformation (RAEB-t, comprised of 20–30% blasts), and chronic myelomonocytic leukemia (CMML). RAEB and RAEB-t can be considered preleukemic conditions because of a very high risk of transforming to acute leukemia. Childhood MDS are heterogeneous myeloid disorders that are more difficult to classify (7). To summarize, the FAB definitions for AML and MDS are based on two major features: the presence of trilineage dysplasia and the percentage of blasts.

Non-randomly occurring cytogenetic changes have been identified in AML, MDS, and CML. The Philadelphia chromosome (Ph), the hallmark of CML, was the first recognized of these abnormalities (8). The Ph chromosome is the consequence of a reciprocal translocation in which the *ABL* oncogene from chromosome 9 is transposed to chromosome 22 within the breakpoint cluster region of the *BCR* gene at band q11. The resulting *BCR-ABL* fusion gene is associated with elevated protein tyrosine kinase activity, and a CML-like disease is produced in mice receiving P210 bcr-abl transduced bone marrow cells (9). The murine CML model recapitulates important features of human CML, including transformation to AML and acute lymphocytic leukemia (ALL), suggesting that it is a true stem cell disorder. Further, recent data are consistent with *BCR-ABL* being the sole genetic change needed for the establishment of the chronic phase of CML (10). The presence of the Ph chromosome characterizes more than 90% of CML (1), 30% of ALL (11), and 1–4% of AML cases (12). It is not yet clear whether unifying aspects of the Ph chromosome are etiologically meaningful.

Cytogenetic studies of AML and MDS have shown that the majority of patients have acquired chromosome aberrations, including:

  recurrent balanced rearrangements, most commonly t(15;17), t(8;21), and inv(16)
  partial deletions (e.g., del(5q) or del(7q)), loss of whole chromosomes (e.g., −5, −7), or gains of whole chromosomes (e.g., trisomy 21 and trisomy 8)

These chromosome aberrations may be epidemiologically meaningful if determined to be related to specific exposures and not evidence of genomic instability. (Chapter 5 discusses cytogenetic aspects of MDS in detail.)

Three balanced chromosome rearrangements in particular are commonly seen in AML. The abnormality t(15;17), seen almost exclusively in acute promyelocytic leukemia (AML subtype M3) (13), results from fusion of the *PML* gene from chromosome 15 to the *RAR*-α gene from chromosome 17 to generate the *PML/RAR*-α fusion gene. This gene abnormality occurs in about 90% of AML-M3 cases (14). The abnormality t(8;21), most often associated with AML M2, occurs when the *ETO* gene from chromosome 8 is fused to the *AML1* gene from chromosome 21 (15). The inv(16) abnormality, often linked with trisomy 22 in myelomonocytic leukemia or M4 (16), results from an inversion of the telomeric sequences of chromosome 16 that generates a fusion gene of *MYH11* and *CBFb*. The molecular mechanisms responsible for translocations may provide important clues about environmental exposures. For example, breakpoints in the *MLL* gene resulting in t(11q23) differ in de novo and topoisomerase II inhibitor-induced leukemias (17).

Partial deletions and losses or gains of whole chromosomes are also seen in cytogenetic analyses of patients with AML and MDS. Interstitial deletions of the long arms or even loss of a whole copy of chromosome 5 and 7 in AML and MDS is likely to result from involvement of multiple genes. Monosomy of chromosome 7 can also be a congenital condition and is associated with a high risk of childhood MDS. Trisomy of chromosome 8 has been linked with MDS, and appears to predispose affected MDS patients to a higher risk of acute leukemic transformation (18). Similar cytogenetic abnormalities characterize de novo AML occurring in elderly persons and secondary MDS and AML (19), perhaps suggesting overlapping pathogenic and/or etiological factors. Other molecular abnormalities seen in AML and MDS include *RAS* and *P53* mutations, microsatellite instability, and endoduplications of the Flt 3 receptor (20).

## III.  DESCRIPTIVE EPIDEMIOLOGY OF AML AND MDS

### A.  Age-Specific Incidence Patterns

As depicted in Figure 1, AML incidence rates peak slightly in infancy, but then decline until age 10 when incidence begins to rise again. After age 40, incidence rises more rapidly until approximately age 70; a slower rise is then observed in incidence rates for the >70 age group. During infancy, childhood, and early adulthood, AML incidence rates are similar for males and females. However, beginning at age 40, incidence rises more rapidly among males, with rates consistently higher for males than females from middle age onward (21,22).

Incidence data for MDS are limited, since these disorders are not routinely included in most population-based cancer registries (see Chapter 2). Population-based data from regions in the United Kingdom reveal very low and flat incidence rates for MDS, all types combined, during childhood and early adolescence, with rates rising linearly during later adolescence and then increasing exponentially after age 50–60; see Figure 1 (22). Incidence rates are higher for males than females during childhood, but from midadolescence until age 50, rates for females surpass those of males. After age 50, rates for males rise exponentially, surpassing rates in females at older ages (22).

### B.  International, Racial, and Geographic Patterns

The highest age-standardized incidence rates for AML occur among Caucasian populations in northern and western Europe, North America, and Oceania, and the lowest rates are seen among Asians. Incidence rates for infants reveal that AML occurs more frequently among Caucasians than African-American infants. However, incidence rates for children are higher in African-Americans than Caucasians. From adolescence until late middle age, AML rates are similar for both sexes and all races; thereafter, incidence is higher among Caucasian and African-American males than among Caucasian and African-American females, and rates

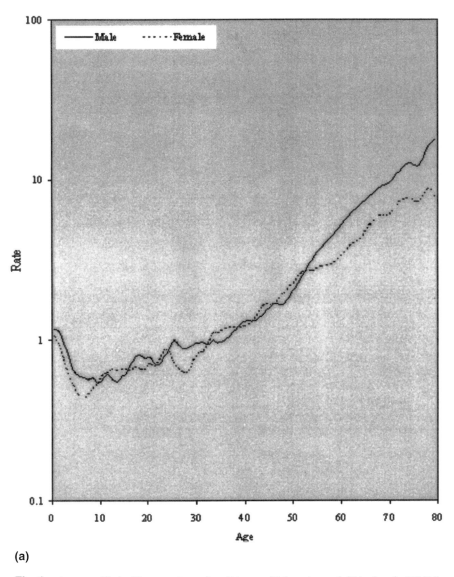

(a)

**Fig. 1**  Age-specific incidence patterns for all types of (a) acute myeloid leukemia (AML) and (b) myelodysplastic syndromes. Both frames show incidence rates per 100,000 population-years based on population data for parts of England and Wales, 1984–1993. [Reprinted courtesy of Leukemia Research Fund (22).]

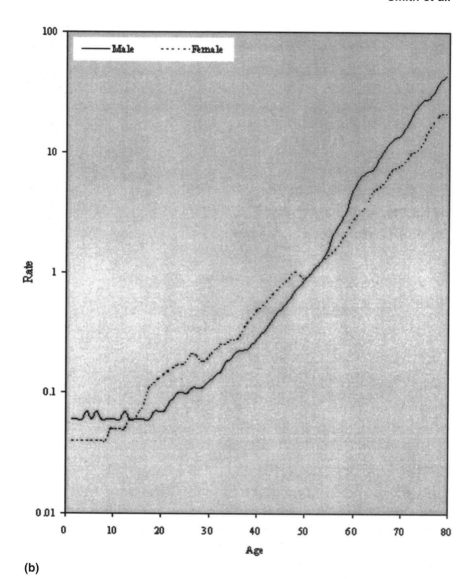

**(b)**

**Fig. 1** Continued

are higher among Caucasians than African-Americans regardless of gender. Although the limited availability of population-based incidence data for MDS precludes comprehensive international comparisons, relevant studies are highlighted in Chapter 2.

## IV.  CAUSES OF AML AND MDS

Because AML and MDS are often evaluated together (and sometimes are considered a single entity) in the same epidemiological study and because there are few epidemiological studies focusing solely on MDS, the analytical epidemiological literature on causative agents is therefore summarized together. The list of established risk factors for AML and MDS includes:

> genetic components (e.g., excess of t(15;17) among adults of Hispanic origin) (23)
>
> exposure to ionizing radiation (which directly or indirectly induces DNA strand breaks that may lead to chromosomal translocations and deletions) (24)
>
> treatment with alkylating chemotherapeutic agents (which apparently increase susceptibility to breakage at the centromere and may cause whole rather than partial chromosomal deletions in tMDS/tAML (25)
>
> exposure to benzene (with healthy exposed workers showing similar types of cytogenetic abnormalities, such as long-arm deletions of chromosomes 5 and 7, and the t(8;21) (26,27), such as those observed in tMDS and tAML (2))

Limited data from small, case-controlled studies of MDS/AML have also linked specific karyotypic abnormalities with reported exposure to paint, cigarette smoking, and alcohol (28,29). Larger studies have been difficult to interpret when risks of MDS cases with all types of cytogenetic abnormalities combined were evaluated in relation to heterogeneous exposure groupings such as all organic chemicals or all inorganic dusts (30). Similarly, it has been difficult to interpret studies of AML cases characterized by *RAS* mutations that were linked with all forms of solvent exposures combined (31) in the absence of exposure validation and replication (32).

## V.  FAMILIAL AND GENETIC FACTORS

Clinical reports of families with multiple members in different generations developing AML, MDS, or both are rare, but data support the contribution of highly penetrant mutations in leukemia susceptibility genes. Familial AML appears to be a heterogeneous disease since there is not a single karyotypic abnormality or molecular defect nor a typical age or age range at onset common to affected persons in all such families (33). Some familial AML is characterized by mono-somy 7 (34,35), whereas affected members in other families are karotypically characterized by loss of the long arm of chromosome 5 (36,37), while still others have other karyotypic abnormalities or none at all (38). The molecular mecha-nism(s) underlying occurrence of familial AML (even those with apparent autoso-mal dominant transmission) have not been elucidated. In a multiply affected fam-ily with apparent autosomal transmission of AML and loss of the long arm of chromosome 5, the susceptibility gene was not localized to the portion of 5q that is commonly deleted (39).

Similar detailed studies of the molecular features of familial MDS/AML may shed further light on the genetic mechanisms underlying hematopoietic tran-scription and hematopoietic function. Additionally, molecular abnormalities char-acterizing familial cases may also be useful in identifying genetic and environ-mental factors that predispose individuals to what appear to be sporadic cases of MDS/AML. Although a substantial proportion of children with MDS are thought to have familial MDS, data from a population-based linked registry study in Den-mark did not support this conclusion nor did the data demonstrate a higher-than-expected occurrence of all types of cancers among first- and second-degree rela-tives of children with MDS, AML, or CML (40).

It has been estimated that approximately 5% of AML/MDS cases may be associated with inherited genetic syndromes (41). Children with Down syndrome are at increased risk of developing acute leukemia, particularly AML M7, perhaps owing to a functional role of mutant *P53* in the evolution from a transient form of leukemia to acute megakaryoblastic leukemia (42,43). Several types of bone marrow failure syndromes are linked with increased risk of developing AML, including Fanconi anemia (44), Bloom syndrome (45), Diamond-Blackfan syn-drome, and amegakaryocytic thrombocytopenia.

## VI.  EXPOSURE TO IONIZING RADIATION

To date, ionizing radiation is the best-studied risk factor for the leukemias. Ioniz-ing radiation is a clastogen that randomly deposits energy in tissues, inducing DNA strand breaks that may lead to chromosomal translocations and deletions (24). Strand breaks may occur directly from the radiation or indirectly from the generation of free radicals of oxygen. Susceptibility to radiation-induced malig-nancy appears to vary widely among different subsets of marrow-derived cells, thus highlighting the need to consider lineage-specific developmental processes (46). It is important to recognize the different forms of ionizing radiation, since biological effects depend not only on dose, but also on the type of radiation (e.g., linear energy transfer, a measure of the energy loss per unit distance traveled, which depends on the velocity, charge, and mass of a particle or the energy from x-rays or gamma rays) and the relative biological effectiveness (e.g., the ability to produce a given adverse effect in man). Recently, it has been suggested that the *AML1* gene (a transcriptional activator essential for normal hematopoietic development) may be a target for radiation-induced AML (47).

## A. Atomic Bomb Survivors

Follow-up studies of the Japanese atomic bomb survivors have provided much of our understanding about the dose-response relationship between radiation exposure and risk of developing leukemia (48–51), and to a lesser extent, MDS (52). Based on incidence data for the period 1950–1987, the AML dose-response function was nonlinear. When averaged over the follow-up period, the excess absolute risk was 1.1 per $10^4$ person-years per sievert (Sv), and the corresponding estimated average excess relative risk at 1 Sv exposure was 3.3 (51). Males had similar relative risks as females but twofold higher absolute excess risks. Persons exposed before age 20 had absolute excess risks of AML peaking within 10 years, then falling rapidly, with the survivors who were youngest at exposure having the highest average absolute excess risks and those exposed at ages 20–35 having less pronounced peaks. No significant effects on the risk were found for such variables as time-since-exposure, gender, or city.

A detailed histopathological review using the FAB classification revealed a considerable proportion of MDS cases among survivors with myeloid disorders in the high-dose-exposure group (53). A quantitative evaluation of the dose-response relationship for MDS, albeit based on only 13 cases, suggested a higher average excess relative risk per Sv (ERR) of 13.0 compared with that estimated for AML (ERR = 3.3) (52). By conventional G-banding, cytogenetic characterization of MDS/AML cases exposed to 1 gray (Gy) (1 Gy = 100 rad) compared with nonexposed de novo AML cases revealed a higher incidence of structural and numerical cytogenetic abnormalities without any specific recurrent abnormality among the exposed (54). However, cytogenetic characterization using fluorescence in situ hybridization (FISH) demonstrated a significantly higher incidence of subclones with monosomy 7 and deletion of the 20q13.2 region among the exposed (54). Quantitative dose-response data for MDS among the survivors have not been reported. In a pooled analysis of Japanese atomic bomb survivors, women treated for cervical cancer, and patients irradiated for ankylosing spondylitis, Little et al. (55) found that the relative risk of AML rose within a few years after exposure, then decreased with increasing time after exposure. No difference among the three populations was detected in the relative risk of AML (or of CML or ALL, each considered separately) and its pattern as a function of radiation dose, age, and time (55).

## B. Other Environmental Sources of Radiation

Although ecological studies have suggested correlations between radon or other natural background radiation sources and myeloid leukemia (56), there is little evidence of a link between AML in adults (57) or children (58) and measured levels of radon or gamma radiation in subjects' homes.

## C. Radiation Therapy for Malignant Conditions

Patients treated with radiation therapy for several types of malignancy have consistently shown two- to threefold excess risks of sAML (46). The excess risks of AML subsequent to non-Hodgkin's lymphoma, breast cancer, uterine cervix cancer, uterine corpus cancer, and Ewing's sarcoma are likely due to treatment with radiation therapy (59,60), whereas the elevated risks of sAML associated with Hodgkin's disease, ovarian cancer, and testicular cancer are likely due to treatment with alkylating agents or other chemotherapy (60–62). Similar to findings from the studies of the Japanese atomic bomb survivors (51), the excesses of leukemia subsequent to radiotherapy are generally apparent within the first 5 years following radiation therapy: most radiogenic leukemia arises within 10 years following first exposure, and generally not beyond 15 years (46,60). AML excesses have been associated with estimated bone marrow doses ranging from 1 to 15 Gy for adults and often higher for children (60). Risk of radiation-induced leukemia appears to be greater when large volumes of bone marrow are treated with lower doses or dose fractions. It has been postulated that the low risk of sAML associated with high partial-body radiation exposures is due to radiation-induced apoptosis in exposed cells (60).

## D. Radiation Therapy for Benign Conditions

Increased risk of AML has also been linked with radiation treatment for benign conditions, including ankylosing spondylitis (associated with a relative risk of 7.0 for leukemia up to 25 years after exposure to a uniform dose of 1 Gy) (63). Risks for AML ranging from 1.2- to 3.0-fold increases have been linked with radiation therapy treatments for benign gynecological disorders (64), menorrhagia not associated with malignancy (65,66), peptic ulcer (67), and tinea capitis (68).

## E. Occupational Exposures

It is generally acknowledged that four major categories of workers are exposed to ionizing radiation. Radiologists and x-ray technicians employed in the first half of the twentieth century were found to be at increased risk of leukemia, ranging from 6- to 8.8-fold excesses in leukemia mortality among British (65) and U.S. (69,70) radiologists joining specialty societies during 1897–1921 and 1920–1929, respectively. Subsequently, no significant excess (British radiologists entering after 1921) or declining (U.S. radiologists entering in 1940 or later) risks were observed. (U.S. radiologists entering in 1930–1939 had a 3.4-fold increase, whereas those entering in 1940 or later had no significant excess risk.) With one exception (chronic lymphocytic leukemia, CLL), leukemia incidence was significantly elevated among 27,911 diagnostic x-ray workers followed during 1950–1980 in China (71), but not among U.S. Army x-ray technicians followed during 1946–1974 (72) or among U.S. x-ray technologists employed during 1926–1990 (73).

Many studies of nuclear industry workers have generally showed no excess risk or only very small increases in leukemia (reviewed in Ref. 46). Recent combined analyses of 95,673 British, Canadian, and U.S. nuclear workers employed for 6 months or longer found a relative risk of 1.2 for leukemia mortality (excluding CLL) associated with a cumulative protracted dose of 100 mSv compared with 0 mSv, and an ERR of 2.2 for leukemia incidence (74). A small excess relative risk for leukemia (excluding CLL) of borderline significance was found in a cohort of 124,743 U.K. radiation workers (75).

No significant excess of leukemia has been observed among cohorts of U.S. or U.K. radium dial workers (76–78) or among uranium miners (79). A 2.5-fold leukemia excess (primarily AML and CML) was seen among 3741 U.S. servicemen exposed to one above-ground 1957 nuclear detonation (80), but no increased risk was noted for 46,186 U.S. military participants in several other atmospheric nuclear tests conducted between 1951 and 1958 (81). Elevated leukemia incidence and mortality were noted in a follow-up of 528 New Zealand military participants in British atomic weapons tests (82). An excess mortality for leukemia and multiple myeloma was ascertained among 22,347 British participants in nuclear tests (83), although the unexposed comparison group was determined to have a substantially lower rate of hematopoietic neoplasms compared with national mortality rates (46).

## VII. AML AND MDS SECONDARY TO CANCER CHEMOTHERAPY

Numerous chemotherapeutic agents used in the treatment of an initial cancer diagnosis have been linked with the subsequent development of AML and MDS (2). In more than 70% of patients with tAML, there was a preceding MDS (84). Alkylating agents, in particular, have been associated with increased risks of MDS and/or tAML (85). Typically MDS and tAML occur 5–7 years following treatment for the initial cancer and risk is related to the cumulative alkylating drug dose. Both conditions are frequently characterized by a preleukemic phase, trilineage dysplasia, and cytogenetic abnormalities involving partial deletions of chromosomes 5 and 7. Certain common chemotherapeutic alkylating agents, such as melphalan, pose a higher risk than others, such as cyclophosphamide, for reasons that are unclear (86,87). Therapy-related MDS and tAML have been reported subsequent to treatment for Hodgkin's disease, non-Hodgkin's lymphoma, multiple myeloma, polycythemia vera, and breast, ovarian, and testicular cancers (59,61,62,86–88).

A second group of tAML is linked with topoisomerase II inhibitors, specifically epipodophyllotoxins. When tAML is associated with treatment with epipodophyllotoxins, the condition is often not preceded by a preleukemic phase and develops after a shorter latency period (typically 2 years) but apparently is not related to cumulative dose (89). The pattern of cytogenetic abnormalities is also different, with balanced translocations involving 11q23 being the most characteristic abnormality; less often, other balanced translocations are seen (90,91). Increasing doses of platinum-based chemotherapy for ovarian cancer have been quantitatively associated with increasing risks for tAML (92). A 10-fold higher risk of tMDS/AML has been observed in breast cancer patients treated with mitoxantrone and methotrexate or methotrexate and mitomycin C (93). Recent analyses of predictors for tMDS/AML also show an association with high-dose chemotherapy and autologous stem cell transplantation for malignant diseases, particularly when total-body irradiation (94) or VP-16 (the latter used for priming lymphoma patients for stem cell mobilization) (87) were used in the preparative region for the autologous stem cell transplant. Recent efforts have begun to be directed at identifying host-related genetic variables that may influence risk of developing tAML (95,96).

## VIII.  EXPOSURE TO BENZENE

### A.  Association with Leukemias and MDS

Benzene, the oldest and best-known chemical leukemogen (97), has been the subject of numerous mechanistic and epidemiological studies over the years. The first cases of benzene-induced hematotoxicity were described in 1897, and the first case of leukemia associated with benzene exposure was reported in 1928 (97). Prior to the last few decades, workplace exposures were the primary source of general population exposures, but recognition of the leukemogenicity of benzene exposure led to notable reduction in workplace use, at least in Western industrialized nations. Yet, the sources of small but measurable levels of benzene consistently identified in blood samples of the general population have not been completely traced, but include cigarette smoke (significantly higher levels of both benzene and its genotoxic intermediates in blood and urine of smokers) and unleaded gasoline (98,99). The contribution of internally generated sources (as opposed to external exposures) and genetic factors to measurable levels of benzene in humans has not been well delineated.

Leukemia (mostly AML) has been reported to be 1.9- to >10.0-fold increased in cohort and case-controlled studies of benzene-exposed painters, printers, and workers employed in petroleum refining and in chemical, rubber, Pliofilm, and shoe manufacturing (100–104). Although benzene has been most strongly associated with AML and aplastic anemia, there is evidence to suggest that other subtypes of leukemia, MDS, non-Hodgkin's lymphoma, and possibly other hematopoietic and lymphoproliferative malignancies and related disorders are linked with exposure to this chemical as well (100,103–111).

Early descriptions of preleukemias associated with benzene exposure (102) were likely cases of MDS. For example, significantly elevated risks of MDS were found in the China benzene cohort (103), although each worker ultimately determined to have MDS was initially diagnosed as having acute nonlymphocytic leukemia (ANLL). Only upon review by expert hematologists affiliated with the National Cancer Institute, the Chinese Academy of Preventive Medicine, the Peking Union Medical College Hospital, and the Mayo Clinic was it recognized that the correct diagnosis was MDS (112). The cytogenetic abnormalities seen in benzene-exposed workers (26,27) have also been identified among persons with tMDS (2), suggesting a similar pathogenesis.

Much debate has surrounded the evaluation of risks of AML at low levels of benzene exposure and the dose-response pattern, the relevant exposure metric(s) (e.g., average exposure level, duration of exposure, and/or cumulative exposure), and exposure latency (113–117). Overall, the data support the linear extrapolation of high-exposure data to effects at low doses (116,117) and a recent risk assessment shows that similar carcinogenic potency values for benzene are obtained from both Chinese and U.S. cohort studies (117).

Peripheral lymphocyte levels appear to represent a sensitive marker of benzene exposure levels (118,119), with decreased lymphocyte counts serving as a biomarker to validate benzene exposure level estimates (120). Recent evidence also suggests that the CD4+ T lymphocytes are the primary target, resulting in a lowering of the CD4/CD8 ratio, an immunosuppressive pattern similar to that seen with the onset of acquired immunodeficiency syndrome (AIDS) (121).

## B.   Metabolism of Benzene

It has been clearly demonstrated that benzene must be metabolized for induction of its hematotoxic and leukemogenic effects (122). Initial metabolism of benzene takes place in the liver (123) where cytochrome P450 enzymes, in particular the CYP2E1 isozyme (122), convert it to a number of reactive intermediates (Fig. 2). The initial metabolite of benzene is benzene oxide, which spontaneously re-

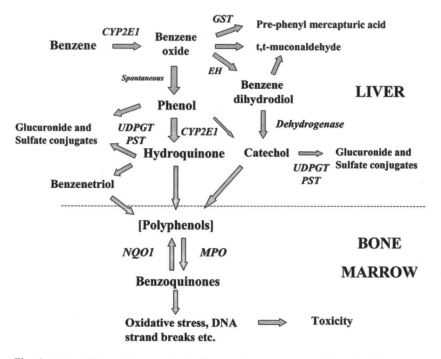

**Fig. 2** Metabolism of benzene in the liver and bone marrow. GST: glutathione S-transferase; EH: epoxide hydrolase; UDPGT, uridine diphosphate glucuronyl transferase; PST, phenol sulfotransferase; NQO1, NAD(P)H: quinone oxidoreductase 1; MPO, myeloperoxidase.

arranges mainly to phenol, but it may also be conjugated with glutathione by glutathione S-transferases (GST) to form pre-phenyl mercapturic acid or metabolized by epoxide hydrolase to benzene dihydrodiol (123). Benzene dihydrodiol can then undergo dehydrogenation to form catechol, which can be conjugated with sulfate or glucuronic acid and excreted in the urine. Benzene oxide can also form an oxepin, whose ring structure opens to *trans,trans*-muconaldehyde, a highly reactive compound that may have toxic effects. However, the primary metabolite of benzene is phenol, which can be further metabolized by CYP2E1 to hydroquinone, which in turn can be further hydroxylated to 1,2,4-benzenetriol. The three polyphenols, namely hydroquinone, catechol, and benzenetriol, accumulate in bone marrow and are readily oxidized to highly toxic benzoquinones by peroxidase enzymes such as bone marrow myeloperoxidase (MPO), a process enhanced by the presence of phenol (124).

The main protection against the toxic effects of these benzoquinones is NAD(P)H: quinone oxidoreductase 1 (NQO1), originally called DT-diaphorase (125) (Fig. 2). Thus, individuals who have high CYP2E1 activity and low NQO1 activity would potentially be more susceptible to the toxic effects of benzene than individuals with low CYP2E1 and high NQO1 activities. In a case-controlled study of benzene-poisoned workers in China, Rothman et al. (126) showed that such an increased susceptibility was indeed observed, with individuals lacking NQO1 activity being about 2.5-fold more susceptible to benzene's hematotoxicity and that high-versus-low CYP2E1 activity conferred an additional 2.5-fold increased susceptibility. Individuals with the combination of high CYP2E1 activity and null NQO1 activity had the highest risk of benzene poisoning [odds ratio (OR): 7.6] (126). In the study, CYP2E1 activity was measured phenotypically using hydroxylation of the drug chlorzoxazone as the biomarker. Unfortunately, this phenotypic measurement of CYP2E1 activity may not correlate with any of the multiple *CYP2E1* genotypes. None of the multiple polymorphisms in the *CYP2E1* gene appear to have any significant effect on enzyme activity (M. Ingelman-Sundberg, personal communication). Thus, it may not be worthwhile to study these polymorphisms in the context of leukemia risk.

Unlike CYP2E1, NQO1 activity is closely correlated with genotype. A single nucleotide polymorphism (cytosine $\rightarrow$ thymidine) at position 609 in the *NQO1* gene was first identified in a human colon cancer cell line with very low NQO1 activity (127). This mutation produces a proline to serine substitution that inactivates NQO1 enzyme activity. People who are homozygous for the variant allele completely lack NQO1 activity, whereas heterozygotes have low-to-intermediate activity compared with the wild-type allele (128). The incidence of the polymorphism varies widely by race and associations have been made between the presence of variant alleles and lung and urological cancers (125). Given that the *NQO1* C609T polymorphism was related to benzene-induced hematotoxicity and leukemia, one of the authors (MTS), in collaboration with others, investigated whether or not this polymorphism conferred an increased risk of leukemia in general, as discussed below.

## IX. LOW NAD(P)H:QUINONE OXIDOREDUCTASE ACTIVITY IS ASSOCIATED WITH ACUTE LEUKEMIA

In a series of 104 cases of AML and MDS, the laboratory of Martyn Smith in Berkeley, with Richard Larson's group in Chicago, examined the evidence that the *NQO1* C609T variant allele was overrepresented in therapy-related myeloid leukemias and in individuals with specific chromosome aberrations (95). Together these investigators found that having low or null NQO1 activity conferred an increased risk of tAML, especially in persons harboring changes in chromosomes 5 and 7. These studies encouraged Smith, Morgan, and colleagues to examine the effects of the *NQO1* polymorphism in de novo acute leukemias in the general population (129).

In a population-based, case-controlled study conducted in England, DNA samples from 493 adult de novo acute leukemia patients and 838 unaffected age-, sex-, and geographically matched controls were genotyped for the *NQO1* C609T allele. The frequency of cases with low or null NQO1 activity (heterozygote + homozygous mutant) was significantly higher among total acute leukemia cases compared with matched controls [OR: 1.49; 95% confidence interval (CI): 1.17–1.89]. Both ALL (OR: 1.93; 95% CI: 0.96–3.87) and AML cases (OR: 1.47; 95% CI: 1.13–1.90) exhibited a higher ratio of low/null *NQO1* genotypes compared with controls (129). Among de novo AML cases, low/null NQO1 activity was significantly associated with cases harboring translocations and inversions (OR: 2.39; 95% CI: 1.34–4.27), especially those having inv (16). These findings were confirmed in a second group of 217 de novo AML cases with known cytogenetic profiles (129).

By inference, these data suggest that environmental agents that are normally detoxified by NQO1 are risk factors for producing ALL and AML in the general population. Thus, benzene exposure from gasoline, cigarette smoking, and air pollution may be a risk factor for some forms of leukemia in the general population. However, it is likely that environmental benzene exposures are too low to be considered a significant risk factor for most people.

As discussed above, NQO1 is thought to protect against benzene by maintaining its phenolic metabolites in their reduced form, preventing quinone formation, and reducing oxidative stress. Recently, it has been suggested that a more likely source of phenol, hydroquinone, and catechol may be the diet and the intestinal breakdown of excess dietary protein (130). These dietary sources far outweigh environmental benzene exposures and, therefore, it is possible that phenols derived mainly from diet are important risk factors for acute leukemia (130). However, many other compounds are substrates for NQO1—including quinones, quinone-epoxides, quinone-imines, naphthoquinones, methylene blue, and azo- and nitro-compounds—and it is possible that all these may be involved in leukemia induction (125). Others, probably metabolized by NQO1, include dietary flavonoids, which are topoisomerase II inhibitors and have been linked with infant leukemia (131), as has the *NQO1* C609T polymorphism (132). NQO1 also protects cells from the effects of chronic oxidative stress by maintaining antioxidant forms of ubiquinone and vitamin E (133). Thus, agents that induce chronic oxidative stress through inflammation or other mechanisms may also play a role in producing acute leukemia.

## A.  Other Enzyme Variants

By reviewing Figure 2, it is clear that other enzyme variants may be relevant to susceptibilities to benzene toxicity. For example, the main pathway for removal of the phenolic metabolites from the body is conjugation with sulfate or glucuronic acid. These conjugation reactions are catalyzed by phenol sulfotransferase (PST) and uridine diphosphate glucuronyl transferase (UDPGT), respectively. Smith, Morgan, et al. are currently investigating the role, if any, that polymorphisms in *PST* and *UDPGT* genes play in susceptibility to benzene toxicity and acute leukemia in general.

Another key enzyme shown in Figure 2 is MPO. Variants of MPO could affect the generation of quinones from phenolic derivatives in the bone marrow. One small study, involving only 20 subjects, has looked at the association of MPO polymorphic variants with the M3 subtype of AML and found a positive association (134). The association was subsequently studied in a larger group that included 45 cases of acute promyelocytic and 62 cases of myelomonocytic leukemia. In this larger study, no difference was found in variant allele frequency between the cases and matched controls (135).

## X.  EXPOSURE TO OTHER CHEMICALS

Table 1 lists specific occupational groups reported to have an increased risk of AML and/or MDS (136–148). In addition to occupational exposures to various chemicals, proximity to industrial facilities that release chemicals in the air (either

**Table 1**  Occupational Groups at Risk for Acute Myeloid Leukemia and/or Myelodysplastic Syndromes

| Occupation | Ref. |
|---|---|
| Painters | 136,137 |
| Plant and machine operators and assemblers | 138 |
| Coal miners | 138 |
| Embalmers | 139,140 |
| Garage and transport workers | 141,142 |
| Shoe workers | 143 |
| Hairdressers and cosmetologists | 144,145 |
| Seamen on tankers | 146 |
| Clinical laboratory and research science technicians | 147 |
| Other occupational and industrial groups | 148 |

routinely or after an accident) has also been recognized as a risk factor for leukemias. Myeloid leukemia was increased among 20,000 persons under age 19 residing in Seveso, Italy, within 10 years after an industrial accident caused contamination of the region with 2,3,7,8-tetrachlorobibenzo-*p*-dioxin (149), and a 40% increased risk was observed for AML among adults who reported living within 8 km of an industrial plant in the United States (150).

Another chemical that has been linked to the induction of leukemia is 1,3-butadiene (BD), which was first produced in large volumes during World War II and is still commonly used in the production of rubber and thermoplastic resins (151,152). BD has also been found in automobile exhaust, in cigarette smoke, and in community air at the perimeter of manufacturing plants. BD was recently classified by the International Agency for Research on Cancer as a probable human carcinogen (Group 2A), based upon sufficient evidence for carcinogenicity in animals and limited evidence in humans (152). Although several smaller investigations were carried out, the evidence of carcinogenicity in humans is based largely on one epidemiological study of the U.S. and Canada styrene-butadiene rubber industry (153,154). The study showed excesses of leukemia in these workers and that those with apparently higher BD exposure had a higher risk than those with lower exposure.

To provide a mechanistic underpinning for the human carcinogenicity studies, various groups have investigated genotoxic effects in workers exposed to BD (155–161). In a study at a polybutadiene production facility in China, Hayes et al. (157) examined a broad spectrum of genotoxic and other potential effects of BD. Overall, this investigation in China demonstrated that exposure to butadiene, quantified by a variety of short- and long-term measures, did not show specific genotoxic effects related to the exposure (157). This study and others have cast doubt on the genotoxic potential of butadiene at low levels of occupational exposure (162), such that the leukemogenic potential of BD in man now appears questionable and requires further investigation.

## XI. FARMING, AGRICULTURAL, AND RELATED EXPOSURES

Some studies of farmers and farm workers have shown modest excesses of AML (163) as well as virtually all other subtypes of leukemia (risks ranging from 1.1- to 1.4-fold elevated), whereas others have shown no increase in risk (164–166). Perhaps because agriculture-related exposures are not uniform across the globe (differing with different farming practices), risks vary to a certain extent internationally (167–170). Suspected leukemogens include pesticides (particularly animal insecticides and herbicides), fertilizers, diesel fuel and exhaust, infectious agents, and possibly other exposures associated with livestock (171). Only a few of the earlier studies evaluated specific pesticide exposures in relation to AML or other leukemia subtypes (172,173), but recent studies are increasingly incorporating newer approaches and biological measurements to evaluate specific agricultural exposures (174–176). AML was also increased among New Zealand abattoir workers (177), workers in the U.S. meat industry (178), and U.S. veterinarians (179), all of which may be consistent with a viral etiology.

## XII. LIFESTYLE EXPOSURES, INCLUDING SMOKING, ALCOHOL, AND HAIR DYES

### A. Cigarette Smoking

Several large studies (180–182), but not all (183,184), have found small excesses of adult acute leukemia associated with cigarette smoking. Summary assessments have concluded that cigarette smoking is weakly associated (relative risks estimated as 1.3–1.5) with elevated risks of adult myeloid leukemia (185,186). Limited data also suggest that cigarette smoking appears to be a risk factor for several types of MDS, with risk related to intensity and duration of smoking (187).

### B. Alcohol

Several studies have linked alcohol consumption with adult leukemia (188–192), and in a limited epidemiological investigation Ido et al. have assessed the role of alcohol consumption in MDS (193).

### C. Hair Dyes

Hair dye use, particularly dark hair dyes, has been weakly linked with adult AML and MDS (194–196).

## XIII. INFECTIOUS AGENTS

### A. Viruses

AML in adults has been linked with seropositivity to human herpes virus-6 (HHV-6), the risk of AML rising with increasing geometric mean titer in one study (197). A nonsignificant increase in hepatitis B surface antigen (198) among AML cases compared with controls is difficult to interpret as is a statistical association between a past history of measles (ascertained by questionnaire) and an elevated risk of AML in adults (199). The rarity of AML and MDS generally requires use of the case-control study design to investigate postulated risk factors; however, the potential etiological role of infectious agents is particularly difficult to evaluate epidemiologically using case-control study designs because evidence of a prior infection ascertained after diagnosis of AML/MDS is not conclusive.

Raza (200,201) has proposed that MDS can begin as a viral disease. She suggests the causative virus may be a dormant lentivirus that is made oncogenic by "promoting events" such as immunosuppression or a second viral infection. The infected cell may not be a stem cell, but a cell belonging to the stroma or to the immune system. Raza contends that circumstantial evidence supports the possibility that the initial transforming event in MDS is a viral insult. It may be useful to consider studying the interrelationship between postulated viruses and immunological dysfunction in populations with elevated risks of AML/MDS that may be linked with viral exposures (179), namely farmers, veterinarians, and abattoir workers.

## XIV. DIETARY FACTORS, INFLAMMATORY BOWEL DISEASE, AND LEUKEMIA RISK

Only a few studies have evaluated the relationship between dietary factors and AML/MDS (202,203) despite the fact that diet is one of the most important causes of cancer overall (204). Given the association between NQO1 and leukemia (discussed above) and the potential importance of phenol and its metabolite hydroquinone in benzene-induced leukemia, it seems logical to hypothesize that dietary intake and secondary production of phenol by the gut flora are contributing factors to leukemia risk (130).

Phenol and hydroquinone are derived from the diet both directly and indirectly. Many common foods and beverages contain phenol and hydroquinone. A major source of phenol stems from the catabolism of protein and other compounds by gut bacteria, which appears to depend highly on the metabolic activity of the intestinal bacterial microflora (130). Individuals consuming high-meat diets have increased populations of phenol-producing anaerobic *Bacteroides* spp. compared with individuals on vegetarian diets. Comparisons of Western and Eastern populations indicate that individuals who consume a typical British and American high-meat diet have a higher ratio of anaerobic to aerobic microflora than persons from Japan, Uganda, or India, whose diets are largely vegetarian. Thus, Westerners have higher phenol production in their intestines. A potentially significant source of hydroquinone comes from ingestion of foods containing glycoside arbutin, a naturally occurring plant product that is converted to hydroquinone by stomach acids. Wheat is an arbutin-rich food staple, and rice is not. The differences in arbutin intake and microflora production of phenol may therefore explain the higher risk of AML seen in the West described earlier in this chapter (see Sections VIII and IX, above).

Further support for the hypothesis that diet and phenol production are linked to leukemia risk comes from the study of Crohn's disease, a common type of inflammatory bowel disease. Numerous case reports and reviews suggest that Crohn's disease patients have an increased risk of AML and MDS (205–210). Interestingly, urinary phenol levels among Crohn's disease patients are approximately four- to 30-fold higher than levels among healthy subjects, further implicating gut microflora phenol production in the development of leukemia (130). An attractive feature of this hypothesis is that it may explain why many people who have no known occupational chemical exposures, prior radiation or chemotherapeutic treatment, or significant smoking history develop leukemia. The hypothesis predicts that susceptibility to AML and MDS is related to diet, genetics, and gut-flora composition. The latter two predictors are largely beyond any individual's control, and thus dietary modification may be one of the best intervention strategies for lowering leukemia risk. Further examination of dietary risk factors in producing MDS is necessary before such intervention strategies can be proposed to the general public.

## XV. CONCLUDING REMARKS

As documented here, a wide variety of exposures have been linked with increased risk of MDS and AML, but the majority of cases in the general population remain unexplained. Obviously, much still needs to be learned about the causes of MDS and leukemia. One area that remains relatively unexplored is the role of diet. However, it is difficult to examine dietary factors retrospectively and this is further complicated for MDS since there are few or no incidence data and classification and diagnosis problems make performing a population-based epidemiological study extremely difficult. These problems are not insurmountable, however, and studies could be done if patients from several major clinical centers, which capture most of the MDS and AML patients in a given region, were enrolled in a large case-controlled study. This would allow, for example, studies to be performed into why certain patients with MDS progress to AML and others do not and for sophisticated biological sample collection. The latter would allow molecular epidemiological studies of genetic susceptibility to MDS and AML to be carried out along with molecular pathological analysis of the cases. Such studies could provide new insights into potential causative factors that could be explored further by more traditional methodologies.

## ACKNOWLEDGMENTS

MTS was supported by the National Institute of Environmental Health Sciences (grants P42ES04705, P30ES01896, and R01ES06721) and the National Foundation for Cancer Research. MSL is an investigator in the intramural program of the National Cancer Institute. GJM is supported by the Leukaemia Research Fund of Great Britain.

## REFERENCES

1. Lee GR, Foerster J, Lukens J, Paraskevas F, Greer JP, Rodgers GM, eds. Wintrobe's Clinical Hematology. 10th ed. Philadelphia: Lippincott Williams & Wilkins, 1999:56–71, 2209–2373.
2. van Leeuwen FE. Risk of acute myelogenous leukaemia and myelodysplasia following cancer treatment (review). Baillieres Clinical Haematol 1996; 9:57–85.
3. Bhatia M, Wang JC, Kapp U, Bonnet D, Dick FE. Purification of primitive human hematopoietic cells capable of repopulating immune-deficient cells in mice. Proc Natl Acad Sci USA 1997; 94:5320–5325.
4. Bennett JM, Catovsky D, Daniel MT, Flandrin G, Galton DA, Gralnick HR, Sultan C. Proposals for the classification of the acute leukemias. French-American-British (FAB) Cooperative Group. Br J Haematol 1997; 33:451–458.
5. Bennett JM, Catovsky D, Daniel MT, Flandrin G, Galton DA, Gralnick HR, Sultan C. Criteria for the diagnosis of acute leukemia of megakaryocyte lineage (M7). A report of the French-American-British Cooperative Group. Ann Intern Med 1985; 103:460–462.
6. Cheson BD, Cassileth PA, Head DR, Schiffer CA, Bennett JM, Bloomfield CD, Brunning R, Gale RP, Grever MR, Keating MJ, et al. Report on the National Cancer Institute-sponsored workshop on definitions of diagnosis and response in acute myeloid leukemia (review). J Clin Oncol 1990; 8:813–819.
7. Groupe Francais de Cytogenetique Hematologique: Forty-four cases of childhood myelodysplasia with cytogenetics, documented by the Groupe Francais de Cytogenetique Hematologique. Leukemia 1997; 11:1478–1485.
8. Kurzrock R, Talpaz M. The molecular pathology of chronic myelogenous leukaemia (review). Br J Haematol 1991; 79(suppl 1):34–37.
9. Pear WS, Miller JP, Xu L, Pui JC, Soffer B, Quackenbush RC, Pendergast AM, Bronson R, Aster JC, Scott ML, Baltimore D. Efficient and rapid induction of a chronic myelogenous leukemia-like myeloproliferative disease in mice receiving P210 bcr/abl-transduced bone marrow. Blood 1998; 92:3780–3792.
10. Era T, Witte ON. Regulated expression of P210 Bcr-Abl during embryonic stem cell differentiation stimulates multipotential progenitor expansion and myeloid cell fate. Proc Natl Acad Sci USA 2000; 97:1737–1742.
11. Faderl S, Kantarjian HM, Thomas DA, Cortes J, Giles F, Pierce S, Albitar M, Estrov Z. Outcome of Philadelphia chromosome-positive adult acute lymphoblastic leukemia. Leuk Lymphoma 2000; 36:263–273.
12. Paietta E, Racevskis J, Bennett JM, Neuberg D, Cassileth PA, Rowe JM, Wiernik PH. Biologic heterogeneity in Philadelphia chromosome-positive acute leukemia with myeloid morphology: the Eastern Cooperative Oncology Group experience. Leukemia 1998; 12:1881–1885.

13. Grignani F, Valtieri M, Gabbianelli M, Gelmetti V, Botta R, Luchetti L, Masella B, Morsilli O, Pelosi E, Samoggia P, Pelicci PG, Peschle C. PML/RAR alpha fusion protein expression in normal human hematopoietic progenitors dictates myeloid commitment and the promyelocytic phenotype. Blood 2000; 96:1531–1537.

14. Sainty D, Liso V, Cantu-Rajnoldi A, Head D, Mozziconacci MJ, Arnoulet C, Benattar L, Fenu S, Mancini M, Duchayne E, Mahon FX, Gutierrez N, Birg F, Biondi A, Grimwade D, Lafage-Pochitaloff M, Hagemeijer A, Flandrin G. A new morphologic classification system for acute promyelocytic leukemia distinguishes cases with underlying PLZF/RARA gene rearrangements. Group Francais de Cytogenetique Hematologique, UK Cancer Cytogenetics Group and BIOMED 1 European Community-Concerted Action "Molecular Cytogenetic Diagnosis in Haematological Malignancies." Blood 2000; 96:1287–1296.

15. Hagemeijer A, de Klein A, Wijsman J, van Meerten E, de Greef GE, Sacchi N. Development of an interphase fluorescent in situ hybridization (FISH) test to detect t(8;21) in AML patients. Leukemia 1998; 12:96–101.

16. Wong KF, Kwong YL. Trisomy 22 in acute myeloid leukemia: a marker for myeloid leukemia with monocytic features and cytogenetically cryptic inversion 16. Cancer Genet Cytogenet 1999; 109:131–133.

17. Broeker PL, Super HG, Thirman MJ, Pomykala H, Yonebayashi Y, Tanabe S, Zeleznik-Le N, Rowley JD. Distribution of 11q23 breakpoints within the MLL breakpoint cluster region in de novo acute leukemia and in treatment-related acute myeloid leukemia: correlation with scaffold attachment regions and topoisomerase II consensus binding sites. Blood 1996; 87:1912–1922.

18. Sole F, Espinet B, Sanz GF, Cervera J, Calasanz MJ, Luno E, Prieto F, Granada I, Hernandez JM, Cigudosa JC, Diez JL, Bureo E, Marques ML, Arranz E, Rios R, Martinez Climent JA, Vallespi T, Florensa L, Woessner S. Incidence, characterization and prognostic significance of chromosomal abnormalities in 640 patients with primary myelodysplastic syndromes. Grupo Cooperativo Espanol de Citogenetica Hematologica. Br J Haematol 2000; 108:346–356.

19. Rossi G, Pelizzari AM, Bellotti D, Tonelli M, Barlati S. Cytogenetic analogy between myelodysplastic syndrome and acute myeloid leukemia of elderly patients. Leukemia 2000; 14:636–641.

20. Willman CL. Molecular evaluation of acute myeloid leukemias (review). Semin Hematol 1999; 36:390–400.

21. Groves FD, Linet MS, Devesa SS. Epidemiology of leukemia: overview and patterns of occurrence. In: Henderson ES, Lister TA, Greaves MF, eds. Leukemia. 6th ed. Philadelphia: WB Saunders, 1996:145–159.

22. Cartwright RA, McNally RJQ, Rowland DJ, Thomas J. The Descriptive Epidemiology of Leukaemia and Related Conditions in Parts of the United Kingdom, 1984–1993. London: Leukaemia Research Fund, 1997.

23. Douer D, Preston-Martin S, Chang E, Nichols PW, Watkins KJ, Levine AM. High frequency of acute promyelocytic leukemia among Latinos with acute myeloid leukemia. Blood 1996; 87:308–313.

24. Little JB. Cellular, molecular, and carcinogenic effects of radiation (review). Hematol Oncol Clin North Am 1993; 7:337–352.

25. Andersen MK, Pedersen-Bjergaard J. Increased frequency of dicentric chromo-

somes in therapy-related MDS and AML compared to de novo disease is significantly related to previous treatment with alkylating agents and suggests a specific susceptibility to chromosome breakage at the centromere. Leukemia 2000; 14:105–111.

26. Zhang L, Wang Y, Shang N, Smith MT. Benzene metabolites induce the loss and long arm deletion of chromosomes 5 and 7 in human lymphocytes. Leuk Res 1998; 22:105–113.

27. Smith MT, Zhang L, Wang Y, Hayes RB, Li G, Wiemels J, Dosemeci M, Titenko-Holland N, Xi L, Kolachana P, Yin S, Rothman N. Increased translocations and aneusomy in chromosomes 8 and 21 among workers exposed to benzene. Cancer Res 1998; 58:2176–2181.

28. Crane MM, Strom SS, Halabi S, Berman EL, Fueger JJ, Spitz MR, Keating MJ. Correlation between selected environmental exposures and karyotype in acute myelocytic leukemia. Cancer Epidemiol Biomarkers Prev 1996; 8:639–644.

29. Davico L, Sacerdote C, Ciccone G, Pegoraro L, Kerim S, Ponzio G, Vineis P. Chromosome 8, occupational exposures, smoking, and acute nonlymphocytic leukemias: a population-based study. Cancer Epidemiol Biomarkers Prev 1998; 12:1123–1125.

30. West RR, Stafford DA, White AD, Bowen DT, Padua RA. Cytogenetic abnormalities in the myelodysplastic syndromes and occupational or environmental exposure. Blood 2000; 95:2093–2097.

31. Taylor JA, Sandler DP, Bloomfield CD, Shore DL, Ball ED, Neubauer A, McIntyre OR, Liu E. Ras oncogene activation and occupational exposures in acute myeloid leukemia. J Natl Cancer Inst 1992; 84:1626–1632.

32. Smith MT, Wiemels J, Rothman N, Linet MS. Chemical exposure, ras oncogene activation, and acute myeloid leukemia. J Natl Cancer Inst 1992; 84:1614–1615.

33. Horowitz M. The genetics of familial leukemia. Leukemia 1997; 11:1347–1359.

34. Gilchrist DM, Friedman JM, Rogers PC, Creighton SP. Myelodysplasia and leukemia syndrome with monosomy 7: a genetic perspective. Am J Med Genet 1990; 35:437–441.

35. Kwong YL, Ng MH, Ma SK. Familial acute myeloid leukemia with monosomy 7: late onset and involvement of a multipotential progenitor cell. Cancer Genet Cytogenet 2000; 116:170–173.

36. Grimwade DJ, Stephenson J, De Silva C, Dalton RG, Mufti GJ. Familial MDS with 5q-abnormality. Br J Haematol 1993; 84:536–538.

37. Olopade OI, Roulston D, Baker T, Narvid S, Le Beau MM, Freireich EJ, Larson RA, Golomb HM. Familial myeloid leukemia associated with loss of the long arm of chromosome 5. Leukemia 1996; 10:669–674.

38. Mandla SG, Goobie S, Kumar RT, Hayne O, Zayed E, Guernsey DL, Greer WL. Genetic analysis of familial myelodysplastic syndrome: absence of linkage to chromobosomes 5q31 and 7q22. Cancer Genet Cytogenet 1998; 105:113–118.

39. Gao Q, Horwitz M, Roulston D, Hagos F, Zhao N, Freireich EJ, Golomb HM, Olopade OI. Susceptibility gene for familial acute myeloid leukemia associated with loss of 5q and/or 7q is not localized on the commonly deleted portion of 5q. Genes Chromosomes Cancer 2000; 28:164–172.

40. Hasle H, Olsen JH. Cancer in relatives of children with myelodysplastic syndrome, acute and chronic myeloid leukaemia. Br J Haematol 1997; 97:127–131.
41. Taylor GM, Birch JM. The hereditary basis of human leukemia. In: Henderson ES, Lister TA, Greaves MJ, eds. Leukemia. 6th ed. Philadelphia: WB Saunders, 1996: 210–245.
42. Malkin D, Brown EJ, Zipursky A. The role of p53 in megakaryoctye differentiation and the megakaryocytic leukemias of Down syndrome. Cancer Genet Cytogenet 2000; 116:1–5.
43. Hasle H, Clemmensen IH, Mikkelsen M. Risks of leukaemia and solid tumours in individuals with Down's syndrome. Lancet 2000; 355:165–169.
44. Alter BP. Fanconi's anemia and malignancies (review). Am J Hematol 1996; 53: 99–110.
45. Bloom GE, Warner S, Gerald PS, Diamond LK. Chromosome abnormalities in constitutional aplastic anemia. N Engl J Med 1966; 274:8–14.
46. Boice JD Jr, Land CE, Preston DL. Ionizing radiation. In: Schottenfeld D, Fraumeni JF Jr, eds. Cancer Epidemiology and Prevention. 2nd ed. New York: Oxford University Press, 1996:319–354.
47. Hromas R, Shopnick R, Jumean HG, Bowers C, Varella-Garcia M, Richkind K. A novel syndrome of radiation-associated acute myeloid leukemia involving *AML1* gene translocations. Blood 2000; 95:4011–4013.
48. Shimizu Y, Schull WJ, Kato H. Cancer risk among atomic bomb survivors. The RERF Life Span Study. Radiation Effects Research Foundation. JAMA 1990; 264: 601–604.
49. UNSCEAR. Sources and Effects of Ionizing Radiation. United National Publ No E.94.IX. 11. New York: United Nations Scientific Committee on the Effects of Atomic Radiation, 1994.
50. Pierce DA, Shimizu Y, Preston DL, Vaeth M, Mabuchi K. Studies of the mortality of atomic bomb survivors. Report 12, Part I. Cancer: 1950–1990. Radiat Res 1996; 146:1–27.
51. Preston DL, Kusumi S, Tomonaga M, Izumi S, Ron E, Kuramoto A, Kamada N, Dohy H, Matsuo T, Matsui T [corrected to Matsuo T], et al. Cancer incidence in atomic bomb survivors. Part III. Leukemia, lymphoma and multiple myeloma, 1950–1987. Radiat Res 1994; 137(suppl 2):S68–S97.
52. Shimizu Y, Pierce DA, Preston DL, Mabuchi K. Studies of the mortality of atomic bomb survivors. Report 12, part II. Noncancer mortality: 1950–1990. Radiat Res 1999; 152:374–389.
53. Matsuo T, Tomonaga M, Bennett JM, Kuriyama K, Imanaka F, Kuramoto A, Kamada N, Ichimaru M, Finch SC, Pisciotta AV, et al. Reclassification of leukemia among A-bomb survivors in Nagasaki using French-American-British (FAB) classification for acute leukemia. Jpn J Clin Oncol 1988; 18:91–96.
54. Nakanishi M, Tanaka K, Shintani T, Takahashi T, Kamada N. Chromosomal instability in acute myelocytic leukemia and myelodysplastic syndrome patients among atomic bomb survivors. J Radiat Res (Tokyo) 1999; 40:159–167.
55. Little MP, Weiss HA, Boice JD Jr, Darby SC, Day NE, Muirhead CR. Risks of leukemia in Japanese atomic bomb survivors, in women treated for cervical cancer, and in patients treated for ankylosing spondylitis. Radiat Res 1999; 152:280–292.

56. Henshaw DL, Eatough JP, Richardson RB. Radon as a causative factor in induction of myeloid leukaemia and other cancers (review). Lancet 1990; 335:1008–1012.
57. Forastiere F, Sperati A, Cherubini G, Miceli M, Biggeri A, Axelson O. Adult myeloid leukaemia, geology, and domestic exposure to radon and gamma radiation: a case control study in central Italy. Occup Environ Med 1998; 55:106–110.
58. Steinbuch M, Weinberg CR, Buckley JD, Robison LL, Sandler DP. Indoor residential radon exposure and risk of childhood acute myeloid leukaemia. Br J Cancer 1999; 81:900–906.
59. Travis LB, Curtis RE, Stovall M, Holowaty EJ, van Leeuwen FE, Glimelius B, Lynch CF, Hagenbeek A, Li CY, Banks PM, et al. Risk of leukemia following treatment for non-Hodgkin's lymphoma. J Natl Cancer Inst 1994; 86:1450–1457.
60. Inskip PD. Second cancers following radiotherapy. In: Neugut AI, Meadows AT, eds. Multiple Primary Cancers. Philadelphia: Lippincott Williams & Wilkins, 1999: 91–135.
61. Kaldor JM, Day NE, Clarke EA, Van Leeuwen FE, Henry-Amar M, Fiorentino MV, Bell J, Pedersen D, Band P, Assouline D, et al. Leukemia following Hodgkin's disease. N Engl J Med 1990; 322:7–13.
62. Kaldor JM, Day NE, Pettersson F, Clark EA, Pedersen D, Mehnert W, Bell J, Host H, Prior P, Karjalainen S, et al. Leukemia following chemotherapy for ovarian cancer. N Engl J Med 1990; 322:1–6.
63. Weiss HA, Darby SC, Fearn T, Doll R. Leukemia mortality after x-ray treatment for ankylosing spondylitis. Radiat Res 1995; 142:1–11.
64. Inskip PD, Kleinerman RA, Stovall M, Cookfair DL, Hadjimichael O, Moloney WC, Monson RR, Thompson WD, Wactawski-Wende J, Wagoner JK, et al. Leukemia, lymphoma, and multiple myeloma after pelvic radiotherapy for benign diseases. Radiat Res 1993; 135:108–124.
65. Smith PG, Doll R. Late effects of x irradiation in patients treated for metropathia hemorrhagica. Br J Radiol 1976; 49:224–232.
66. Inskip PD, Monson RR, Wagoner JK, Stovall M, Davis FG, Kleinerman RA, Boice JD Jr. Leukemia following radiotherapy for uterine bleeding. Radiat Res 1990; 122: 107–119.
67. Griem ML, Kleinerman RA, Boice JD Jr, Stovall M, Shefner D, Lubin JH. Cancer following radiotherapy for peptic ulcer. J Natl Cancer Inst 1994; 86:842–849.
68. Shore DL, Sandler DP, Davey FR, McIntyre OR, Bloomfield CD. Acute leukemia and residential proximity to potential sources of environmental pollutants. Arch Environ Health 1993; 48:414–420.
69. Seltser R, Sartwell PE. The influence of occupational exposure on the mortality of American radiologists and other medical specialists. Am J Epidemiol 1965; 101: 188–198.
70. Matanoski GM, Sartwell P, Elliott E, et al. Cancer risks in radiologists and radiation workers. In: Boice JD Jr, Fraumeni JF Jr, eds. Radiation Carcinogenesis: Epidemiology and Biological Significance. New York: Raven Press, 1984:83–96.
71. Wang JX, Inskip PD, Boice JD Jr, Li BX, Zhang JY, Fraumeni JF Jr. Cancer incidence among medical diagnostic x-ray workers in China, 1950 to 1985. Int J Cancer 1990; 45:889–95.

72. Jablon S, Miller RW. Army technologists: 29-year follow up for cause of death. Radiology 1978; 126:677–679.

73. Doody MM, Mandel JS, Lubin JH, Boice JD Jr. Mortality among United States radiologic technologists, 1926–90. Cancer Causes Control 1998; 9:67–75.

74. Cardis E, Gilbert ES, Carpenter L, Howe G, Kato I, Armstrong BK, Beral V, Cowper G, Douglas A, Fix J, et al. Effects of low doses and low dose rates of external ionizing radiation: cancer mortality among nuclear industry workers in three countries. Radiat Res 1995; 142:117–132.

75. Muirhead CR, Goodill AA, Haylock RG, Vokes J, Little MP, Jackson DA, O'Hagan JA, Thomas JM, Kendall GM, Silk TJ, Bingham D, Berridge GL. Occupational radiation exposure and mortality: second analysis of the National Registry for Radiation Workers. J Radiol Prot 1999; 19:3–26.

76. Spiers FW, Lucas HF, Rundo J, Anast GA. Leukemia incidence in the U.S. dial workers. Health Physics 1983; 44(suppl 1):65–72.

77. Stebbings JH, Lucas HF, Stehney AF. Mortality from cancers of major sites in female radium dial workers. Am J Indust Med 1984; 5:435–459.

78. Baverstock KF, Papworth DG. The UK radium luminiser survey. In: Gossner W, Gerber GB, eds. The Radiobiology of Radium. Munich: Urban, 1986:22–28.

79. National Research Council. Health Effects of Exposure to Radon. BEIR VI. Washington, DC: National Academy of Sciences, 1999:(18–20).

80. Caldwell GG, Kelley D, Zack M, Falk H, Heath CW Jr. Mortality and cancer frequency among military nuclear test (Smoky) participants, 1957 through 1979. JAMA 1983; 250:620–624.

81. Robinette DC. Studies of Participants in Nuclear Tests: Final Report, 1 September 1978–31 October 1984. Washington, DC: Defense Nuclear Agency, 1985. OCLC 17231691. NTIS# ADA1 55245. [Also known as Mortality of Nuclear Weapons Test Participants.]

82. Pearce N, Prior I, Methven D, Culling C, Marshall S, Auld J, de Boer G, Bethwaite P. Follow up of New Zealand participants in British atmospheric nuclear weapons tests in the Pacific. Br Med J 1990; 300:1161–1166.

83. Darby SC, Kendall GM, Fell TP, O'Hagan JA, Muirhead CR, Ennis JR, Ball AM, Dennis JA, Doll R. A summary of mortality and incidence of cancer in men from the United Kingdom who participated in the United Kingdom's atmospheric nuclear weapons tests and experimental programmes. Br Med J (Clin Res Ed) 1988; 296: 332–338.

84. Giles FJ, Koeffler HP. Secondary myelodysplastic syndromes and leukemias (review). Curr Opin Hematol 1994; 1:256–260.

85. Leone G, Mele L, Pulsoni A, Equitani F, Pagano L. The incidence of secondary leukemias (review). Haematologica 1999; 84:937–945.

86. Curtis RE, Boice JD Jr, Stovall M, Bernstein L, Greenberg RS, Flannery JT, Schwartz AG, Weyer P, Moloney WC, Hoover RN. Risk of leukemia after chemotherapy and radiation treatment for breast cancer. N Engl J Med 1992; 326:1745–1751.

87. Krishnan A, Bhatia S, Slovak ML, Arber DA, Niland JC, Nademanee A, Fung H, Bhatia R, Kashyap A, Molina A, O'Donnell MR, Parker PA, Sniecinski I, Snyder DS, Spielberger R, Stein A, Forman SJ. Predictors of therapy-related leukemia and

myelodysplasia following autologous transplantation for lymphoma: an assessment of risk factors. Blood 2000; 95:1588–1593.

88. van Leeuwen FE, Chorus AM, van den Belt-Dusebout AW, Hagenbeek A, Noyon R, van Kerkhoff EH, Pinedo HM, Somers R. Leukemia risk following Hodgkin's disease: relation to cumulative dose of alkylating agents, treatment with teniposide combinations, number of episodes of chemotherapy, and bone marrow damage. J Clin Oncol 1994; 12:1063–1073.

89. Smith MA, Rubinstein L, Anderson JR, Arthur D, Catalano PJ, Freidlin B, Heyn R, Khayat A, Krailo M, Land VJ, Miser J, Shuster J, Vena D. Secondary leukemia or myelodysplastic syndrome after treatment with epipodophyllotoxins. J Clin Oncol 1999; 17:569–577.

90. Felix CA. Secondary leukemias induced by topoisomerase-targeted drugs (review). Biochim Biophys Acta 1998; 1400:233–235.

91. Andersen MK, Johansson B, Larsen SO, Pedersen-Bjergaard J. Chromosomal abnormalities in secondary MDS and AML. Relationship to drugs and radiation with specific emphasis on the balanced rearrangements. Haematologica 1998; 83:483–488.

92. Travis LB, Andersson M, Gospodarowicz M, van Leeuwen FE, Bergfeldt K, Lynch CF, Curtis RE, Kohler BA, Wiklund T, Storm H, Holowaty E, Hall P, Pukkala E, Sleijfer DT, Clarke EA, Boice JD Jr, Stovall M, Gilbert E. Treatment-associated leukemia following testicular cancer. J Natl Cancer Inst 2000; 92:1165–1171.

93. Saso R, Kulkarni S, Mitchell P, Treleaven J, Swansbury GJ, Mehta J, Powles R, Ashley S, Kuan A, Powles T. Secondary myelodysplastic syndrome/acute myeloid leukaemia following mitoxantrone-based therapy for breast carcinoma. Br J Cancer 2000; 83:91–94.

94. Pedersen-Bjergaard J, Andersen MK, Christiansen DH. Therapy-related acute myeloid leukemia and myelodysplasia after high-dose chemotherapy and autologous stem cell transplantation (review). Blood 2000; 95:3273–3279.

95. Larson RA, Wang Y, Banerjee M, Wiemels J, Hartford C, Le Beau MM, Smith MT. Prevalence of the inactivating 609C → T polymorphism in the NAD(P)H: quinone oxidoreductase (NQO1) gene in patients with primary and therapy-related myeloid leukemia. Blood 1999; 94:803–807.

96. Woo MH, Shuster JJ, Chen C, Bash RO, Behm FG, Camitta B, Felix CA, Kamen BA, Pui CH, Raimondi SC, Winick NJ, Amylon MD, Relling MV. Glutathione S-transferase genotypes in children who develop treatment-related acute myeloid malignancies. Leukemia 2000; 14:232–237.

97. Delore P, Borgomano C. Leukemia aigue un cour de l'intoxication benzenique, sur l'origine toxique de certains leukemias aigues et leurs relations avec les anemies graves. J Med Lyon 1928; 9:227–233.

98. Brugnone F, Perbellini L, Giuliari C, Cerpelloni M, Soave M. Blood and urine concentrations of chemical pollutants in the general population. Med Lav 1994; 85:370–89.

99. Kok PW, Ong CN. Blood and urinary benzene determined by headspace gas chromatography with photoionization detection: application in biological monitoring of low-level nonoccupational exposure. Int Arch Occup Environ Health 1994; 66:195–201.

100. Rinsky RA, Smith AB, Hornung R, Filloon TG, Young RJ, Okun AH, Landrigan PJ. Benzene and leukemia. An epidemiologic risk assessment. N Engl J Med 1987; 316:1044–1050.

101. Wong O. An industrywide mortality study of chemical workers occupationally exposed to benzene. II. Dose response analyses. Br J Indust Med 1987; 44:382–395.

102. Aksoy M. Benzene as a leukemogenic and carcinogenic agent. Am J Indust Med 1985; 8:9–20.

103. Yin SN, Hayes RB, Linet MS, Li GL, Dosemeci M, Travis LB, Li CY, Zhang ZH, Li DG, Chow WH, Wacholder S, Wang YZ, Jiang ZL, Dai TR, Zhang WY, Chao XJ, Ye PZ, Kou QR, Zhang XC, Lin XF, Meng JF, Ding CY, Zho JS, Blot WJ. A cohort study of cancer among benzene-exposed workers in China: overall results. Am J Indust Med 1996; 29:227–235.

104. Hayes RB, Yin SN, Dosemeci M, Li GL, Wacholder S, Travis LB, Li CY, Rothman N, Hoover RN, Linet MS. Benzene and the dose-related incidence of hematologic neoplasms in China. Chinese Academy of Preventive Medicine–National Cancer Institute Benzene Study Group. J Natl Cancer Inst 1997; 89:1065–1071.

105. Schnatter AR, Theriault G, Katz AM, Thompson FS, Donaleski D, Murray N. A retrospective mortality study within operating segments of a petroleum company. Am J Indust Med 1992; 22:209–229.

106. Schnatter AR, Armstrong TW, Thompson LS, Nicolich MJ, Katz AM, Huebner WW, Pearlman ED. The relationship between low-level benzene exposure and leukemia in Canadian petroleum distribution workers. Environ Health Perspect 1996; 104(suppl 6):1375–1379.

107. Schnatter AR, Armstrong TW, Nicolich MJ, Thompson FS, Katz AM, Huebner WW, Pearlman ED. Lymphohaematopoietic malignancies and quantitative estimates of exposure to benzene in Canadian petroleum distribution workers. Occup Environ Med 1996; 53:773–781.

108. Huebner WW, Schnatter AR, Nicolich MJ, Jorgensen G. Mortality experience of a young petrochemical industry cohort. 1979–1992 follow-up study of US-based employees. J Occup Environ Med 1997; 39:970–982.

109. Ireland B, Collins JJ, Buckley CF, Riordan SG. Cancer mortality among workers with benzene exposure. Epidemiology 1997; 8:318–320.

110. Rushton L, Romaniuk H. A case-control study to investigate the risk of leukaemia associated with exposure to benzene in petroleum marketing and distribution workers in the United Kingdom. Occup Environ Med 1997; 54:152–166.

111. Savitz DA, Andrews KW. Review of epidemiologic evidence on benzene and lymphatic and hematopoietic cancers (review). Am J Indust Med 1997; 31:287–295.

112. Travis LB, Li CY, Zhang ZN Li DG, Yin SN, Chow WH, Li GL, Dosemeci M, Blot W, Fraumeni JF Jr, et al. Hematopoietic malignancies and related disorders in benzene-exposed workers in China (review). Leuk Lymphoma 1994; 14:91–102.

113. Paustenbach DJ, Price PS, Ollison W, Blank C, Jernigan JD, Bass RD, Peterson HD. Reevaluation of benzene exposure for the Pliofilm (rubberworker) cohort (1936–1976) (review). J Toxicol Environ Health 1992; 36:177–231.

114. Utterback DF, Rinsky RA. Benzene exposure assessment in rubber hydrochloride workers: a critical evaluation of previous estimates. Am J Indust Med 1995; 27: 661–676.

115. Crump KS. Risk of benzene-induced leukemia predicted from the Pliofilm cohort. Environ Health Perspect 1996; 104(suppl 6):1437–1441.
116. Smith MT. Mechanistic studies of benzene toxicity—implications for risk assessment (review). Adv Exp Med Biol 1996; 387:259–266.
117. Zeise L, McDonald TA. California perspective on the assessment of benzene toxicological risks (review). J Toxicol Environ Health A 2000; 61:479–483.
118. Ward E, Hornung R, Morris J, Rinsky R, Wild D, Halperin W, Guthrie W. Risk of low red or white blood cell count related to estimated benzene exposure in a rubberworker cohort (1940–1975). Am J Indust Med 1996; 29:247–257.
119. Rothman N, Li GL, Dosemeci M, Bechtold WE, Marti GE, Wang YZ, Linet M, Xi LQ, Lu W, Smith MT, Titenko-Holland N, Zhang LP, Blot W, Yin SN, Hayes RB. Hematotoxicity among Chinese workers heavily exposed to benzene. Am J Indust Med 1996; 29:236–246.
120. Dosemeci M, Yin SN, Linet M, Wacholder S, Rothman N, Li GL, Chow WH, Wang YZ, Jiang ZL, Dai TR, Zhang WU, Chao XJ, Ye PZ, Kou QR, Fan YH, Zhang XC, Lin XF, Meng JF, Zho JS, Blot WJ, Hayes RB. Indirect validation of benzene exposure assessment by association with benzene poisoning. Environ Health Perspect 1996; 104(suppl 6):1343–1347.
121. Lan Q, Li G-L., Zhang L, Dosemeci M, Smith MT, Yin S, Rabkin C, Rappaport SC, HayesRB, Linet M, Rothman N. Analysis of lymphocyte subsets among workers exposed to benzene in China. Proc Am Assoc Cancer Res 2001 [Abstract 818].
122. Valentine JL, Lee SS, Seaton MJ, Asgharian B, Farris G, Corton JC, Gonzalez FJ, Medinsky MA. Reduction of benzene metabolism and toxicity in mice that lack CYP2E1 expression. Toxicol Appl Pharmacol 1996; 141:205–213.
123. Ross D. Metabolic basis of benzene toxicity (review). Eur J Haematol 1996; 60(suppl):111–118.
124. Smith MT, Yager JW, Steinmetz KL, Eastmond DA. Peroxidase-dependent metabolism of benzene's phenolic metabolites and its potential role in benzene toxicity and carcinogenicity (review). Environ Health Perspect 1989; 82:23–29.
125. Smith MT. Benzene, NQO1, and genetic susceptibility to cancer (review). Proc Natl Acad Sci USA 1999; 96:7624–7626.
126. Rothman N, Smith MT, Hayes RB, Traver RD, Hoener B, Campleman S, Li GL, Dosemeci M, Linet M, Zhang L, Xi L, Wacholder S, Lu W, Meyer KB, Titenko-Holland N, Stewart JT, Yin S, Ross D. Benzene poisoning, a risk factor for hematological malignancy, is associated with the NQO1 609C → T mutation and rapid fractional excretion of chlorzoxazone. Cancer Res 1997; 57:2839–2842.
127. Traver RD, Horikoshi T, Danenberg KD, Stadlbauer TH, Danenberg PV, Ross D, Gibson NW. NAD(P)H:quinone oxidoreductase gene expression in human colon carcinoma cells: characterization of a mutation which modulates DT-diaphorase activity and mitomycin sensitivity. Cancer Res 1992; 52:797–802.
128. Siegel D, McGuinness SM, Winski SL, Ross D. Genotype-phenotype relationships in studies of a polymorphism in NAD(P)H: quinone oxidoreductase 1. Pharmacogenetics 1999; 9:113–121.
129. Smith MT, Wang Y, Kane E, Rollinson S, Wiemels JL, Roman E, Roddam P, Cartwright R, Morgan G. NAD(P)H:quinone oxidoreductase 1 activity is associated with increased risk of acute leukemia in adults. Blood 2001; 97:1422–1426.

130. McDonald TA, Holland NT, Skibola C, Duramad P, Smith MT. Hypothesis: Phenol and hydroquinone derived mainly from diet and gastrointestinal flora activity are causal factors in leukemia (review). Leukemia 2001; 15:10–20.
131. Ross JA. Maternal diet and infant leukemia: a role for DNA topoisomerase II inhibitors? Int J Cancer 1998; 11(suppl):26–28.
132. Wiemels JL, Pagnamenta A, Taylor GM, Eden OB, Alexander FE, Greaves MF. A lack of a functional NAD(P)H:quinone oxidoreductase allele is selectively associated with pediatric leukemias that have MLL fusions. United Kingdom Childhood Cancer Study Investigators. Cancer Res 1999; 59:4095–4099.
133. Siegel D, Bolton EM, Burr JA, Liebler DC, Ross D. The reduction of alpha-tocopherolquinone by human NAD(P)H: quinone oxidoreductase: the role of alpha-tocopherolhydroquinone as a cellular antioxidant. Mol Pharmacol 1997; 52:300–305.
134. Reynolds WF, Chang E, Douer D, Ball ED, Kanda V. An allelic association implicates myeloperoxidase in the etiology of acute promyelocytic leukemia. Blood 1997; 90:2730–2737.
135. Smith MT, Ryan E, Rollinson S, Roddam P, Dring A, Roman E, Morgan GJ. The myeloperoxidase polymorphism at −463 is not associated with the M3 and M4 FAB subtypes of acute myeloid leukemia (unpublished data).
136. Matanoski GM, Stockwell HG, Diamond EL, Haring-Sweeney M, Joffe RD, Mele LM, Johnson ML. A cohort mortality study of painters and allied tradesmen. Scand J Work Environ Health 1986; 12:16–21.
137. Chen R, Seaton A. A meta-analysis of painting exposure and cancer mortality. Cancer Detect Prev 1998; 22:533–539.
138. Nisse C, Lorthois C, Dorp V, Eloy E, Haguenoer JM, Fenaux P. Exposure to occupational and environmental factors in myelodysplastic syndromes. Preliminary results of a case-control study. Leukemia 1995; 9:693–699.
139. Hayes RB, Blair A, Stewart PA, Herrick RF, Mahar H. Mortality of U.S. embalmers and funeral directors. Am J Indust Med 1990; 18:641–652.
140. Linos A, Blair A, Cantor KP, Burmeister L, VanLier S, Gibson RW, Schuman L, Everett G. Leukemia and non-Hodgkin's lymphoma among embalmers and funeral directors. J Natl Cancer Inst 1990; 82:66.
141. Hunting KL, Longbottom H, Kalavar SS, Stern F, Schwartz E, Welch LS. Haematopoietic cancer mortality among vehicle mechanics. Occup Environ Med 1995; 52: 673–678.
142. Hotz P, Lauwerys RR. Hematopoietic and lymphatic malignancies in vehicle mechanics (review). Crit Rev Toxicol 1997; 27:443–494.
143. Bulbulyan MA, Changuina OV, Zaridze DG, Astashevsky SV, Colin D, Boffetta P. Cancer mortality among Moscow shoe workers exposed to chloroprene (Russia). Cancer Causes Control 1998; 9:381–387.
144. Lynge E. Danish Cancer Registry as a resource for occupational research. J Occup Med 1994; 36:1169–1173.
145. Miligi L, Seniori Costantini A, Crosignani P, Fontana A, Masala G, Nanni O, Ramazzotti V, Rodella S, Stagnaro E, Tumino R, Vigano C, Vindigni C, Vineis P. Occupational, environmental, and life-style factors associated with the risk of hematolymphopoietic malignancies in women. Am J Indust Med 1999; 36: 60–69.

146. Nilsson RI, Nordlinder R, Horte LG, Jarvholm B. Leukaemia, lymphoma, and multiple myeloma in seamen on tankers. Occup Environ Med 1998; 55:517–521.

147. Burnett C, Robison C, Walker J. Cancer mortality in health and science technicians. Am J Indust Med 1999; 36:155–158.

148. Linet MS, Cartwright RA. The leukemias. In: Schottenfeld DM, Fraumeni JF, eds. Cancer Epidemiology and Prevention. 2nd ed. New York: Oxford University Press, 1996:841–892.

149. Pesatori AC, Consonni D, Tironi A, Zocchetti C, Fini A, Bertazzi PA. Cancer in a young population in a dioxin-contaminated area. Int J Epidemiol 1993; 22:1010–1013.

150. Shore DL, Sandler DP, Davey FR, McIntyre OR, Bloomfield CD. Acute leukemia and residential proximity to potential sources of environmental pollutants. Arch Environ Health 1993; 48:414–420.

151. Morrow NL. The industrial production and use of 1,3-butadiene (review). Environ Health Perspect 1990; 86:7–8.

152. International Agency for Research on Cancer. 1,3-Butadiene. Lyon, France: IARC, 1998.

153. Delzell E, Sathiakumar N, Hovinga M, Macaluso M, Julian J, Larson R, Cole P, Muir DC. A follow-up study of synthetic rubber workers. Toxicology 1996; 113: 182–189.

154. Sathiakumar N, Delzell E, Hovinga M, Macaluso M, Julian JA, Larson R, Cole P, Muir DC. Mortality from cancer and other causes of death among synthetic rubber workers. Occup Environ Med 1998; 55:230–235.

155. Ward JB Jr, Ammenheuser MM, Bechtold WE, Whorton EB Jr, Legator MS. Hprt mutant lymphocyte frequencies in workers at a 1,3-butadiene production plant. Environ Health Perspect 1994; 102(suppl 9):79–85.

156. Ward JB, Ammenheuser MM, Whorton EB Jr, Bechtold WE, Kelsey KT, Legator MS. Biological monitoring for mutagenic effects of occupational exposure to butadiene. Toxicology 1996; 113:84–90.

157. Hayes RB, Xi L, Bechtold WE, Rothman N, Yao M, Henderson R, Zhang L, Smith MT, Zhang D, Wiemels J, Dosemeci M, Yin S, O'Neil JP. Hprt mutation frequency among workers exposed to 1,3-butadiene in China. Toxicology 1996; 113:100–105.

158. Sorsa M, Autio J, Demopoulus NA, Jarventaus H, Rossner P, Sram RJ, Stephanou G, Vlachodimitropoulos D. Human cytogenetic biomonitoring of occupational exposure to 1,3-butadiene. Mutat Res 1994; 309:321–326.

159. Sorsa M, Peltonen K, Anderson D, Demopoulus NA, Neuman HG, Osterman-Golkar S. Assessment of environmental and occupational exposures to butadiene as a model for risk estimation of petrochemical emissions. Mutagenesis 1996; 11: 9–17.

160. Sram RJ, Rossner P, Peltonen K, Podrazilova K, Mrackova G, Demopoulus NA, Stephanou G, Vlachodimitropoulos D, Darroudi F, Tates AD. Chromosomal aberrations, sister-chromatid exchanges, cells with high frequency of SCE, micronuclei, and comet assay parameters in 1,3-butadiene-exposed workers. Mutat Res 1998; 419:145–154.

161. Tates AD, van Dam FJ, de Zwart FA, Darroudi F, Natarajan AT, Rossner P, Pe-

terkova K, Peltonen K, Demopoulus NA, Stephanou G, Vlachodimitropoulos D, Sram RJ. Biological effect monitoring in the industrial workers from the Czech Republic exposed to low levels of butadiene. Toxicology 1996; 113:91–99.

162. Bond JA, Recio L, Andjelkovich D. Epidemiological and mechanistic data suggest that 1,3-butadiene will not be carcinogenic to humans at exposures likely to be encountered in the environment or workplace (review). Carcinogenesis 1995; 16: 165–171.

163. Pearce NE, Smith AH, Howard JK, Sheppard RA, Giles HJ, Teague CA. Case-control study of multiple myeloma and farming. Br J Cancer 1986; 54:493–500.

164. Blair A, Zahm SH. Agricultural exposures and cancer (review). Environ Health Perspect 1995; 103(suppl 8):205–208.

165. Keller-Byrne JE, Khuder SA, Schaub EA. Meta-analysis of leukemia and farming. Environ Res 1995; 71:1–10.

166. Zahm SH, Ward MH, Blair A. Pesticides and cancer (review). Occup Med 1997; 12:269–289.

167. Wiklund K, Holm LE. Trends in cancer risks among Swedish agricultural workers. J Natl Cancer Inst 1986; 77:657–664.

168. Dean G. Deaths from primary brain cancers, lymphatic and haematopoietic cancers in agricultural workers in the Republic of Ireland. J Epidemiol Community Health 1994; 48:364–368.

169. Avnon L, Oryan I, Kordysh E, Goldsmith J, Sobel R, Friger M. Cancer incidence and risks in selected agricultural settlements in the Negev of Israel. Arch Environ Health 1998; 53:336–343.

170. Kristensen P, Andersen A, Irgens LM, Laake P, Bye AS. Incidence and risk factors of cancer among men and women in Norwegian agriculture. Scand J Work Environ Health 1996; 22:14–26.

171. Blair A, Zahm SH, Pearce NE, Heineman EF, Fraumeni JR Jr. Clues to cancer etiology from studies of farmers. Scand J Work Environ Health 1992; 18:209–215.

172. Brown LM, Blair A, Gibson R, Everett GD, Cantor KP, Schuman LM, Burmeister LF, Van Lier SF, Dick F. Pesticide exposures and other agricultural risk factors for leukemia among men in Iowa and Minnesota. Cancer Res 1990; 50:6585–6591.

173. Sathiakumar N, Delzell E. A review of epidemiologic studies of triazine herbicides and cancer (review). Crit Rev Toxicol 1997; 27:599–612.

174. Alavanja MC, Sandler DP, McMaster SB, Zahm SH, McDonnell CJ, Lynch CF, Pennybacker M, Rothman N, Dosemeci M, Bond AE, Blair A. The Agricultural Health Study. Environ Health Perspect 1996; 104:362–369.

175. Stewart PA, Fears T, Kross B, Ogilvie L, Blair A. Exposure of farmers to phosmet, a swine insecticide. Scand J Work Environ Health 1999; 25:33–38.

176. Stewart PA, Stewart WF, Heineman EF, Dosemeci M, Linet M, Inskip PD. A novel approach to data collection in a case-control study of cancer and occupational exposures. Int J Epidemiol 1996; 25:744–752.

177. Pearce N, Smith AH, Reif JS. Increased risks of soft tissue sarcoma, malignant lymphoma, and acute myeloid leukemia in abattoir workers. Am J Indust Med 1988; 14:63–72.

178. Metayer C, Johnson ES, Rice JC. Nested case-control study of tumors of the hema-

topoietic and lymphatic systems among workers in the meat industry. Am J Epidemiol 1998; 147:727–738.

179. Pearce N and Reif JS. Epidemiologic studies of cancer in agricultural workers (review). Am J Indust Med 1990; 18:133–148.

180. Sandler DP, Shore DL, Anderson JR, Davey FR, Arthur D, Mayer RJ, Silver RT, Weiss RB, Moore JO, Schiffer CA, et al. Cigarette smoking and risk of acute leukemia: associations with morphology and cytogenetic abnormalities in bone marrow. J Natl Cancer Inst 1993; 85:1994–2003.

181. Garfinkel L and Boffetta P. Association between smoking and leukemia in two American Cancer Society prospective studies. Cancer 1990; 65:2356–2360.

182. Kane EV, Roman E, Cartwright R, Parker J, Morgan G. Tobacco and the risk of acute leukaemia in adults. Br J Cancer 1999; 81:1228–1233.

183. Engeland A, Andersen A, Haldorsen T, Tretli S. Smoking habits and risk of cancers other than lung cancer. 28 years' follow-up of 6,000 Norwegian men and women. Cancer Causes Control 1996; 7:497–506.

184. Adami J, Nyrén O, Berström R, Ekbom A, Engholm G, Englund A, Glimelius B. Smoking and the risk of leukemia, lymphoma, and multiple myeloma (Sweden). Cancer Causes Control 1998; 9:49–56.

185. Brownson RC, Novotny TE, Perry MC. Cigarette smoking and adult leukemia. A meta-analysis. Arch Intern Med 1993; 153:469–475.

186. Doll R. Cancers weakly related to smoking (review). Br Med Bull 1996; 52:35–49.

187. Bjork J, Albin M, Mauritzson N, Stromberg U, Johansson B, Hagmar L. Smoking and myelodysplastic syndromes. Epidemiology 2000; 11:285–291.

188. Williams RR, Horm JW. Association of cancer sites with tobacco and alcohol consumption and socioeconomic status of patients: interview study from the Third National Cancer Survey. J Natl Cancer Inst 1977; 58:525–547.

189. Blackwelder WC, Yano K, Rhoads GG, Kagan A, Gordon T, Palesch Y. Alcohol and mortality: the Honolulu Heart Study. Am J Med 1980; 68:164–169.

190. Hinds MW, Kolonel LN, Lee T, Hirohata T. Associations between cancer incidence and alcohol/cigarette consumption among five ethnic groups in Hawaii. Br J Cancer 1980; 41:929–940.

191. Carstensen JM, Bygren LO, Hatschek T. Cancer incidence among Swedish brewery workers (review). Int J Cancer 1990; 45:393–396.

192. Brown LM, Gibson R, Burmeister LF, Schuman LM, Everett GD, Blair A. Alcohol consumption and risk of leukemia, non-Hodgkin's lymphoma, and multiple myeloma. Leuk Res 1992; 16:979–984.

193. Ido M, Nagata C, Kawakami N, Shimizu H, Yoshida Y, Nomura T, Mizoguchi H. A case-control study of myelodysplastic syndromes among Japanese men and women. Leuk Res 1996; 20:727–731.

194. Mele A, Szklo M, Visani G, Stazi MA, Castelli G, Pasquini P, Mandelli F. Hair dye use and other risk factors for leukemia and pre-leukemia: a case-control study. Italian Leukemia Study Group. Am J Epidemiol 1994; 139:609–619.

195. Nagata C, Shimizu H, Hirashima K, Kakishita E, Fujimura K, Niho Y, Karasawa M, Oguma S, Yoshida Y, Mizoguchi H. Hair dye use and occupational exposure

to organic solvents as risk factors for myelodysplastic syndrome. Leuk Res 1999; 23:57–62.

196. Correa A, Mohan A, Jackson L, Perry H, Helzlsouer K. Use of hair dyes, hematopoietic neoplasms, and lymphomas: a literature review (review). I. Leukemias and myelodysplastic syndromes. Cancer Invest 2000; 18:366–380.

197. Gentile G, Mele A, Ragona G, Faggioni A, Zompetta C, Tosti ME, Visani G, Castelli G, Pulsoni A, Monarca B, Martino P, Mandelli F. Human herpes virus-6 seroprevalence and leukaemias: a case-control study. GIMEMA (Gruppo Italiano Malattie Ematologiche dell' Adulto). Br J Cancer 1999; 80:1103–1106.

198. Gentile G, Mele A, Monarco B, Vitale A, Pulsoni A, Visani G, Castelli G, Rapicetta M, Verani P, Martino P, Mandelli F. Hepatitis B and C viruses, human T-cell lymphotropic virus types I and II, and leukemias: a case-control study. The Italian Leukemia Study Group. Cancer Epidemiol Biomarkers Prev 1996; 5:227–230.

199. Cooper GS, Kamel F, Sandler DP, Davey FR, Bloomfield CD. Risk of adult acute leukemia in relation to prior immune-related conditions. Cancer Epidemiol Biomarkers Prev 1996; 5:867–872.

200. Raza A. Hypothesis: myelodysplastic syndromes may have a viral etiology (review). Int J Hematol 1998; 68:245–256.

201. Raza A. Myelodysplastic syndromes may have an infectious etiology. J Toxicol Environ Health A 2000; 61:387–390.

202. Hursting SD, Margolin BH, Switzer BR. Diet and human leukemia: an analysis of international data (review). Prev Med 1993; 22:409–422.

203. Kwiatkowski A. Dietary and other environmental risk factors in acute leukemias: a case-control study of 119 patients. Eur J Cancer Prev 1993; 2:139–146.

204. Doll R and Peto R. The causes of cancer: quantitative estimates of avoidable risks of cancer in the United States today (review). J Natl Cancer Inst 1981; 66:1191–1308.

205. Caspi O, Polliack A, Klar R, Ben-Yehuda D: The association of inflammatory bowel disease and leukemia—coincidence or not? (review). Leuk Lymphoma 1995; 17:255–262.

206. Dombret H, Marolleau JP. De novo acute myeloid leukemia in patients with Crohn's disease. Nouv Rev Fr Hematol 1995; 37:193–196.

207. Harewood GC, Loftus EV Jr, Tefferi A, Tremaine WJ, Sandborn WJ. Concurrent inflammatory bowel disease and myelodysplastic syndromes. Inflamm Bowel Dis 1999; 5:98–103.

208. Hatake K, Tanaka M, Muroi K, Miura Y. Leukaemia risk in Crohn's disease. Lancet 1996; 347:1049–1050.

209. Harewood G, Markovic S. Treatment of acute myeloid leukemia M3 in a patient with Crohn's disease. Cancer Invest 2000; 18:98.

210. Tani T, Sakai Y, Shirai Y, Ohtake M, Hatakeyama K. Simultaneous development of Crohn's disease and myelodysplastic syndrome progressing to acute myelocytic leukemia in a patient with a normal karyotype (review). J Gastroenterol 1996; 31:599–602.

# 4
# Immunology of the Myelodysplastic Syndromes

**Terry J. Hamblin**
*South Hampton University and Royal Bournemouth Hospital,
Bournemouth, England*

## I. INTRODUCTION

There is little doubt that the immune system is abnormal in myelodysplastic syndromes (MDS), but exactly how it is impaired and why remains in dispute. Some evidence points to a fundamental defect at a stem cell level that permeates the lymphoid system in the same way that the myeloid system is affected. However, it is possible that all the immune system abnormalities can be explained by defects in the effector functions of phagocytic cells or by dysfunctional antigenic presentation by dendritic cells of myelomonocytic origin. This is the fourth in a series of reviews that this author has written on this subject (1–3) and in order to avoid duplicate publication, extensive reference to the first three articles is made. This chapter concentrates on new information and insights since 1995.

Evidence of impaired immunity in MDS is threefold: an increased susceptibility to infection; autoimmunity; and an increased incidence of malignant neoplasms, especially lymphoid neoplasms. In this chapter, the clinical and laboratory evidence for impaired immunity is presented first, followed by the attempts that have been made to demonstrate that the lymphoid system is part of the MDS clone. The newer immunological treatments for MDS are detailed, with a concentration on how this aids in understanding the condition. Finally, the last section of this chapter examines the most satisfactory explanation of the phenomenon that best fits the available evidence.

## II. INFECTION

Approximately 10% of MDS patients present with infection (1), and in 20–35% of patients infection is the major cause of death (1,3). Low neutrophil counts and/or impaired neutrophil function appear to be involved in some but certainly not all types of infection. For example, gram-negative septicemias and bacterial bronchopneumonias are usually attributed to neutropenia, but bacterial infections may also occur in the absence of neutropenia, especially in chronic myelomonocytic leukemia (CMML) where a neutrophil leukocytosis is the rule (3). In a series of patients with clinically silent abscesses (perinephric, paracolic, intramuscular), neutrophil counts were normal but impaired neutrophil function was likely responsible for both the accumulation of pus and the observed limited systemic effect (1).

Fungal infections are rare manifestations of MDS, although they may be seen as a consequence of intensive treatment. However, atypical mycobacterial infections have frequently been reported (3). Recent publications have detailed a case of drug-resistant tuberculous uveitis associated with MDS (4) and a case of hemophagocytic syndrome (5). The latter case was resistant to treatment with steroids, but was responsive to plasma exchange. It is tempting to attribute these findings to disordered macrophage function, perhaps enhanced by treatment with corticosteroids. Not only may macrophages be poorly phagocytic, but they may secrete an abnormal spectrum of cytokines as well (3). Infection with the fungi-like protozoan *Pneumocystis carinii* has also been reported in patients with MDS (3).

Viral infections are also rare in MDS, although a single case of chronic herpes encephalitis has been reported (3). An Epstein-Barr virus–associated B-cell lymphoma of the brain has been recently reported in an HIV-negative patient with MDS (6). Infection with human immunodeficiency virus (3) and parvovirus (7) may mimic the marrow morphology of MDS. Raza has hypothesized that MDS itself might have a viral etiology (8). In patients with MDS, Raza et al. were able to demonstrate the presence of actively replicating herpesviruses [Epstein-Barr virus (EBV) and cytomegalovirus (CMV)] in the bone marrow mononuclear cells; they also demonstrated the ability of MDS bone marrow stroma to support viral activation (9). Human T-cell leukemia virus-1 (HTLV-1) has also been implicated in the etiology of MDS. Karlic et al. found polymerase chain reaction (PCR) and/or serological evidence of HTLV-1 in 11 of 65 cases of MDS in Austria, a nonendemic area (10). No relationship with blood transfusion was found.

## III. AUTOIMMUNE DISEASE IN MDS

Tissue-specific autoantibodies are not found any more frequently in MDS patients than they are in age-matched controls (11). However, rashes are particularly common in MDS and might have an autoimmune etiology. Cutaneous vasculitis was first reported in MDS by French investigators (12) and has since been regularly observed and reported.

It should be noted that the term "cutaneous vasculitis," as used here, refers very specifically to the response of small blood vessels in the skin to injury. With such a broad definition, perhaps it is not surprising that cutaneous vasculitis encompasses a wide variety of reactions—from a transient increase in permeability to coagulation and necrosis with ulceration. Among the reactions included are the following conditions: Henoch-Schönlein purpura, polyarteritis nodosa, nodular vasculitis, leukocytoclastic vasculitis, allergic granulomatosis, Behçet's syndrome, purpura fulminans, pyoderma gangrenosum, thromboangiitis obliterans, erythema nodosum, chilblains, livedo reticularis, and white atrophy (atrophie blanche) (3).

Injury to a blood vessel invokes an immune response designed to remove the cause of the injury and repair the damage. This inflammatory response is complex and its nature depends on several factors, including the intensity of the injury, the efficiency of the inflammation, and the effectiveness of the repair, as well as a number of local and host factors. The exact pattern of the resultant rash will therefore vary and the vasculitis may not be confined to the skin. Even the aorta may be involved (13). The wide variety of vasculitic conditions seen with MDS may well have a common etiology. Table 1 lists the inflammatory diseases that have been associated with MDS.

Acute febrile neutrophilic dermatosis (Sweet's syndrome) is the most commonly reported vasculitic condition in MDS. Multiple edematous, beefy-red papules or plaques, which may become pustular, are found in association with fever, high erythrocyte sedimentation rate (ESR), and leukocytosis (14,15). The rash is typically on the face, neck, or arms, but can be found anywhere on the skin.

**Table 1**  Inflammatory Diseases Associated with MDS

Acute febrile neutrophilic dermatosis (Sweet's syndrome)
Allergic granulomatosis
Behçet's syndrome
Chronic nonsuppurative panniculitis
Cutaneous vasculitis
Desquamative interstitial pneumonitis
Eosinophilic fasciitis
Erythema elevatum diutinum
Erythema nodosum
Leukocytoclastic vasculitis
Pyoderma gangrenosum
Relapsing polychondritis
Subcorneal pustular dermatosis

Histologically, the rash consists of a diffuse or perivascular infiltrate of polymorphs in the dermis. Sweet himself recognized that the syndrome might have systemic manifestations and described joint and muscle pains, conjunctivitis, and episcleritis (16) whereas others have described renal (15), hepatic (17), and pulmonary involvement (18). A recent report has detailed a sterile, neutrophilic myositis (19). Cardiac muscle may also be involved (20), and the orbital inflammation reported by Rouhiainen et al. may well have been another manifestation of neutrophilic dermatosis (21).

A useful review of skin lesions in MDS (22) has detailed several case reports not included in previous reviews by this author (1–3). Avivi et al. recognized 23 cases in the literature. A total of 10 further case reports have since appeared (20,21,23–30). It is very likely that other cases have escaped mention in any of these reviews.

Pyoderma gangrenosum is another neutrophilic dermatosis associated with MDS (3). This condition is characterized by painful nodules or pustules that break down to form ulcers that progressively enlarge. The nodules or pustules have raised, tender, undermined borders that occur on the abdomen, buttocks, or legs. This obscure condition is a reaction pattern in which venous and capillary engorgement, hemorrhage, and coagulation feature prominently together with an intense neutrophilic infiltrate. A bullous variety is reportedly associated with hematological conditions and has been seen in MDS (31). Avivi et al. (22) detailed nine cases of MDS and pyoderma gangrenosum in their literature review, but again this is probably an underestimate of its prevalence. Journal referees show a marked reluctance to accept such case reports for publication unless novel features can be demonstrated.

Two less common forms of neutrophilic dermatosis have also been associated with MDS. Subcorneal pustular dermatosis is characterized by annular plaques located in skin folds (32). In erythema elevatum diutinum, symmetrical nodules, papules, or plaques develop on the extensor surfaces of hands, elbows, or knees (14,33). The histological picture is of leukocytoclastic vasculitis with a dense dermal infiltrate of neutrophils (34).

Other similar syndromes reported in association with MDS include eosinophilic fasciitis, a syndrome of sclerodermatous change in the skin of the limbs and trunk, sparing the hands and feet, and a transient pemphigus-like syndrome with acantholysis (3).

It is thought that Behçet's syndrome represents an immunological reaction to chronic infections with *Streptococcus viridans*, with endothelial injury being caused by the products of activated neutrophils. Five cases of Behçet's syndrome in association with MDS have previously been reported (3). A review by Ohno et al. (35) identified four other cases and contributed one of their own. Subsequently, three other cases have been reported (36–38). With one exception—an Italian case—all the reports have been of Japanese or Korean nationals. Two of the patients had intestinal involvement while most had trisomy 8.

Chronic, nonsuppurative panniculitis, or Weber-Christian disease, is characterized by bouts of fever and crops of subcutaneous nodules. Histological analysis shows necrosis of fat with neutrophils and lipid-filled macrophages. Five cases of Weber-Christian disease associated with MDS have been reported (3,39).

Relapsing polychondritis is a rare disorder of uncertain origin characterized by recurrent inflammation of the cartilage associated with a polyarteritis, a non-erosive polyarthritis, and inflammation of the eye. It has been reported on 15 occasions in association with MDS (40). One group estimated that 0.6% of all patients with MDS suffer from relapsing polychondritis, and that these patients represent 28% of all cases of polychondritis. Since this estimation of incidence, five further cases have been reported (41–43).

The diagnosis of cutaneous vasculitis is rather common in MDS. In 1996, a literature review by this author identified 16 cases (3). One year later, Pirayesh et al. identified 44 cases, including the 16 characterized in the 1996 review (44). Many cases of cutaneous vasculitis in MDS also have features of other connective tissue disorders. Maeda et al. (45), for example, reported a patient who also had polymyositis. Chandran et al. (46) recognized an overlap between cutaneous vasculitis and seronegative arthritis, which had previously been noted to be common in MDS (47). A case with vasculitis and seropositive rheumatoid arthritis (48) has also been reported.

Enright et al. (49) reported pulmonary infiltrates in five of seven MDS patients with an acute syndrome of vasculitic rash, fever, and arthritis, and a case of MDS with desquamative interstitial pneumonitis has been described in great detail (50). In Bournemouth, from a series of cases that now amounts to more than 800, six patients with MDS have been seen with a restrictive lung defect accompanied by pulmonary infiltrates. Three of these patients responded to treatment with corticosteroids, as did all three of the patients with pulmonary disorders reported by Matsushima et al. (51). The patients described by Matsushima et al. had bone marrow eosinophilia and a similar cytogenetic abnormality involving a 1q;7p translocation.

Renal disease is common in systemic vasculitides, but rare in vasculitides that accompany MDS. Saito et al. (52) identified five of 125 patients with MDS who had glomerular disease, three of whom had formal nephritic syndrome. Patients with CMML were particularly susceptible. A single patient with crescentic glomerulonephritis accompanied by antineutrophil cytoplasmic antibodies (ANCA) has been identified (53), but generally most patients with vasculitis are ANCA-negative. Hamidou et al. (54) described 13 of 60 patients with MDS who had various types of vasculitis, and only one was ANCA-positive.

Although the vasculitides are commonly regarded as autoimmune conditions, there is little to suggest that these conditions are the result of autoantibody activity or T-cell attack on blood vessels. It is more likely that the vasculitides are consequences of granulocyte and/or macrophage dysfunction. Immune complexes, which are normally disposed of by a properly operating phagocytic system, are the normal consequence of exposure to food or bacterial antigens. In MDS, phagocytic dysfunction impairs this process so that immune complexes are deposited in small blood vessels allowing the local activation of inflammatory mediators. Neutrophil dysfunction (55) or abnormal cytokine production (32) may play a part in the inappropriate and exaggerated response. Sweet's syndrome sometimes occurs as a result of treatment of MDS with granulocyte colony-stimulating factor (G-CSF) (25,56).

## IV.  NEOPLASMS IN MDS

Cancer is so common in late middle age that it is difficult to establish whether it is any more common among MDS patients. With the exception of lymphoid malignancies, there is no firm evidence that cancer is more prevalent among MDS patients than the general population (3). Almost all patients with cancer get a blood test and since having a blood test is a prerequisite for diagnosing MDS, a diagnosis of cancer is more likely in MDS patients than in the general population. Although there are case series that suggest that cancer is more common than in the general population, these series all suffer from an indeterminate denominator (3).

However, there seems little doubt that lymphoid malignancies are more common in MDS than in the general population. The occurrence of cancer among MDS patients has been extensively reviewed previously (1–3). All types of lymphoid tumors have been found in association with MDS, and since the 1996 review article (3), several other lymphoid cancers have been reported: adult T-cell leukemia (ATL) (57), T-cell large granular lymphocytic leukemia [T-LGL] (58), and hairy cell leukemia (59).

The patient with ATL (57) was the first reported case of this type of leukemia in association with MDS. HTLV-1 DNA was not integrated into the DNA of the patient's bone marrow myeloid cells. According to reports in 1987 and 1994, T-LGL and MDS were previously noted to have an association (60,61). Nine of 76 patients with MDS referred to the U.S. National Institutes of Health (NIH) also had T-LGL; conversely, nine of 33 patients with T-LGL also had MDS. However, it should not be assumed that such a relationship represents either a malignancy clonally related to MDS or even a malignancy. Molldrem et al. (62) have demonstrated oligoclonal T-cell expansions that suppress autologous progenitor cell growth. Because of the limited T-cell receptor V beta repertoire, such proliferations may be taken for neoplasms.

## V.  LABORATORY EVIDENCE FOR IMMUNOLOGICAL ABNORMALITIES IN MDS

As outlined in Table 2, immunological abnormalities associated with MDS have diverse effects on several immune cell types and immunoglobulins.

## A.  Abnormalities of B Cells

Seven independent groups of investigators have reported evidence of polyclonal hypergammaglobulinemia in a high proportion of patients with MDS, especially in patients with CMML (3,63). Hypogammaglobulinemia is also occasionally seen (3,64), particularly in refractory anemia with ringed sideroblasts (RARS) and in children. Monoclonal immunoglobulins were found in approximately 12% of patient populations in three studies (3), about twice the prevalence in age-matched controls.

Using standard immunofluorescent screening, two studies have found both organ-specific and non-organ-specific autoantibodies to be no more common than in age-matched controls, except in CMML where they were twice as common (3). As noted above, ANCA positivity is not common, even in patients with vasculitis. Three studies have found a higher than-expected prevalence of autoantibodies to red cells (3). Katsuki et al. (65) reported two cases of MDS with extramedullary, polyclonal plasma cell proliferation and autoantibody production (antinuclear factor and anti-red cell antibodies). Using quantitative immunoblotting, Stahl et al. (66) analyzed the global antibody repertoires of immunoglobulin M (lgM) and immunoglobulin G (lgG) antibodies in the plasma of 10 MDS patients. These investigators demonstrated significantly altered patterns of self-reactivity among patients compared with healthy controls.

Normal absolute numbers of circulating B cells have been reported by a

**Table 2**  Immunological Abnormalities Associated with MDS

| Immunoglobulins | B cells | T cells | Natural killer (NK) cells |
|---|---|---|---|
| Polyclonal hypergammaglobulinemia | Normal in number | T-cell lymphopenia | Reduced in number |
| Hypogammaglobulinemia | Functionally immature | Reduced CD4+ cells | Functionally immature |
| Monoclonal gammopathy | | Impaired T-cell function | |
| Anti-red cell antibodies | | | |

number of groups, although two studies found reduced B-cell numbers (3,64). By contrast, bone marrow B lymphocytes were increased in 19% of cases of RAEB and RAEB-t (67). Minor functional abnormalities have also been found (3).

## B.  Abnormalities of T Cells

Although little clinical evidence for a T-cell defect in MDS can be cited, there is ample laboratory evidence. There is usually an absolute lymphopenia that is almost entirely due to reduced numbers of T cells (1–3). In most studies, the greatest reduction occurred in the CD4+ subset of T cells, although reductions in the CD8+ subset were also seen (3,63). Further analysis of T-cell subsets demonstrates that $T_H1$ and $T_C1$ subtypes predominate (68), correlating with raised levels of soluble interleukin-2 (IL-2) in the serum (69). Interestingly, T-cell numbers in bone marrow trephine biopsies were normal (67).

Abnormalities of T-cell function have also been widely reported. Among these are poor lymphoproliferative responses to phytohemagglutinin, concanavalin A, and anti-CD3 (3,70,71). Because the lymphoproliferative defect could not be corrected in vitro by cimetidine, indomethacin, or isoprinosine, it is unlikely that the impairment is due to suppressor T-cell activity, monocyte suppression, or deficient helper/inducer function, respectively (71). However, T cells from MDS patients respond normally when stimulated by phorbol myristate acetate plus a $Ca^{2+}$ ionophore (70). Other abnormalities of T-cell function include impaired cloning efficiency in a T-cell-colony assay and increased lymphocyte sensitivity to x-rays (3).

## C.  Abnormalities of Natural Killer Cells

Natural killer (NK) activity may be defined as the ability of NK cells to kill certain tumor target cells without requiring the target cells to express class I or II molecules of the major histocompatibility complex (MHC) (2). Large granular lymphocytes of neither B-cell nor T-cell lineage are the major population of blood cells able to mediate this activity. These granular lymphocytes have their origin in the bone marrow and characteristically express CD56 and CD16 cell surface proteins. A minor fraction of CD3+T lymphocytes are also able to mediate NK activity. Impaired NK activity in MDS is assessed by killing of the K562, 1301, and MOLT-4 cell lines (2). Other NK cell functions, such as antibody-dependent cellular cytotoxicity, interferon-α production, and inhibition of myeloid progenitor cell growth, have also been shown to be defective (2). Many NK cell functions may be restored by incubation with α-, but not γ-, interferon (3).

In the laboratory, it has proved difficult to count NK cells. Early studies used the HNK-1 (CD57) monoclonal antibody, identifying reduced numbers.

More recently, the NKH-1 (CD56) and CD16 antibodies have been used and normal numbers of NK cells were obtained (3).

## D. Abnormalities of the Mononuclear Phagocytic System

The numbers of macrophages in the bone marrow are thought to be increased in all types of MDS, not just in CMML (72,73). Approximately 20% of patients with MDS have increased numbers of circulating monocytes, even though the increases do not reach levels seen in CMML (74). While there is doubt as to whether lymphocytes derive from the MDS clone, it is known that monocytes are certainly derived from the MDS clone.

Many authors have assumed that the monocyte/macrophage system functions abnormally in MDS, and that this accounts for abnormalities in antibody production, suggesting that antigen presentation and secretion of cytokines are disordered (3,75). Monocyte-derived cytokines, such as tumor necrosis factor-$\alpha$, interferon-$\gamma$, interleukin-1$\beta$, and transforming growth factor-$\beta$, are increased in MDS (76–80). Many of these cytokines are important in inducing apoptosis and therefore may play a crucial role in the pathogenesis of MDS (78).

Incubation of peripheral blood monocytes with granulocyte-macrophage colony-stimulating factor (GM-CSF) and interleukin-4 in vivo results in the production of dendritic cells. In MDS, dendritic cells produced in this way are derived from the malignant clone and have deficient antigen uptake and presentation (81).

It is important to note that many functions of monocytes have been demonstrated to be normal in most cases of MDS, including phagocytosis of opsonized bacteria, pinocytosis of dextran sulphate, and phagocytosis and intracellular killing of *Candida albicans* (3). Receptors for Fc and C3b have been found to be normal in number in most cases, but some investigators have found activation-associated changes of cell surface markers in infection-free MDS patients. In particular, Fc receptors, complement receptors, CD67, and M5 were all present with increased density (3). Cytochemical staining shows low levels of nonspecific esterase in blood monocytes and low levels of peroxidase in blood and bone marrow monocytes and promonocytes (3).

Phagocytosis of IgG-coated sheep red blood cells by both blood and bone marrow monocytes has been found to be suboptimal in CMML; skin window techniques demonstrated normal emigration of blood monocytes into the tissues but delayed acquisition of lysosomal enzymes (3). Perhaps involved in the poor immune function in MDS is the down-regulation of CD43, a sialylated glycoprotein involved in cell adhesion and signaling, which has been implicated in the immunodeficiency of Wiskott-Aldrich syndrome (82).

In summary, monocyte numbers are generally increased in MDS, and some functions of monocytes and macrophages are abnormal. Increased or inappropriate activity in cytokine production may play a part in the pathogenesis of MDS and in the abnormal immunological activity.

## VI.  IS THE LYMPHOID SYSTEM INVOLVED IN THE DYSPLASTIC PROCESS?

Does the MDS follow the chronic myeloid leukemia paradigm of deriving from a pluripotential stem cell capable of differentiating into lymphoid and myeloid lineages? It is by no means clear that it does or that it does so in every case; see Table 3.

### A.  Transformation to Acute Lymphoblastic Leukemia

Lymphoid transformations in MDS are surpassingly rare. In a 1996 review, evidence was presented for 19 reported cases where acute lymphoblastic leukemia (ALL) followed the development of MDS (3). In three of these cases, T-cell ALL was diagnosed. Seven further cases have since been published (83–89). In three of the seven cases, the linkage between MDS and ALL was confirmed by a common karyotypic abnormality [del(7), trisomy 8, and del(20q)] (84,86,89). Of the 19 cases discussed in the review article mentioned above, in only two of the cases could the MDS and ALL be linked cytogenetically (3). Of the remaining 17 cases, two were transformations from juvenile myelomonocytic leukemia (JMML)(86,87) and one was a transformation from CMML (88). In one case, the transformation was marked by the acquisition of a Philadelphia chromosome and a p190 BCR/ABL transcript (89). Interestingly, Leseve et al. (90) have described two cases of RAEB without transformation that also had the p190 BCR/

**Table 3**  Evidence of Lymphoid Involvement in Myelodysplastic Syndromes

---

Transformation of MDS to acute lymphoblastic leukaemia
Comment: Very few well-documented cases
Coexistent MDS and lymphoid malignancies
Comment: Particularly associated with myeloma
Inactivation of same X chromosome in lymphoid and myeloid cells
Comment: Well-known index cases, but most workers do not find it
Same cytogenetic abnormality in lymphoid and myeloid cells
Comment: Almost never found
Same oncogene mutations in lymphoid and myeloid cells
Comment: Very few reports

---

ABL version of the Philadelphia chromosome. This is a phenomenon that merits watching. In 1972, before molecular biology had emerged as a biological science, this author saw two patients with MDS (RARS and RAEB) who had the Philadelphia chromosome, but medical journals were not interested in publishing the case reports.

Early cases of ALL were diagnosed on morphological grounds alone, but later cases were better documented by cell markers and cytochemistry, and indeed by response to vincristine and prednisolone. In addition, 14 cases of bilineal and seven cases of biphenotypic leukemia have been reported in association with MDS (3). In the former, two distinct types of blast with different cell markers are seen, and in the latter, one kind of blast cell has both lymphoid and myeloid markers. It has become well recognized that markers previously thought to be confined to lymphoblasts (e.g., TdT) are frequently found in myeloblastic leukemias (3). Unusual coexpression of surface markers is very common and should not be taken as evidence of an ALL transformation of MDS (3). A study from Houston (91) identified nine cases in their adult leukemia database with evidence of an ALL transformation from MDS, but mixed myeloid and lymphoid markers were often found, which confounds the understanding of the phenomenon.

## B. Clonal Markers in Lymphoid and Myeloid Populations

Two classic experiments making use of the Mary Lyon hypothesis underpin the whole science of the origin of hemopoietic lineages. The majority of the genes on one or the other X chromosome in females are inactivated, and in any particular cell this inactivation randomly affects either the maternal or paternal X. Where a gene carried on the X chromosome is polymorphic, it can act as a clonal marker since all of the progeny in a particular clone will have the same X chromosome inactivated. The gene first used in this way to study clonal populations has been that of the enzyme glucose 6-phosphate dehydrogenase (G-6-PD), since the isoenzymes may be distinguished electrophoretically with relative ease.

Prchal et al. (92) studied a woman with RARS who was heterozygous for the A and B variants of G-6-PD. Cultured fibroblasts contained both types of the isoenzyme, but erythrocytes, platelets, granulocytes, and macrophages all contained only the type A isotype. T and B lymphocytes also contained only the type A isoenzyme, confirming that in this case a clonal disorder existed at a primitive progenitor cell level.

Raskind et al. (93) studied a woman with refractory anemia (RA). Examination of fibroblasts cultured from her skin revealed that she was heterozygous for the A and B isoenzymes of G-6-PD. Studies of blood cell fractions and hematopoietic colonies indicated that granulocytes, platelets, and red cells were clonal, expressing type B isozyme of G-6-PD exclusively. B-lymphoblastoid cell lines were generated by EBV transformation. Of 24 lines with a single G-6-PD isozyme, 21 were type B and three were type A. The ratio of cell lines producing κ and λ immunoglobulin light chains was 14:10.

On different occasions, two separate karyotypic abnormalities were found in direct preparations of bone marrow cells. Trisomy 8 was found twice, and del(11)(q23) on three occasions. Both abnormalities are found in MDS, but on no occasion was a cell found that contained both abnormalities. All of the cells examined from the B-lymphoblastoid cell lines were karyotypically normal. This is an important observation, not only because it demonstrates that B cells may be clonally related to the hematopoietic cells in MDS, but also because at least three separate "events" must have taken place to produce cells of the same G-6-PD phenotype with three different karyotypes.

G-6-PD isoenzymes are of limited use since their polymorphism is restricted to certain racial groups. Molecular technology allows us to probe for other polymorphisms, including those of hypoxanthine phosphoribosyl transferase (HPRT) and phosphoglycerate kinase (PGK). Using these polymorphisms, seven of eight patients showed a monoclonal pattern of X inactivation in peripheral blood or bone marrow leukocytes thought to contain at least 40% lymphocytes. The sensitivity of the technique should have detected a major heterogeneous population (3).

The human androgen receptor (HUMARA) gene shows an even greater degree of polymorphism and is widely available in research laboratories. It is surprising, therefore, that more evidence of the involvement of lymphoid cells in the dysplastic process has not been forthcoming. A single case report of a patient developing secondary MDS 5 years after a renal transplant utilized HUMARA to suggest B-cell involvement (94).

Skewed X inactivation is by its nature unable to detect minor subpopulations that are clonal. Furthermore, it appears that abnormal skewing of X-chromosome inactivation is relatively common, especially in the elderly, making it difficult to interpret apparently monoclonal patterns in individuals. Among larger populations, such skewing may be informative. A study by Okada et al. (95) suggested that the B cells were more likely to have a skewed pattern in cases of MDS that showed evidence of immunological abnormalities.

Cytogenetic abnormalities may be used as clonal markers in both sexes. Karyotypic abnormalities are found in the bone marrow cells of upward of 30% of patients with MDS. In most instances, the abnormalities have been found on direct preparations of bone marrow and not in lymphocytes stimulated to divide by mitogens. In a small number of cases there has been evidence that the same chromosomal abnormality has been found in both myeloid and lymphoid cells (1–3), but the limiting factor has been the difficulty in obtaining readable karyotypes and in ensuring that an abnormal karyotype came from a particular lineage.

Fluorescence in situ hybridization (FISH) enables the investigator to look for major chromosomal abnormalities in interphase cells, and this technique can be combined with immunophenotyping to definitively identify the abnormal cell. Using this combination of techniques with probes for chromosomes 7, 8, and Y, Soenen et al. (96) were able to exclude lymphoid involvement in 15 MDS cases, a result confirmed in individual cases by Abruzzese et al. (97) and Fugazza et al. (98).

However, two other groups found that one of three cases had B-cell, but not T-cell, involvement (99,100). Billstrom et al. (101) found a minor population of CD5+ B cells with trisomy 8 in a patient who had trisomy 8 in 55% of his myeloid cells and an associated vasculitis, again raising the possibility that an abnormal B-cell clone was responsible for the immune abnormality. Mongkonsritragoon et al. (102) found bone marrow lymphoid aggregates in a patient with MDS and monosomy 7. Although the aggregates were mixtures of T and B cells, they also showed clonal rearrangements of B- and T-cell receptors and monosomy 7 in the lymphoid cells by FISH. Finally, Miura et al. (103) used FISH to demonstrate monosomy 7 in the NK cells and NK progenitors in three of four patients with MDS. One of the problems with the FISH technique is the presence of a low level of background monosomies in normal cells. Thus, the threshold for identifying monosomies in myeloid and lymphoid cells as an abnormality has to be set rather high to account for the background noise.

Another means of linking myeloid and lymphoid cells is the identification of abnormal oncogenes in different populations. Using such an approach, it has been possible to identify N-*ras* mutations in granulocytes, monocytes, and B and T lymphocytes of patients with MDS (3). More recently, Cooper et al. (104) have studied a child with neurofibromatosis type 1 who developed both JMML and a T-cell lymphoma. Such children have a constitutional inactivation of one allele of the *NF1* gene on chromosome 17. The development of JMML in such children involves the somatic loss of the normal *NF1* allele. In this case, the loss of the normal *NF1* gene and 50Mb of flanking sequence in both JMML cells and T-cell lymphoma cells suggests that both tumors derived from a common cell.

## VII. EVIDENCE FROM THE IMMUNOTHERAPY OF MDS

In 1988, the Basel group diagnosed RAEB as the cause of pancytopenia in a young boy who had previously responded to antilymphocyte globulin as a treatment for his aplastic anemia (105). His condition greatly improved, raising the suspicion that MDS might have an immune etiology. Litzow and Kyle reported on a similar patient who continued to respond to cyclosporine despite transforming from aplastic anemia to MDS (106). Motoji et al. (107) and Muller et al. (108) reported responses in low-grade MDS to treatment with moderate-dose or high-dose corticosteroids. Biesma et al. (109) described two patients with hypoplastic MDS who responded to treatment with antithymocyte globulin (ATG) or cyclosporine or a combination of the two, and in the same year Molldrem et al. (110) described responses to ATG in 11 of 25 patients with MDS. Responses were especially seen in RA, but also in RAEB.

A Czech group (111) reported responses in 14 of 17 patients with hypoplastic MDS treated with cyclosporine, and others have reported similar responses (112–114). According to Catalano et al. (115), who saw responses in seven of nine patients with hypoplastic MDS, the responses are long-lasting and free of toxicity.

How immunosuppressive therapy works remains under investigation. Killick et al. (116) demonstrated a rise in bone marrow CD34+ cells and an increase in colony-forming units-granulocyte/monocyte (CFU-GM) colonies. Molldrem et al. (62) suggested that patients who respond to ATG have CD8+ T-cell clones that suppress CFU-GM colonies, and that these are replaced by nonsuppressive polyclonal CD8+ cells after treatment.

## VIII. MODELS FOR LYMPHOID INVOLVEMENT IN MDS

There is evidence that, at least in some cases, the lymphoid cells in MDS are part of the same clone as the hematopoietic cells. Like the myeloid cells, they are reduced in number and impaired in function in MDS. Although morphological changes have not been described, such changes in morphology might be difficult to demonstrate in lymphocytes. There is evidence of impaired expression of surface antigens appropriate to a particular stage of maturation. Thus, one model that can explain all of the findings described above would be to assume that MDS begins as a series of genetic mistakes in the common progenitor cell for lymphoid and myeloid maturation.

The same model is proposed for chronic myeloid leukemia (CML), but lymphoid involvement in the malignant clone results in quite different patterns of disease: lymphoblastic transformations are much more common and associated myeloma or monoclonal immunoglobulins from other causes are much more rare. In addition, disorders of immune function are not a feature of CML.

Monocyte/macrophages are clearly part of the abnormal clone in MDS. They are increased in number and functionally abnormal. Quite apart from their abnormal phagocytic function, which might be implicated in some of the infectious complications of MDS, there are two distinct ways in which they might be involved in the pathogenesis of MDS and its complications.

> They are potent secretors of cytokines. Proinflammatory and proapoptotic cytokines are frequently up-regulated in MDS and might account for cytopenias, neutrophilic dermatoses, and CD8+ T-cell proliferations.

Monocytes are progenitors of dendritic cells, which are crucial for antigenic presentation to the immune system. It is possible to propose that disordered dendritic cell function leads to abnormal antibody production with resultant hypergammaglobulinemia and autoantibodies. The proliferating B cells would then be subject to a greater risk of genetic error leading to neoplastic and eventually malignant change.

The initiating event in MDS is unknown, although it would be unwise at this time to discard the suspicion of Raza that it might be a virus (8). The feline leukemia virus is capable of causing both MDS and lymphoid tumors in cats (117).

## IX.  CONCLUDING REMARKS

Although immunological abnormalities undoubtedly occur in MDS, attempts to establish that the lymphoid system is part of the malignant clone because of the involvement of a common stem cell have been generally unsuccessful. On the contrary, it is more likely that the immune system functions in an abnormal way owing to the presence of the MDS clone. The mononuclear phagocytic system almost certainly derives from the myelomonocytic progenitor cell. Many of the so-called autoimmune manifestations seen in association with MDS are disorders of phagocytosis. Professional antigen-presenting cells are derived, at least in part, from monocytes, and dendritic cell function is abnormal in MDS . The influence of monocyte-derived cytokines on hematopoiesis undoubtedly accounts for some of the imbalances in lymphocyte subsets, and a chronically active immune stimulation is likely to cause raised levels of immunoglobulins.

The lymphoid tumors seen in MDS probably arise from chronic immune stimulation. Just how much the progressive nature of MDS itself derives from a cytokine imbalance is moot, but the response of MDS to therapeutic immune modulation at least hints that the early phases of the syndrome may be a transient phase still subject to regulation by cytokines.

## REFERENCES

1.  Hamblin TJ. Immunological abnormalities in MDS. In: Galton DAG, Mufti GJ, eds. The Myelodysplastic Syndromes. Edinburgh: Churchill Livingstone, 1991:97–114.
2.  Hamblin TJ. Immunological abnormalities in myelodysplastic syndromes. Hematol Oncol Clin North Am 1992; 6:571–586.

3. Hamblin TJ. Immunological abnormalities in myelodysplastic syndromes (review). Semin Hematol 1996; 33:150–162.

4. Aomatsu I, Isano K, Iizuka S, Mori T, Ohara HM, Ishii Y. A case of tuberculous uveitis complicated by myelodysplastic syndrome. Nippon Ganka Gakkai Zasshi 2000; 104:183–188 [Japanese].

5. Satomi A, Nagai S, Nagai T, Niikura K, Ideura T, Ogata H, Akizaw T. Effect of plasma exchange on refractory hemophagocytic syndrome complicated with myelo-dysplastic syndrome. Ther Apher 1999; 3:317–319.

6. Kuwahara Y, Hirata A, Miwa H, Munakata S, Ueda S, Kanakura Y, Maruno M, Hongyo T, Nomura T, Aozasa K. Epstein-Barr virus associated B-cell lymphoma of brain developing in myelodysplastic syndrome with c-kit mutation (Tyr-577 → stop). Am J Hematol 2000; 65:234–238.

7. Yetgin S, Cetin M, Yenicesu I, Ozaltin F, Uckan D. Acute parvovirus B19 infection mimicking juvenile myelomonocytic leukemia. Eur J Haematol 2000; 65:276–278.

8. Raza A. Initial transforming event in myelodysplastic syndromes may be viral: case for cytomegalovirus. Med Oncol 1998; 15:165–173.

9. Mundle S, Allampallam K, Aftab Rashid K, Dangerfield B, Cartlidge J, Zeitler D, Afenya E, Alvi S, Shetty V, Venugopal P, Raza A. Presence of activation-related m-RNA for EBV and CMV in the bone marrow of patients with myelodysplastic syndromes. Cancer Lett 2001; 164:197–205.

10. Karlic H, Mostl M, Mucke H, Pavlova B, Pfeilstocker M, Heinz R. Association of human T-cell leukemia virus and myelodysplastic syndrome in a central European population. Cancer Res 1997; 57:4718–4721.

11. Mufti GJ, Figes A, Hamblin TJ, Oscier DG, Copplestone JA. Immunological abnor-malities in myelodysplastic syndromes. I. Serum immunoglobulins and autoanti-bodies. Br J Haematol 1986; 63:143–147.

12. Dreyfus B, Vernant JP, Wechsler J, Imbert M, de Pprost Y, Reyes F, Sobel A, Rochant H, Galacteros F, Farcet JP. Anemie refractaire avec exces de myeloblastes et vascularite cutanee. Nouv Rev Fr Hematol 1981; 21:115–121.

13. Lopez FF, Vaidyan PB, Mega AE, Schiffman FJ. Aortitis as a manifestation of myelodysplastic syndrome. Postgrad Med J 2001; 77:116–118.

14. Aractingi S, Bachmeyer C, Dombret H, Vignon-Pennamen D, Degos L, Dubertret L. Simultaneous occurrence of two rare cutaneous markers of poor prognosis in myelodysplastic syndrome: erythema elevatum diutinum and specific lesions (re-view). Br J Dermatol 1994; 113:112–117.

15. Kurzrock R, Cohen PR. Mucocutaneous paraneoplastic manifestations of hemato-logic malignancies (review). Am J Med 1995; 99:207–216.

16. Sweet RD. Acute febrile neutrophilic dermatosis—1978. Br J Dermatol 1979; 100: 93–99.

17. Krolikowski FJ, Reuter K, Shultis EW. Acute febrile neutrophilic dermatosis (Sweet's syndrome) associated with lymphoma. Hum Pathol 1985; 16:520–522.

18. Lazarus AA, McMillan M, Miramadi A. Pulmonary involvement in Sweet's syn-drome (acute febrile neutrophilic dermatosis). Preleukemic and leukemic phases of acute myelogenous leukaemia. Chest 1986; 90:922–924.

19. Marie I, Levesque H, Joly P, Reumont G, Courville P, Baudrimont M, Baubion

D, Cailleux N, Courtois H. Neutrophilic myositis as an extracutaneous manifestation of neutrophilic dermatosis. J Am Acad Dermatol 2001; 44:137–139.

20. Rouhiainen HJ. Orbital inflammation as a presenting sign for myelodysplastic syndrome. Acta Ophthalmol (Copenh) 1989; 67:109–111.

21. Shimizu K. Neutrophilic infiltration of the myocardium in a patient with myelodysplastic syndrome. Am J Hematol 1998; 58:337–338.

22. Avivi I, Rosenbaum H, Levy Y, Rowe J. Myelodysplastic syndrome and associated skin lesions: a review of the literature (review). Leuk Res 1999; 23:323–330.

23. DasGupta R, Fairham SA, Womack C, Burton C, Sivakumaran M. An unusual cutaneous manifestation of myelodysplastic syndrome: "pseudo-Koebner phenomenon." J Clin Pathol 1998; 51:860–861.

24. Grune S, Panizzon R, Egli F, Siegenthaler W, Greminger P. The appearance of Sweet's syndrome during the transition from a myelodysplastic syndrome to erythroleukemia (review). Dtsch Med Wochenschr 1996; 121:939–942 [German].

25. Arbetter KR, Hubbard KW, Markovic SN, Gibson LE, Phyliky RL. Case of granulocyte colony-stimulating factor-induced Sweet's syndrome. Am J Hematol 1999; 61:126–129.

26. Equitani F, Mele L, Rutella S, Belli P, Paciaroni K, Piscitelli R, Pagano L. Atypical Sweet's syndrome in a neutropenic patient with acute myeloid leukemia, secondary to RAEB-T, simulating thrombophlebitis. Panminerva Med 1999; 41:261–263.

27. Megarbane B, Bodemer C, Valensi F, Radford-Weiss I, Fraitag S, MacIntyre E, Bletry O, Varet B, Hermine O. Association of acute neutrophilic dermatosis and myelodysplastic syndrome with (6;9) chromosome translocation: a case report and review of the literature (review). Br J Dermatol 2000; 143:1322–1324.

28. Watari K, Tojo A, Ngamura-Inoue T, Matsuoka M, Irie S, Tani K, Yamada Y, Asano S. Hyperfunction of neutrophils in a patient with BCR/ABL negative chronic myeloid leukemia: a case report with in vitro studies. Cancer 2000; 89:551–560.

29. Zappasodi P, Corso A, del Forno C. Sweet's syndrome and myelodysplasia: two entities with a common pathogenetic mechanism? A case report. Haematologica 2000; 85:868–869.

30. Tomasini C, Aloi F, Osella-Abate S, Dapavo P, Pippione M. Immature myeloid precursors in chronic neutrophilic dermatosis associated with myelodysplastic syndrome. Am J Dermatopathol 2000; 22:429–433.

31. Keoster G, Tarnower A, Levisohn D, Burgdorf W. Bullous pyoderma gangrenosum (review). J Am Acad Dermatol 1993; 29:875–878.

32. Reuss-Borst MA, Pawelec G, Saal JG, Horny HP, Muller CA, Waller HD. Sweet's syndrome associated with myelodysplasia: a possible role of cytokines in the pathogenesis of the disease. Br J Haematol 1993; 84:356–358.

33. Quiepo de Llano MP, Yerba M, Cabrera R, Suarez E. Myelodysplastic syndrome in association erythema elevatum diutinum. J Rheumatol 1992; 19:1005–1006.

34. Katz SI, Gallin JL, Hertz KC, Fauci AS, Lawley TS. Erythema elevatum diutinum: skin and systemic manifestations, immunologic studies and successful treatment with dapsone. Medicine (Baltimore) 1977; 56:443–455.

35. Ohno E, Ohtsuka E, Watanabe K, Kohono T, Takeoka K, Saburi Y, Kikuchi H, Nasu M. Behçet's disease associated with myelodysplastic syndromes. A case report and review of the literature (review). Cancer 1997; 79:262–268.

36. Oh EJ, Yoon JS, Park YJ, Cho CS, Kim BK. Behçet's disease associated with myelodysplastic syndrome: a case report. J Korean Med Sci 1999; 14:685–687.

37. Della Rossa A, Tavoni A, Tognetti A, Testi C, Bombardieri S. Behçet's disease with gastrointestinal involvement associated with myelodysplasia in a patient with congenital panhypopituitarism. Clin Rheumatol 1998; 17:515–517.

38. Tanaka E. Nishinarita M, Uesato M, Kamatani N. A case of intestinal Behçet's disease with abnormal ossification complicated by myelodysplastic syndrome, symptoms revealed after the perforation of ileum ulcer (review). Ryumachi 2000; 40:711–718 [Japanese].

39. Billstrom R, Johansson H, Johansson B, Mitelman F. Immune-mediated complications in patients with myelodysplastic syndromes—clinical and cytogenetic features. Eur J Haematol 1995; 55:42–48.

40. Hebbar M, Brouillard M, Wattel E, Decoulx M, Hatron PY, Devulder B, Fenaux P. Association of myelodysplastic syndrome and relapsing polychondritis: further evidence (review). Leukemia 1995; 9:731–733.

41. Loeffler KU, McLean IW. Bilateral necrotizing scleritis and blindness in the myelodysplastic syndrome presumably due to relapsing polychondritis. Acta Ophthalmol Scand 2000; 78:228–231.

42. Diebold L, Rauh G, Jager K, Lohrs U. Bone marrow pathology in relapsing polychondritis: high frequency of myelodysplastic syndromes. Br J Haematol 1995; 89: 820–830.

43. Hall R, Hopkinson N, Hamblin TJ. Relapsing polychondritis, smouldering nonsecretory myeloma and early myelodysplastic syndrome in the same patient: three difficult diagnoses produce a life threatening illness. Leuk Res 2000; 24:91–93.

44. Pirayesh A, Verbunt RJ, Kluin PM, Meinders AE, De Meijer PH. Myelodysplastic syndrome with vasculitic manifestations (review). J Intern Med 1997; 242:425–431.

45. Maeda Y, Arakawa K, Araki E, Kikuchi H, Ikezoe K, Taniwaki T, Kira J. Polymyositis and cutaneous vasculitis in a patient with myelodysplastic syndrome. Rinsho Shinkeigaku 1999; 39:639–642 [Japanese].

46. Chandran G, Ahern MJ, Seshadri P, Coghlan D. Rheumatic manifestations of the myelodysplastic syndrome: a comparative study. Aust NZ J Med 1996; 26:683–688.

47. George SW, Newman ED. Seronegative inflammatory arthritis in the myelodysplastic syndromes (review). Semin Arthritis Rheum 1992; 21:345–354.

48. Hisakawa N, Nishiya K, Hashimoto K, Tanaka Y. A case of malignant rheumatoid arthritis associated with myelodysplastic syndrome (review). Ryumachi 1997; 37: 30–35 [Japanese].

49. Enright H, Jacob HS, Vercellotti G, Howe R, Belzer M, Miller W. Paraneoplastic autoimmune phenomena in patients with myelodysplastic syndromes: response to immunosuppressive therapy. Br J Haematol 1995; 91:403–408.

50. Scully RE, Mark EJ, McNely WF, Ebeling SH, Phillips LD. Case records of the Massachusetts General Hospital Case 5-1998. N Engl J Med 1998; 338:453–461.

51. Matsushima T, Murakami H, Kim K, Uchiumi H, Murata N, Tamura J, Sawamura M, Karasawa M, Naruse T, Tsuchiya J. Steroid-responsive pulmonary disorders

associated with myelodysplastic syndromes with der(1q;7p) chromosomal abnormality. Am J Hematol 1995; 50:110–115.

52. Saito T, Murakami H, Uchiumi H, Moridaira K, Maehara T, Matsushima T, Tsukamoto N, Tamura J, Karasawa M, Naruse T, Tsuchiya J. Myelodysplastic syndromes with nephritic syndrome. Am J Hematol 1999; 60:200–204.

53. Komatsuda A, Miura I, Ohtani H, Hamai K, Wakui H, Imai H, Kobayashi Y, Miura A. Crescentic glomerulonephritis accompanied by myeloperoxidase antineutrophil cytoplasmic antibodies in a patient having myelodysplastic syndrome with trisomy 7. Am J Kidney Dis 1998; 31:336–340.

54. Hamidou MA, Derenne S, Audrain MA, Berthelot JM, Boumalassa A, Grolleau JY. Prevalence of rheumatic manifestations and antineutrophil cytoplasmic antibodies in haematological malignancies. A prospective study. Rheumatology (Oxford) 2000; 39:417–420.

55. Komiya I, Tanoue K, Kakinuma K, Kaneda M, Shinohara T, Kuriya S, Nomura T, Saito Y. Superoxide anion hyperproduction by neutrophils in a case of myelodysplastic syndrome. Association with Sweet's syndrome and interstitial pneumonia. Cancer 1991; 67:2337–2341.

56. Matsumura T, Kami M. Sweet's syndrome after granulocyte colony-stimulating factor administration for refractory myelodysplastic syndrome. Medical Images. Br J Haematol 2001; 113:1.

57. Kawabata H, Utsunomiya A, Hanada S, Makino T, Takatsuka Y, Takeuchi S, Suzuki S, Suzumiya J, Ohshima K, Horiike S. Myelodysplastic syndrome in a patient with adult T-cell leukaemia. Br J Haematol 1999; 106:702–705.

58. Saunthararajah Y, Molldrem JL, Rivera M, Williams A, Stetler-Stevenson M, Sorbara L, Young NS, Barrett JA. Coincident myelodysplastic syndrome and T-cell large granular lymphocytic disease: clinical and pathophysiological features. Br J Haematol 2001; 112:195–200.

59. Lorand-Metze I, Lima CS, Cardinalli IA, Vassallo J. Association of a myelodysplastic syndrome with hairy cell leukaemia. Eur J Haematol 1995; 55:341–343.

60. Bassan R, Marini B, Allavena P, Pirelli A, Barbui T. RAEB in a patient with chronic granulated T-lymphocytosis. Br J Haematol 1987; 65:503–504.

61. Dhodapkar MV, Li CY, Lust JA, Tefferi A, Phyliky RL. Clinical spectrum of clonal proliferations of T-large granular lymphocytes: a T-cell clonopathy of undetermined significance? Blood 1994; 84:1620–1627.

62. Molldrem JJ, Jiang YZ, Stetler-Stevenson M, Mavroudis D, Hensel N, Barrett JA. Haematological response of patients with myelodysplastic syndrome to antithymocyte globulin is associated with a loss of lymphocyte-mediated inhibition of CFU-GM and alterations in T-cell receptor V beta profiles. Br J Haematol 1998; 102: 1314–1322.

63. Luraschi A, Saglietti G, Fedeli P, Gioria A, Della Vedova A, Ferrari V, Borgotti P. Immunological indices in myelodysplastic syndromes. Minerva Med 1994; 85: 145–153 [Italian].

64. Srivannaboon K, Conley ME, Coustan-Smith E, Wang WC. Hypogammaglobulinemia and reduced numbers of B-cells in children with myelodysplastic syndrome. Am J Pediatr Hematol Oncol 2001; 23:122 125.

65. Katsuki K, Shinohara K, Kameda N, Yamada T, Takeda K, Kamei T. Two cases

of myelodysplastic syndrome with extramedullary polyclonal plasma cell proliferation and autoantibody production: possible role of soluble Fas antigen for production of excessive self-reactive B cells. Intern Med 1998; 37:973–977.

66. Stahl D, Egerer G, Goldschmidt H, Sibrowski W, Kazatchkine MD, Kaveri SV. Altered self-reactive antibody repertoires are a general feature of patients with myelodysplastic syndrome. J Autoimmune Dis 2001; 16:77–86.

67. Hilbe W, Eisterer W, Schmid C, Starz I, Silly H, Duba C, Ludescher C, Thaler J. Bone marrow lymphocyte subsets in myelodysplastic syndromes. J Clin Pathol 1994; 47:505–507.

68. Tsuda H, Yamasaki H. Type I and type II T-cell profiles in aplastic anemia and refractory anemia. Am J Hematol 2000; 64:271–274.

69. Yokose N, Ogata K, Ito T, An E, Tamura H, Dan K, Hamaguchi H, Sakamaki H, Onozawa Y, Nomura T. Elevated plasma soluble interleukin-2 receptor level correlates with defective natural killer and CD8+ T-cells in myelodysplastic syndromes. Leuk Res 1994; 18:777–782.

70. Tsuchida T, Sakane T, Ishikura H, Tsunematsu T. Impairment of lymphocyte function in patients with myelodysplastic syndrome and its correction by addition of Ca2+ ionophore and phorbol myristate acetate. Int J Hematol 1991; 54:505–513.

71. Baumann MA, Milson TJ, Patrick CW, Libnoch JA, Keller RH. Immunoregulatory abnormalities in myelodysplastic disorders. Am J Hematol 1986; 22:17–26.

72. Thiele J, Romatowski C, Wagner S, Dienemann D, Stein H, Fischer R, Falini B. Macrophages (phagocytic-histiocytic reticular cells) in reactive-inflammatory lesions in the bone marrow and in myelodysplastic syndromes (MDS). Pathol Res Pract 1992; 188:995–1001.

73. Kitagawa M, Kamiyama R, Kasuga T. Increase in number of bone marrow macrophages in patients with myelodysplastic syndromes. Eur J Haematol 1993; 51:56–58.

74. Rigolin GM, Cuneo A, Roberti MG, Bardi A, Castoldi G. Myelodysplastic syndromes with monocytic component: hematologic and cytogenetic characterization. Haematologica 1997; 82:25–30.

75. Ohmori M, Ohmori S, Ueda Y, Tohyama K, Yoshida Y, Uchino H. Myelodysplastic syndrome (MDS)-associated inhibitory activity on haemopoietic progenitor cells. Br J Haematol 1990; 74:179–184.

76. Zoumbos N, Symeonidis A, Kourakli A, Katevas P, Matsouka P, Peraki M, Georgoulias V. Increased levels of soluble interleukin-2 receptors and tumor necrosis factor in serum of patients with myelodysplastic syndromes. Blood 1991; 77:413–414.

77. Kitagawa M, Saito I, Yoshida S, Yamaguchi S, Takahashi M, Tanizawa I, Kamiyama R, Hirokawa K. Overexpression of tumor necrosis factor (TNF) alpha and interferon (IFN) gamma by bone marrow cells from patients with myelodysplastic syndromes. Leukemia 1997; 11:2049–2054.

78. Shetty V, Mundle S, Alvi S, Showel M, Broady-Robinson L, Dar S, Borok R, Showel J, Gregory S, Rifkin S, Gezer S, Parcharidou A, Venugopal P, Shah R, Hernandez B, Klein M, Alston V, Robin E, Dominque C, Raza A. Measurement of apoptosis proliferation and three cytokines in 46 patients with myelodysplastic syndromes. Leuk Res 1996; 20:891–900.

79. Verhoef GE, De Schouwer P, Ceuppens JL, Van Damme J, Goossens W, Boogaerts MA. Measurement of serum cytokine levels in patients with myelodysplastic syndromes. Leukemia 1992; 6:1268–1272.

80. Menconi M, Castello G, Lerza R, Haupt R, Ballarino P, Cerruti A, Bogliolo G, Pannacciulli I. Production of tumor necrosis factor and granulocyte colony stimulating factor by bone marrow accessory cells in myelodysplastic patients. Eur J Haematol 1996; 56:148–152.

81. Matteo Rigolin G, Howard J, Buggins A, Sneddon C, Castoldi G, Hirst WJ, Mufti GJ. Phenotypic and functional characteristics of monocyte-derived dendritic cells from patients with myelodysplastic syndromes. Br J Haematol 1999; 107:844–850.

82. Kyriakou D, Liapi D, Kyriakou E, Alexandrakis M, Vlachonikolis IG, Mavromanolakis M, Eliakis P, Eliopoulos GD. Aberrant expression of the major sialoglycoprotein (CD43) on the monocytes of patients with myelodysplastic syndromes. Ann Hematol 2000; 79:198–205.

83. Pajor L, Matolcsy A, Vass JA, Mehes G, Marton E, Szabo F, Ivanyi JL. Phenotypic and genotypic analyses of blastic cell population suggest that pure B-lymphoblastic leukemia may arise from myelodysplastic syndrome. Leuk Res 1998; 22:13–17.

84. Abruzzese E, Buss D, Rainer R, Pettenati MJ, Rao PN. Progression of a myelodysplastic syndrome to pre-B acute lymphoblastic leukemia: a case report and cell lineage study. Ann Hematol 1966; 73:35–38.

85. Lima CS, deSouza CA, Cardinalli IA, Lorand-Metze I. Lymphoblastic transformation of myelodysplastic syndrome. Rev Paul Med 1997; 115:1508–1512.

86. Lau RC, Squire J, Brisson L, Kamel-Ried S, Grunberger T, Dube I, Letarte M, Shannon K, Freedman MH. Lymphoid blast crisis of a B-lineage phenotype with monosomy 7 in a patient with juvenile chronic myelogenous leukemia (JCML). Leukemia 1994; 8:903–908.

87. Yamamoto M, Nakagawa M, Ichimura N, Ohtsuki F, Ohtsuka Y, Tsujino Y, Tanaka A, Kamiya T, Wada H. Lymphoblastic transformation of chronic myelomonocytic leukemia in an infant. Am J Hematol 1996; 52:212–214.

88. Kouides PA, Bennett JM. Transformation of chronic myelomonocytic leukemia to acute lymphoblastic leukemia: case report and review of the literature of lymphoblastic transformation of myelodysplastic syndrome (review). Am J Hematol 1995; 49:157–162.

89. Kohno T, Amenomori T, Atogami S, Sasagawa I, Nakamura H, Kuriyama K, Tomonaga M. Progression from myelodysplastic syndrome to acute lymphoblastic leukaemia with Philadelphia chromosome and p190 BCR-ABL transcript. Br J Haematol 1996; 93:389–391.

90. Leseve JF, Troussard X, Bastard C, Hurst JP, Nouet D, Callat MP, Lenormand B, Piguet H, Flandrin G, Macintyre E. p190bcr/abl rearrangement in myelodysplastic syndromes: two reports and review of the literature (review). Br J Haematol 1996; 95:372–375.

91. Escudier SM, Albitar M, Robertson LE, Andereef M, Pierce S, Kantarjian HM. Acute lymphoblastic leukemia following preleukemic syndromes in adults. Leukemia 1996, 10:473–477.

92. Prchal JT, Throckmorton DW, Carroll AJ III, Fuson EW, Gams RA, Prchal JF A

common progenitor for human myeloid and lymphoid cells. Nature 1978; 274:590–591.

93. Raskind WH, Tirumali N, Jacobson R, Singer J, Fialkow PJ. Evidence for a multistep pathogenesis of a myelodysplastic syndrome. Blood 1984; 63:1318–1323.

94. Okamoto T, Okada M, Itoh T, Mori A, Saheki K, Takatsuka H, Wada H, Tamura A, Fujimori Y, Takemoto Y, Kanamaru A, Kakishita E. Myelodysplastic syndrome with B cell clonality in a patient five years after renal transplantation. Int J Hematol 1998; 68:61–65.

95. Okada M, Okamoto T, Takemoto Y, Kanamaru A, Kakishita E. Function and X chromosome inactivation analysis of B lymphocytes in myelodysplastic syndromes with immunological abnormalities. Acta Haematol 2000; 102:124–130.

96. Soenen V, Fenaux P, Flactif M, Lepelley P, Lai JL, Cosson A, Predhomme C. Combined immunophenotyping and in situ hybridization (FICTION): a rapid method to study cell lineage involvement in myelodysplastic syndromes. Br J Haematol 1995; 90:701–706.

97. Abruzzese E, Buss D, Rainer R, Rao PN, Pettenati MJ. Study of clonality in myelodysplastic syndromes: detection of trisomy 8 in bone marrow cell smears by fluorescence in situ hybridisation. Leuk Res 1996; 20:551–557.

98. Fugazza G, Lerza R, Bruzzone R, Sessarego M. Clonality study by fluorescence in situ hybridisation of a patient with refractory anemia with ringed sideroblasts and monosomy 7. Haematologica 1995; 80:54–57.

99. Jaju RJ, Jones M, Boultwood J, Kelly S, Mason DY, Wainscoat JS, Kearney L. Combined immunophenotyping and FISH identifies the involvement of B-cells in the 5q-syndrome. Genes Chromosomes Cancer 2000; 29:276–280.

100. van Lom K, Hagemeijer A, Smit E, Hahlen K, Groeneveld K, Lowenberg B. Cytogenetic clonality analysis in myelodysplastic syndrome: monosomy 7 can be demonstrated in the myeloid and lymphoid lineage. Leukemia 1995; 9:1818–1821.

101. Billstrom R, Johansson B, Strombeck B, el-Rifai W, Larramendy M, Olofsson T, Mitelman F, Knuutila S. Clonal CD5-positive B lymphocytes in myelodysplastic syndrome with systemic vasculitis and trisomy 8. Ann Hematol 1997; 74:37–40.

102. Mongkonsritragoon W, Letendre L, Li CY. Multiple lymphoid nodules in bone marrow have the same clonality as underlying myelodysplastic syndrome recognized with fluorescent in situ hybridisation technique. Am J Hematol 1998; 59: 252–257.

103. Miura I, Kobayashi Y, Takahashi N, Saitoh K, Miura AB. Involvement of natural killer cells in patients with myelodysplastic syndrome carrying monosomy 7 revealed by the application of fluorescent in situ hybridization to cells collected by means of fluorescence-activated cell sorting. Br J Haematol 2000; 110:876–879.

104. Cooper LJ, Shannon KM, Loken MR, Weaver M, Stephens K, Sievers EL. Evidence that juvenile myelomonocytic leukemia can arise from a pluripotential stem cell. Blood 2000; 96:2310–2313.

105. Tichelli A, Gratwohl A, Wuersch A, Nissen C, Speck B. Antilymphocyte globulin for myelodysplastic syndrome. Br J Haematol 1988; 68:139–140.

106. Litzow MR, Kyle RA. Multiple responses of aplastic anemia to low-dose

cyclosporine therapy despite development of a myelodysplastic syndrome. Am J Hematol 1989; 32:226–229.

107.  Motoji T, Teramura M, Takahashi M, Oshimi K, Okada M, Kusakabe K, Mizoguchi H. Successful treatment of refractory anemia with high-dose methylprednisolone. Am J Hematol 1990; 33:8–12.

108.  Muller EW, de Wolf JT, Vellenga E. Successful immunosuppressive treatment after failure of erythropoietin therapy in two subjects with refractory anaemia. Br J Haematol 1993; 83:171–172.

109.  Biesma DH, van den Tweel JG, Verdonck LF. Immunosuppressive therapy for hypoplastic myelodysplastic syndrome. Cancer 1997; 79:1548–1551.

110.  Molldrem JJ, Caples M, Mavroudis D, Plante M, Young NS, Barrett AJ. Antithymocyte globulin for patients with myelodysplastic syndrome. Br J Haematol 1997; 99:699–705.

111.  Jonasova A, Neuwirtova R, Cermak J, Vozobulova V, Mocikova K, Siskova M, Hochova I. Cyclosporin A therapy in hypoplastic MDS patients and certain refractory anaemias without hypoplastic bone marrow. Br J Haematol 1998; 100:304–309.

112.  Berer A, Ohler L, Simonitsch I, Thalhammer R, Lechner K, Geissler K. Longterm improvement of hematopoiesis following cyclosporine treatment in a patient with myelodysplastic syndrome. Wien Klin Wochenschr 1999; 111:815–818.

113.  Samuelsson J, Larfars G. Unusual clinical presentation in a patient with myelodysplastic syndrome, with subsequent haematological remission and suppression of malignant clone following treatment with cyclosporine A, erythropoietin and granulocyte colony-stimulating factor. Leuk Res 1999; 23:513–517.

114.  Takanashi M, Kadono Y, Tabata Y, Hibi S. Successful immunosuppressive therapy for a patient with hypoplastic myelodysplastic syndrome. Rinsho Ketsueki 1999; 40:1093–1099 [Japanese].

115.  Catalano L, Selleri C, Califano C, Luciano L, Volpicelli M, Rocco S, Varriale G, Ricci P, Rotoli B. Prolonged response to cyclosporin-A in hypoplastic anemia and correlation with in vitro studies. Haematologica 2000; 85:133–138.

116.  Killick SB, Marsh JC, Gordon-Smith EC, Sorlin L, Gibson FM. Effects of antithymocyte globulin on bone marrow CD34+ cells in aplastic anaemia and myelodysplasia. Br J Haematol 2000; 108:582–591.

117.  Jarrett O, Onions DE. Retroviruses in leukaemia of animals. In: Goldman JM, Preisler HD, eds. Butterworths' International Medical Reviews of Haematology. 1, Leukaemias. London: Butterworths, 1984:1–34.

# 5

# The Cytogenetics and Molecular Biology of Myelodysplastic Syndromes

**Harold J. Olney**
*Centre Hospitalier de l'Université de Montreal, Montreal, Quebec, Canada*

**Michelle M. Le Beau**
*The University of Chicago, Chicago, Illinois*

## I. INTRODUCTION

Today, the myelodysplastic syndromes (MDS) are recognized as a collection of five clinicopathological entities that describe a wide spectrum of clinical manifestations and survival. It was in 1982 that the French-American-British (FAB) cooperative group proposed the five modern entities of MDS based on a structured clinicopathological approach (1). These clinicopathological entities, described in detail in Chapter 1, are: refractory anemia (RA), refractory anemia with ringed sideroblasts (RARS), refractory anemia with excess blasts (RAEB), refractory anemia with excess blasts in transformation (RAEB-t), and chronic myelomonocytic leukemia (CMML). Prior to the FAB classification system, the lack of a uniform nomenclature for myeloid disorders contributed to the confusion surrounding these diseases (2). Although not perfect, the FAB system has allowed clinicians and researchers to advance the understanding of the pathogenesis and prognosis of MDS as well as to evaluate the utility of therapeutic interventions.

Following the introduction of the FAB classification, several authors reported the added value of cytogenetic analysis in predicting survival and determining the risk of leukemic transformation during a patient's clinical course (3–6). At the time of diagnosis, recurring chromosomal abnormalities are found in 40–70% of patients with primary MDS and in 95% of patients with therapy-related MDS (tMDS) (7). The frequency of cytogenetic abnormalities increases with the severity of disease and the risk of leukemic transformation, ranging from

15–20% of cases in RA and RARS to 75% in RAEB and RAEB-t. The abnormal clones may evolve with disease progression, and typically resolve following treatment, indicative of disease remission. The most common cytogenetic abnormalities encountered in MDS are del(5q), −7, and +8 (Table 1), which have been included in subsequent prognostic scoring systems of MDS. Clones with unrelated abnormalities, one of which typically has a gain of chromosome 8, are seen at a greater frequency in patients with MDS than in patients with AML: ~5% versus ~1%, respectively. Among the few independent variables identified that predict clinical outcomes in MDS, cytogenetic findings form the cornerstone of successful prognostic scoring systems (8).

The proposed World Health Organization (WHO) classification, currently gaining acceptance, requires cytogenetic data for diagnostic purposes; thus, cytogenetic analysis will be a mandatory step in the full evaluation of a newly diagnosed patient (9,10). This proposal eliminates RAEB-t, redefining such cases as AML; reclassifies CMML as a hybrid between MDS and myeloproliferative diseases (MPD); separates the 5q− syndrome as a distinct MDS entity; and introduces the new entity of refractory cytopenias with multilineage dysplasia (RCMD).

In summarizing our current understanding of the recurring chromosomal alternations and molecular biological findings in MDS, this chapter reveals how cytogenetic and molecular analyses have been instrumental in refining the prognosis of MDS patients; predicting the likelihood of progression to acute myeloid

**Table 1**  Recurring Chromosomal Abnormalities in Myelodysplastic Syndromes

|                    | Abnormality              | Frequency |
|--------------------|--------------------------|-----------|
| De novo MDS        | −5/del(5q)               | 10–20%    |
|                    | +8                       | 10%       |
|                    | −7/del(7q)               | 5–10%     |
|                    | −Y                       | 10%       |
|                    | 17p−                     | 7%        |
|                    | del(20q)                 | 5%        |
|                    | t(11q23)                 | 5–6%      |
|                    | Complex karyotypes       | 10–20%    |
| CMML               | t(5;12)(q33;p12)         | <1%       |
| Therapy-related MDS | −5/del(5q) or −7/del(7q) | 90%       |
|                    | +8                       | 10%       |
|                    | t(11q23)                 | 3%        |
|                    | Complex karyotypes       | 90%       |

CMML: chronic myelomonocytic leukemia.

leukemia (AML); predicting survival; establishing clonality of these diseases; and clarifying some of the pathobiology involved in the genesis of the entities now recognized as MDS. The authors emphasize the most current literature, and extend acknowledgment to the many investigators who contributed to our early understanding of MDS.

## II. DIFFERENTIAL DIAGNOSIS

Classification of a hematological malignant disease can be a challenging undertaking, but it is crucial for the appropriate management of a patient. In difficult cases in particular, the detection of a cytogenetic abnormality may be useful in establishing the diagnosis of MDS, or in distinguishing between a benign, reactive lymphoid or myeloid hyperplasia and a malignant monoclonal proliferation.

In general, the recurring abnormalities found in MDS are unbalanced, with chromosomal loss and deletions as well as unbalanced translocations commonly observed (Table 1). Although less common, recurring balanced translocations have been reported in some cases. A few specific cytogenetic abnormalities have been recognized that are closely associated with morphologically and clinically distinct subsets of MDS, including the 5q − syndrome (11), the 17p − syndrome (12), and the isodicentric X chromosome associated with RARS (which has a high likelihood of transformation to AML) (13). (See below for detailed discussions on 5q − syndrome and 17p − syndrome.) Other abnormalities, such as the t(15; 17), inv(16), and t(8;21), are usually restricted to acute leukemia (14). The t(9; 22) is characteristic of chronic myelogenous leukemia (CML) and a subtype of acute lymphoblastic leukemia (ALL), but has only rarely been reported in MDS (15). Many other findings, including loss or deletions of chromosomes 5 or 7, trisomy 8, and complex karyotypes, are common to both MDS and AML, including the new RCMD subtype of the WHO classification. The detection of one of these recurring abnormalities can be quite helpful in establishing the correct diagnosis, and can add important prognostic information permitting tailored treatment planning. Serial evaluations can also be informative, particularly when there is a change in the clinical picture. The identification of new abnormalities in the karyotype often signals a change in the pace of the disease, usually to a more aggressive course and may herald incipient leukemia.

## III. PROGNOSIS

The initial FAB classification provided the first systematic prognostic classification. The RA and RARS subtypes were generally more favorable (''low risk'')

**Table 2**  International Prognosis Scoring System

|                   | Cytogenetic findings | Median survival | 25% AML progression |
|-------------------|----------------------|-----------------|---------------------|
| Favorable risk    | Normal karyotype     | 3.8 years       | 5.6 years           |
|                   | Isolated del(5q)     |                 |                     |
|                   | Isolated del(20q)    |                 |                     |
|                   | Isolated −Y          |                 |                     |
| Intermediate risk | Other abnormalities  | 2.4 years       | 1.6 years           |
| Poor risk         | −7                   | 0.8 years       | 0.9 years           |
|                   | del(7q)              |                 |                     |
|                   | Complex karyotypes   |                 |                     |

AML: acute myeloid leukemia.

than CMML ("intermediate risk"), with RAEB and RAEB-t having the poorest prognosis ("high risk"). The Spanish (16), Dusseldorf (17), Lille (3), and Bournemouth (18) classification systems were proposed subsequently, each adding clinical or laboratory information to the basic morphological descriptions of the FAB subtypes. More recently, the International MDS Risk Analysis Workshop combined cytogenetic, morphological, and clinical data from seven large, risk-based studies to describe an International Prognostic Scoring System (IPSS) for MDS (8). The IPSS combines cytogenetic abnormalities (outlined in Table 2), percentage of marrow blasts, and number of peripheral cytopenias to define three risk groups: good, intermediate, and poor outcome, with a median survival of 3.8, 2.4, and 0.8 years, respectively. The IPSS has been found to be highly reproducible in predicting survival and the risk of leukemic transformation (6,19,20).

## IV.  KARYOTYPIC EVOLUTION

Clonal cytogenetic evolution is the acquisition of an abnormal clone where only karyotypically normal cells have been seen previously, or the progression from the presence of a single clone (often with a simple karyotype) to multiple related abnormal clones. In most published series, the majority of MDS patients succumb to bone marrow failure, half progress to acute leukemia, and a few die of intercurrent illness. In general, there are three disease patterns in MDS:

a gradual increase in marrow blast count associated with worsening pancytopenia;

    a relatively stable clinical course followed by an abrupt change with a clear
    leukemic transformation; and

    a stable course over many years without any increase in marrow blast
    counts upon reinvestigation (21).

In the first group, the karyotype typically remains stable, and the progression to
leukemia is based on the relatively arbitrary finding of greater than 30% blasts
in the marrow (20% in the newly proposed WHO classification (9)), making the
transition to AML a relatively ill-defined event. In the second group, an abrupt
change in the karyotype with the gain of secondary clones and complex karyotypes is typically observed. The karyotype as well as disease tends to remain
stable in the third group. Few series with sequential cytogenetic studies have been
published, and most series are small with short follow-up (22–24). Nonetheless,
karyotypic evolution in MDS is associated with a transformation to acute leukemia in about 60% of cases and reduced survival, particularly for those patients
whose karyotype evolves within a short period (less than 100 days) (23).

## V.  EVIDENCE FOR CLONALITY

Monoclonality is a key feature of neoplastic diseases. Given the varied pathological and clinical picture of MDS, some authors have proposed that MDS is characterized by multifactorial, nonclonal cell dysfunction. However, cytogenetic analysis has confirmed the clonal nature of MDS.

    Initial work with isotypes of the enzyme glucose-6-phosphate dehydroge-
nase (G-6-PD), which varies with X-chromosome inactivation patterns in heterozygous females, suggested that MDS was a clonal disorder (25). Obviously, the
application of the G-6-PD technique is limited to heterozygous females; furthermore, the results can be difficult to interpret in some cases with random imbalances in X inactivation (26). Amplifying a polymorphic short tandem repeat in
the human androgen receptor gene (HUMARA) on the X chromosome with polymerase chain reaction (PCR) techniques is an extension of this rationale (27).
Taken together, X-inactivation patterns, recurring chromosomal abnormalities,
analysis of restriction fragments length polymorphisms, and mutated oncogenes
and tumor suppressor genes (discussed below) indicate that MDS is a clonal
neoplastic disease (28). In light of these findings, it can be concluded that some
poorly defined initiating event(s) affects a pluripotent, or at least multipotent,
progenitor cell in the bone marrow, conferring this cell with a growth advantage
(increased proliferation, apoptotic defect, or both), which allows it to establish
clonal, but ineffective hematopoiesis. The dysplasia in MDS indicates that there
is also a defect in normal differentiation; see Chapter 3.

## VI.  B-CELL LINEAGE INVOLVEMENT

MDS is usually thought of as a disease of myeloid cells; however, the earliest report of clonality analysis in MDS suggested the involvement of a pluripotent cell capable of contributing to both myeloid and lymphoid lineages (25). Cytogenetic evidence of recurring abnormalities in lymphoid cells, particularly B cells, has since confirmed the involvement of both myeloid and in rare cases lymphoid cells (29–31). It is not known whether the transforming event(s) occurs in a very early progenitor cell with no manifested defect in B cells in most cases, or whether the transforming event(s) involves a myeloid-restricted progenitor cell.

## VII.  ALTERATIONS IN GENE FUNCTION

A growing body of evidence suggests that mutations of multiple genes mediate the pathogenesis and progression of MDS. A detailed review of these genes is beyond the scope of this chapter. Table 3 provides a partial list of these genes and an overview summary of some of their salient features in relation to MDS.

The most extensively studied gene family in MDS is the *RAS* family. RAS proteins are a critical component of the signaling pathways leading from cell-surface receptors to the nucleus, where these signal transduction pathways result in the control of cellular proliferation, differentiation, and cell death. RAS proteins bind guanine nucleotides, and their function is controlled by cycling between the guanosine triphosphate (GTP)-bound (active) and guanosine diphosphate (GDP)-bound (inactive) forms (32). Once activated by a cell-surface receptor, RAS proteins induce a cascade of kinase activity, resulting in the transduction of the signals to the nucleus. Mutant RAS proteins retain the active GTP-bound form, promoting constitutive activation. The most frequent mutation is a single base change at codon 12 (resulting in an amino acid substitution in the protein), but codons 13 and 61 are also frequently mutated. Codons 12 and 13 are located within the pocket that binds GTP, and mutant proteins have decreased phosphatase activity. Normal phosphatase activity results in a reversion of RAS binding to the inactive GDP form (33,34). A wide variety of human malignancies have been found to harbor mutations in *RAS* genes.

Constitutively activating point mutations of *NRAS* have been detected at high frequency in hematological malignancies. In MDS, *NRAS* mutations have been detected in 10–40% of cases. These mutations have been associated with a poor prognosis: a higher incidence of transformation to AML and shorter survival. Patients with abnormal karyotypes and *NRAS* mutations have the highest likelihood of transformation (33,35–38).

**Table 3** Partial List of Genes Altered in Myelodysplastic Syndromes

| Gene | Alteration | Associated features | Ref. |
|---|---|---|---|
| BCL2 | Overexpressed in all FAB subtypes | Encodes a protein product that suppresses apoptosis | (41,42,103) |
| | | No correlation with survival | |
| | | Highest levels in higher-risk entities where apoptosis is reduced | |
| CSF1R/FMS | Mutated in 12–20%, increased with higher risk MDS | Encodes the macrophage colony-stimulating factor receptor with tyrosine kinase activity | (36,104) |
| | | Karyotype predominantly normal | |
| | | Increased frequency of transformation to AML and poor survival | |
| FLT3 | Mutated (internal tandem duplication) in ~0% of MDS and AML with trilineage dysplasia | Encodes a class III receptor tyrosine kinase playing a role in stem cell differentiation | (105,106) |
| | | Elongation of gene causes activation of product | |
| | | Associated with progression to AML and poor prognosis | |
| | | Frequently observed with normal karyotype in AML | |
| KIT | Overexpressed; no mutations found | Encodes the stem cell factor receptor | (107,108) |
| | | May provide an autocrine growth pathway | |
| MDR1 | Expressed in ~60% | Encodes a transmembrane drug efflux pump | (109) |
| | | May be involved in resistance of MDS to drug therapy | |
| | | Associated with monosomy 7 | |

**Table 3** Continued

| Gene | Alteration | Associated features | Ref. |
|---|---|---|---|
| MDM2 | Overexpressed in ~70% | Encodes a protein product (murine double min-utes-2) that abrogates the function of the p53 tumor suppressor protein<br>Gene amplification not detected<br>Associated with unfavorable cytogenetic abnormalities<br>Shorter remission duration | (110,111) |
| MPL | Overexpressed in ~45% of CMML, and ~40% of RAEB, RAEB-t patients; underexpressed (~50% of normal) in most MDS patients, especially RA | Encodes the thrombopoietin receptor<br>Higher expression in RAEB and RAEB-t associated with poor prognosis, increased progression to AML<br>Correlated with dysmegakaryocytopoiesis | (112,113) |
| GCSFR | Point mutations identified | Encodes the G-CSR receptor<br>Severe congenital neutropenia (SCN) patients with G-CSF receptor defects can progress to MDS and/or AML<br>Mutation alone is not sufficient for transformation<br>Progression to leukemia in SCN associated with loss of chromosome 7 and RAS mutations | (114) |
| NF1 | Loss and mutations identified, particularly in pediatric MDS/MPS | Encodes neurofibromin, a tumor suppressor gene product, that functions as a GTPase-activating (GAP) protein to down-regulate RAS function<br>High incidence of MDS and AML in children with neurofibromatosis type I<br>No structural alteration in homologous allele in adults with loss of one chromosome 17 | (115,116) |

| | | |
|---|---|---|
| *NRAS* | Mutated in 20–40%; overexpressed in RA, RARS | Encodes a component of various cell surface signal transduction pathways<br>Activating mutations result in constitutive signaling<br>Associated with monocytic component<br>Increased risk of progression to AML<br>Overexpression may represent an early event in the multistep process of transformation | (117) |
| Telomerase (including *hTERT*, *hTR*, and *TPI*) | Increased activity late in disease, particularly *hTERT* | Enzyme complex responsible for chromosome telomere maintenance and replication<br>Variable levels of activity<br>Abnormal telomere maintenance may be an early indication of genetic instability<br>Telomeres shortened with disease progression | (118–121) |
| *TP53* | Mutated in 5–25%; higher frequency in tMDS | Encodes G1 and G2 checkpoint protein product that monitors integrity of genome; arrests cell cycle in response to DNA damage,<br>Loss of wild-type allele<br>Associated with weak BCL2 expression<br>Observed as both early and late genetic event in MDS<br>Associated with rapid progression and poor outcome seen with loss of 17p, −5/del(5q), −7/del(7q) suggesting pathogenic exposure to carcinogens | (36,122) |

FAB: French-American-British cooperative group; AML: acute myeloid leukemia; CMML: chronic myelomonocytic leukemia; RA: refractory anemia; RAEB: refractory anemia with excess blasts; RAEB-t: refractory anemia with excess blasts in transformation; RARS: refractory anemia with ringed sideroblasts.

## VIII.  PROLIFERATION AND PROGRAMMED CELL DEATH
IN MDS

One of the paradoxes associated with MDS is the presence of peripheral cytopenias, frequently involving all three blood cell lineages (granulocytic, erythroid, and megakaryocytic) and a hypercellular bone marrow. Cells in both the peripheral blood and bone marrow exhibit varying degrees of dysmorphic features, frequently with high proportions of immature cells. Neoplastic disease results from disruption of the normal balance between cell proliferation, cell differentiation, and cell survival. The tightly regulated and complex process of cellular death—apoptosis—plays an important role in maintaining normal homeostasis by removing immature and dysmorphic cells. The apoptotic process is highly conserved throughout evolution and involves a cascade of proteins that effectively monitors both extracellular and intracellular conditions (39). Apoptosis is immunologically silent and does not produce inflammation; these characteristics distinguish apoptosis from the well-known phenomenon of necrosis (also seen in neoplastic disease), in which the cells are highly proliferative and have outgrown supportive stromal elements.

The efforts to decipher this paradox have been intensive. Although some of the findings are conflicting, there is consensus on a number of points. Measurements of cell cycle kinetics by biochemical (bromo- and/or iododeoxyuridine) and immunophenotypic (Ki-67 positivity) methodologies demonstrate an increase in the proliferation of all hematopoietic cell lineages, particularly the myeloid cell line (40,41). This proliferation is balanced by an increase in apoptosis in MDS. Interestingly, the lower-risk MDS entities (RA and RARS) seem to have a greater apoptotic rate than the higher-risk entities (RAEB, RAEB-t), which remain elevated but approach the mildly elevated levels seen in AML. Levels of the antiapoptotic proteins (BCL2 and related family members) seem to parallel this increase (41,42). It is not known whether the intrinsic defect producing the hyperproliferative, dysplastic hematopoietic cells directly results in the apoptosis of these same cells, or whether the apoptosis is a compensatory homeostatic response to this hyperproliferation through indirect means.

It is well documented that altered cytokine levels play a pivotal role in the apoptotic process. The proapoptotic cytokines—tumor necrosis factor-alpha (TNF-$\alpha$), transforming growth factor-alpha (TGF-$\alpha$), interferon-gamma (IFN-$\gamma$), and interleukin-1 beta (IL-1$\beta$)—are increased in MDS (43,44). They may function to suppress the growth of hematopoietic progenitors and induce expression of the FAS receptor, which, when appropriately triggered, can initiate the apoptotic pathways. The prominent role of some cytokines has been examined in clinical studies. For example, strategies to neutralize TNF-$\alpha$ with pentoxifylline to decrease its production and with soluble TNF-$\alpha$ receptors (to competitively bind the excess TNF) have resulted in clinical responses in a minority of MDS patients (45).

## IX. MOLECULAR MODELS FOR CHROMOSOME ABNORMALITIES IN MDS

As described earlier, many of the recurring chromosomal abnormalities in MDS lead to the loss of genetic material, which is the hallmark of tumor suppressor genes. Tumor suppressor genes normally function to control cell growth and/or cell death by regulating the cell cycle, response to DNA damage, and apoptosis.

A simple, "two-hit" model involving a single target tumor suppressor gene (Knudson's model) predicts that loss of function of both alleles must occur for manifestation of the malignant phenotype (46). Loss of gene function may occur in a number of ways, including chromosomal loss or deletion, point mutations, or by transcriptional silencing via methylation of the control elements of the gene. A clinical example, which illustrates this principle, is the occurrence of MDS or AML following cytotoxic therapy (tMDS and tAML, respectively). A relatively long latency period between the time of exposure and bone marrow dysfunction in many of these patients is compatible with a two-step mechanism in which two mutations within a target gene must occur in a myeloid progenitor cell. These patients may have two normal alleles at the tumor suppressor gene locus initially, one of which becomes mutated as a result of therapy. Subsequent loss of the second allele in a bone marrow stem cell would permit leukemia development. The cytotoxic therapy may induce visible chromosomal abnormalities or submicroscopic mutations (or both) in bone marrow cells of tAML patients. Alternatively, because AML develops in only 5–15% of patients who are treated for a primary tumor, these individuals may have inherited a predisposing mutant allele; subsequent exposure to cytotoxic therapy may induce the second mutation, giving rise to leukemia. In these cases, characterization of the predisposing mutations will be important in identifying individuals who are at risk of developing tAML and in the selection of the appropriate therapy for the primary malignant disease.

In an alternative model, loss of only a single copy of a gene may result in a reduction in the level of one or more critical gene products (haploinsufficiency). Several recent reports implicate haploinsufficiency of the *Tp53* and *p27Kip1* genes in the pathogenesis of tumors in mice, where a substantial percentage of tumors retain a functional copy of *Tp53* or *p27Kip1*. The *Tp53* gene is an important tumor suppressor gene that functions to arrest cell cycling after DNA damage. In humans, haploinsufficiency of the *RUNX1* (runt-related transcription factor 1, also known as *AML1*) gene results in a familial platelet disorder with a predisposition to AML (47). Importantly, the few leukemias available for analysis from affected family members appear to retain one normal *RUNX1* allele. With respect to the deletions of 5q, 7q, and 20q in MDS and AML, homozygous deletions have not been detected, an observation that is compatible with a haploinsufficiency model in which loss of one allele of the relevant gene (or genes) perturbs cell fate. However, the presence of one or more genes required for cell viability in close proximity to a tumor suppressor gene locus may preclude the existence of large, homozygous structural deletions. At present, there is little experimental evidence favoring one or the other of these models in the pathogenesis of MDS.

## X.  CYTOGENETIC SUBGROUPS IN MDS

### A.  Normal Karyotype

As noted above, between 30 and 60% of MDS patients have a normal karyotype. It is likely that this subgroup is heterogeneous, consisting of patients in whom the genetic alterations responsible for neoplastic transformation are not detectable by standard cytogenetic methods, or in whom chromosomally abnormal cells were not detected owing to technical factors. Regardless of the etiology, these cases are found to have a better prognosis than some cases of MDS with readily detectable cytogenetic abnormalities and serve as a reference for comparison of outcomes. The median survival for these IPSS good-risk patients is 3.8 years. The time to progression to AML for 25% of good-risk patients is 5.6 years (8).

### B.  Deletion of the Long Arm of Chromosome 20: del(20q)

A del(20q) is a common, recurring abnormality in malignant myeloid disorders. Although initially described in polycythemia vera, del(20q) was soon detected in other myeloid disorders including MDS, AML, and other MPD cases (31). The abnormality is seen in approximately 5% of MDS cases and 7% of tMDS cases (7).

A number of consistent features have been described in MDS patients with del(20q), including low-risk disease (usually RA), low rate of progression to AML, and prolonged survival (median of 45 months vs. 28 months for other MDS patients) (48). Morphologically, the presence of a del(20q) is associated with prominent dysplasia in the erythroid and megakaryocytic lineages (49). The International MDS Risk Analysis Workshop found that patients with a del(20q), observed in association with a complex karyotype, constituted a poor-risk group with a median survival of 9.6 months, whereas the prognosis for patients with an isolated del(20q) was favorable (8). Taken together, these data suggest that the del(20q) in MDS may be associated with a favorable outcome when noted as the sole abnormality, but with a less favorable prognosis in the setting of a complex karyotype. This phenomenon is analogous to that observed for the del(5q) in MDS (discussed below).

Cytogenetic analysis of the deleted chromosome 20 homologs has revealed that the deletions are variable in size, but the majority are large with loss of most of 20q (50,51). By using fluorescence in situ hybridization (FISH) with a panel of probes from 20q, combined with loss-of-heterozygosity (LOH) studies, investigators have identified an interstitial commonly deleted segment (CDS) within 20q12 that is flanked by D20S206 on the proximal side and D20S424 on the distal side. This CDS is ~4 Mb and is gene-rich (52,53). At present, the identity of a myeloid tumor suppressor gene on 20q is unknown. Several research groups have identified interesting candidate genes by generating a detailed physical map as well as a transcriptional map of the CDS (52,53). The functions of candidate genes within the CDS are diverse, and include transcription factors, components of signal transduction pathways, an RNA transcription modulator, and a regulator of apoptosis (53).

## C. Loss of the Y Chromosome: −Y

The clinical and biological significance of −Y is unknown. A −Y chromosome has been noted in a number of malignant diseases, but has also been reported to be a phenomenon of aging (54). The United Kingdom Cancer Cytogenetics Group undertook a comprehensive analysis of this abnormality in both normal and neoplastic bone marrows (55). They found that −Y could be identified in 7.7% of patients without a hematological malignant disease and in 10.7% of patients with MDS; thus, the presence of −Y could not be used to document a malignant process. The International MDS Risk Analysis Workshop found that whereas −Y may not be diagnostic of MDS, once the disease is identified by clinical and pathological means, the loss of a Y chromosome as the sole cytogenetic abnormality conferred a favorable outcome (8). More recently, Wiktor et al. reported on a large series of 215 male patients, noting that patients with a hematological disease had a significantly higher percentage of cells with −Y (52% vs. 37%, $p = 0.036$). In this series, the presence of −Y in >75% of metaphase cells accurately predicted a malignant hematological disease (56). Wiktor et al. also noted a neutral or favorable prognosis for an isolated −Y.

## D. Loss of Chromosome 5 or del(5q): −5/del(5q)

Loss of a whole chromosome 5 or a deletion of the long arm of this chromosome, designated as −5/del(5q), is observed in 10–20% of patients with MDS or AML arising de novo, and in 40% of patients with tMDS/tAML (Fig. 1) (7,57). Notably, many patients with de novo AML or MDS and either −5/del(5q) or −7/del(7q) (discussed below) have a significant occupational exposure to po-

**del(5)(q14q33)**                                 **del(7)(q11q36)**

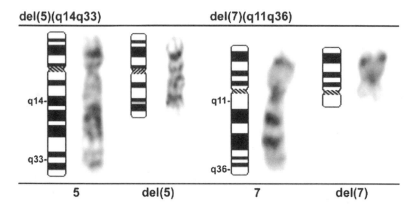

|       |        |       |        |
|:-----:|:------:|:-----:|:------:|
|   5   | del(5) |   7   | del(7) |

**Fig. 1** In this del(5q), breakpoints occur in q14 and q33 resulting in interstitial loss of the intervening chromosomal material. In this del(7q), breakpoints occur in q11 and q36. In both cases, the critical commonly deleted segments are lost. Normal chromosome 5 and 7 homologs are shown for comparison.

tential carcinogens, suggesting that abnormalities of chromosome 5 or 7 may be a marker of mutagen-induced malignant hematological disease (58).

In primary MDS, abnormalities of chromosome 5 are observed in the 5q − syndrome (described below) or, more commonly, in RAEB or RAEB-t in association with a complex karyotype. Clinically, patients with del(5q) and additional cytogenetic abnormalities have a poor prognosis with early progression to leukemia, development of treatment resistance, and short survival. Abnormalities of 5q are associated with previous exposure to standard and high-dose alkylating agent therapy, including use in immunosuppressive regimens (59–62). Exposure to benzene (63) and therapeutic ionizing radiation (64) have recently emerged as risks for MDS (see also Chapter 3).

## 1. 5q − Syndrome

The identification of a del(5q) as the sole karyotypic abnormality is associated with a distinct clinical syndrome (11,65). This syndrome features an overrepresentation of females (2:1), which is in contrast to the male preponderance of MDS in general. The initial finding is usually macrocytic anemia combined with a normal or elevated platelet count. The diagnosis is usually RA (~67% of cases) or RAEB (~33% of cases). The presence of abnormalities in the megakaryocytic lineage (particularly micromegakaryocytes) is the predominant finding in the bone marrow. Patients with 5q − syndrome have a favorable outcome, in fact the best of any MDS subgroup, with low rates of leukemic transformation and a relatively long survival of several years' duration (8,65).

## 2.   Molecular Analysis of the del(5q)

Several groups of investigators have defined a CDS on the long arm of chromosome 5 (Fig. 2) (66–69). It is predicted that this CDS contains a myeloid tumor suppressor gene. Using cytogenetic and FISH analysis of the chromosomes of 177 patients with de novo MDS/AML or tMDS/AML, Le Beau and colleagues defined a 1.5-Mb CDS within 5q31 flanked by D5S479 and D5S500 (67,70). To identify candidate tumor suppressor genes, these investigators developed a transcript map of the CDS, which contains 18 known genes and 12 expressed sequence tags (ESTs) (67). The function of these genes covers a spectrum of activities, including regulation of mitosis and the G2 checkpoint, transcriptional

# Commonly Deleted Segment of 5q

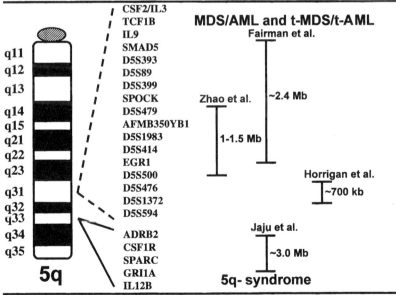

**Fig. 2**   Ideogram of the long arm of chromosome 5 showing chromosome markers and candidate genes within commonly deleted segments (CDS) as reported by various investigators. The proximal CDS (dashed lines) in 5q31 was identified in MDS, AML, and tMDS/AML, whereas the distal CDS (solid lines) in 5q33 was identified in the 5q − syndrome.

and translational regulators, and cell-surface receptors. Analysis of myeloid leukemia cells for inactivating mutations has eliminated the 18 genes within the CDS, suggesting that a novel myeloid tumor suppressor gene located in this interval might be involved in the pathogenesis of these disorders (67, and Le Beau unpublished data).

Molecular analysis of the del(5q) in patients with the 5q − syndrome suggests that a different region, and hence a different gene, is involved. Boultwood and colleagues examined three patients with the 5q − syndrome with small deletions extending from 5q31–33, and identified a 3-Mb CDS within 5q33 between *ADRB2* and *IL12B* (71). This region is distal to the CDS in 5q31 found in the patients with RAEB, RAEB-t, and AML who have a del(5q). Whether all patients with the 5q − syndrome have involvement of a gene in this distal region and whether this gene plays a role in the pathogenesis of other subtypes of MDS or AML is unknown.

In summary, the existing data suggest that there are two nonoverlapping CDS in 5q31 and 5q33. The proximal segment in 5q31 is likely to contain a tumor suppressor gene involved in the pathogenesis of both de novo and tMDS/tAML. Band 5q33 is likely to contain a second myeloid tumor suppressor gene involved in the pathogenesis of the 5q − syndrome.

## E. Loss of Chromosome 7 or del(7q): −7/del(7q)

In approximately 5% and 55% of patients with de novo MDS (5,6) and tMDS (57), respectively, a −7/del(7q) is observed as the sole abnormality (Fig. 1). The loss or deletion can occur in three general contexts:

> de novo MDS and AML;
> myeloid leukemia associated with constitutional predisposition; and
> tMDS/tAML (reviewed in Ref. 72).

The similar clinical and biological features of the myeloid disorders associated with −7/del(7q) suggest that the same gene(s) is altered in each of these contexts. An entity designated "monosomy 7 syndrome" has been described in young children, and is characterized by a preponderance of males (~4:1), hepatosplenomegaly, leukocytosis, thrombocytopenia, and poor prognosis (73,74). Juvenile myelomonocytic leukemia (JMML, previously known as juvenile chronic myelogenous leukemia) shares many features with monosomy 7 syndrome, and bone marrow examination from patients with JMML often reveals −7 either at diagnosis or as a new cytogenetic finding associated with disease acceleration (72). In fact, most authors now consider the monosomy 7 syndrome a subset of JMML. A −7/del(7q) is the most frequent cytogenetic abnormality detected in the bone marrow of patients with constitutional predispositions to myeloid neoplasms, including Fanconi anemia, neurofibromatosis type 1, and severe congenital neutropenia. As with −5/del(5q), occupational or environmental exposure to mutagens including chemotherapy, radiotherapy, benzene exposure, and smoking (75), as well as severe aplastic anemia (regularly treated with immunosuppressive agents alone), have been associated with −7/del(7q).

## 1. Molecular Analysis of the −7/del(7q)

As with the −5/del(5q), investigators have examined the breakpoints and extent of the deletions of 7q in patients to identify a CDS (Fig. 3) (76–81). Le Beau et al. examined 81 patients with de novo and tMDS/AML, and identified two distinct CDSs. In 65 of the patients, the CDS was within q22, whereas in the 16 other patients, interstitial deletions of a more distal segment were detected with a CDS of q32–33 (78). Using FISH, an ~2-Mb CDS in 7q22 was identified, a finding that is consistent with most published data (76,79,82,83). Tosi et al. evaluated patients with 7q abnormalities and identified an interesting patient with a complex karyotype and a t(7;7); the patient had a deletion associated with the

# Commonly Deleted Segment of 7q

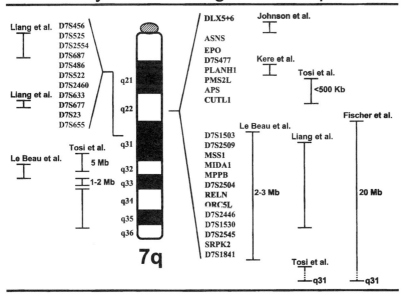

**Fig. 3**  Ideogram of the long arm of chromosome 7 showing chromosome markers and candidate genes within commonly deleted segments (CDS) as reported by various investigators. The information on the left of the ideogram illustrate the more distal CDS identified in 7q31–7q36 and the information on the right represents the CDSs identified in 7q22

translocation breakpoint of 150 kb proximal to the CDS defined by Le Beau et al. (81). A number of candidate genes have been identified and evaluated for mutations within the CDS at 7q22, including extracellular (or extracellular-like) proteins, replication and transcriptional control elements, a splicing factor kinase, and a mitochondrial-processing peptidase. None have disclosed mutations in the remaining allele.

Data from cytogenetic, FISH, and LOH studies performed in a number of laboratories paint a complex picture of 7q deletions in myeloid malignancies. There is general agreement that 7q22 is involved in a majority of cases. Defining a consistent CDS has been complicated by several factors, namely the relatively low frequency of del(7q) versus complete loss of chromosome 7; the use of different techniques to investigate marrow samples (e.g., FISH vs. LOH); the wide spectrum of myeloid disorders with alterations in chromosome 7, suggesting genetic heterogeneity; and the existence of multiple and sometimes complex cytogenetic abnormalities in some cases.

## F. 17p− Syndrome

Abnormalities resulting in the loss of the short arm of chromosome 17 (17p−) have been reported in up to 5% of patients with MDS (84). These include simple deletions, unbalanced translocations, dicentric rearrangements (particularly with chromosome 5), or less often −17, or isochromosome formation. A frequent recurring rearrangement is the dic(5;17)(q11–13;p11–13) (85,86). Approximately one-third of these patients have tMDS (87), and most have additional cytogenetic abnormalities. The most common additional changes are unbalanced translocations involving chromosomes 5 or 7.

Morphologically, the 17p − syndrome is associated with a typical form of dysgranulopoiesis, combining pseudo-Pelger-Hüet hypolobulation and the presence of small granules in granulocytes. Clinically, the disease is aggressive with resistance to treatment and short survival. The *TP53* gene is located at 17p13.1. One allele of *TP53* is typically lost as a result of the abnormality of 17p in these cases; an inactivating mutation in the second allele on the remaining, normal chromosome 17 occurs in ~70% of cases (85,86). Sankar et al. mapped a CDS in leukemia and lymphoma patients to 17p13.3, suggesting the existence of a novel tumor suppressor gene distal to *TP53* (88).

## G. 11q23

The *MLL* (mixed lineage leukemia) gene (also known as *ALL1*, *Htrx*, *HRX*) is involved in more than 40 reciprocal translocations in acute leukemia (89). In a recent European workshop that investigated 550 patients with 11q23 abnormalities, 28 cases (5.1%) were noted to present with a MDS and five others had evolved from tMDS to tAML prior to cytogenetic study, accounting for up to 6% of the total cases examined. Seven of these 33 cases were tMDS (90). In both de novo and tMDS, the 11q23 abnormalities were frequently accompanied by additional abnormalities, including complex karyotypes and −7/del(7q). No association with FAB subgroup was identified, but RA was overrepresented and RARS underrepresented as compared with most series of MDS patients. The median survival was short (19 months), with leukemic transformation observed in ~20% of cases. This workshop did not find the classic association of prior exposure to topoisomerase II inhibitors in their examination of 40 cases of tMDS and tAML, but this negative finding may simply reflect the relatively small number ($n = 23$) of cases with full treatment details (91).

An International Workshop on Leukemia Karyotype and Prior Treatment, held in June 2000, evaluated 511 patients with tMDS/tAML and balanced chromosomal aberrations, such as translocations (balanced aberrations are found in 20–33% of tMDS/tAML cases). Of the 162 patients with 11q23 involvement, just under 12% presented with a tMDS (personal communication, J.D. Rowley). One-third of these patients (six of 19) had progression to an acute leukemia (five AML, one ALL), but no clear association with FAB subtype was identified. The most common translocations were t(9;11) in five cases; t(11;19) in four cases (three of which involved 19p13.1); and t(11;16) in three cases.

## H.  Gain of Chromosome 8: +8

In MDS, the incidence of +8—an abnormality observed in all FAB subgroups (3,7,8)—is ~10%. However, the significance of the gain of chromosome 8 in MDS patients is not fully characterized as a risk factor. The situation is complicated in that +8 is often associated with other recurring abnormalities known to have prognostic significance, and may be seen in isolation as a separate clone unrelated to the primary clone in up to 5% of cases. The International MDS Risk Analysis Workshop ranked this abnormality in the intermediate-risk group (8).

## I.  Complex Karyotypes

Complex karyotypes have been variably defined, but generally involve the presence of ≥3 abnormalities. The majority of cases with complex karyotypes involve unbalanced chromosomal abnormalities leading to the loss of genetic material. Complex karyotypes are observed in ~20% of patients with primary MDS, and in as many as 90% of patients with tMDS (57,92). Abnormalities involving chromosomes 5, 7, or both are identified in most cases with complex karyotypes. There is general agreement that a complex karyotype carries a poor prognosis (8,21).

## XI.  THERAPY-RELATED MDS (tMDS)

Evolving management strategies for oncology patients have led to a dramatic improvement in the survival of some cancer patients, many of whom now survive the acute toxicities of therapy, living long enough to develop late toxic complications. Techniques in supportive care, including stem cell transplantation, have reduced the once-lethal complications of treatment strategies, and not only have permitted dose escalation, but also have allowed the testing of significantly more toxic agents and combinations of agents.

One of the most serious consequences of cancer therapy is the development of a second cancer of myeloid origin. In patients treated with high-dose therapy for breast cancer, lymphoma, leukemias, and multiple myeloma, the reported incidences of tMDS/tAML is 1–24% of treated patients (61). Increasing numbers of patients with benign disease, particularly rheumatology and dermatology patients as well as organ transplant recipients, are also being exposed to cytotoxic agents for immunosuppression, placing them at risk for some of the same late complications.

Cytogenetic aberrations are detected in up to 90% of patients with tMDS (57). Common cytogenetic findings are listed in Table 1. Several clinical-morphological-cytogenetic subsets of tMDS/tAML have been identified, which are closely associated with the type of prior therapy. Patients exposed to alkylating agents, for example, typically have a longer latency period to bone marrow dysfunction (median 5–7 years); the tMDS that ensues is characterized by trilineage dysplasia, which often progresses to tAML. Abnormalities of chromosomes 5 and/or 7 and complex karyotypes predominate. Patients exposed to topoisomerase II inhibitors are more likely to present with tAML, have a shorter latency period to bone marrow dysfunction (~2 years or less), and have abnormalities involving *MLL* at 11q23 or *RUNX1* (*AML1*) at 21q22 (93,94).

## XII.  RARE RECURRING TRANSLOCATIONS

The identification of genes involved in recurring cytogenetic abnormalities has been extremely useful in gaining insights into their normal functions and their role in leukemogenesis (89,95). The consequence of the recurring translocations is the deregulation of gene expression, with quantitatively altered production of a normal protein product or the generation of a novel fusion gene and production of a fusion protein. In MDS, several such translocations have been identified and examined by molecular analysis. A few examples are described below.

## A. The t(5;12) Translocation

The t(5;12)(q33;p12) is observed in ~1% of patients with CMML. In 1994, the molecular consequences of this translocation were elucidated. The gene encoding the beta chain of the platelet-derived growth factor receptor (*PDGFRB*) resides on chromosome 5. A novel *ETS*-like (*e*rythroblastosis virus *t*ransforming *s*equence) transcription factor, *TEL*, also known as *ETV6* (*t*ranslocated *ETS* in *l*eukemia), is the gene affected on chromosome 12. The translocation creates a fusion gene and fusion protein containing the 5' portion of *TEL* and the 3' portion of *PDGFRB* (96). It is believed that the PDGFRB kinase activity is perturbed, resulting in the transformed phenotype. *TEL* encodes a transcriptional repressor, and is promiscuously involved in translocations with some 40 genes known to be involved in hematological malignancies (89).

## B. The t(3;21) Translocation

The t(3;21)(q26.2;q22.1) has been linked to acute leukemia arising after cytotoxic therapy. This abnormality was first recognized in CML in blast crisis (97) and later in tMDS/tAML (98). The *EAP* gene (*E*pstein-Barr virus small RNAs *a*ssociated *p*rotein) at 3q26 encodes a highly expressed, small nuclear protein associated with EBV small RNA (EBER1). *EAP* was found to be fused with the *RUNX1* gene at 21q22, retaining the DNA-binding sequences of EAP. The fusion is out-of-frame, such that the *RUNX1* gene is truncated and loses its functional activity. Further work has identified two additional genes 400–750 kb centromeric to *EAP*, also at 3q26, namely *MDS1/EVI1* (MDS-associated sequences) and *EVI1* (ecotropic virus insertion site) (99). Both genes encode nuclear transcription factors containing DNA-binding zinc finger domains, which are identical except for an N-terminal extension of 12 amino acids in the MDS1/EVI1 protein, representing a splicing variant. Each gene has independent and tightly controlled expression during differentiation (100). The MDS1/EVI1 and EVI1 proteins have opposite functions. EVI1 inhibits both granulocyte colony-stimulating factor (G-CSF)-mediated differentiation and TGFβ1 growth-inhibitory effect, whereas MDS1/EVI1 has no effect on G-CSF differentiation and enhances TGFβ1 growth-inhibition (100). *RUNX1* fuses with *MDS1/EVI1*, in frame, resulting in the loss of the first 12 amino acids, producing a novel EVI1 protein, and a phenotype of arrested differentiation that leads to apoptosis in vitro (101).

## C. The t(11;16) Translocation

The t(11;16)(q23;p13.3) occurs primarily in tMDS, but some cases have presented as tAML (Fig. 4) (102). Among the more than 40 recurring translocations

**t(11;16)(q23;p13.3)**

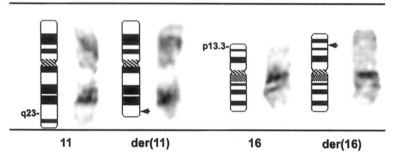

**11            der(11)            16            der(16)**

**Fig. 4**   In the t(11;16), breakpoints occur in 11q23 and 16p13.3 followed by a reciprocal exchange of chromosomal material. The 5′ end of the *MLL* gene at 11q23 is fused to the 3′ end of the *CBP* gene from 16p13.3 to form the *MLL/CBP* fusion gene on the der(11). Arrowheads indicate the breakpoints. Normal chromosome 11 and 16 homologs are shown for comparison.

involving *MLL* in myeloid neoplasms (with AML predominating), the t(11;16) is unique in that most patients have tMDS. The *MLL* gene on chromosome 11 is fused with *CBP* (CREB-binding protein gene) on chromosome 16. The MLL protein is likely to be multifunctional, and is known to regulate *HOX* gene expression during development. CBP is an adapter protein involved in transcription control via histone acetylation, which mediates chromosome decondensation, thereby facilitating transcription. Both genes have multiple translocation partners in various hematological disorders, and elucidating their function will undoubtedly lead to significant progress in leukemia research.

## XIII.   CONCLUDING REMARKS

The role of cytogenetic analysis in the diagnosis, prognosis, and follow-up of patients with MDS has been defined clearly. Other molecular cytogenetic methods, such as FISH, have been shown to be complementary, without replacing the information that is obtained by conventional cytogenetic analysis. Further observations and investigations with the various molecular techniques will undoubtedly contribute to improved understanding and management of patients with MDS.

# REFERENCES

1. Bennett JM, Catovsky D, Daniel MT, Flandrin G, Galton DA, Gralnick HR, Sultan C. Proposals for the classification of the myelodysplastic syndromes. Br J Haematol 1982; 51:189–199.
2. Bagby GC, Jr. The concept of preleukemia: clinical and laboratory studies (review). Crit Rev Oncol Hematol 1986; 4:203–220.
3. Morel P, Hebbar M, Lai JL, Duhamel A, Preudhomme C, Wattel E, Bauters F, Fenaux P. Cytogenetic analysis has strong independent prognostic value in de novo myelodysplastic syndromes and can be incorporated in a new scoring system: a report on 408 cases. Leukemia 1993; 7:1315–1323.
4. Jotterand M, Parlier V. Diagnostic and prognostic significance of cytogenetics in adult primary myelodysplastic syndromes. Leuk Lymphoma 1996; 23(3–4):253–266.
5. Toyama K, Ohyashiki K, Yoshida Y, Abe T, Asano S, Hirai H, Hirashima K, Hotta T, Kuramot A, Kurix S, et al. Clinical implications of chromosomal abnormalities in 401 patients with myelodysplastic syndromes: a multicentric study in Japan. Leukemia 1993; 7:499–508.
6. Sole F, Espinet B, Sanz GF, Cervera J, Calasanz MJ, Luno E, Prieto F, Granada I, Hernandez JM, Cigudosa JC, Diez JL, Bureo E, Marques ML, Arranz E, Rios R, Martinez, Climent JA, Vallespi T, Florensa L, Woessner S. Incidence, characterization and prognostic significance of chromosomal abnormalities in 640 patients with primary myelodysplastic syndromes. Grupo Cooperativo Espanol de Citogenetica Hematologica. Br J Haematol 2000; 108:346–356.
7. Vallespi T, Imbert M, Mecucci C, Preudhomme C, Fenaux P. Diagnosis, classification, and cytogenetics of myelodysplastic syndromes (review). Haematologica 1998; 83:258–275.
8. Greenberg P, Cox C, Le Beau MM, Fenaux P, Morel P, Sanz G, Sanz M, Vallespi T, Hamblin T, Oscier D, Obyashiki K, Toyama K, Aul C, Mufti G, Bennett J. International scoring system for evaluating prognosis in myelodysplastic syndromes. Blood 1997; 89:2079–2088.
9. Bennett JM. World Health Organization classification of the acute leukemias and myelodysplastic syndrome (review). Int J Hematol 2000; 72:131–133.
10. Harris NL, Jaffe ES, Diebold J, Flandrin G, Muller-Hermelink HK, Vardiman J, Lister TA, Bloomfield CD. World Health Organization classification of neoplastic diseases of the hematopoietic and lymphoid tissues: report of the Clinical Advisory Committee meeting, Airlie House, Virginia, November 1997. J Clin Oncol 1999; 17:3835–3849.
11. Van den Berghe H, Michaux L. 5q-, twenty-five years later: a synopsis. Cancer Genet Cytogenet 1997; 94:1–7.
12. Jary L, Mossafa H, Fourcade C, Genet P, Pulik M, Flandrin G. The 17p- syndrome: a distinct myelodysplastic syndrome entity? Leuk Lymphoma 1997; 25:163–168.
13. Dewald GW, Pierre RV, Phyliky RL. Three patients with structurally abnormal X chromosomes, each with Xq13 breakpoints and a history of idiopathic acquired sideroblastic anemia. Blood 1982; 59:100–105.

14. Rowley JD. The role of chromosome translocations in leukemogenesis (review). Semin Hematol 1999; 36(Suppl 7):59–72.

15. Smadja N, Krulik M, Hagemeijer A, van der Plas DC, Gonzalez Canali G, de Gramont A. Cytogenetic and molecular studies of the Philadelphia translocation t(9;22) observed in a patient with myelodysplastic syndrome. Leukemia 1989; 3:236–238.

16. Sanz GF, Sanz MA, Vallespi T, Canizo MC, Torrabadella M, Garcia S, Irriguible D, San Miguel JF. Two regression models and a scoring system for predicting survival and planning treatment in myelodysplastic syndromes: a multivariate analysis of prognostic factors in 370 patients. Blood 1989; 74:395–408.

17. Aul C, Gattermann N, Germing U, Runde V, Heyll A, Schneider W. Risk assessment in primary myelodysplastic syndromes: validation of the Dusseldorf score. Leukemia 1994; 8:1906–13.

18. Parlier V, van Melle G, Beris P, Schmidt PM, Tobler A, Haller E, Bellomo MJ. Prediction of 18-month survival in patients with primary myelodysplastic syndrome. A regression model and scoring system based on the combination of chromosome findings and the Bournemouth score. Cancer Genet Cytogenet 1995; 81: 158–165.

19. Sanz GF, Sanz MA, Greenberg PL. Prognostic factors and scoring systems in myelodysplastic syndromes (review). Haematologica 1998; 83:358–368.

20. Nevill TJ, Fung HC, Shepherd JD, Horsman DE, Nantel SH, Klingemann HG, Forrest DL, Toze CL, Sutherland HJ, Hogge DE, Naiman SC, Le A, Brockington DA, Barnett MJ. Cytogenetic abnormalities in primary myelodysplastic syndrome are highly predictive of outcome after allogeneic bone marrow transplantation. Blood 1998; 96:1910–1917.

21. Hamblin TJ, Oscier DG. The myelodysplastic syndrome—a practical guide (review). Hematol Oncol 1987; 5:19–34.

22. Horiike S, Taniwaki M, Misawa S, Abe T. Chromosome abnormalities and karyotypic evolution in 83 patients with myelodysplastic syndrome and predictive value for prognosis. Cancer 1988; 62:1129–1138.

23. Geddes AA, Bowen DT, Jacobs A. Clonal karyotype abnormalities and clinical progress in the myelodysplastic syndrome. Br J Haematol 1990; 76:194–202.

24. de Souza Fernandez T, Ornellas MH, Otero de Carvalho L, Tabak D, Abdelhay E. Chromosomal alterations associated with evolution from myelodysplastic syndrome to acute myeloid leukemia. Leuk Res 2000; 24:839–848.

25. Prchal JT, Throckmorton DW, Carroll AJ 3rd, Fuson EW, Gams RA, Prchal JF. A common progenitor for human myeloid and lymphoid cells. Nature 1978; 274: 590–591.

26. Busque L, Gilliland DG. X-inactivation analysis in the 1990s: promise and potential problems (review). Leukemia 1998; 12:128–135.

27. Okamoto T, Okada M, Wada H, Kanamaru A, Kakishita E, Hashimoto T, Furuyama J. Clonal analysis of hematopoietic cells using a novel polymorphic site of the X chromosome. Am J Hematol 1998; 58:263–266.

28. Weimar IS, Bourhis JH, De Gast GC, Gerritsen WR. Clonality in myelodysplastic syndromes (review). Leuk Lymphoma 1994; 13:215–221.

29. Lawrence HJ, Broudy VC, Magenis RE, Olson S, Tomar D, Barton S, Fitchen JH, Bagby GC Jr. Cytogenetic evidence for involvement of B lymphocytes in acquired idiopathic sideroblastic anemias. Blood 1987; 70:1003–1005.

30. Nilsson L, Astrand-Grundstrom I, Arvidsson I, Jacobsson B, Hellstrom-Lindberg E, Hast R, Jacobsen SE. Isolation and characterization of hematopoietic progenitor/ stem cells in 5q-deleted myelodysplastic syndromes: evidence for involvement at the hematopoietic stem cell level. Blood 2000; 96:2012–2021.

31. Asimakopoulos FA, Green AR. Deletions of chromosome 20q and the pathogenesis of myeloproliferative disorders (review). Br J Haematol 1996; 95:219–226.

32. Rebollo A, Martinez-A C. Ras proteins: recent advances and new functions (review). Blood 1999; 94:2971–2980.

33. Neubauer A, Dodge RK, George SL, Davey FR, Silver RT, Schiffer CA, Mayer RJ, Ball ED, Wurster-Hill D, Bloomfield CD, et al. Prognostic importance of mutations in the ras proto-oncogenes in de novo acute myeloid leukemia. Blood 1994; 83:1603–1611.

34. Gallagher A, Darley R, Padua RA. RAS and the myelodysplastic syndromes (review). Pathol Biol (Paris) 1997; 45:561–568.

35. Beaupre DM, Kurzrock R. RAS and leukemia: from basic mechanisms to gene-directed therapy (review). J Clin Oncol 1999; 17:1071–1079.

36. Padua RA, Guinn BA, Al-Sabah AI, Smith M, Taylor C, Pettersson T, Ridge S, Carter G, White D, Oscier D, Chevret S, West R. RAS, FMS and p53 mutations and poor clinical outcome in myelodysplasias: a 10-year follow-up. Leukemia 1998; 12: 887–892.

37. de Souza Fernandez T, Menezes de Souza J, Macedo Silva ML, Tabak D, Abdelhay E. Correlation of N-ras point mutations with specific chromosomal abnormalities in primary myelodysplastic syndrome. Leuk Res 1998; 22:125–134.

38. Tien HF, Wang CH, Chuang SM, Chow JM, Lee FY, Liu MC, Chen YC, Shen MC, Lin DT, Lin KH. Cytogenetic studies, ras mutation, and clinical characteristics in primary myelodysplastic syndrome. A study on 68 Chinese patients in Taiwan. Cancer Genet Cytogenet 1994; 74:40–49.

39. Vander Heiden MG, Thompson CB. Bcl-2 proteins: regulators of apoptosis or of mitochondrial homeostasis? (review). Nat Cell Biol 1999; 1:E209–E216.

40. Raza A, Mundle S, Iftikhar A, Gregory S, Marcus B, Khan Z, Alvi S, Shetty V, Dameron S, Wright V, et al. Simultaneous assessment of cell kinetics and programmed cell death in bone marrow biopsies of myelodysplastics reveals extensive apoptosis as the probable basis for ineffective hematopoiesis. Am J Hematol 1995; 48:143–154.

41. Parker JE, Mufti GJ, Rasool F, Mijovic A, Devereux S, Pagliuca A. The role of apoptosis, proliferation, and the Bcl-2-related proteins in the myelodysplastic syndromes and acute myeloid leukemia secondary to MDS. Blood 2000; 96:3932–3938.

42. Kurotaki H, Tsushima Y, Nagai K, Yagihashi S. Apoptosis, bcl-2 expression and p53 accumulation in myelodysplastic syndrome, myelodysplastic-syndrome-derived acute myelogenous leukemia and de novo acute myelogenous leukemia. Acta Haematol 2000; 102:115–123.

43. Reza S, Dar S, Andric T, Qawi H, Mundle S, Shetty V, Venugopal P, Ali I, Lisak L, Raza A. Biologic characteristics of 164 patients with myelodysplastic syndromes. Leuk Lymphoma 1999; 33:281–287.

44. Yoshida Y, Mufti GJ. Apoptosis and its significance in MDS: controversies revisited (review). Leuk Res 1999; 23:777–785.

45. Raza A, Mundle S, Shetty V, Alvi S, Chopra H, Span L, Parcharidou A, Dar S, Venugopal P, Borok R, Gezer S, Showel J, Loew J, Robin E, Rifkin S, Alston D, Hernandez B, Shah R, Kaizer H, Gregory S. Novel insights into the biology of myelodysplastic syndromes: excessive apoptosis and the role of cytokines (review). Int J Hematol 1996; 63:265–278.

46. Knudson AG Jr. Mutation and cancer: statistical study of retinoblastoma. Proc Natl Acad Sci USA 1971; 68:820–823.

47. Song WJ, Sullivan MG, Legare RD, Hutchings S, Tan X, Kufrin D, Ratajczak J, Resende IC, Haworth C, Hock R, Loh M, Felix C, Roy DC, Busque L, Kurnit D, Willman C, Gewirtz AM, Speck NA, Bushweller JH, Li FP, Gardiner K, Poncz M, Maris JM, Gilliland DG. Haploinsufficiency of *CBFA2* causes familial thrombocytopenia with propensity to develop acute myelogenous leukaemia. Nat Genet 1999; 23:166–175.

48. Wattel E, Lai JL, Hebbar M, Preudhomme C, Grahek D, Morel P, Bauters F, Fenaux P. De novo myelodysplastic syndrome (MDS) with deletion of the long arm of chromosome 20: a subtype of MDS with distinct hematological and prognostic features? (review). Leuk Res 1993; 17:921–926.

49. Kurtin PJ, Dewald GW, Shields DJ, Hanson CA. Hematologic disorders associated with deletions of chromosome 20q: a clinicopathologic study of 107 patients. Am J Clin Pathol 1996; 106:680–688.

50. Davis MP, Dewald GW, Pierre RV, Hoagland HC. Hematologic manifestations associated with deletions of the long arm of chromosome 20. Cancer Genet Cytogenet 1984; 12:63–71.

51. Aatola M, Armstrong E, Teerenhovi L, Borgström GH. Clinical significance of the del(20q) chromosome in hematologic disorders. Cancer Genet Cytogenet 1992; 62: 75–80.

52. Bench AJ, Nacheva EP, Hood TL, Holden JL, French L, Swanton S, et al. Chromosome 20 deletions in myeloid malignancies: reduction of the common deleted region, generation of a PAC/BAC contig and identification of candidate genes. UK Cancer Cytogenetics Group (UKCCG). Oncogene 2000; 19:3902–3913.

53. Wang PW, Eisenbart JD, Espinosa R 3rd, Davis EM, Larson RA, Le Beau MM. Refinement of the smallest commonly deleted segment of chromosome 20 in malignant myeloid diseases and development of a PAC-based physical and transcription map. Genomics 2000; 67:28–39.

54. Pierre RV, Hoagland HC. Age-associated aneuploidy: loss of Y chromosome from human bone marrow cells with aging. Cancer 1972; 30:889–894.

55. United Kingdom Cancer Cytogenetics Group (UKCCG). Loss of the Y chromosome from normal and neoplastic bone marrows. Genes Chromosomes Cancer 1992; 5:83–88.

56. Wiktor A, Rybicki BA, Piao ZS, Shurafa M, Barthel B, Maeda K, Van Dyke DL.

Clinical significance of Y chromosome loss in hematologic disease. Genes Chromosomes Cancer 2000; 27:11–16.

57. Thirman MJ, Larson RA. Therapy-related myeloid leukemia (review). Hematol Oncol Clin North Am 1996; 10:293–320.

58. West RR, Stafford DA, White AD, Bowen DT, Padua RA. Cytogenetic abnormalities in the myelodysplastic syndromes and occupational or environmental exposure. Blood 2000; 95:2093–2097.

59. Larson RA, LeBeau MM, Vardiman JW, Rowley JD. Myeloid leukemia after hematotoxins. Environ Health Perspect 1996; 104(suppl 6):1303–1307.

60. Aul C, Bowen DT, Yoshida Y. Pathogenesis, etiology and epidemiology of myelodysplastic syndromes (review). Haematologica 1998; 83:71–86.

61. Pedersen-Bjergaard J, Andersen MK, Christiansen DH. Therapy-related acute myeloid leukemia and myelodysplasia after high-dose chemotherapy and autologous stem cell transplantation (review). Blood 2000; 95:3273–3279.

62. McCarthy CJ, Sheldon S, Ross CW, McCune WJ. Cytogenetic abnormalities and therapy-related myelodysplastic syndromes in rheumatic disease. Arthritis Rheum 1998; 41:1493–1496.

63. Hayes RB, Yin SN, Dosemeci M, Li GL, Wacholder S, Travis LB, Li CY, Rothman N, Hoover RN, Linet MS. Benzene and the dose-related incidence of hematologic neoplasms in China. Chinese Academy of Preventive Medicine—National Cancer Institute Benzene Study Group. J Natl Cancer Inst 1997; 89:1065–1071.

64. Fenaux P, Lucidarme D, Lai JL, Bauters F. Favorable cytogenetic abnormalities in secondary leukemia. Cancer 1989; 63:2505–2508.

65. Boultwood J, Lewis S, Wainscoat JS. The 5q- syndrome (review). Blood 1994; 84:3253–3260.

66. Fairman J, Chumakov I, Chinault AC, Nowell PC, Nagarajan L. Physical mapping of the minimal region of loss in 5q- chromosome. Proc Natl Acad Sci USA 1995; 92:7406–7410.

67. Zhao N, Stoffel A, Wang PW, Eisenbart JD, Espinosa R 3rd, Larson RA, Le Beau MM. Molecular delineation of the smallest commonly deleted region of chromosome 5 in malignant myeloid diseases to 1–1.5 Mb and preparation of a PAC-based physical map. Proc Natl Acad Sci USA 1997; 94:6948–6953.

68. Jaju RJ, Boultwood J, Oliver FJ, Kostrzewa M, Fidler C, Parker N, McPherson JD, Morris SG, Muller U, Wainscoat JS, Kearney L. Molecular cytogenetic delineation of the critical deleted region in the 5q- syndrome. Genes Chromosomes Cancer 1998; 22:251–256.

69. Horrigan SK, Arbieva ZH, Xie HY, Kravarusic J, Fulton NC, Naik H, Le TT, Westbrook CA. Delineation of a minimal interval and identification of 9 candidates for a tumor suppressor gene in malignant myeloid disorders on 5q31. Blood 2000; 95:2372–2377.

70. Le Beau MM, Espinosa R 3rd, Neuman WL, Stock W, Roulston D, Larson RA, Keinanen M, Westbrook C. Cytogenetic and molecular delineation of the smallest commonly deleted region of chromosome 5 in malignant myeloid diseases. Proc Natl Acad Sci USA 1993; 90:5484–5488.

71. Boultwood J, Fidler C, Strickson AJ, Watkins F, Kostrzewa M, Jaju RJ, Muller U,

Wainscoat JS. Transcription mapping of the 5q- syndrome critical region: cloning of two novel genes and sequencing, expression, and mapping of a further six novel cDNAs. Genomics 2000; 66:26–34.

72. Luna-Fineman S, Shannon KM, Lange BJ. Childhood monosomy 7: epidemiology, biology, and mechanistic implications (review). Blood 1995; 85:1985–1999.

73. Emanuel PD. Myelodysplasia and myeloproliferative disorders in childhood: an update (review). Br J Haematol 1999; 105:852–863.

74. Martinez-Climent JA, Garcia-Conde J. Chromosomal rearrangements in childhood acute myeloid leukemia and myelodysplastic syndromes (review). J Pediatr Hematol Oncol 1999; 21:91–102.

75. Bjork J, Albin M, Mauritzson N, Stromberg U, Johansson B, Hagmar L. Smoking and myelodysplastic syndromes. Epidemiology 2000; 11:285–291.

76. Kere J. Chromosome 7 long arm deletion breakpoints in preleukemia: mapping by pulsed field gel electrophoresis. Nucleic Acids Res 1989; 17:1511–1520.

77. Johnson EJ, Scherer SW, Osborne L, Tsui LC, Oscier D, Mould S, Cotter FE. Molecular definition of a narrow interval at 7q22.1 associated with myelodysplasia. Blood 1996; 87:3579–3586.

78. Le Beau MM, Espinosa R 3rd, Davis EM, Eisenbart JD, Larson RA, Green ED. Cytogenetic and molecular delineation of a region of chromosome 7 commonly deleted in malignant myeloid diseases. Blood 1996; 88:1930–1935.

79. Fischer K, Frohling S, Scherer SW, McAllister Brown J, Scholl C, Stilgenbauer S, Tsui LC, Lichter P, Dohner H. Molecular cytogenetic delineation of deletions and translocations involving chromosome band 7q22 in myeloid leukemias. Blood 1997; 89:2036–2041.

80. Liang H, Fairman J, Claxton DF, Nowell PC, Green ED, Nagarajan L. Molecular anatomy of chromosome 7q deletions in myeloid neoplasms: evidence for multiple critical loci. Proc Natl Acad Sci USA 1998; 95:3781–3785.

81. Tosi S, Scherer SW, Giudici G, Czepulkowski B, Biondi A, Kearney L. Delineation of multiple deleted regions in 7q in myeloid disorders. Genes Chromosomes Cancer 1999; 25:384–392.

82. Döhner K, Brown J, Hehmann U, Hetzel C, Stewart J, Lowther G, Scholl C, Frohling S, Cuneo A, Tsui LC, Lichter P, Scherer SW, Dohner H. Molecular cytogenetic characterization of a critical region in bands 7q35–q36 commonly deleted in malignant myeloid disorders. Blood 1998; 92:4031–4035.

83. Lewis S, Abrahamson G, Boultwood J, Fidler C, Potter A, Wainscoat JS. Molecular characterization of the 7q deletion in myeloid disorders. Br J Haematol 1996; 93: 75–80.

84. Johansson B, Mertens F, Mitelman F. Cytogenetic deletion maps of hematologic neoplasms: circumstantial evidence for tumor suppressor loci (review). Genes Chromosomes Cancer 1993; 8:205–218.

85. Wang P, Spielberger RT, Thangavelu M, Zhao N, Davis EM, Iannantuoni K, Larson RA, Le Beau MM. Dic(5;17): a recurring abnormality in malignant myeloid disorders associated with mutations of TP53. Genes Chromosomes Cancer 1997; 20: 282–291.

86. Lai JL, Preudhomme C, Zandecki M, Flactif M, Vanrumbeke M, Lepelley P, Wattel E, Fenaux P. Myelodysplastic syndromes and acute myeloid leukemia with 17p

deletion. An entity characterized by specific dysgranulopoiesis and a high incidence of P53 mutations. Leukemia 1995; 9:370–381.

87. Merlat A, Lai JL, Sterkers Y, Demory JL, Bauters F, Preudhomme C, Fenaux P. Therapy-related myelodysplastic syndrome and acute myeloid leukemia with 17p deletion. A report on 25 cases. Leukemia 1999; 13:250–257.

88. Sankar M, Tanaka K, Kumaravel TS, Arif M, Shintani T, Yagi S, Kyo T, Dohy H, Kamada N. Identification of a commonly deleted region at 17p13.3 in leukemia and lymphoma associated with 17p abnormality. Leukemia 1998; 12:510–516.

89. Rowley JD. Molecular genetics in acute leukemia. Leukemia 2000; 14:513–517.

90. Bain BJ, Moorman AV, Johansson B, Mehta AB, Secker-Walker LM. Myelodysplastic syndromes associated with 11q23 abnormalities. European 11q23 Workshop participants. Leukemia 1998; 12:834–839.

91. Secker-Walker LM, Moorman AV, Bain BJ, Mehta AB. Secondary acute leukemia and myelodysplastic syndrome with 11q23 abnormalities. EU Concerted Action 11q23 Workshop. Leukemia 1998; 12:840–844.

92. Le Beau MM, Albain KS, Larson RA, Vardiman JW, Davis EM, Blough RR, Golomb HM, Rowley JD. Clinical and cytogenetic correlations in 63 patients with therapy-related myelodysplastic syndromes and acute nonlymphocytic leukemia: further evidence for characteristic abnormalities of chromosomes no. 5 and 7. J Clin Oncol 1986; 4:325–345.

93. Cortes J, O'Brien S, Kantarjian H, Cork A, Stass S, Freireich EJ, Keating M, Pierce S, Estey E. Abnormalities in the long arm of chromosome 11 (11q) in patients with de novo and secondary acute myelogenous leukemias and myelodysplastic syndromes. Leukemia 1994; 8:2174–2178.

94. Super HJ, McCabe NR, Thirman MJ, Larson RA, Le Beau MM, Pedersen-Bjergaard J, Philip P, Diaz MO, Rowley JD. Rearrangements of the MLL gene in therapy-related acute myeloid leukemia in patients previously treated with agents targeting DNA–topoisomerase II. Blood 1993; 82:3705–3711.

95. Look AT. Oncogenic transcription factors in the human acute leukemias (review). Science 1997; 278:1059–1064.

96. Golub TR, Barker GF, Lovett M, Gilliland DG. Fusion of PDGF receptor beta to a novel ets-like gene, tel, in chronic myelomonocytic leukemia with t(5;12) chromosomal translocation. Cell 1994; 77:307–316.

97. Rubin CM, Larson RA, Bitter MA, Carrino JJ, Le Beau MM, Diaz MO, Rowley JD. Association of a chromosomal 3;21 translocation with the blast phase of chronic myelogenous leukemia. Blood 1987; 70:1338–1342.

98. Rubin CM, Larson RA, Anastasi J, Winter JN, Thangavelu M, Vardiman JW, Rowley JD, Le Beau MM. t(3;21)(q26;q22): a recurring chromosomal abnormality in therapy-related myelodysplastic syndrome and acute myeloid leukemia. Blood 1990; 76:2594–2598.

99. Nucifora G, Begy CR, Kobayashi H, Roulston D, Claxton D, Pedersen-Bjergaard J, Parganas E, Ihle JN, Rowley JD. Consistent intergenic splicing and production of multiple transcripts between AML1 at 21q22 and unrelated genes at 3q26 in (3; 21)(q26;q22) translocations. Proc Natl Acad Sci USA 1994; 91:4004–4008.

100. Sitailo S, Sood R, Barton K, Nucifora G. Forced expression of the leukemia-associ-

ated gene EVI1 in ES cells: a model for myeloid leukemia with 3q26 rearrangements. Leukemia 1999; 13:1639–1645.

101. Sood R, Talwar-Trikha A, Chakrabarti SR, Nucifora G. MDS1/EVI1 enhances TGF-beta 1 signaling and strengthens its growth-inhibitory effect but the leukemia-associated fusion protein AML1/MDS1/EVI1, product of the t(3;21), abrogates growth-inhibition in response to TGF-beta1. Leukemia 1999; 13:348–357.

102. Rowley JD, Reshmi S, Sobulo O, Musvee T, Anastasi J, Raimondi S, Schneider NR, Barredo JC, Cantu ES, Schlegelberger B, Behm F, Doggett NA, Borrow J, Zeleznik-Le N. All patients with the T(11;16)(q23;p13.3) that involves MLL and CBP have treatment-related hematologic disorders. Blood 1997; 90:535–541.

103. Lepelley P, Soenen V, Preudhomme C, Merlat A, Cosson A, Fenaux P. bcl-2 expression in myelodysplastic syndromes and its correlation with hematological features, p53 mutations and prognosis. Leukemia 1995; 9:726–730.

104. Ridge SA, Worwood M, Oscier D, Jacobs A, Padua RA. FMS mutations in myelodysplastic, leukemic, and normal subjects. Proc Natl Acad Sci USA 1990; 87:1377–1380.

105. Kiyoi H, Towatari M, Yokota S, Hamaguchi M, Ohno R, Saito H, Naoe T. Internal tandem duplication of the FLT3 gene is a novel modality of elongation mutation which causes constitutive activation of the product. Leukemia 1998; 12:1333–1337.

106. Horiike S, Yokota S, Nakao M, Iwai T, Sasai Y, Kaneko H, Taniwaki M, Kashima K, Fujii H, Abe T, Misawa S. Tandem duplications of the FLT3 receptor gene are associated with leukemic transformation of myelodysplasia. Leukemia 1997; 11: 1442–1446.

107. Arland M, Fiedler W, Samalecos A, Hossfeld DK. Absence of point mutations in a functionally important part of the extracellular domain of the c-kit proto-oncogene in a series of patients with acute myeloid leukemia (AML). Leukemia 1994; 8: 498–501.

108. Siitonen T, Savolainen ER, Koistinen P. Expression of the c-kit proto-oncogene in myeloproliferative disorders and myelodysplastic syndromes. Leukemia 1994; 8: 631–637.

109. Zochbauer S, Gsur A, Gotzl M, Wallner J, Lechner K, Pirker R. MDR1 gene expression in myelodysplastic syndrome and in acute myeloid leukemia evolving from myelodysplastic syndrome. Anticancer Res 1994; 14:1293–1295.

110. Bueso-Ramos CE, Manshouri T, Haidar MA, Huh YO, Keating MJ, Albitar M. Multiple patterns of MDM-2 deregulation in human leukemias: implications in leukemogenesis and prognosis (review). Leuk Lymphoma 1995; 17:13–18.

111. Faderl S, Kantarjian HM, Estey E, Manshouri T, Chan CY, Rahman Elsaied A, Komblau SM, Cortes J, Thomas DA, Pierce S, Keating MJ, Estrov Z, Albitar M. The prognostic significance of p16(INK4a)/p14(ARF) locus deletion and MDM-2 protein expression in adult acute myelogenous leukemia. Cancer 2000; 89:1976–1982.

112. Ogata K, Tamura H. Thrombopoietin and myelodysplastic syndromes (review). Int J Hematol 2000; 72:173–177.

113. Bouscary D, Preudhomme C, Ribrag V, Melle J, Viguie F, Picard F, Guesnu M,

Fenaux P, Gisselbrecht S, Dreyfus F. Prognostic value of c-mpl expression in myelodysplastic syndromes. Leukemia 1995; 9:783–788.

114. Tidow N, Kasper B, Welte K. Clinical implications of G-CSF receptor mutations. Crit Rev Oncol Hematol 1998; 28:1–6.

115. Shannon KM, O'Connell P, Martin GA, Paderanga D, Olson K, Dinndorf P, McCormick F. Loss of the normal NF1 allele from the bone marrow of children with type 1 neurofibromatosis and malignant myeloid disorders. N Engl J Med 1994; 330:597–601.

116. Gallagher A, Darley RL, Padua R. The molecular basis of myelodysplastic syndromes (review). Haematologica 1997; 82:191–204.

117. Padua RA, West RR. Oncogene mutation and prognosis in the myelodysplastic syndromes. Br J Haematol 2000; 111:873–874.

118. Counter CM, Gupta J, Harley CB, Leber B, Bacchetti S. Telomerase activity in normal leukocytes and in hematologic malignancies. Blood 1995; 85:2315–2320.

119. Norrback KF, Roos G. Telomeres and telomerase in normal and malignant haematopoietic cells (review). Eur J Cancer 1997; 33:774–780.

120. Xu D, Gruber A, Peterson C, Pisa P. Telomerase activity and the expression of telomerase components in acute myelogenous leukaemia. Br J Haematol 1998; 102: 1367–1375.

121. Li B, Yang J, Andrews C, Chen YX, Toofanfard P, Huang RW, Horvath E, Chopra H, Raza A, Preisler HD. Telomerase activity in preleukemia and acute myelogenous leukemia. Leuk Lymphoma 2000; 36:579–587.

122. Misawa S, Horiike S. TP53 mutations in myelodysplastic syndrome (review). Leuk Lymphoma 1996; 23:417–422.

# 6
# Hypocellular Myelodysplastic Syndromes and Hypocellular Acute Myeloid Leukemia: Relationship to Aplastic Anemia

**Masao Tomonaga and Kazuhiro Nagai**
*Nagasaki University School of Medicine, Nagasaki, Japan*

## I. INTRODUCTION

Myelodysplastic syndromes (MDS) (1) and acute myeloid leukemia (AML) (2) usually manifest in cellular bone marrow as a proliferation of abnormal clones. The clones of MDS, although abnormal, are capable of differentiation whereas the AML clones are characterized by an increased amount of blast cells* owing to maturation arrest. Rather than a proliferation of clones, abnormal clones in hypocellular or hypoplastic bone marrow has been reported in about 8–20% of MDS cases (4–8) and 7.7–15% of AML cases (9–14). MDS cases with hypocellular bone marrow (hypo-MDS) can be difficult to distinguish from aplastic anemia (AA) whereas AML cases with hypocellular bone marrow (hypo-AML) can be difficult to distinguish from refractory anemia with excess blasts (RAEB). Whether these minor subgroups of MDS or AML cases are distinct clinical entities has been a matter of long debate.

In this chapter we describe clinical and hematological features of these ill-defined categories of clonal hemopathies. In addition, we discuss the status of hypo-MDS and hypo-AML as clinical entities and in relation to AA.

---

* A criterion of >30% blasts, according to the French-American-British classification system, indicates a diagnosis of AML but the criterion has recently changed to ≥20% with publication of the World Health Organization's (WHO) classification system (1,3).

**121**

## II. METHODS TO EVALUATE BONE MARROW CELLULARITY

### A. Histological Evaluation

In clinical diagnostic settings, histological sections of bone marrow biopsy specimens from an iliac crest or clot specimens of aspirated bone marrow are usually used to evaluate the cellularity of a given case. Clot sections can be obtained only when bone marrow is easily aspirated either from the sternum or from the posterior iliac crest.

The ratio of hematopoietic tissue to fat tissue has been used to evaluate bone marrow cellularity, usually by point-counting technique. Some investigators use a criterion of 40% as the lower limit of normocellular bone marrow and others use a criterion of 30%. As stated clearly by Hartsock et al. (15), bone marrow cellularity declines with aging, especially after age 70. So while it is necessary to take into account an age factor in evaluating bone marrow cellularity, the lack of a standardized age-correcting formula makes it difficult for clinicians to have a correct diagnosis of hypocellularity. To improve the assessment of cellularity, Tuzuner and Bennett provided simple reference standards by preparing and publishing 11 histological photographs that demonstrate 1–100% cellular marrow (16).

By using many histological samples of clonal disorders, Tuzuner et al. showed that certain proportions of MDS and AML cases have hypocellular bone marrow whereas there are no such hypocellular cases in myeloproliferative disorders (MPD), including chronic myeloid leukemia (17). Interestingly, they observed that the AML cases with hypocellular bone marrow were mostly those of elderly patients whereas hypocellular MDS cases were observed in all age groups.

### B. Cytological Evaluation

Bone marrow aspirate smears stained with May-Grunwald Giemsa (MGG) are also used by experienced hematologists for routine evaluation of cellularity. However, an excessive tap dilutes the aspirates with peripheral blood, producing erroneous interpretation of hypocellularity. In some hospitals hematologists prefer particle smears to aspirate smears. In addition, bone marrow fibrosis, which occurs with some frequency in MDS and AML, also limits the reliability of aspirate smears for evaluation of cellularity.

### C. Magnetic Resonance Imaging

Magnetic resonance imaging (MRI) is the most powerful radiological method for visualizing the systemic distribution of hematopoietic tissues in flat bones, especially the vertebrae. Visualization of bone marrow cellularity depends on the absorption difference, a function of the water content, between the fatty tissue and hematopoietic tissue. Short inversion-time inversion-recovery (STIR) is a particularly effective pulse sequence for visualizing bone marrow.

Kusumoto et al. proposed a system for classifying into four types the STIR images of vertebral bone marrow in patients with MDS or AA (18). Type I is characterized by a diffuse, low-signal intensity and is most representative of hypocellular bone marrow (Fig. 1A). Type II represents normal bone marrow and is characterized by a marginally high signal intensity (Fig. 1B). Type III has an inhomogeneous signal intensity that results from a mixture of cellular and fatty tissues and is most frequently seen in MDS, especially refractory anemia (RA), and less frequently observed in AA (Fig. 1C). Type IV is characterized by a diffuse, high-signal intensity and is most compatible with a diagnosis of hypercellular acute leukemia or MPD, including chronic myelomonocytic leukemia (Fig. 1D).

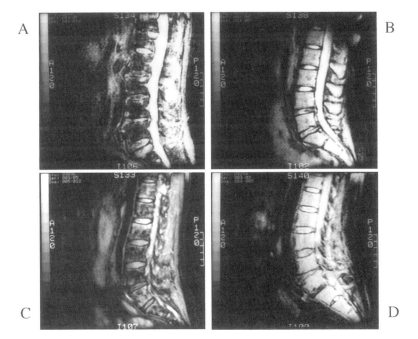

**Fig. 1** Four MRI-STIR signal intensity patterns classified according to Kusumoto et al. [18]: Type I; diffuse low-intensity signal representative of hypocellular bone marrow (A). Type II; marginally high intensity representative of normocellular bone marrow (B). Type III; inhomogeneous signal intensity suggestive of uneven distribution of cellular bone marrow (C). Type IV; diffuse high-signal intensity representative of hypercellular bone marrow (D).

**Table 1**  A Combined Histology/MRI Study of the Response of Myelodysplastic Syndromes and Aplastic Anemia to Immunosuppressive Therapy

| Case no. | Age | Sex | Diagnosis | BM cellularity | | Karyotype | Response | | |
|---|---|---|---|---|---|---|---|---|---|
| | | | | Histology | MRI | | Hb | Neutrophil | Platelet |
| 1 | 58 | M | AA | Hypo | Hypo (I) | Normal | NR | NR | NR |
| 2 | 54 | M | AA | Hypo | Hypo (I) | Normal | GR | GR | PR |
| 3 | 59 | F | AA | Hypo | Hypo (I) | Normal | GR | GR | GR |
| 4 | 65 | F | AA | Hypo | Hypo (I) | Normal | NR | NR | NR |
| 5 | 16 | F | AA | Hypo | NA | Normal | GR | GR[a] | MR |
| 6 | 59 | F | AA | Hypo | Hypo (I) | Normal | GR | GR[a] | MR |
| 7 | 52 | F | AA | Hypo | NA | Normal | GR | GR[a] | GR |
| 8 | 65 | F | AA | Hypo | Hypo (I) | Normal | GR | PR | GR |
| 9 | 70 | M | AA | Hypo | Hypo (I) | Normal | GR | GR[a] | GR |
| 10 | 58 | M | AA | Hypo | NA | Normal | GR | GR | GR |
| 11 | 61 | F | AA | Hypo | Normo (II) | Normal | GR | GR | GR |
| 12 | 73 | F | AA | Hypo | Hypo (I) | Normal | GR | GR[a] | PR |
| 13 | 15 | M | AA | Hypo | Hypo (I) | Normal | GR | GR[a] | MR |
| 14 | 58 | F | AA | Hypo | Hypo (I) | NA | GR | GR | PR |
| 15 | 54 | F | AA | Hypo | Hypo (I) | Normal | GR | GR | PR |
| 16 | 63 | F | MDS | Normo | Hyper (IV) | Normal | NR | NR | NR |

| No. | Age | Sex | Type | Cellularity | MRI (type) | Karyotype | | | |
|---|---|---|---|---|---|---|---|---|---|
| 17 | 53 | F | MDS | Hyper | Normo (II) | 48XX, +8, +9 (12/20) | NR | NR | NR |
| 18 | 18 | F | MDS | Hypo | Hyper (IV) | Normal | NR | NR | NR |
| 19 | 65 | F | MDS | Hypo | Inhomogeneous (III) | 45XX, −7 (7/20) | NR | NR | NR |
| 20 | 58 | M | MDS | Normo | Inhomogeneous (III) | Normal | GR | NE | NR |
| 21 | 50 | F | MDS | Hyper | NA | Normal | GR | MR | MR |
| 22 | 69 | M | MDS | Hyper | Hyper (IV) | Normal | NR | NE | NR |
| 23 | 48 | F | MDS | Hyper | Hyper (IV) | Normal | GR | NR | MR |
| 24 | 57 | M | MDS | NA | Inhomogeneous (III) | Normal | GR | NR | MR |
| 25 | 64 | F | MDS | Normo | Normo (II) | 46XX, add(3) (q21) (4/20) | PR | MR | MR |
| 26 | 68 | M | MDS | Normo | NA | Normal | GR | MR | PR |
| 27 | 64 | M | HMDS | Hypo | Hypo (I) | Normal | GR | GR[a] | PR |
| 28 | 65 | F | HMDS | Hypo | NA | Normal | GR | NR | MR |
| 29 | 58 | M | HMDS | Hypo | Hypo (I) | Normal | GR | GR | PR |
| 30 | 41 | M | HMDS | Hypo | Hypo (I) | Normal | GR | MR | GR |
| 31 | 17 | F | HMDS | Hypo | Hypo (I) | Normal | GR | GR | GR |
| 32 | 59 | M | HMDS | Hypo | Inhomogeneous (III) | 46XY, t(12;15) (q23;q12) (3/19) | GR | GR | PR |
| 33 | 60 | M | HMDS | Hypo | Inhomogeneous (III) | 47XY, +8 (13/20) | NR | NR | NR |

[a] While all MDS cases were treated with CSA and all AA cases were treated with CSA and ATG, these cases were concomitantly treated with G-CSF.
AA, aplastic anemia; MDS, myelodysplastic syndrome; HMDS, hypoplastic MDS; BM, bone marrow; No., number; I. II, III, IV, type according to MRI analysis; MRI, magnetic resonance imaging; M. male; F, female; Hb, hemoglobin; GR, good response; PR, partial response; MR, minimal response; NR, no response; NE, not evaluable; N.A, not available; CSA, cyclosporine A; ATG, antithymocyte globulin; G-CSF, granulocyte colony-stimulating factor.

We analyzed MDS and AA cases by comparing biopsy-proven histological classification with classification according to the MRI-STIR images. Histological classification was based on biopsies at two sites, one from the sternum as a clot section biopsy and the other from the iliac crest as a needle biopsy. Histological diagnosis of less than 40% cellularity in at least one of the biopsies was required to classify the case as hypocellular. As shown in Table 1, Type I, Type II, and Type IV correlated with the histologically determined hypocellularity, normocellularity, and hypercellularity, respectively. However, Type III classifications were somewhat inconsistent in histological pattern; most Type III cases showed hypocellular bone marrow in at least one biopsy site and one MDS case (No. 20) showed normocellular bone marrow at two sites. These results may indicate genuine inhomogeneous distributions of hematopoietic tissue in Type III cases. Therefore, histological diagnosis in single-site biopsy does not necessarily reflect the bone marrow cellularity as a whole. A similar inhomogeneous finding in MRI with discrepant histology (hypocellularity) has been reported in a single MDS case (19). Lorand-Metze et al. also pointed out that scattered or uniform patterns of MRI in femoral bone marrow are signs of more aggressive disease (20).

## III.  DEFINITION OF HYPOCELLULAR BONE MARROW

From the results of MRI analysis, it is likely that a single-site biopsy is not sufficient to assess systemic distribution of hematopoietic tissue since many MDS cases with RA actually show a Type III inhomogeneous pattern. This discrepancy gives the hematologists considerable difficulty in identifying hypocellular bone marrow in routine clinical practice. It might be possible to overcome this difficulty if clinicians could obtain a more precise sum of hematopoietic tissue based on MRI figures; for example, such a method might provide a basis for further subdividing Type III pattern into hypocellular type and normo- or hypercellular type. This approach is currently not feasible owing to the lack of such summation technology.

Biopsy at two sites of bone marrow is currently the best approach for identifying hypocellular marrow. If two sites equally show, for example, less than 40% cellular marrow, systemic hypocellular bone marrow may be indicated. If two sites split into hypocellular and normo- or hypercellular marrows, the whole marrow may be inhomogeneous with a tendency toward being hypocellular. In this context, single-site biopsy does not necessarily represent whole marrow status and may lead to underestimations of the frequency of hypocellular cases.

In defining the lower limit of histologically determined normocellularity, the age factor is important, as already mentioned. A level of 40% may be reasonable in the age range from adolescence through the sixties, but 30% or even 20%

may be better for ages above seventy. Tuzuner et al. tried to adjust for this age factor in their analysis of hypocellular MDS cases but they had limited success (6).

Because the age effect is not clearly established, we have arbitrarily employed 40% as the lower limit of normocellular bone marrow irrespective of patient's age. This decision was based upon the earlier observation that among clonal hemopathies, only cases with MDS and AML had shown hypocellular bone marrow while MPD cases never did, even for patients over 70 years of age. Thus, the 40% criterion adequately defines cases useful for the comparison of hypercellular MDS/AML (the majority of the cases) with the less common hypocellular MDS/AML.

## IV. HYPOCELLULAR MYELODYSPLASTIC SYNDROMES: A CLINICAL ENTITY?

### A. Clinical and Hematological Features of Hypo-MDS

Single-site biopsy and a 30% or 40% criterion for diagnosing hypo-MDS have been the procedures used for most studies, including those reported by Tuzuner et al. In these studies, about 20% of the MDS cases could be interpreted as hypo-MDS (6,17). Although the sensitivity of the single-site histology is not as high as two-sites biopsy combined with MRI typing, the series analyzed by Tuzuner et al. is the largest ever reported and so provides some of the best data currently available (17).

For this series, various clinical and hematological parameters as well as patient survival were compared between hypo-MDS and normo- or hypercellular MDS. There were no differences in the degrees of cytopenias for the three cell lines, in cytogenetic abnormalities, in overall survival, and in the rate of leukemic transformation. These findings suggest that histological discrimination between hypo-MDS and normo- or hypercellular MDS does not necessarily mean basic difference in the pathophysiology of MDS. Similar results were reported in other studies (4,5). If true, the classical definition of MDS, being that the bone marrow is normo- or hypercellular despite peripheral blood bi-or pancytopenias and which together indicate ineffective hematopoiesis (1), would need to be changed; the revised definition would need to state that bone marrow of MDS patients exhibits a wide range of cellularity, from hypocellular to normo- or hypercellular.

Our preliminary study indicates the necessity of reevaluation of hypo-MDS cases by employing both histology and MRI to improve the accuracy of subclassification of bone marrow cellularity. Perhaps with improved subclassification, differences in the pathophysiology of hypo-MDS and normo/hypercellular MDS will become apparent.

## B. Immunosuppressive Therapy for MDS

Molldrem et al. showed for the first time a considerably high response rate (64%) to immunosuppressive therapy with antithymocyte globulin (ATG) for patients with RA (21). Molldrem et al. observed the response not only in cases of hypo-MDS but also in ordinary cases of MDS. In some responding cases, pretreatment profiles of T-cell receptor $V_\beta$ were clonal and changed to polyclonal after ATG treatment, suggesting an appearance of one or more cytotoxic T-cell clones against hematopoietic stem cells (22). Jonasova et al. also observed good response (14 out of 16 cases) to cyclosporine A (CSA) in RA patients regardless of bone marrow cellularity (23). As shown in Table 1, our clinical trial in which the response to immunosuppressive therapy by MDS patients was compared with that of AA patients also revealed that both hypo-MDS cases and normo- or hypercellular MDS cases responded. In this series, MDS cases were treated primarily with CSA while AA cases were treated with a combination of CSA and ATG; so while direct comparison is not appropriate, the overall response rate was as high as 60% in MDS cases and was slightly lower than in the AA cases (80%). (Grades of response in three cell lines were also inferior for MDS cases as compared with the AA cases.) Interestingly, these studies indicated that RA cases preferentially responded while only a few RAEB cases responded. More recently, Barrett et al. suggested that a significant difference in response rate to ATG seemed to occur for hypo-MDS (52%) as compared with ordinary MDS (28%) in their series of 61 cases (24).

There has been no report of combination immunosuppressive therapy utilizing both CSA and ATG for MDS patients. This is in contrast to AA cases, for which this combination is commonly used. Thus, it might be possible to obtain better results for MDS cases by using such a combination.

## C. Hypo-MDS Cases that Mimic Severe AA

In some cases of hypo-MDS, the hypocellularity is as marked as in cases with severe AA as judged from both histology and MRI survey. These cases must be carefully differentiated since hypo-MDS, like AA, often shows a good response to immunosuppressive treatment. In Figure 2, a typical case (No. 32 in Table 1) of hypo-MDS mimicking severe AA is illustrated; this case showed severe hypocellularity at two sites of bone marrow, Type III MRI pattern (inhomogeneous with much low-signal intensity) as shown in Figure 2A, apparent trilineage dysplasias in a small amount of residual myeloid cells including megakaryocytes, and a nonrandom chromosome translocation—t(12;15). Combined immunosuppressive treatment with CSA, methylprednisolone, and antilymphocyte globulin (ALG) resulted in good clinical response of the trilineage cytopenias. Interest-

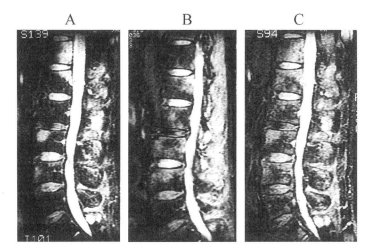

**Fig. 2** Changes of MRI-STIR (magnetic resonance imaging: short inversion-time inversion-recovery) pattern along with immunosuppressive therapy in a patient with hypocellular MDS (case No. 32 in Table 1); although the STIR pattern of each figure was classified into Type III (inhomogeneous pattern), signal intensity was apparently increased from low (A) before therapy, to intermediate (B), and high (C) after a good hematological response was obtained (Fig. 3).

ingly, the translocation disappeared after good response was obtained (25). The inhomogeneous pattern persisted but with an apparent increase in signal intensity as shown in Figures 2B and 2C. The remission, with a hemoglobin value around 15 g/dl, has been maintained for over 4 years with maintenance by CSA but the morphological dysplasia has also persisted. The clinical course in this case is illustrated in Figure 3.

Besides hypo-MDS mimicking AA, there have also been reported cases of severe AA that progressed to MDS after clinical response to immunosuppressive therapy (26). Often, these cases exhibited a coincidental appearance of nonrandom chromosome abnormalities such as monosomy 7. Thus, there are small populations of MDS cases and AA cases that can develop a clonal hemopathy under the condition of bone marrow hypocellularity.

## D. Why Do Many Cases of MDS Show an Inhomogeneous Distribution of Cellular Bone Marrow?

At present there is no reasonable explanation for the inhomogeneous distribution of cellular bone marrow that is observed in many cases of MDS. Our earlier

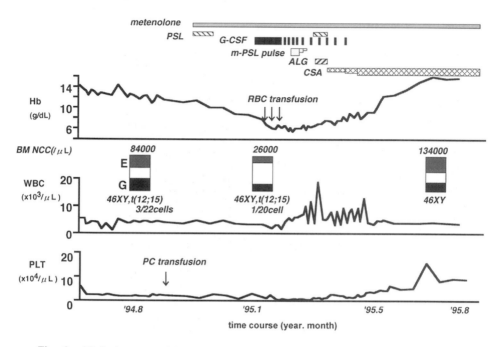

**Fig. 3** Clinical course of immunosuppressive therapy in a patient with hypocellular MDS carrying a chromosome abnormality (case No. 32 in Table 1). BM NCC, bone marrow nucleated cell count; PSL, prednisolone; m-PSL, methylprednisolone; G-CSF, granulocyte colony-stimulating factor; ALG, antithymocyte globulin; CSA, cyclosporine A; Hb, hemoglobin; RBC, red blood cells; E, erythrocytes; G, granulocytes; WBC, white blood cells; plt, platelets; PC, platelet concentrate.

study showed that the absolute number of CD34+ primitive progenitor cells in peripheral blood was markedly reduced in almost all cases of RA in addition to all cases of severe AA (27). In contrast, cases of RAEB and RAEB in transformation (RAEB-t) had markedly increased, usually by more than 100-fold, numbers of CD34+ cells and these cells were apparently larger in size (similar to blasts) than CD34+ cells from normal or RA patients. These observations may indicate a pathological state of MDS (especially RA) stem cells for migration into the peripheral blood and homing to the bone marrow; this assumes that migration and homing are required for maintenance of an even distribution of hematopoietic tissues in systemic bones. A similar finding of low numbers of primitive progenitor cells in the peripheral blood of MDS patients was reported by Sato et al. by using a modified long-term culture-initiating cell assay (28).

## V.  HYPOCELLULAR ACUTE MYELOID LEUKEMIA

### A.  Definition of Hypo-AML

Because of the technical difficulty in assessing bone marrow cellularity, we again used the criterion of less than 40% cellularity to distinguish hypo-AML from overt AML (13). Hypo-AML comprised about 15% of total AML cases at our institute and the age of these patients ranged from 45 to 82 years with a median age of 65 years. Because the median age is about 60 for whole cases of AML, these data indicate that hypo-AML is actually a subtype of elderly AML.

For hypocellular bone marrow, counting of blasts is difficult. In our series of 32 cases of hypo-AML, the blast percentage ranged from 20 to 70% (mean of 34%) of total mononuclear cells of the bone marrow. By excluding lymphocytes, which are relatively increased in percentage in hypocellular bone marrow, the blast percentage ranged from 38 to 94% (mean of 58%). Exclusion of erythroblasts in addition to lymphocytes increased the blast percentage further, to a mean of 78%. The actual blast percentage in hypo-AML is, then, almost the same as that of usual AML. Thus, the maturation arrest in myeloid differentiation is as complete in hypo-AML as in overt AML.

Hypo-AML is often confused with RAEB or RAEB-t because some cases of hypo-AML show morphological trilineage dysplasias in mature cells. These diseases can be distinguished, however, by maturation arrest, which is incomplete in RAEB/RAEB-t. Exclusion of lymphocytes and erythrocytes does not increase the blast percentage for cases of RAEB and RAEB-t due to abundant intermediate granulocytes and erythroblasts in the bone marrow.

In summary, hypo-AML can be diagnosed for cases with bone marrow cellularity at less than 40% and blast percentage at more than 30% of the bone marrow mononuclear cells when lymphocytes and erythroblasts are excluded.

### B.  Clinical Features of Hypo-AML

Our study (13) and others (9–12,14) have indicated that about 15% of AML cases show hypocellular bone marrow and that most of them are elderly cases. In addition, peripheral blood findings are characterized by a severe pancytopenia with an appearance of only a few blasts. For these cases, conventional intensive chemotherapy with multiple drugs can induce remission with some frequency but the remissions are not durable and are without long-term survivors (10). Our study also indicated that low-dose cytarabine therapy can induce a similar remission rate (about 60%) but again failed to prolong survival of hypo-AML cases owing to early relapse.

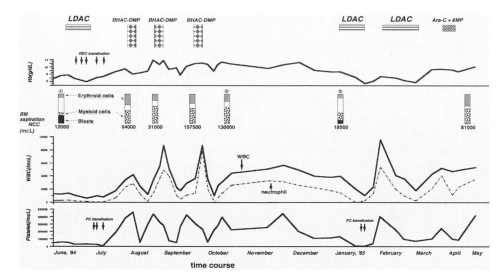

**Fig. 4** Clinical course of low-dose cytarabine therapy in a patient with hypocellular AML. BHAC, behenoyl cytosine arabinoside; LDAC, low-dose cytarabine; DMP, daunomycin + 6-mercaputopurine + prednisolone; Ara-C, cytosine arabinoside; 6MP, 6-mercaptopurine + prednisolone; RBC, red blood cells; Hb, hemoglobin; WBC, white blood cells; PC, platelet concentrate; NCC, nucleated cell count.

## C.  Relationship of Hypo-AML to RAEB and RAEB-t

We consider that hypo-AML is not equivalent to RAEB or RAEB-t. The latter MDS subtypes rarely present with hypocellular marrow and these cases are fairly resistant to low-dose cytarabine therapy, having a remission rate of less than 30%. In contrast, hypo-AML can be rather easily induced into remission, at a rate of 60%, with this type of chemotherapy. Furthermore, the remission state in hypo-AML is characterized by a return to normocellular bone marrow with full recovery of morphologically normal trilineage hematopoiesis and is characterized by the disappearance of cytogenetic abnormalities such as trisomy 8 (Fig. 4) (29). Interestingly, when these complete-remission patients relapse, hypocellular bone marrow again appears. In contrast, RAEB/RAEB-t patients who achieve remission with chemotherapy often return to a MDS(RA) state.

## D.  Pathophysiology of Hypo-AML

There may be some particular pathophysiology in hypo-AML that induces hypocellular leukemic hematopoiesis. One theory is that hypo-AML is associated with an immune mechanism similar to that of AA and MDS. Another theory is that blasts in hypo-AML are genuine leukemia blasts that, although in a low-prolifera- tive state, are able to induce full leukemic suppression of normal stem cells (he- matopoiesis). We prefer the latter hypothesis because, if the blast count is reduced to <5%, treatment of hypo-AML with low-dose cytarabine (which suppresses DNA synthesis but not the immune system) can render full recovery of normal hematopoiesis (30,31).

Hypo-AML cases have blasts with immature myeloid features, such as low or negative myeloperoxidase, but also have CD13+ or CD33+ blasts like those in AML-M0 (minimally differentiated AML) (5).

A rare case of acute lymphocytic leukemia (ALL) showed hypocellular bone marrow. The hypocellularity was most apparent in the early phase of ALL development (32).

Thus, hypo-AML seems to be a clinical subtype of AML of the elderly and shows primitive myeloid phenotypes and primary resistance to conventional antileukemia agents. For elderly patients with hypo-AML, treatments of novel modality, such as nonmyeloablative hematopoietic stem cell transplantation (minitransplant), should be used.

## VI. RELATIONSHIP BETWEEN HYPO-MDS, HYPO-AML, AND AA

### A. Leukemic Change in AA and MDS

AA and MDS are both hematopoietic disorders with preleukemic features, al- though the incidence of leukemic evolution is much lower in AA. We have not observed cases with AA or MDS that have progressed to hypo-AML; rather, AA and MDS transform into overt AML, often through RAEB/RAEB-t with normo- or hypercellular bone marrow. This observation suggests that hypo-AML, al- though sometimes difficult to distinguish from RAEB/RAEB-t, has different pathophysiology from AA and MDS.

### B. AA Cases that Progress to MDS

The similarities of AA to hypo-MDS or overt MDS apply not only to adult cases but also to pediatric cases, although most children with AA evolving to MDS develop a monosomy 7 clone (33–36). Whether this transformation has been enhanced by immunosuppressive therapy and/or administration of granulocyte colony-stimulating factor (G-CSF) has long been a matter of debate. This issue is currently being investigated through prospective randomized controlled trials (37).

Other studies are needed to clarify whether ordinary MDS and AA that progresses to MDS are, in fact, the same disease that presents with different phenotypes. In addition to these studies, sensitive techniques such as two-probe FISH (fluorescence in situ hybridization) for detection of a minimal population of an abnormal clone (such as a monosomy 7 clone in the severe AA stage) would improve such clinical trials.

## C.  Immune-Mediated Pathology in AA and MDS

Although AA has been known as a heterogeneous disease complex, recent studies revealed that around 80% of cases respond to immunosuppressive therapy (26,38). Even cases with posthepatitis AA responded, although some of these cases developed monosomy 7–positive MDS (35). Thus, AA seems to include a minor proportion of cases that have predisposition toward MDS/AML; in other words, AA stem cells may have some genetic abnormality responsible for the transformation to MDS/AML. The relationship between immune suppression in AA stem cells and such putative genetic predisposition toward MDS/AML must be intensively studied in the near future.

Our experience with immunosuppressive therapy for MDS cases has indicated that both hypo-MDS and overt MDS cases respond, although Barrett et al. suggested that there might have been a difference in sensitivity to ATG between the two groups (24). Our results and also those of Molldrem et al. (21) indicated that the response rate (less than 60%) and response degree among MDS (particularly RA) cases were apparently inferior to the response rate of 80% and good trilineage response in severe AA cases. These differences suggest further heterogeneity in immune pathology between AA and MDS.

The appearance of cytogenetic abnormalities is not a hallmark of MDS. Geary et al. reported 13 cases of AA with cytogenetic abnormalities; most of the abnormalities were similar to those observed in MDS (39). Interestingly, these AA patients showed a high response rate (eight out of 13) to ATG/CSA therapy and, in four cases, the cytogenetic abnormalities disappeared after a good response was obtained. None of these 13 cases developed to MDS/AML during the follow-up time of 4.1 years. This observation suggests that AA cases include a minor group of patients with an apparent cytogenetic abnormality but lacking morphological dysplasias. Currently, there is no reasonable explanation for the relation between the chromosome abnormalities in AA and those in MDS.

## VII.  SUMMARY

Irrespective of clonal and nonclonal disorders, bone marrow hypocellularity is an interesting pathology, yet difficult to evaluate correctly owing to whole-body distribution of hematopoiesis. While hypo-AML has distinct features, characteristics of AA and MDS overlap with each other. In some cases with apparent MDS clones, bone marrow shows marked hypocellularity equivalent to that in severe AA. There might be varied pathophysiology in MDS and AA stem cells as yet to be elucidated; immune-mediated growth suppression (even in normo- or hypercellular cases) and preleukemic gene abnormalities are two major aspects.

Further development of techniques for quantifying bone marrow cellularity are necessary to provide for better understanding of hypo-MDS. Specifically, Type III MRI pattern must be further evaluated in terms of pathological distribution of MDS hematopoiesis and stem cell function. In addition, molecular techniques that allow analysis of CD34+ stem cells are essential to understanding the similarities and dissimilarities of the pathophysiology of AA and MDS. In this respect, it is interesting that Elghetany et al. reported significantly elevated p53 expression in MDS (RA) bone marrow cells regardless of cellularity, but not in AA (40).

Although hypo-AML is sometimes difficult to distinguish from hypo-MDS (particularly RAEB/RAEB-t) because of low blast count, the hypocellular marrow of AML seems to be induced by a particular feature of genuine leukemia blasts. These blasts are characterized by slow growth but induce full suppression of normal hematopoiesis. The leukemia burden is apparently small in hypo-AML and this subtype, which is prevalent in the elderly, is one of the most refractory subtypes of AML.

Molecular analysis employing new techniques such as DNA microarray will allow researchers to elucidate the specific nature of the blasts of hypo-AML and to compare the nature of these blasts with those of ordinary AML and RAEB/RAEB-t. These new developments will bring about a novel therapeutic approach to each disease entity with hypocellular bone marrow.

## REFERENCES

1. Bennett JM, Catovsky D, Daniel MT, Flandrin G, Galton DA, Gralnick HR, Sultan C. Proposals for the classification of the myelodysplastic syndromes. Br J Haematol 1982; 51:189–199.
2. Bennett JM, Catovsky D, Daniel MT, Flandrin G, Galton DA, Gralnick HR, Sultan C. Proposals for the classification of the acute leukaemias. French-American-British (FAB) co-operative group. Br J Haematol 1976; 33:451–458.
3. Harris NL, Jaffe ES, Diebold J, Flandrin G, Muller-Hermelink HK, Vardiman J, Lister TA, Bloomfield CD. World Health Organization classification of neoplastic diseases of the hematopoietic and lymphoid tissues. Report of the Clinical Advisory Committee meeting—Airlie House, Virginia, November 1997. J Clin Oncol 1999; 17:3835–3849.
4. Yoshida Y, Oguma S, Uchino H, Maekawa T. Refractory myelodysplastic anaemias with hypocellular bone marrow. J Clin Pathol 1988; 41:763–767.
5. Toyama K, Ohyashiki K, Yoshida Y, Abe T, Asano S, Hirai H, Hirashima K, Hotta

T, Kuramoto A, Kuriya S, Miyazaki T, Kakishita E, Mizoguchi H, Mori M, Shirakawa S, Takaku F, Tomonaga M, Uchino H, Urabe A, Yasunaga K, Nomura T. Clinical and cytogenetic findings of myelodysplastic syndromes showing hypocellular bone marrow or minimal dysplasia, in comparison with typical myelodysplastic syndromes. Int J Hematol 1993; 58:53–61.

6. Tuzuner N, Cox C, Rowe JM, Watrous D, Bennett JM. Hypocelluler myelodysplastic syndromes (MDS): new proposals. Br J Haematol 1995; 91:612–617.

7. Elghetany MT, Hudnall SD, Gardner FH. Peripheral blood picture in primary hypocellular refractory anemia and idiopathic acquired aplastic anemia: an additional tool for differential diagnosis (review). Haematologica 1997; 82:21–24.

8. Goyal R, Qawi H, Ali I, Dar S, Mundle S, Shetty V, Mativi Y, Allampallam K, Lisak L, Loew J, Venugopal P, Gezer S, Robin E, Rifkin S, Raza A. Biologic characteristics of patients with hypocellular myelodysplastic syndromes. Leuk Res 1999; 23:357–364.

9. Beard MEJ; Bateman CJT, Crowther DC, Wrigley PFM, Whitehouse JMA, Fairley GH, Scott RB. Hypoplastic acute myelogenous leukaemia. Br J Haematol 1975; 31: 167–176.

10. Howe RB, Bloomfield CD, McKenna RW. Hypocellular acute leukemia. Am J Med 1982; 72:391–395.

11. Needleman SW, Burns CP, Dick FR, Armitage JO. Hypoplastic acute leukemia. Cancer 1981; 48:1410–1414.

12. Gladson CL, Naeim F. Hypocellular bone marrow with increased blasts. Am J Hematol 1986; 21:15–22.

13. Nagai K, Kohno T, Chen YX, Tsushima H, Mori H, Nakamura H, Jinnai I, Matsuo T, Kuriyama K, Tomonaga M, Bennett JM. Diagnostic criteria for hypocellular acute leukemia: a clinical entity distinct from overt acute leukemia and myelodysplastic syndrome. Leuk Res 1996; 20:563–574.

14. Tuzuner N, Cox C, Rowe JM, Bennett JM. Hypocellular acute myeloid leukemia: the Rochester (New York) experience. Hematol Pathol 1995; 9:195–203.

15. Hartsock RJ, Smith EB, Petty CS. Normal variations with aging of the amount of hematopoietic tissue in bone marrow from the anterior iliac crest. Am J Clin Pathol 1965; 43:326–331.

16. Tuzuner N, Bennett JM. Reference standards for bone marrow cellularity. Leuk Res 1994; 18:645–647.

17. Tuzuner N, Cox C, Rowe JM, Bennett JM. Bone marrow cellularity in myeloid stem cell disorders: impact of age correction. Leuk Res 1994; 18:559–564.

18. Kusumoto S, Jinnai I, Matsuda A, Murohashi I, Bessho M, Saito M, Hirashima K, Heshiki A, Minamihisamatsu M. Bone marrow patterns in patients with aplastic anaemia and myelodysplastic syndrome: observations with magnetic resonance imaging. Eur J Haematol 1997; 59:155–161.

19. Schick F, Weiss B, Einsele H. Magnetic resonance imaging reveals a markedly inhomogeneous distribution of marrow cellularity in a patient with myelodysplasia. Ann Hematol 1995; 71:143–146.

20. Lorand-Metze I, Santiago GF, Lima CS, Zanardi VA, Torriani M. Magnetic resonance imaging of femoral marrow cellularity in hypocellular haemopoietic disorders. Clin Radiol 2001; 56:107–110.

21. Molldrem JJ, Caples M, Mavroudis D, Plante M, Young NS, Barrett AJ. Antithymocyte globulin for patients with myelodysplastic syndrome. Br J Haematol 1997; 99: 699–705.

22. Molldrem JJ, Jiang YZ, Stetler-Stevenson M, Mavroudis D, Hensel N, Barrett AJ. Haematological response of patients with myelodysplastic syndrome to antithymocyte globulin is associated with a loss of lymphocyte-mediated inhibition of CFU-GM and alterations in T-cell receptor Vbeta profiles. Br J Haematol 1998; 102: 1314–1322.

23. Jonasova A, Neuwirtova R, Cermak J, Vozobulova V, Mocikova K, Siskoua M, Hochova I. Cyclosporin A therapy in hypoplastic MDS patients and certain refractory anaemias without hypoplastic bone marrow. Br J Haematol 1998; 100:304–309.

24. Barrett J, Sauntharararajah Y, Molldrem J. Myelodysplastic syndrome and aplastic anemia: distinct entities or diseases linked by a common pathophysiology? (review). Semin Hematol 2000; 37:15–29.

25. Iwanaga M, Sadamori N, Amenomori T, Kawaguchi Y, Nakamura H, Matsuo T, Kuriyama K, Tomonaga M. A new translocation (4;12)(q21;q15) after combined immunosuppressive therapy in a case of hypoplastic myelodysplastic syndrome with translocation (12; 15)(q23; q12). Cancer Genet Cytogenet 1998; 107:82–84.

26. Socie G, Henry-Amar M, Bacigalupo A, Hows J, Tichelli A, Ljungman P, McCann SR, Frickhofen N, Van't Veer-Korthof E, Gluckman E. Malignant tumors occurring after treatment of aplastic anemia. European Bone Marrow Transplantation-Severe Aplastic Anaemia Working Party. N Engl J Med 1993; 329:1152–1157.

27. Fuchigami K, Mori H, Matsuo T, Iwanaga M, Nagai K, Kuriyama K, Tomonaga M. Absolute number of circulating CD34+ cells is abnormally low in refractory anemias and extremely high in RAEB and RAEB-t; novel pathologic features of myelodysplastic syndromes identified by highly sensitive flow cytometry. Leuk Res 2000; 24:163–174.

28. Sato T, Kim S, Selleri C, Young NS, Maciejewski JP. Measurement of secondary colony formation after 5 weeks in long-term cultures in patients with myelodysplastic syndrome. Leukemia 1999; 12:1187–1194.

29. Tagawa M, Shibata J, Tomonaga M, Amenomori T, Yoshida Y, Kuriyama K, Matsuo T, Sadamori N, Ichimaru M. Low-dose cytosine arabinoside regimen induced a complete remission with normal karyotypes in a case with hypoplastic acute myeloid leukaemia with No. 8-trisomy: in vitro and in vivo evidence for normal haematopoietic recovery. Br J Haematol 1985; 60:449–455.

30. Kohno T, Nagai K, Tsukasaki K, Jinnai I, Tomonaga M, Ichimaru M, Tagawa M. [Effects of low dose Ara-C regimen in acute leukemias and RAEB.] Rinsho Ketsueki 1989; 30:638–643 [Japanese].

31. Kanamori H, Maruta A, Miyashita H, Harano H, Fukawa H, Matsuzaki M, Motomura S, Mohri H, Kodama F, Okubo T. Low-dose cytosine arabinoside for treating hypocellular acute leukemia in the elderly. Am J Hematol 1992; 39:52–55.

32. Suzan F, Terre C, Garcia I, Bastie JN, Baumelou E, Gluckman E, Castaigne S. Three cases of typical aplastic anaemia associated with a Philadelphia chromosome. Br J Haematol 2001; 112:385–387.

33. Kojima S, Tsuchida M, Matsuyama T. Myelodysplasia and leukemia after treatment of aplastic anemia with G-CSF. N Engl J Med 1992; 326:1294–1295.

34.  Kojima S, Hibi S, Kosaka Y, Yamamoto M, Tsuchida M, Mugishima H, Sugita K, Yabe H, Ohara A, Tsukimoto I. Immunosuppressive therapy using antithymocyte globulin, cyclosporine, and danazol with or without human granulocyte colony-stimulating factor in children with acquired aplastic anemia. Blood 2000; 96:2049–2054.

35.  Ohara A, Kojima S, Hamajima N, Tsuchida M, Imashuku S, Ohta S, Sasaki H, Okamura J, Sugita K, Kigasawa H, Kiriyama Y, Akatsuka J, Tsukimoto I. Myelodysplastic syndrome and acute myelogenous leukemia as a late clonal complication in children with acquired aplastic anemia. Blood 1997; 90:1009–1013.

36.  Kaito K, Kobayashi M, Katayama T, Masuoka H, Shimada T, Nishiwaki K, Sekita T, Otsubo H, Ogasawara Y, Hosoya T. Long-term administration of G-CSF for aplastic anaemia is closely related to the early evolution of monosomy 7 MDS in adults. Br J Haematol 1998; 103:297–303.

37.  Kojima S, Nakao S, Tomonaga M, Hows J, Marsh J, Gerard S, Bacigalupo A, Mizoguchi H. Consensus conference on the treatment of aplastic anemia (review). Int J Hematol 2000; 72:118–123.

38.  Matsuo Y, Iwanaga M, Mori H, Yoshida S, Kawaguchi Y, Yakata Y, Murata K, Nagai K, Jinnai I, Matsuo T, Kuriyama K, Tomonaga M. Recovery of hematopoietic progenitor cells in patients with severe aplastic anemia who obtained good clinical response with a combination therapy of immunosuppressive agents and recombinant human granulocyte colony-stimulating factor. Int J Hematol 2000; 72:37–43.

39.  Geary CG, Harrison CJ, Philpott NJ, Hows JM, Gordon-Smith EC, Marsh JC. Abnormal cytogenetic clones in patients with aplastic anaemia: response to immunosuppressive therapy. Br J Haematol 1999; 104:271–274.

40.  Elghetany MT, Vyas S, Yuoh G. Significance of p53 overexpression in bone marrow biopsies from patients with bone marrow failure: aplastic anemia, hypocellular refractory anemia, and hypercellular refractory anemia. Ann Hematol 1998; 77:261–264.

# 7

# The Syndrome of Therapy-Related Myelodysplasia and Myeloid Leukemia

**Lucy A. Godley and Richard A. Larson**
*The University of Chicago, Chicago, Illinois*

## I. INTRODUCTION

Patients who have received cytotoxic therapy with chemotherapy drugs and/or radiotherapy are at risk for long-term complications from their treatment. One of the most grave of these is the development of myelodysplasia or acute myeloid leukemia. Although a causal link has not yet been proven, these neoplasms are thought to be a direct consequence of mutational events caused by cytotoxic therapy and to be independent of the primary disease. Thus, they have been termed "therapy-related myelodysplastic syndrome" (t-MDS) and "therapy-related acute myeloid leukemia" (t-AML).

These therapy-related diseases, which have a spectrum of clinical presentations, morphologics, and outcomes, represent distinct entities that differ from their counterparts that occur de novo. Sadly, the prognosis for patients with the therapy-related diseases is often worse. A deeper understanding of the factors that predispose patients to the development of t-MDS and t-AML may help clinicians focus their monitoring on patients at highest risk after treatment for a primary malignancy. Already, aggressive treatment strategies for primary cancers such as Hodgkin's disease, non-Hodgkin's lymphoma, breast cancer, ovarian cancer, testicular cancer, and germ cell tumors have been modified to minimize the subsequent development of t-MDS or t-AML. Preventive interventions remain to be developed.

The terms "t-MDS" and "t-AML" are used specifically to describe myeloid neoplasms that arise in individuals previously treated with cytotoxic chemotherapy, ionizing radiation, or both. The use of the term "therapy-related" implies a causal relationship between the primary therapy and the development of leukemia, although the precise sequence of mutational events remains to be determined. The primary disease for which cytotoxic therapy was given could have been any malignant or nonmalignant disease, but primary MDS and AML de novo are usually excluded from these groupings because of the difficulty in separating a relapse or progression of the primary disease from the emergence of a true therapy-related one. Additionally, the term "secondary leukemia" is best reserved for situations in which leukemia has developed as part of the natural history of a hematological disorder, e.g., AML that evolves in a patient with a primary MDS or as the terminal phase of a chronic myeloproliferative disorder such as polycythemia vera or essential thrombocythemia. In addition to t-AML, therapy-related acute lymphoblastic leukemia (t-ALL) has been described.

Importantly, some individuals may develop leukemia serendipitously following prior treatment for cancer, but independent of the prior cytotoxic therapy. These cases may be very difficult to distinguish from true therapy-related cases; the concept of "post hoc, ergo propter hoc" is not always correct. However, certain aspects of their presentation, such as the latency from primary therapy or the clinical features of the myeloid disease, may yield clues that these cases are not the typical therapy-related leukemic diseases as presented here. Further exploration for evidence of another cancer predisposition, such as a familial predisposition, should be undertaken.

## II. CLINICAL AND BIOLOGICAL FEATURES

The diagnosis of therapy-related leukemia is usually straightforward, especially in a patient who is otherwise free of disease and off therapy. The presentation may be confusing, however, in a patient who is still under treatment or who has persistent primary cancer involving the bone marrow. Symptoms related to bone marrow failure are usually the first indication of t-MDS/t-AML. Fatigue and weakness due to anemia and occasionally fever related to neutropenia are the most frequent complaints. Bleeding complications caused by thrombocytopenia are also common. Notably absent are some features of acute leukemia de novo such as splenomegaly, lymphadenopathy, hepatomegaly, gingival hyperplasia, skin infiltrates, or central neurological complications.

On laboratory evaluation, one of the earliest detectable signs of t-MDS can be anemia with oval macrocytes and an increased mean corpuscular volume (MCV). Anemia, thrombocytopenia, and occasionally leukopenia are common. Trilineage dysplasia is a hallmark of the therapy-related hematopoietic disorders and implies a multipotent stem cell origin (Table 1). The bone marrow is some-

**Table 1** Morphological Features of Blood and Bone Marrow in Classic Alkylator Therapy-Related Myeloid Leukemia

| | Erythroid series | Granulocytic series | Megakaryocytic series |
|---|---|---|---|
| Peripheral blood | Anemia, an sopoikilocytosis including teardrops, spherocytes, and spiculated RBCs, nucleated RBCs, basophilic stippling, circulating erythroblasts, macrocytosis, polychromasia | Hypogranular neutrophils, hypo- or hyperlobulated nuclei, nuclear excrescences, psuedo-Pelger-Huet nuclei, basophilia, neutropenia, monocytosis, immature myeloid cells with blasts appearing eventually; rarely Auer rods | Giant platelets, degranulated platelets. thrombocytopenia, circulating micromegakaryocytes, megakaryoblasts, and megakaryocyte fragments |
| Bone marrow | Erythroblasts, periodic acid-Schiff-positive normoblasts, dyserythropoiesis, erythroid hyperplasia, megaloblastoid features, ringed sideroblasts, nuclear budding, karyorrhexis, binuclearity, nuclear bridging | Nuclear hyposegmentation, cytoplasmic hypogranulation | Megakaryocytic hyperplasia with atypical forms, micromegakaryocytes, abnormal nuclear contours and sizes, widely spaced nuclear lobes, mononuclear forms, giant compound granules, hypogranular cytoplasm |

**Table 2** The Syndromes of Therapy-Related Myelodysplasia and Myeloid Leukemia

| Type of cytotoxic agents received | Prelukemic phase | Morphology of t-AML | Typical cytogenetic abnormalities | Latency | Response to induction chemotherapy | Long-term survival |
|---|---|---|---|---|---|---|
| Alkylating agents (melphalan, mechloreth-amine, chloram-bucil, cyclo-phosphamide, carmustine, lo-mustine, semus-tine, procarbaz-ine, dacarbazine, mitolactol) | MDS (RCMD, RAEB) | M1, M2, M4 | del(5q) −5 del(7q) −7 | 5–7 years | Poor | Poor |
| Radiation | | | | | | |
| Topoisomerase II inhibitors (eto-poside, tenipo-side, actinomy-cin D, doxorubicin, 4 epidoxorubicin, mitoxantrone) | None | M4, M5 Less commonly: M1, M2, ALL-L1 | Translocations in-volving 11q23 and 21q22 | 6 months–5 years | Good | Fair |
| Other agents (for example, bimo-lane or radiation alone) | None None | M3 M4Eo | t(15;17) inv(16) | 2–3 years <3 years | Good Good | Good Good |

times hypercellular despite cytopenias in the blood, but hypocellular and even nearly aplastic marrow samples are also observed on trephine biopsies. Some degree of marrow fibrosis with increased reticulin fibers is also common.

Neither t-MDS nor t-AML is easily categorized according to the French-American-British (FAB) classification scheme but together they represent their own entity in the newly proposed World Health Organization (WHO) classification (1). (By current convention, t-MDS denotes fewer than 30% blasts in the marrow; once the blast count rises above 30%, the malignancy has been considered to be an overt leukemia. The new WHO classification lowers the transition point from MDS to AML to a blast count $\geq 20\%$.) The t-MDS cases most often resemble refractory cytopenia with multilineage dysplasia (RCMD) or refractory anemia with excess blasts (RAEB). t-AML that develops after exposure to alkylating agents most closely resembles FAB M1, M2, or M4 acute leukemias. When AML occurs de novo, FAB M1 designates a malignancy with minimal maturation and scant granules within myeloblasts; M2 leukemia represents a malignancy with greater maturation and partial differentiation; M4 leukemia is a malignancy of myelomonocytic blasts. As described later, t-AML cases with specific cytogenetic abnormalities such as balanced translocations have the same morphologies as do AML de novo cases with the identical chromosomal rearrangements.

The presenting stage of therapy-related disease is in part related to the clinician's astuteness in suspecting the diagnosis of a therapy-related bone marrow disorder. Because of the rapid progression of t-MDS to t-AML, a median time of about 6 months, approximately one-third of the patients already have overt leukemia when therapy-related disease is first recognized. Further complicating diagnosis is that there are different morphological subtypes of t-MDS/t-AML. These disease subtypes are associated with the type of primary chemotherapy or radiotherapy that was received and the cytogenetic abnormalities that are subsequently detected (Table 2).

## III. EPIDEMIOLOGY

Two paths of investigation have led to our understanding of the patients at risk for the development of t-MDS/t-AML. First, meticulous clinicopathological and cytogenetic analyses of individual cases have defined several subtypes of disease (Table 2). Second, large-scale epidemiological surveys have defined high-risk patient populations. Patients with Hodgkin's disease were the first large cohort of relatively uniformly treated cancer patients who experienced prolonged survival. After long-term follow-up, hundreds of cases of therapy-related leukemia have now been reported on and analyzed (2–17). It soon became clear that patients with other cancers, such as breast cancer, multiple myeloma, and germ cell tumors, and even nonmalignant disorders, shared the risk of therapy-related leukemia if they had received cytotoxic treatment (18–34). Among the 560 patients recently examined at an international workshop evaluating balanced chromosomal translocations in therapy-related leukemia, the primary disease was a solid tumor in 277 (52%), a hematological malignancy in 250 (47%), and a nonmalignant disorder in 7 (1.3%) (35).

Both ionizing radiation and many chemotherapy drugs alter cellular DNA. If not repaired, this damage is most often lethal to cells. This, of course, is the desired consequence if the target cell were a tumor cell. Occasionally, however, nonlethal and heritable mutations occur in single somatic cells (36). Such an alteration in DNA might involve a single base change (as in the *RAS* genes), deletion or inactivation of a growth suppressor gene (such as the *RB1* gene in retinoblastoma), or changes in the expression of certain critical genes (such as oncogenes or growth factor genes). Alkylating agents, in particular, and radiation both possess strong mutagenic activity in vitro plus carcinogenic potency in vivo. In contrast, equally cytotoxic agents such as antimetabolites or vinca alkaloids lack both mutagenicity and significant carcinogenic potential.

Ionizing radiation is a classic genotoxic agent (37). Radiation causes a variety of DNA lesions such as specific base alterations, but the primary mutagenic and carcinogenic effects result from unrejoined or misrepaired DNA double-strand breaks. Medical radiation therapy is a relatively weak mutagen because it is highly lethal to cells. Thus, it would be expected that the adjunctive use of low or intermediate doses of radiation therapy might be more leukemogenic than high treatment doses.

The repair of double-strand breaks following radiation therapy is complex and involves recombinational events. While unrejoined DNA breaks are lethal to cells, incorrectly rejoined segments are likely to be mutagenic. These are generally large-scale changes leading to loss of entire genes through deletions or rearrangements. Loss of heterozygosity may result (38).

In contrast to ionizing radiation, alkylating agents primarily lead to point mutations through damage to individual bases via adduct formation and interstrand or intrastrand cross-linking. Activation of oncogenes such as *RAS* has been shown to occur in this manner (39). In addition, chromosomal deletions or unbalanced translocations also occur. Loss of genetic material leads to inactivation of tumor suppressor genes. Finally, the agents etoposide, teniposide, and doxorubicin are potent inhibitors of topoisomerase II, a critical enzyme involved in DNA replication, and are associated with illegitimate chromosomal recombination events. These events, balanced translocations without loss of genomic DNA, lead to chimeric fusion genes that eventually transform the hematopoietic target. The translocations most commonly identified involve chromosome bands 11q23 (32%) or 21q22 (15%), or an inv(16) (9%), or t(15;17) (8%) (35).

## A. Exposure to Specific Agents

Prior exposure to alkylating agents is commonly associated with the development of t-MDS with characteristic deletions or losses of chromosomes 5 and/or 7, followed several months later by progression to t-AML (Tables 2 and 3) (40,41) (see Chapter 5). The alkylators vary in their likelihood of causing the development of leukemia (nitrogen mustard > melphalan > nitrosoureas > cyclophosphamide > chlorambucil) (24,32), and there is a clear dose-response relationship between the amount of alkylating agent received and the risk of leukemia (2,9,11,18–20,22,23). This syndrome of t-MDS/t-AML typically occurs within 5–7 years after initial exposure to chemotherapy or radiotherapy (Table 4). The risk appears to diminish considerably if patients have survived more than 10 years after the last exposure (7,9). It has been observed more frequently when prolonged courses of alkylating agents have been used often at relatively low doses, or when multiple courses of chemotherapy and/or radiotherapy have been administered intermittently over time. This observation suggests that leukemia develops from cells that undergo mutations due to sublethal treatment and that these cells are unable to repair damaged DNA. Perhaps because it arises in the milieu of cytotoxic therapy, t-MDS/t-AML is itself poorly responsive to antileu-

**Table 3** Cytogenetic Features of t-MDS/t-AML (University of Chicago series)

| | |
|---|---|
| Number of patients | 297 |
| Number of patients with clonal abnormalities | 275 (93%) |
| Abnormalities of chromosomes 5 and 7 | 209 (70%) |
| Chromosome 5 only | 61 (20%) |
| Chromosome 7 only | 84 (28%) |
| Chromosomes 5 and 7 | 64 (21%) |
| t(11q23) | 10 (3%) |
| t(3;21) or t(8;21) or t(21q22) | 8 (3%)[a] |
| t(15;17) | 6 (2%) |
| +8 | 8 (3%) |
| inv(16) | 5 (2%) |
| −13 or del(13q) | 3 (1%) |
| del(20q) | 1 (0.3%) |
| del(11q) | 1 (0.3%) |
| +11 | 1 (0.3%) |
| +21 | 1 (0.3%) |
| −Y | 1 (0.3%) |
| Other abnormalities | 22 (7%) |

[a] One patient had both a del(5q) and t(3;21).
*Source*: Data kindly provided by M.M. Le Beau (2000).

**Table 4**   Prior Therapy, Latency Period, and Clinical Features of Therapy-Related Myeloid Leukemia

| Ref. | No. patients with prior RT | No. patients with prior CT | No. patients with prior RT and CT | Median latency (range) | Median age (range) | No. patients with t-MDS | No. patients with t-AML | Progression from t-MDS to t-AML (median) | Median survival (mo) |
|---|---|---|---|---|---|---|---|---|---|
| 130 | 8 | 25 | 22 | 48 mo (12–131 mo) | 62 (22–75) | 44 | 11 | 84% (5 mo) | 7 |
| 131 | 15 | 17 | | 50 mo | About 50 | 20 | 35 | | 4–8 |
| 132 | | | 24 | 60 mo (1–204 mo) | 58 (18–90) | 0 | 56 | | 5 |
| 133 | 11 | 21 | 31 | 56 mo (10–192 mo) | 55 (6–76) | 48 | 15 | 60% (5 mo) | 8 |
| 134 | 14 | 25 | 26 | 58 mo (11–192 mo) | 53 (1–81) | 39 | 26 | 28% (4 mo) | 4 |
| 8 | 2 | 7 | 66 | 34 mo from CR | | 55 | 20 | 73% (7 mo) | 4–10 |
| 117 | 26 | 37 | 49 | 71 mo (7–331 mo) | 65 (20–82) | 57 | 55 | 55% | 8 |
| 135 | 10 | 29 | 37 | 6 yr (1–21 yr) | 58 (18–89) | 29 | 47 | 57% (6 mo) | 7 |

No., number; mo, months; yr, years; RT, radiotherapy; CT, chemotherapy; CR, complete remission.

kemia chemotherapy. Consequently, the prognosis for these patients is poor (see Section V).

A second and distinctly different form of t-AML arises after chemotherapy using topoisomerase II inhibitors. This syndrome often involves translocations involving chromosome bands 11q23 or 21q22 (Tables 2 and 3; see Chapter 5) (42–55). Andersen et al. reported on 422 cases of t-MDS/t-AML with balanced translocations and found that balanced translocations involving 11q23, 21q22, inv(16), t(15;17), and t(9;22) are often associated with prior use of DNA topoisomerase II inhibitors (55). Patients with uncharacteristic balanced translocations had received alkylating agents most commonly (55). Recently, 560 t-MDS/t-AML patients who displayed clonal balanced translocations (about 25% of all t-MDS/t-AML) were described (35). Among these, 32% of the translocations involved band 11q23, and 15% involved band 21q22. Typically, translocations with a breakpoint in band 11q23 involve the *MLL* (mixed lineage leukemia) gene and those with a breakpoint in band 21q22 involve the *AML1* gene (56). Among those patients with balanced rearrangements involving bands 11q23, 21q22, inv(16), and t(15;17), 82% 74%, 56%, and 46%, respectively, had received some form of topoisomerase II–inhibiting drug, but often this was given in combination with other cytotoxic agents (35). These same rearrangements were also seen in some patients who had received only radiotherapy for their primary treatment. Within the same four cytogenetic subgroups, radiotherapy was observed as the sole modality of prior treatment in 5%, 6%, 21%, and 28%, respectively (35). Some of these patients may have developed AML spontaneously and unrelated to their prior radiotherapy, but this cannot yet be known.

Leukemias arising following the use of topoisomerase II inhibitors were first described in survivors of non–small cell lung cancer (43) and in children who had received epipodophyllotoxins for the treatment of acute lymphoblastic leukemia (ALL) (42,45,48). In the former group, the risk was related to the cumulative dose of etoposide, and in the latter group, the highest risk correlated with the use of prolonged weekly or twice-weekly etoposide or teniposide exposure.

These therapy-related leukemias differ from those associated with alkylating agents in several regards. First, these leukemias are often not preceded by a preleukemic myelodysplastic phase, but rather they present with rapidly progressive leukemia and high white blood cell counts. Second, they occur with a shorter latency, often within 2–3 years of first cytotoxic therapy and in some cases within 12 months. Third, their initial response to antileukemia chemotherapy is good, although their prognosis overall is only fair. Approximately 20% of these patients survive, but the use of bone marrow stem cell transplantation (SCT) is often required.

More rarely, other forms of t-AML have been described. Some of these have occurred after treatment with antimetabolite drugs that have not generally been thought to be leukemogenic. For example, a case of t-AML following sole treatment with 5-fluorouracil (5-FU) was recently described (57). Others may be examples of a second independent neoplasm. Saitoh et al. reported a case of therapy-related megakaryoblastic leukemia in a 66-year-old Japanese man who had been treated 6 years previously with alkylating agents for non-Hodgkin's lymphoma (58). This patient presented with myelodysplasia and myelofibrosis in the bone marrow. At autopsy, he was found to have leukemic infiltration of multiple organs, including the posterior pituitary gland. Finally, a case of therapy-related myeloid/natural killer cell precursor leukemia has been reported in a patient with essential thrombocythemia (59). The patient had received a nitrosourea for his primary malignancy for 8.5 years. The leukemic blasts expressed the cell surface markers CD5, CD7, CD33, CD34, and CD56.

Recently, two cases of t-MDS that progressed into t-AML were described following standard chemotherapy for acute promyelocytic leukemia (APL) (60). Although neither patient received alkylating agents during their APL treatment, both patients developed cytogenetic abnormalities with losses of chromosomes 5 and 7. In one patient, cytogenetic analysis of the t-MDS failed to identify the pathognomonic 15;17 translocation, which characterizes APL de novo, although analysis by fluorescent in situ hybridization (FISH) demonstrated the t(15;17) in 11% of mitoses. In the second case, however, neither cytogenetic analysis nor FISH could detect t(15;17) in the therapy-related malignancy. Both patients developed their t-AML within 2.5 years after achieving a complete remission (CR) from APL, timing consistent with the development of therapy-related disease. The authors postulate that the causative chemotherapy agents may have been an anthracycline, 6-mercaptopurine, or methotrexate. Both patients had also received tretinoin.

The appearance of therapy-related APL (t-APL) following treatment of psoriasis with bimolane underscores the association with prior therapy and makes it clear that t-AML can occur in individuals without a prior malignant disease (33,34). Bimolane is a dioxopiperazine derivative that interacts with topoisomerase II in a mechanism different from the epipodophyllotoxins and anthracyclines. In the report by Xue et al., 14 patients were described: eight had a t(15;17), four had a t(8;21), and two had a del(7q) (33). The median latency was 30 months, with a range from 12 to 96 months. A larger study of 140 cases of bimolane-related leukemia reported that t-APL was the most common phenotype, with an average latency of 46 months (34).

The use of etoposide for the treatment of Langerhans cell histiocytosis has also been associated with the development of t-APL (61). Although these leukemias usually contain t(15;17), the breakpoints in the *RARα* gene differed from those in APL de novo (62). The breakpoints were clustered in a 670-bp fragment of intron 2 in three t-APL patients examined. Intron 2 of the *RARα* gene is 10 kb in size, and breakpoints in the de novo disease are scattered throughout its length. Interestingly, no topoisomerase II cleavage sites were found at the breakpoints of the *RAR*α gene in t-APL cases, suggesting that chromatin structure may be critical in the development of this therapy-related disease.

Although this chapter focuses on therapy-related myeloid disorders, brief mention should be made of t-ALL. Numerous case reports have described this entity, which often involves translocations of chromosome 11, usually with re-arrangements of the *MLL* gene (63–66). In 1985, Secker-Walker et al. reported on a child with neuroblastoma who was treated with a regimen that included doxorubicin and teniposide and who developed t-ALL with t(4;11) within 12 months of completing chemotherapy (63). Two patients who were treated for breast cancer with doxorubicin-containing chemotherapy developed t-ALL, also with t(4;11) (64). Jonveaux et al. described a patient who initially presented with acute monoblastic leukemia de novo with a t(6;11) (q27;q23) and developed t-ALL after chemotherapy (66). Cytogenetic analysis of the t-ALL revealed a new translocation, t(4;11), involving a novel *MLL* gene rearrangement not present in the original disease. In a molecular analysis of 10 t-ALL cases following treatment with topoisomerase II inhibitors, MLL rearrangements were observed in 7/7 cases with detectable 11q23 translocations and in 2/2 cases with unsuccessful karyotypes (65). Whereas the incidence of 11q23 translocations in ALL de novo exceeds that observed in AML de novo, the ratios are reversed in the therapy-related setting. This may reflect the increased cycling of myeloid precursor cells following chemotherapy.

## B. Genetic Predisposition to t-MDS/t-AML

It has not yet been possible to determine whether the development of t-MDS/t-AML is a stochastic event (occurring by chance) or whether certain individuals are at higher risk (perhaps due to a DNA-repair deficiency or a heritable predisposition such as altered drug metabolism) and thus might be identifiable in advance. The identification of such an underlying preexisting condition would help the screening and counseling of patients at the time of treatment of their primary disease (Table 5).

For example, investigators at the University of Chicago and the University of California at Berkeley have found that patients with t-MDS/t-AML have a disproportionately high frequency of mutations in a benzene-detoxifying enzyme, NAD(P)H:quinone oxidoreductase (NQO1) (67). Benzene is a known hemato-toxin and has been associated with primary MDS and AML. The NQO1 enzyme (also known as DT-diaphorase) converts quinones derived from benzene into hydroquinones, which are less toxic. A point mutation at codon 187 changes a proline to a serine and results in a completely inactivated enzyme. Larson et al. examined 56 patients with t-AML and found that six (11%) were homozygous and 23 (41%) were heterozygous for the mutant allele (67). These gene frequencies were higher than expected for the ethnic mix of the patients studied; only

**Table 5**  Genes Involved in the Development of t-MDS/t-AML

| Gene | Associated protein's function | Possible role in t-AML | Ref. |
|------|-------------------------------|------------------------|------|
| NQO1 | Detoxifies benzene derivatives | Increased risk due to an inactivating mutation in the homozygous and heterozygous states | 67 68 |
| CYP3A | Component of the cytochrome P450 system | Increased risk with wild-type promoter sequence | 70 |
| MDR1 | Drug efflux pump | Overexpression confers multidrug resistance | 74 |
| p53 | Tumor suppressor | Mutated in approximately 40% of t-AML cases | 73 |
| Gene on 5q | Presumed tumor suppressor | Deleted in approximately 20% of t-AML cases | 41 |
| Gene on 7q | Presumed tumor suppressor | Deleted in approximately 30% of t-AML cases | 40 |

three homozygotes (5%) and 19 heterozygotes (34%) had been expected. Of 45 patients with either t-MDS/t-AML or primary MDS or AML de novo who had abnormalities of chromosomes 5 or 7, 16% were homozygous and 38% were heterozygous for the mutant NQO1 allele, again both higher than expected. The authors speculated that individuals heterozygous for the mutant NQO1 allele (who have reduced but not absent enzyme activity) might be represented among the t-MDS/t-AML patients at a higher-than-expected frequency if the normal allele underwent mutation or gene silencing in a hematopoietic stem cell. Thus, homozygotes and heterozygotes would be less able to defend against mutations from chemoradiotherapy.

Similar results have been obtained recently by Naoe et al., who studied the frequencies of NQO1 loss-of-function mutations in leukemias from Japanese individuals (68). The frequency of a homozygous loss of function mutation at codon 187 was 24% in t-MDS/t-AML patients (14/58) compared with only 16% in AML de novo cases. The mutation was seen in only 11% (16/150) of normal controls. The different allele frequencies of NQO1 suggest that patients with a nonfunctional NQO1 allele are at increased genetic risk for the development of therapy-related leukemia. Furthermore, Wiemels et al. have demonstrated an increased incidence of NQO1 loss of function alleles in pediatric ALL de novo cases with MLL gene rearrangements (69). The authors of this study postulate that infants with less efficient NQO1 enzymes are predisposed to the development of ALL with MLL gene rearrangements through genotoxic exposure in utero.

Further evidence for the importance of drug-detoxifying enzymes in the development of t-AML comes from an analysis of the *CYP3A4* gene (70). CYP3A metabolizes epipodophyllotoxins, generating catechol and quinone metabolites, which can damage DNA. In this study, a comparison was made between the incidence of a promoter variant and wild-type alleles. Nineteen percent (19/99) of patients with AML de novo and 21% (9/42) of patients with AML de novo and *MLL* gene rearrangements possessed the variant promoter allele. In contrast, only 3% (1/30) of patients with t-AML and none of 22 patients with t-AML and *MLL* gene rearrangements had the variant allele. Unfortunately, in this study, no control population without cancer was examined. Also, whether the promoter variant has any functional consequence for the expression of the *CYP3A* gene (e.g., decreased production of *CYP3A*, leading to diminished intracellular drug oxidation and the production of fewer DNA-damaging intermediates) has not been determined. Nevertheless, this study suggests that patients with the wild-type *CYP3A* promoter may have an increased risk for the development of t-AML and that increased epipodophyllotoxin metabolism by CYP3A may be important in the etiology of t-AML. Notably in the Naoe study (68), no such correlation between leukemia susceptibility and *CYP3A* genotype was seen within the Japanese population.

The likely role of tumor suppressor genes in the development of t-MDS/t-AML has been suggested from numerous studies. The frequent loss of an entire chromosome 5 or 7 or the long arms of these chromosomes [del(5q) or del(7q)] suggests the locations of tumor suppressor genes at these loci that are important for the development of t-MDS/t-AML (40,41). The involvement of known tumor suppressor genes has been the subject of considerable research. Nagai et al. have established a granulocyte-macrophage colony-stimulating factor (GM-CSF)-dependent cell line from a patient who developed t-MDS and later t-AML after treatment for Hodgkin's disease (71). This cell line, OHN-GM, has a deletion of chromosome 5q as well as a translocation involving t(10;13)(q24;q14). The translocation resulted in the deletion of the *RB1* gene, and Western blotting has confirmed that the cell line lacks RB protein. Furthermore, the cell line has two missense mutations of the *p53* gene.

There are other examples of *p53* mutation. A 15-year-old girl with osteosarcoma developed t-MDS/t-AML with abnormalities of chromosomes 5, 7, and 17 (72). This patient was found to have two germline mutations in the *p53* gene; thus, the question was raised whether the patient had Li-Fraumeni syndrome, which is known to confer an increased risk for the development of leukemia. Ben-Yehuda et al. analyzed the status of the *p53* gene in 21 patients with t-AML and found mutations in 38% of cases (73). Importantly, these mutations were confined to the leukemia cells and were not found in nonmalignant tissues. Furthermore, 94% of the patients studied demonstrated microsatellite instability, evidence that t-AML blast cells exhibit defects in DNA repair. As such, these cells may accumulate genetic changes more readily than normal cells. This is called a mutator phenotype. Over time, such mutations could allow tumor cells to divide more rapidly or to escape normal controls on cell growth and also to resist chemotherapy drugs.

Damiani et al. studied t-AML blast cells in vitro to assess the expression and functional significance of P-glycoprotein overexpression (74). P-glycoprotein is a membrane-bound drug efflux pump that confers multidrug resistance by transporting many chemotherapy drugs outward from the cellular cytosol. P-glycoprotein is encoded by the *MDR1* gene and is known to be overexpressed in many AML de novo cases, especially those observed in older individuals or those evolving from a known MDS where a stem cell origin has been inferred. In this study, P-glycoprotein was overexpressed in 40/54 (74%) t-AML cases. Blasts expressing P-glycoprotein showed an increased ability to efflux daunorubicin from the cytosol and consequently accumulated lower intracellular concentrations of daunorubicin. Coincubation with PSC 833, an inhibitor of P-glycoprotein, resulted in significantly higher levels of intracellular daunorubicin. Expression of P-glycoprotein was associated with poor clinical outcome. Only 2/27 (7%) patients who had expression of P-glycoprotein by blast cells achieved a CR after chemotherapy compared to 8/10 (80%) of patients whose blasts did not express P-glycoprotein.

## IV.  THERAPY-RELATED LEUKEMIA AFTER PRIMARY CANCERS

The development of therapy-related second neoplasms provides a unique and ethically acceptable environment for studying the effects of mutagens on carcinogenesis in humans. As the survival after treatment for primary cancers has improved in recent years, more patients have been available to follow for long-term complications. Large numbers of patients who have been treated for specific diseases have been studied to assess the incidence and severity of therapy-related myeloid disorders.

### A.  After Primary Treatment for Hodgkin's Disease

Survivors of Hodgkin's disease represent one of the largest groups studied for long-term complications, including the onset of t-MDS/t-AML (2–17,26,75,76). The incidence of t-MDS/t-AML ranges from less than 1.5% to 10% and varies according to the number of patients studied, their ages, the types of therapies involved, and the length of follow-up. The development of t-MDS/t-AML is rare after treatment with radiation alone, unless the dose exceeds 2000 cGy (16).

Among 5492 Hodgkin's patients who received only radiation, the 15-year cumulative incidence for the development of t-MDS/t-AML has been estimated at 0.4% (76). However, several studies have reported that the incidence increases when extended-field radiation therapy is combined with MOPP (nitrogen mustard/vincristine/prednisone/procarbazine) chemotherapy (6,7,14,76).

The issue of whether splenectomy (often performed in the past for staging of Hodgkin's disease) confers an increased risk for the development of t-AML has been controversial. Some studies show an increased relative risk of 1.3–14 (11–13,16,17,76), but this has never been validated in a randomized, controlled fashion. Other studies have shown splenectomy to be a risk factor with borderline significance (77), or have failed to demonstrate a relationship between the two (78).

## B.   After Treatment for Non-Hodgkin's lymphoma (NHL)

Travis et al. described 35 cases of t-AML among 11,386 patients who had survived at least 2 years after chemotherapy for NHL (79). Compared to 140 matched control patients, the risk of developing t-MDS/t-AML was increased with the use of prednimustine, mechlorethamine, procarbazine, or a cumulative dose of >1300 mg of chlorambucil. Radiotherapy alone was not associated with the development of t-MDS/t-AML in this study.

Pedersen-Bjergaard et al. diagnosed nine cases of t-MDS/t-AML among 602 patients treated for NHL, giving a cumulative incidence of 6.3 ± 2.6% over 7 years (23). All nine patients who developed t-MDS/t-AML had had previous exposure to alkylating agents, especially cyclophosphamide. Other authors report risks ranging from 4.6% to 8% at 10 years (23,24,79–82). Most of the recent analyses have focused on the incidence of t-MDS/t-AML after autologous stem cell transplantation (SCT) for patients with NHL (see below).

## C.   After Treatment for Multiple Myeloma

The Finnish Leukaemia Group studied the incidence of acute leukemia in 432 patients treated with chemotherapy for multiple myeloma (83). Fourteen cases of t-AML were observed, giving an overall incidence of 9.8% at 9 years. Patients were followed for an average of 16 years after the administration of chemotherapy, and no cases of t-AML were seen after 9 years. The incidence of t-MDS was not specified.

## D.   After Treatment for Breast Cancer

The incidence of t-MDS/t-AML has been studied in survivors of breast cancer. Since breast cancer is a common malignancy and adjuvant chemoradiotherapy is commonly used for early-stage disease, these women represent a large population at risk for long-term complications. In 1985, Fisher et al. published the National Surgical Adjuvant Breast Project (NSABP) experience with over 2000 women treated with surgical removal of their primary cancers followed by adjuvant chemotherapy or radiotherapy (21). They found a cumulative incidence of 1.68 ± 0.3% at 10 years for the development of t-MDS/t-AML in patients who received only chemotherapy as adjuvant treatment and an incidence of 1.39 ± 0.5% at 10 years for patients treated with only regional radiation following surgery. Five cases of t-AML studied by the NSABP were classified as FAB M4 or M5 and had short latency periods. Two of these cases displayed 11q23 abnormalities. These patients had participated in a three-armed trial in which all patients had received four monthly courses of doxorubicin and cyclophosphamide at higher-than-standard doses as well as granulocyte colony-stimulating factor (G-CSF) to decrease toxicity from neutropenia. The rapid appearance of several cases of t-AML in this trial prompted a warning by the National Cancer Institute (84). There has been some concern that the use of growth factors may be synergistic with chemotherapy in inducing t-AML, although no data outside of this trial have been published to further support this association.

Tallman et al. reported the follow-up of 2638 patients treated on six Eastern Cooperative Oncology Group (ECOG) clinical trials between 1978 and 1987 (85). Among these patients, three cases of t-MDS and two cases of leukemia were identified. Of the leukemias observed, the first was ALL associated with human T-lymphotropic virus type 1 (HTLV-1), and the second was t-AML that developed in a patient who had received additional cyclophosphamide for metastatic breast cancer. Including all five cases, the authors estimated the incidence of t-MDS/t-AML to be 26 per 100,000 person-years and concluded that this was not greater than the risk for the general population.

Among 13,734 women given initial chemotherapy and followed by the Surveillance, Epidemiology, and End Results Program, 24 developed t-MDS/t-AML, giving a cumulative incidence of 0.7% at 10 years (31). Carli et al. performed a retrospective analysis of patients registered with hematological malignancies and found that 7.7% (12/156) had had a history of breast cancer (86). Ten of these patients had received topoisomerase II inhibitors, and eight of them had received mitoxantrone. Chaplain et al. found a dose-dependent increase in the incidence of t-MDS/t-AML in breast cancer survivors who had received mitoxantrone at a dose of ≥13 mg/m² (87). Overall, they observed 10 cases (0.3%) of t-MDS/t-AML among 3093 women who had been followed for at least 4 years. A similar incidence of 0.7% was calculated in the retrospective study by Linassier et al., who followed 350 patients who had received chemotherapy with mitoxantrone, fluorouracil, and cyclophosphamide along with regional radiotherapy (88). The median latency time was 16 months from beginning chemotherapy and 10.5 months from ending therapy. Within a small series of 24 patients treated with oral etoposide (50 mg or 100 mg/day for 5–7 days at 4-week intervals) for recurrent breast cancer, 3 cases (13%) of t-MDS/t-AML were diagnosed (89). These patients had been previously treated with anthracyclines, cyclophosphamide, or cisplatin as well as radiotherapy prior to receiving the oral etoposide therapy. No cases of t-MDS/t-AML were observed in 119 similar patients who had not received etoposide. The variance in the incidence rates for the development of t-MDS/t-AML in survivors of breast cancer may reflect the heterogeneity of the patients and their prior treatments.

### E.  After Treatment for Ovarian Cancer

The widespread use of alkylating agents in the treatment of ovarian cancer has led to a careful examination of the incidence of t-MDS/t-AML in this patient population. Reimer et al. found 13 cases of t-MDS/t-AML among 5455 patients (0.2%) (18). All of the patients with therapy-related disease had received alkylating agents, and nine had also received radiotherapy. Among 998 women who had received alkylating agents as therapy for ovarian cancer, Greene et al. observed 12 cases of t-MDS/t-AML (1%), an excess risk of 5.8 cases per 1000 women per year (19).

### F.  After Treatment for Germ Cell Tumors

In their original description, Pedersen-Bjergaard et al. observed five cases of t-MDS/t-AML out of 212 patients (2%) treated with etoposide, cisplatin, and bleomycin for germ cell tumors (90). More recently, Schneider et al. followed 1132 patients with malignant germ cell tumors prospectively to determine the incidence of t-MDS/t-AML (91). Among these patients, six cases of t-MDS/t-AML were observed, giving a cumulative incidence of 1% at 10 years for patients treated with chemotherapy alone (3/442) and a cumulative incidence of 4.2% for patients treated with chemoradiotherapy (3/174). Most of those who developed t-MDS/t-AML had received only moderate doses of chemotherapy. Five of these six patients had received epipodophyllotoxins at $<2$ g/m$^2$, and four of the patients had received ifosfamide at $<20$ g/m$^2$.

The incidence of t-MDS/t-AML for survivors of testicular cancer has been estimated at 0.5% at 5 years for patients who have received etoposide at doses of $\leq2$ g/m$^2$, while the incidence increases to 2% for patients who have received etoposide at doses of $>2$ g/m$^2$ (92).

### G.  After Treatment for Childhood Tumors

Recently, the incidence of t-AML has been reported for children who received chemotherapy for Ewing's sarcoma using topoisomerase II inhibitors, alkylating agents, and G-CSF (93). Seventy-three patients had been treated on one of two consecutive protocols. Of the 41 evaluable patients who had been treated with the more chemotherapy-intensive regimen, 7.8% ± 4.7% developed t-AML within 4 years. The disease was preceded by abnormalities of the peripheral blood counts, including an increased MCV and decreased platelet counts. No cases of t-AML were found in the 32 evaluable patients who were treated on the less chemotherapy-intensive protocol. Unfortunately, in this study, the number of patients was insufficient to conclusively demonstrate an association between the use of dose-intensified chemotherapy and the subsequent development of t-MDS/t-AML.

## H. After Autologous Hematopoietic Stem Cell Transplantation

Over the past two decades there has been increasing use of high-dose, short-duration chemotherapy followed by reinfusion of cryopreserved autologous hematopoietic stem cells for the treatment of relapsed primary malignant diseases or for high-risk cancers in first CR. Although intensive, this treatment is not generally myeloablative. The use of SCT has clearly cured some patients who otherwise would have died from their primary disease. However, an alarming rate of t-MDS has been observed among these survivors (Table 6).

Pedersen-Bjergaard et al. recently reviewed the development of t-MDS/ t-AML after the use of high-dose chemotherapy and autologous SCT (94). Various risk factors for the development of t-MDS/t-AML include patient age > 40 years with Hodgkin's disease (77,95) and > 35 years old with non-Hodgkin's lymphoma (96), the amount of alkylating agent therapy received prior to SCT (9,78,97–100), and a history of radiation (99), especially the use of total-body irradiation during the transplant preparative regimen (95,97). Several studies have suggested a higher risk of t-MDS/t-AML for patients who received chemotherapy-primed peripheral blood stem cells rather than bone marrow–derived stem cells obtained without the use of mobilizing chemotherapy (96,101). Whether this reflects chemotherapy damage to the stem cells in the former case or just different populations of stem cells is not yet clear.

Krishnan et al. analyzed the outcomes of 612 patients who underwent high-dose chemotherapy and autologous peripheral blood stem cell rescue for Hodgkin's disease and non-Hodgkin's lymphoma at the City of Hope National Medical Center (102). Twenty-two patients developed t-MDS/t-AML, giving a cumulative risk of 8.6% ± 2.1% at 6 years. The use of etoposide as a means of priming the production of stem cells was found to be an independent risk factor for the development of t-MDS/t-AML. Patients who received etoposide prior to the collection of stem cells had a 12.3-fold increased risk for developing t-AML with abnormalities of chromosome bands 11q23 or 21q22. Multivariate analysis also revealed an association between pretransplant radiation and the development of t-MDS or t-AML.

Pedersen-Bjergaard et al. have summarized the latency periods observed for 80 t-MDS and 20 t-AML patients who had undergone high-dose chemotherapy and autologous stem cell reinfusion (94). Twenty-five percent of t-MDS patients developed their disease within 1 year after SCT, and another 25% had evidence of t-MDS by 2 years. Ninety-four percent of t-MDS patients developed the disease by 5 years. Similarly, 30% of t-AML patients were diagnosed with leukemia within 1 year of SCT, with another 30% developing t-AML by 2 years. All cases of t-AML occurred within 5 years post-SCT.

Similar findings were reported from a study of 230 patients in England who received cyclophosphamide and total-body irradiation followed by autologous stem cell reinfusion as consolidation therapy for non-Hodgkin's lymphoma (103). The vast majority of these patients received bone marrow–derived stem cells, and only nine patients received peripheral blood progenitor cells. After a median follow-up of 6 years, 27 patients (12%) had developed t-MDS/t-AML (16 t-MDS, 10 t-MDS progressing to t-AML, and one t-AML). Using multivariate analysis, prior fludarabine therapy and older age were found to be associated with the development of t-MDS/t-AML. The median latency time to the development of t-MDS/t-AML was 9 years after the diagnosis of lymphoma (range, 2.7–21.6 years) and 4.4 years after autologous SCT (range, 11 months–8.8 years). Karyotype abnormalities were most commonly found for chromosomes 5, 7, 13, 18, and 20.

In their analysis of all 649 patients who underwent autologous bone marrow or peripheral SCT from 1985 until 1997, investigators at the University of Chicago identified six cases of t-MDS/t-AML, an incidence rate of 1% (104). One case of t-ALL was also observed. When analyzed by primary diseases, the incidence of developing t-MDS/t-AML was 0.3% for breast cancer (1/354), 6.3% for Hodgkin's disease (5/79), and 1% for non-Hodgkin's lymphoma (1/103). The median latency periods to develop t-MDS/t-AML after SCT and after initial diagnosis of the primary disease, respectively, were 1.5 years and 5.5 years for both Hodgkin's and non-Hodgkin's lymphoma, and 2.8 years and 4.4 years for breast cancer. Since these therapy-related leukemias developed approximately 4–6 years after primary treatment, i.e., within the same range as the latencies seen for t-AML in other nontransplant settings, it seems most likely that the initial chemotherapy given for the primary malignancy was the predisposing or mutagenic exposure rather than that used for the autologous transplant procedure itself. Alternatively, one might speculate that oligoclonal hematopoiesis occurring during the process of marrow regeneration after autologous SCT increases the likelihood of the emergence of a neoplastic subclone.

Efforts to identify patients at risk for the development of t-MDS/t-AML

**Table 6** Incidence of t-AML After Autologous Stem Cell Transplantation

| Ref. | Primary tumor | No. transplanted | No. t-MDS; No. t-AML; (% affected) | Risk factors identified | Risk estimate (years) |
|---|---|---|---|---|---|
| 101 | HD | 68 | 3; 0; (4%) | | 14.5% (4) |
| | NHL | 138 | 3; 1; (3%) | | |
| 96 | HD, NHL | 258 | 9; 1; (4%) | Age > 35 years | 13.5% (6) |
| 136 | HD | 108 | 2; 2; (4%) | | 9% (3) |
| | NHL | 167 | 5; 1; (4%) | | |
| 102 | HD, NHL | 612 | 24*; (4%) | Use of topoisomerase II inhibitors and the development of 11q23 and 21q22 translocations | 9.4% (9) |
| 95 | HD | 249 | 4; 2; (2%) | Age > 40 years | 4% (5) |
| | NHL | 262 | 6; 0; (2%) | Use of TBI | |
| 97 | NHL | 262 | 18; 2; (8%) | Prolonged time from diagnosis to SCT<br>Duration of prior CT<br>Use of RT, including pelvic irradiation<br>Age > 38 years with thrombocytopenia | 18% (6) |
| 137 | NHL | 552 | 41; 0; (7%) | Lower number of reinfused cells | 20% (10) |
| 138 | HD, NHL | 300 | 6a; (2%) | Prior relapse | 4% (5) |
| 139 | HD | 52 | 0; 1; (2%) | Use of prior RT | 1.1% (1.67) |
| | NHL | 62 | 0; 0; (0%) | | |

| | | | | Risk factors | |
|---|---|---|---|---|---|
| 100 | HD | 27 | 1; 1; (7%) | | 24% (3.6) |
| | NHL | 49 | 3; 1; (8%) | Prior splenectomy | 4% (5) |
| 77 | HD | 467 | 5; 3; (2%) | Prior chemotherapy, especially using MOPP or lomustine | 3% (5) |
| 78 | HD | 595 | 8[a]; (1%) | | |
| 99 | HD, NHL | 4998 | 51; 15; (1%) | Prolonged time from diagnosis to SCT<br>Older age<br>Use of TBI<br>Number of SCTs | H: 5% (5)<br>NHL: 3% (5) |
| 98 | Multiple myeloma | 71<br>117 | Prior treatment with one cycle of CT: 0; 0; (0%)<br>Prior treatment with multiple cycles of CT: 7; 0; (6%) | Timing of SCT relative to prior chemotherapy | 12% (4) |
| 140 | Breast cancer | 864 | 3; 2[b]; (6%) | | 2% (4) |
| 104 | Breast cancer | 354 | 0; 1; (0.3%) | | NR |
| | HD | 79 | 4; 1; (6.3%) | | |
| | NHL | 103 | 1; 0; (1%) | | |
| 92 | Testicular cancer | 302 | 2; 4; (2%) | Prior etoposide (>2.4 g/m$^2$), cisplatin, ifosfamide, and cyclophosphamide | 1% (4.3) |
| 103 | NHL | 230 | 16; 11; (12%) | Prior fludarabine therapy<br>Older age | NR |

[a] Number of t-MDS and t-AML cases not distinguished.
[b] Includes one case of ALL.
HD, Hodgkin's disease; NHL, non-Hodgkin's lymphoma; NR, not reported; TBI, total-body irradiation; RT, radiotherapy; CT, chemotherapy.

after SCT have not as yet yielded many options useful for screening or early detection. Legare et al. reported on the analysis of clonal cell populations as a means of screening patients for the development of t-MDS/t-AML after autologous SCT for lymphoma (105). They reported on one patient whose banked blood samples were analyzed for clonality of the X-linked human androgen receptor. In this one patient, a clonal cell population was identified 6 months after SCT and 1 year prior to the clinical recognition of t-AML. This methodology requires further testing.

A prospective study by Martinez-Climent et al. analyzed the chromosomal abnormalities observed in bone marrow cells of patients with high-risk breast cancer who underwent six courses of FAC/FEC (5-fluorouracil, Adriamycin*/ etoposide, cyclophosphamide) chemotherapy followed by high-dose chemotherapy and autologous peripheral SCT (106). Among 229 women who were followed for 36 months after SCT, no cases of t-AML were seen. Sixty of these women had cytogenetic analysis of bone marrow samples 12–59 months after SCT. Among these women, three (5%) displayed transient, clonal abnormalities, and two (3%) showed nonclonal reciprocal translocations. Thus, cytogenetic surveillance of bone marrow cells was not sensitive. The incidence of t-AML in this series was less than that reported by other groups. This may result from differences in the specific chemotherapy regimens employed.

## V. TREATMENT OF THERAPY-RELATED MYELOID LEUKEMIA

The survival of patients with t-MDS/t-AML is usually poor despite prompt diagnosis and treatment. In a nationwide Japanese study of 256 patients with t-MDS (41%) or t-AML (59%), a poor prognosis was associated with most chromosome 5 abnormalities, hypoproteinemia, high C-reactive protein, thrombocytopenia, and persistence or poor outcome from the primary malignancy (107). The median survival was only 9.7 months. The median age of diagnosis of t-MDS/t-AML was 61 years, and the median latency period from diagnosis of the primary malignancy was 47.9 months. However, the latency period was much shorter for patients who had received topoisomerase II inhibitors for their primary disease.

The majority of the Japanese patients (72%) received antileukemia chemotherapy, either a standard combination using an anthracycline plus cytarabine, or low-dose cytarabine, or tretinoin in the case of seven patients with t-APL (107). A CR was seen in 85 patients (46%). The median and mean durations of these responses were 8.2 and 14.6 months, respectively. Four patients received an allogeneic bone marrow transplant from an HLA-identical sibling. Two of the four

---

* Trademark of Pharmacia & Upjohn, Inc.

transplanted patients maintained their CR, as did four of the seven patients with t-APL.

The outcomes of t-AML patients with an inv(16), t(8;21), or t(15;17) have been more favorable. At the International Workshop on Leukemia Karyotype and Prior Treatment, patients with these recurring abnormalities who were intensively treated had a 70–80% rate of complete remission and a long-term survival of 20–40% (108).

In the series reported by Micallef et al. describing 27 t-MDS/t-AML patients who had received autologous SCT for non-Hodgkin's lymphoma, 21 (78%) died from t-MDS/t-AML or its associated treatment at an average of 10 months following diagnosis (103). Among these 21 patients, 16 died without any evidence remaining of their primary disease. Only supportive treatment had been given to 18 of these 21 patients. Three patients, however, received additional SCT: two with a second autologous SCT and one with an allogeneic SCT. All three died from complications arising from the second transplant. Among the six patients still living at the time of reporting, two were receiving supportive care, three had been treated with antilymphocyte globulin (109), and one had received nonmyeloablative allogeneic SCT.

## A. Supportive Care and the Use of Hematopoietic Growth Factors

Therapy-related leukemia is generally a fatal disease. The life-threatening complications of this disorder are the result of persistent and profound cytopenia due to the failure of normal hematopoiesis regardless of the fraction of myeloblasts accumulating in the bone marrow or blood. Supportive management is still considered the standard of care. Low-dose chemotherapy regimens such as those using cytarabine or 5-azacytidine, which have benefit in primary MDS, have been generally ineffective in therapy-related leukemia. Agents that yield occasional responses in primary MDS, such as hematinic vitamins (folic acid, vitamin $B_{12}$, pyridoxine), immunosuppressive drugs (glucocorticoids, cyclosporine, antithymocyte globulin), and androgens, have not been evaluated in therapy-related leukemia but seem unlikely to alter the disease. Vitamin $D_3$ and retinoids that can induce differentiation of leukemia cells in vitro have yet to be tested.

Hematopoietic growth factors have been investigated in an attempt to preserve and promote normal hematopoiesis while inducing terminal differentiation in the neoplastic clone. Only small numbers of patients with therapy-related leukemia have been reported on, but one of these achieved a complete clinical and cytogenetic response after treatment with GM-CSF (110). Nonclonal hematopoiesis and suppression of the neoplastic clone were observed for 9 months. In a dose-escalation trial at the University of Chicago, 10 patients with t-MDS and severe neutropenia received 14-day courses of GM-CSF (111). Although the neutrophil count increased in most cases, it was rarely sustained. Little stimulation of platelet or red blood cell production was observed, and no evidence was found that GM-CSF preferentially stimulated normal marrow stem cells to proliferate or had the ability to inhibit the cytogenetically abnormal clone by inducing terminal differentiation. Erythropoietin treatment has not been well studied in therapy-related leukemia, but most anemic patients with normal renal function will already have high physiological levels of erythropoietin (112). Few data are yet available regarding G-CSF, interleukin-3, other cytokines, or antiangiogenesis agents in therapy-related leukemia.

## B. Chemotherapy

Poor hematopoietic reserves make the administration of standard AML therapy difficult. Many patients have poor tolerance for the acute toxicity of treatment. The primary cancer may still be present, compromising organ function. Prior transfusions may have led to alloimmunization, and thus patients may be refractory to platelet and red blood cell support. Prior antibiotic use and the immunocompromised state result in colonization by pathogenic flora. Because therapy-related leukemia evolves in the milieu of chemotherapy, the malignant cells are relatively drug-resistant. Expression of the multidrug resistance phenotype is common, as noted earlier.

In a review of 644 t-AML patients treated with standard AML chemotherapy induction programs, 182 (28%) were reported to have achieved a CR (113). Individual small series report CR rates of 40–50% (114–121). This is considerably lower than the 65–80% CR rate observed in patients with AML de novo. Importantly, the small number of patients with t-AML who have a favorable cytogenetic abnormality, such as t(8;21), t(15;17), or inv(16), have a considerably better outcome, not markedly different from the high response rates observed when the same rearrangements are present in AML de novo (52,117,122,123).

Cortes analyzed the outcomes of patients with chromosome band 11q23 abnormalities (124). Twenty of 26 patients (77%) with AML de novo versus five of 12 patients (42%) with t-AML achieved a CR. Median survival was 71 weeks in the de novo group and 6 weeks in the t-AML group. There were no long-term survivors in either group in this study. Because the CR rates appear to be high in both de novo and secondary cases, these patients with 11q23 translocations may be good candidates for more aggressive postremission therapies, such as SCT (see below), or for novel gene therapy approaches.

Gardin et al. described the use of intensive combination chemotherapy in nine patients who had t-AML (125). Idarubicin was given at 12 mg/m$^2$ for 3 days plus cytarabine at 1000 mg/m$^2$ every 12 hr for 5 days (intermediate-dose) for younger patients and at 100 mg/m$^2$ via continuous infusion for 7 days in older patients followed by G-CSF support. Five of the t-AML patients achieved a CR; four had received the intermediate-dose cytarabine. However, only one of these patients survived longer than 1 year.

## C.  Allogeneic Stem Cell Transplantation

The only known curative treatment for patients with t-MDS/t-AML is allogeneic SCT. Several small case series have described the outcomes of these patients, and the survival appears to be about 20–30% (Table 7). The relative drug resistance of t-MDS/t-AML the persistence of the primary malignant disease, and the chronic and cumulative toxicity of prior chemoradiotherapy adversely affect survival. Early deaths from regimen-related toxicity are more common after SCT for therapy-related leukemia than for primary MDS. Autologous SCT for patients who lack an HLA (human leukocyte antigen)–matched donor is currently under investigation.

Anderson et al. compared the outcomes of 17 t-MDS/t-AML patients who underwent allogeneic SCT as an initial treatment versus 12 others who were first shown to have chemotherapy-sensitive disease and then received SCT (126). Compared to patients who underwent allogeneic SCT for secondary AML that had evolved from primary MDS, patients with therapy-related leukemia tended to have shorter disease-free survival and a higher relapse rate, although the numbers were not statistically significant. Survival at 5 years was only 17%.

In an analysis of 70 patients (31 with t-MDS and 39 with t-AML) who underwent allogeneic SCT between 1980 and 1998 in France, poor outcome was associated with age greater than 37 years, male sex, positive cytomegalovirus serology in the recipient, absence of CR at the time of SCT, and the use of intensive conditioning chemotherapy (127). The treatments given were heterogeneous: three patients received peripheral stem cell grafts, 66 received bone marrow-derived stem cells, and one received unrelated cord blood cells. The donors for the allogeneic transplants were also varied: 57 were HLA-identical siblings, two were identical twins, five were HLA-matched but unrelated donors, three were HLA-mismatched related donors, and three were HLA-mismatched unrelated donors. The estimated 2-year survival rate was 30%, event-free survival rate 28%, relapse rate 42%, and SCT-related mortality 49%. Thus, for patients who have chemotherapy-responsive t-AML, allogeneic SCT is a viable option for curative therapy, but it is unfortunately not very successful.

Similar results have been seen in children who have undergone allogeneic SCT for t-AML developing after therapy for ALL. Hale et al. reported on the outcomes of 21 children who had received epipodophyllotoxin-containing regimens for ALL and subsequently developed t-AML (128). Thirteen of these children were treated with induction chemotherapy prior to SCT, whereas seven un-

**Table 7**  Outcome After Allogeneic Stem Cell Transplantation for Patients with t-MDS/t-AML

| Ref. | No. of patients | Median age, years (range) | Preparative regimen[a] | Source of stem cells | Matching of HLA | GVHD prophylaxis[b] | No. with relapse (%) | Percent survival (years) |
|---|---|---|---|---|---|---|---|---|
| 141 | 7 | 42 (27–52) | Cy/TBI | BM | M | MTX/CSA | 3 (43) | 0 |
| 142 | 3 | 9 (7–31) | Bu/AraC/Cy/TBI | BM | MM | T cell depletion/CSA | 0 | 66% (1) |
| 143 | 6 | NR | Cy/TBI; Bu/Cy | BM | Majority M | CSA/MTX/steroids | 1 (17) | 50% (3) |
| 144 | 4 | 22 (14–36) | Bu/Cy | BM | M | CSA/Cy | 0 | 50% (2) |
| 145 | 11 | 28 (3–46) | Cy/TBI; Bu/Cy; AraC/Cy/TBI; Cy/BCNU/E | BM | M | T-cell depletion/CSA/MTX | 2 (18) | 27% (±13%) (5) |
| 146 | 25 | 32 (2–52) | Cy/TBI; Bu/Cy | BM | M | T-cell depletion/other treatment NR | 3 (12) | 18% (±11%)[c] (2) |
| 126 | 17 | NR | Bu/Cy; Cy; BCNU/Cy/E; Cy/TBI; Bu/Cy/TBI | BM | Majority M | MTX/CSA/steroids/FK506 | (43) | 17% (5) |
| 128 | 21 | 11 (3–20) | AraC/Cy/TBI | BM | 11 R, M; 8 MUD; 2 R, MM | ATG (2 patients)/CSA/pentoxyphylline/MTX/T-cell-depleted (HLA-mismatched patients) | 10 (48) | 19% (3) |
| 127 | 70 | 37 (16–55) | Cy/TBI; Cy/Bu; Cy/melphalan; other chemotherapy combinations ± TBI (not otherwise specified) | BM-66 PB-3 CB-1 | 59R, M; 5 MUD; 3 R, MM; 3 UR, MM | CSA/steroids/MTX/ATG | 19 (42) | 30% (2) |

[a] Preparative regimens contained various combinations of the chemotherapy agents listed.
[b] GVHD prophylaxis regimens contained various combinations of the agents listed.
[c] This estimate includes patients with AML evolved from primary MDS. The specific results for therapy-related leukemia are not given.
AraC, cytarabine; ATG, anti-thymocyte globulin; BCNU, carmustine; BM, bone marrow; Bu, busulfan; CB, cord blood; CSA, cyclosporine; Cy, cyclophosphamide; DFS, disease-free survival; E, etoposide; FK506, tacrolimus; GVHD, graft-versus-host disease; M,HLA-matched; MM,HLA-mismatched; MTX, methotrexate; MUD, matched unrelated donor; NR, not reported; PB, peripheral blood; R, related; TBI, total-body irradiation; UR, unrelated.

derwent SCT immediately after diagnosis. One patient received an autologous SCT in first remission from therapy-related disease, but later relapsed, and was subsequently treated at second relapse of his t-AML with an allogeneic SCT. Eleven patients received bone marrow cells from HLA-matched siblings, while eight received bone marrow cells from matched unrelated donors, and two received haploidentical marrow from family members. Three years after SCT, only four patients (19%) were alive. Seven patients died from transplant-related causes, and 10 patients died from relapsed t-AML after a median of 5 months.

Cesaro et al. reported on the use of donor lymphocyte infusion (DLI) in the treatment of one t-AML patient who relapsed after allogeneic SCT (129). After treatment for anaplastic large cell lymphoma, this patient developed t-AML that responded initially to induction chemotherapy and allogeneic peripheral SCT. However, his t-AML relapsed. He was then treated successfully with oral etoposide followed by DLI. The t-AML remained in remission for another 7 months until the patient died from recurrent lymphoma.

## VI. CONCLUSIONS

In recent years, considerable information regarding the predisposing factors and epidemiology of therapy-related myelodysplasia and leukemia has been developed. Prior treatment with alkylating agents predisposes to a myeloid disease characterized by deletions of chromosomes 5 and/or 7, while the use of topoisomerase II inhibitors confers an increased risk of t-AML with balanced translocations involving chromosome bands 11q23 or 21q22. Radiation therapy has been implicated in the cause of the first subtype and is also associated with t-AML with inv(16) or t(15;17). The use of multiagent and multimodality primary treatment programs has made it increasingly likely that additive or perhaps even synergistic effects on leukemogenesis occur. Further, certain patients may have a higher risk than others depending on their genetic constitution. The expression of polymorphic alleles for tumor suppressor genes or genes that encode proteins involved in drug transport, activation, or catabolism may play a large role in determining a patient's individual risk for the development of t-MDS/t-AML. Thus, the future may bring an attempt to sketch a molecular fingerprint for each patient at the time of his or her diagnosis with any cancer. This may allow physicians to choose a particular chemotherapy or radiotherapy regimen that is least likely to lead to a second neoplasm. Current treatment regimens for t-MDS/t-AML are inadequate and need to be markedly improved, especially with regard to decreasing the morbidity of treatment. It is hoped that by understanding more about mechanisms of mutagenesis and the molecular basis of the disease, more directed therapy will emerge. Prevention of this complication of cancer treatment is a clinical and scientific challenge, but it is clearly the appropriate goal.

## ACKNOWLEDGMENT

This work was supported in part by grants PO1 CA-40046 and CA-14599 from the National Institutes of Health.

## REFERENCES

1. Harris NL, Jaffe ES, Diebold J, Flandrin G, Muller-Hermelink HK, Vardiman J, Lister TA, Bloomfield CD. The World Health Organization classification of neoplastic diseases of the hematopoietic and lymphoid tissues. Report of the Clinical Advisory Committee meeting, Airlie House, Virginia, November, 1997. Ann Oncol 1999; 10:1419–1432.
2. Coltman CA Jr, Dixon DO. Second malignancies complicating Hodgkin's disease: a Southwest Oncology Group 10-year followup. Cancer Treat Rep 1982; 66:1023–1033.
3. Glicksman AS, Pajak TF, Gottlieb A, Nissen N, Stutzman L, Cooper MR. Second malignant neoplasms in patients successfully treated for Hodgkin's disease: a Cancer and Leukemia Group B study. Cancer Treat Rep 1982; 66:1035–1044.
4. Pedersen-Bjergaard J, Larsen SO. Incidence of acute nonlymphocytic leukemia, preleukemia, and acute myeloproliferative syndrome up to 10 years after treatment of Hodgkin's disease. N Engl J Med 1982; 307:965–971.
5. Boivin JF, Hutchison GB, Lyden M, Godbold J, Chorosh J, Schottenfeld D. Second primary cancers following treatment of Hodgkin's disease. J Natl Cancer Inst 1984; 72:233–241.
6. Valagussa P, Santoro A, Fossati-Bellani F, Banfi A, Bonadonna G. Second acute leukemia and other malignancies following treatment for Hodgkin's disease. J Clin Oncol 1986; 4:830–837.
7. Blayney DW, Longo DL, Young RC, Greene MH, Hubbard SM, Postal MG, Duffey PL, DeVita VT Jr. Decreasing risk of leukemia with prolonged follow-up after chemotherapy and radiotherapy for Hodgkin's disease. N Engl J Med 1987; 316: 710–714.
8. Brusamolino E, Papa G, Valagussa P, Mandelli F, Bernasconi C, Marmont A, Bonadonna G, Tura S, Bosi A, Mango G, et al. Treatment-related leukemia in Hodgkin's disease: a multi-institution study on 75 cases. Hematol Oncol 1987; 5:83–98.
9. Pedersen-Bjergaard J, Specht L, Larsen SO, Ersboll J, Struck J, Hansen MM, Hansen HH, Nissen NI. Risk of therapy-related leukaemia and preleukaemia after Hodgkin's disease. Relation to age, cumulative dose of alkylating agents, and time from chemotherapy. Lancet 1987; 2:83–88.
10. Tucker MA, Coleman CN, Cox RS, Varghese A, Rosenberg SA. Risk of second cancers after treatment for Hodgkin's disease. N Engl J Med 1988; 318:76–81.
11. van der Velden JW, van Putten WL, Guinee VF, Pfeiffer R, van Leeuwen FE, van der Linden EA, Vardomskaya I, Lane W, Durand M, Lagarde C, et al. Subsequent development of acute non-lymphocytic leukemia in patients treated for Hodgkin's disease. Int J Cancer 1988; 42:252–255.

12. Meadows AT, Obringer AC, Marrero O, Oberlin O, Robinson L, Fossati-Bellani F, Green D, Voute PA, Morris-Jones P, Greenberg M, et al. Second malignant neoplasms following childhood Hodgkin's disease: treatment and splenectomy as risk factors. Med Pediatr Oncol 1989; 17:477–484.

13. van Leeuwen FE, Somers R, Taal BG, van Heerde P, Coster B, Dozeman T, Huisman SJ, Hart AA. Increased risk of lung cancer, non-Hodgkin's lymphoma, and leukemia following Hodgkin's disease. J Clin Oncol 1989; 7:1046–1058.

14. Andrieu JM, Ifrah N, Payen C, Fermanian J, Coscas Y, Flandrin G. Increased risk of secondary acute nonlymphocytic leukemia after extended-field radiation therapy combined with MOPP chemotherapy for Hodgkin's disease. J Clin Oncol 1990; 8: 1148–1154.

15. Devereux S, Selassie TG, Vaughan Hudson G, Vaughan Hudson B, Linch DC. Leukaemia complicating treatment for Hodgkin's disease: the experience of the British National Lymphoma Investigation. Br Med J 1990; 301:1077–1080.

16. Kaldor JM, Day NE, Clarke EA, Van Leeuwen FE, Henry-Amar M, Fiorentino MV, Bell J, Pedersen D, Band P, Assouline D, et al. Leukemia following Hodgkin's disease. N Engl J Med 1990; 322:7–13.

17. Henry-Amar M, Dietrich PY. Acute leukemia after the treatment of Hodgkin's disease. Hematol Oncol Clin North Am 1993; 7:369–387.

18. Reimer RR, Hoover R, Fraumeni JF Jr, Young RC. Acute-leukemia after alkylating-agent therapy of ovarian cancer. N Engl J Med 1977; 297:177–181.

19. Greene MH, Boice JD Jr, Greer BE, Blessing JA, Dembo AJ. Acute nonlymphocytic leukemia after therapy with alkylating agents for ovarian cancer: a study of five randomized clinical trials. N Engl J Med 1982; 307:1416–1421.

20. Greene MH, Young RC, Merrill JM, DeVita VT. Evidence of a treatment dose response in acute nonlymphocytic leukemias which occur after therapy of non-Hodgkin's lymphoma. Cancer Res 1983; 43:1891–1898.

21. Fisher B, Rockette H, Fisher ER, Wickerham DL, Redmond C, Brown A. Leukemia in breast cancer patients following adjuvant chemotherapy or postoperative radiation: the NSABP experience. J Clin Oncol 1985; 3:1640–1658.

22. Greene MH, Boice JD Jr, Strike TA. Carmustine as a cause of acute nonlymphocytic leukemia. N Engl J Med 1985; 313:579.

23. Pedersen-Bjergaard J, Ersboll J, Sorensen HM, Keiding N, Larsen SO, Philip P, Larsen MS, Schultz H, Nissen NI. Risk of acute nonlymphocytic leukemia and preleukemia in patients treated with cyclophosphamide for non-Hodgkin's lymphomas. Comparison with results obtained in patients treated for Hodgkin's disease and ovarian carcinoma with other alkylating agents. Ann Intern Med 1985; 103: 195–200.

24. Greene MH, Harris EL, Gershenson DM, Malkasian GD Jr, Melton LJ, Dembo AJ, Bennett JM, Moloney WC, Boice JD Jr. Melphalan may be a more potent leukemogen than cyclophosphamide. Ann Intern Med 1986; 105:360–367.

25. Coleman MP, Bell CM, Fraser P. Second primary malignancy after Hodgkin's disease, ovarian cancer and cancer of the testis: a population-based cohort study. Br J Cancer 1987; 56:349–355.

26. Kaldor JM, Day NE, Band P, Choi NW, Clarke EA, Coleman MP, Hakama M, Koch M, Langmark F, Neal FE, et al. Second malignancies following testicular

cancer, ovarian cancer and Hodgkin's disease: an international collaborative study among cancer registries. Int J Cancer 1987; 39:571–585.

27. Tucker MA, Meadows AT, Boice JD Jr, Stovall M, Oberlin O, Stone BJ, Birch J, Voute PA, Hoover RN, Fraumeni JF Jr. Leukemia after therapy with alkylating agents for childhood cancer. J Natl Cancer Inst 1987; 78:459–464.

28. Valagussa P, Tancini G, Bonadonna G. Second malignancies after CMF for resectable breast cancer. J Clin Oncol 1987; 5:1138–1142.

29. Curtis RE, Boice JD Jr, Stovall M, Flannery JT, Moloney WC. Leukemia risk following radiotherapy for breast cancer. J Clin Oncol 1989; 7:21–29.

30. Falkson G, Gelman RS, Dreicer R, Tormey DC, Alberts AS, Coccia-Portugal MA, Rushing D, Bennett JM. Myelodysplastic syndrome and acute nonlymphocytic leukemia secondary to mitolactol treatment in patients with breast cancer. J Clin Oncol 1989; 7:1252–1259.

31. Curtis RE, Boice JD Jr, Moloney WC, Ries LG, Flannery JT. Leukemia following chemotherapy for breast cancer. Cancer Res 1990; 50:2741–2746.

32. Curtis RE, Boice JD Jr, Stovall M, Bernstein L, Greenberg RS, Flannery JT, Schwartz AG, Weyer P, Moloney WC, Hoover RN. Risk of leukemia after chemotherapy and radiation treatment for breast cancer. N Engl J Med 1992; 326:1745–1751.

33. Xue Y, Lu D, Guo Y, Lin B. Specific chromosomal translocations and therapy-related leukemia induced by bimolane therapy for psoriasis. Leuk Res 1992; 16: 1113–1123.

34. Zhang MH, Wang XY, Gao LS. [140 cases of acute leukemia caused by bimolane]. Zhonghua Nei Ke Za Zhi 1993; 32:668–672.

35. Rowley JD, Olney H. The relationship of prior therapy to balanced translocations in treatment-related leukemia and myelodysplasia. International Workshop on the Relationship of Prior Therapy to Balanced Chromosome Abberations in Therapy-Related Myelodysplastic Syndromes and Acute Leukemia: Overview Report. Genes, Chromosomes and Cancer 2002; 33: in press.

36. Gerson SL. Molecular epidemiology of therapy-related leukemias. Curr Opin Oncol 1993; 5:136–144.

37. Little JB. Cellular, molecular, and carcinogenic effects of radiation. Hematol Oncol Clin North Am 1993; 7:337–352.

38. Neuman WL, Rubin CM, Rios RB, Larson RA, Le Beau MM, Rowley JD, Vardiman JW, Schwartz JL, Farber RA. Chromosomal loss and deletion are the most common mechanisms for loss of heterozygosity from chromosomes 5 and 7 in malignant myeloid disorders. Blood 1992; 79:1501–1510.

39. Pedersen-Bjergaard J, Janssen WG, Lyons J, Philip P, Bartram CR. Point mutation of the ras protooncogenes and chromosome aberrations in acute nonlymphocytic leukemia and preleukemia related to therapy with alkylating agents. Cancer Res 1988; 48:1812–1817.

40. Le Beau MM, Espinosa R III, Davis EM, Eisenbart JD, Larson RA, Green ED. Cytogenetic and molecular delineation of a region of chromosome 7 commonly deleted in malignant myeloid diseases. Blood 1996; 88:1930–1935.

41. Zhao N, Stoffel A, Wang PW, Eisenbart JD, Espinosa R III, Larson RA, Le Beau MM. Molecular delineation of the smallest commonly deleted region of chromo-

some 5 in malignant myeloid diseases to 1–1.5 Mb and preparation of a PAC-based physical map. Proc Natl Acad Sci USA 1997; 94:6948–69531.

42. Pui CH, Raimondi SC, Behm FG, Ochs J, Furman WL, Bunin NJ, Ribeiro RC, Tinsley PA, Mirro J. Shifts in blast cell phenotype and karyotype at relapse of childhood lymphoblastic leukemia [published erratum appears in Blood 1987; 69: 996]. Blood 1986; 68:1306–1310.

43. Ratain MJ, Kaminer LS, Bitran JD, Larson RA, Le Beau MM, Skosey C, Purl S, Hoffman PC, Wade J, Vardiman JW, et al. Acute nonlymphocytic leukemia following etoposide and cisplatin combination chemotherapy for advanced non-small-cell carcinoma of the lung. Blood 1987; 70:1412–1417.

44. Pedersen-Bjergaard J, Philip P, Ravn V, Hansen SW, Nissen NI. Therapy-related acute nonlymphocytic leukemia of FAB type M4 or M5 with early onset and t(9;11) (p21;q23) or a normal karyotype: a separate entity? J Clin Oncol 1988; 6:395–397.

45. Pui CH, Behm FG, Raimondi SC, Dodge RK, George SL, Rivera GK, Mirro J Jr, Kalwinsky DK, Dahl GV, Murphy SB. Secondary acute myeloid leukemia in children treated for acute lymphoid leukemia. N Engl J Med 1989; 321:136–142.

46. Pedersen-Bjergaard J, Philip P. Balanced translocations involving chromosome bands 11q23 and 21q22 are highly characteristic of myelodysplasia and leukemia following therapy with cytostatic agents targeting at DNA-topoisomerase II. Blood 1991; 78:1147–1148.

47. Pedersen-Bjergaard J, Philip P. Two different classes of therapy-related and de-novo acute myeloid leukemia? Cancer Genet Cytogenet 1991; 55:119–124.

48. Pui CH, Ribeiro RC, Hancock ML, Rivera GK, Evans WE, Raimondi SC, Head DR, Behm FG, Mahmoud MH, Sandlund JT, et al. Acute myeloid leukemia in children treated with epipodophyllotoxins for acute lymphoblastic leukemia. N Engl J Med 1991; 325:1682–1687.

49. Larson RA, Le Beau MM, Ratain MJ, Rowley JD. Balanced translocations involving chromosome bands 11q23 and 21q22 in therapy-related leukemia. Blood 1992; 79:1892–1893.

50. Pedersen-Bjergaard J, Sigsgaard TC, Nielsen D, Gjedde SB, Philip P, Hansen M, Larsen SO, Rorth M, Mouridsen H, Dombernowsky P. Acute monocytic or myelomonocytic leukemia with balanced chromosome translocations to band 11q23 after therapy with 4-epi-doxorubicin and cisplatin or cyclophosphamide for breast cancer (see comments). J Clin Oncol 1992; 10:1444–1451.

51. Ratain MJ, Rowley JD. Therapy-related acute myeloid leukemia secondary to inhibitors of topoisomerase II: from the bedside to the target genes. Ann Oncol 1992; 3:107–111.

52. Quesnel B, Kantarjian H, Bjergaard JP, Brault P, Estey E, Lai JL, Tilly H, Stoppa AM, Archimbaud E, Harousseau JL, et al. Therapy-related acute myeloid leukemia with t(8;21), inv(16), and t(8;16): a report on 25 cases and review of the literature. J Clin Oncol 1993; 11:2370–2379.

53. Pedersen-Bjergaard J, Johansson B, Philip P. Translocation (3;21)(q26;q22) in therapy-related myelodysplasia following drugs targeting DNA-topoisomerase II combined with alkylating agents, and in myeloproliferative disorders undergoing spontaneous leukemic transformation. Cancer Genet Cytogenet 1994; 76:50–55.

54. Pedersen-Bjergaard J, Rowley JD. The balanced and the unbalanced chromosome

aberrations of acute myeloid leukemia may develop in different ways and may contribute differently to malignant transformation. Blood 1994; 83:2780–2786.

55. Andersen MK, Johansson B, Larsen SO, Pedersen-Bjergaard J. Chromosomal abnormalities in secondary MDS and AML. Relationship to drugs and radiation with specific emphasis on the balanced rearrangements. Haematologica 1998; 83:483–488.

56. McCabe NR, Burnett RC, Gill HG, Thirman MJ, Mbangkollo D, Kipiniak M, van Melle E, Ziemin-van der Poel S, Rowley JD, Diaz MO. Cloning of cDNAs of the MLL gene that detect DNA rearrangements and altered RNA transcripts in human leukemic cells with 11q23 translocations. Proc Natl Acad Sci USA 1992; 89: 11794–11798.

57. Turker A, Guler N. Therapy related acute myeloid leukemia after exposure to 5-fluorouracil: a case report. Hematol Cell Ther 1999; 41:195–196.

58. Saitoh T, Morimoto K, Kumagai T, Saiki M, Tanaka M, Aikawa S, Tsuboi I, Sawada U, Horie T. Therapy-related megakaryoblastic leukemia with pituitary involvement following treatment for non-Hodgkin's lymphoma. Intern Med 1999; 38:904–909.

59. Nagai M, Bandoh S, Tasaka T, Fujita M, Yamauchi A, Kuwabara H, Funamoto Y, Yamaoka G, Takahara J. Secondary myeloid/natural killer cell precursor acute leukemia following essential thrombocythemia. Hum Pathol 1999; 30:868–871.

60. Zompi S, Legrand O, Bouscary D, Blanc CM, Picard F, Casadevall N, Dreyfus F, Marie JP, Viguie F. Therapy-related acute myeloid leukaemia after successful therapy for acute promyelocytic leukaemia with t(15;17): a report of two cases and a review of the literature. Br J Haematol 2000; 110:610–613.

61. Kudo K, Yoshida H, Kiyoi H, Numata S, Horibe K, Naoe T. Etoposide-related acute promyelocytic leukemia. Leukemia 1998; 12:1171–1175.

62. Naoe T, Kudo K, Yoshida H, Horibe K, Ohno R. Molecular analysis of the t(15; 17) translocation in de novo and secondary acute promyelocytic leukemia. Leukemia 1997; 11(suppl 3):287–288.

63. Secker-Walker LM, Stewart EL, Todd A. Acute lymphoblastic leukaemia with t(4; 11) follows neuroblastoma: a late effect of treatment? Med Pediatr Oncol 1985; 13:48–50.

64. Archimbaud E, Charrin C, Guyotat D, Magaud JP, Gentilhomme O, Fiere D. Acute leukaemia with t(4;11) in patients previously exposed to carcinogens. Br J Haematol 1988; 69:467–470.

65. Hunger SP, Tkachuk DC, Amylon MD, Link MP, Carroll AJ, Welborn JL, Willman CL, Cleary ML. HRX involvement in de novo and secondary leukemias with diverse chromosome 11q23 abnormalities. Blood 1993; 81:3197–3203.

66. Jonveaux P, Hillion J, Bernard O, Le Coniat M, Derre J, Flexor M, Larsen CJ, Berger R. Distinct MLL gene rearrangements associated with successive acute monocytic and lymphoblastic leukemias in the same patient. Leukemia 1994; 8: 2224–2227.

67. Larson RA, Wang Y, Banerjee M, Wiemels J, Hartford C, Le Beau MM, Smith MT. Prevalence of the inactivating $609^{C \to T}$ polymorphism in the NAD(P)H:quinone oxidoreductase (NQO1) gene in patients with primary and therapy-related myeloid leukemia. Blood 1999; 94:803–807.

68. Naoe T, Takeyama K, Yokozawa T, Kiyoi H, Seto M, Uike N, Ino T, Utsunomiya A, Maruta A, Jin-nai I, Kamada N, Kubota Y, Nakamura H, Shimazaki C, Horiike S, Kodera Y, Saito H, Ueda R, Wiemels J, Ohno R. Analysis of genetic polymorphism in NQO1, GST-M1, GST-T1, and CYP3A4 in 469 Japanese patients with therapy-related leukemia/ myelodysplastic syndrome and de novo acute myeloid leukemia. Clin Cancer Res 2000; 6:4091–4095.

69. Wiemels JL, Pagnamenta A, Taylor GM, Eden OB, Alexander FE, Greaves MF. United Kingdom Childhood Cancer Study Investigators. A lack of a functional NAD(P)H:quinone oxidoreductase allele is selectively associated with pediatric leukemias that have MLL fusions. Cancer Res 1999; 59:4095–4099.

70. Felix CA, Walker AH, Lange BJ, Williams TM, Winick NJ, Cheung NK, Lovett BD, Nowell PC, Blair IA, Rebbeck TR. Association of CYP3A4 genotype with treatment-related leukemia. Proc Natl Acad Sci USA 1998; 95:13176–13181.

71. Nagai M, Fujita M, Ikeda T, Ohmori M, Kuwabara H, Yamaoka G, Tanaka K, Kamada N, Taniwaki M, Inoue T, Irino S, Takahara J. Alterations of p53 and Rb genes in a novel human GM-CSF-dependent myeloid cell line (OHN-GM) established from therapy-related leukaemia. Br J Haematol 1997; 98:392–398.

72. Panizo C, Patino A, Calasanz MJ, Rifon J, Sierrasesumaga L, Rocha E. Emergence of secondary acute leukemia in a patient treated for osteosarcoma: implications of germline TP53 mutations. Med Pediatr Oncol 1998; 30:165–169.

73. Ben-Yehuda D, Krichevsky S, Caspi O, Rund D, Polliack A, Abeliovich D, Zelig O, Yahalom V, Paltiel O, Or R, Peretz T, Ben-Neriah S, Yehuda O, Rachmilewitz EA. Microsatellite instability and p53 mutations in therapy-related leukemia suggest mutator phenotype. Blood 1996; 88:4296–4303.

74. Damiani D, Michieli M, Ermacora A, Candoni A, Raspadori D, Geromin A, Stocchi R, Grimaz S, Masolini P, Michelutti A, Scheper RJ, Baccarani M. P-glycoprotein (PGP), and not lung resistance-related protein (LRP), is a negative prognostic factor in secondary leukemias. Haematologica 1998; 83:290–297.

75. Meadows AT, Baum E, Fossati-Bellani F, Green D, Jenkin RD, Marsden B, Nesbit M, Newton W, Oberlin O, Sallan SG, et al. Second malignant neoplasms in children: an update from the Late Effects Study Group. J Clin Oncol 1985; 3:532–538.

76. Henry-Amar M, Aeppli DM, Anderson J, et al. Section Workshop statistical report. Part IX: Study of second cancer risk. In: Treatment Strategy in Hodgkin's disease. Colloque Inserm. London: Inserm/John Libbey Eurotext, 1990:355.

77. Andre M, Henry-Amar M, Blaise D, Colombat P, Fleury J, Milpied N, Cahn JY, Pico JL, Bastion Y, Kuentz M, Nedellec G, Attal M, Ferme C, Gisselbrecht C. Treatment-related deaths and second cancer risk after autologous stem-cell transplantation for Hodgkin's disease. Blood 1998; 92:1933–1940.

78. Harrison CN, Gregory W, Hudson GV, Devereux S, Goldstone AH, Hancock B, Winfield D, MacMillan AK, Hoskin P, Newland AC, Milligan D, Linch DC. High-dose BEAM chemotherapy with autologous haemopoietic stem cell transplantation for Hodgkin's disease is unlikely to be associated with a major increased risk of secondary MDS/AML. Br J Cancer 1999; 81:476–483.

79. Travis LB, Curtis RE, Stovall M, Holowaty EJ, van Leeuwen FE, Glimelius B, Lynch CF, Hagenbeek A, Li CY, Banks PM, et al. Risk of leukemia following

treatment for non-Hodgkin's lymphoma. J Natl Cancer Inst 1994; 86:1450–1457.

80. Ingram L, Mott MG, Mann JR, Raafat F, Darbyshire PJ, Morris Jones PH. Second malignancies in children treated for non-Hodgkin's lymphoma and T-cell leukaemia with the UKCCSG regimens. Br J Cancer 1987; 55:463–466.

81. Lavey RS, Eby NL, Prosnitz LR. Impact on second malignancy risk of the combined use of radiation and chemotherapy for lymphomas. Cancer 1990; 66:80–88.

82. Pui CH. Therapy-related myeloid leukaemia. Lancet 1990; 336:1130–1131.

83. The Finnish Leukaemia Group. Acute leukaemia and other secondary neoplasms in patients treated with conventional chemotherapy for multiple myeloma: a Finnish Leukaemia Group study. Eur J Haematol 2000; 65:123–127.

84. Abrams J, Smith M. Acute myeloid leukemia following doxorubicin and cyclophosphamide: increased risk for dose-intensive regimens? Physician Data Query, 1994.

85. Tallman MS, Gray R, Bennett JM, Variakojis D, Robert N, Wood WC, Rowe JM, Wiernik PH. Leukemogenic potential of adjuvant chemotherapy for early-stage breast cancer: the Eastern Cooperative Oncology Group experience. J Clin Oncol 1995; 13:1557–1563.

86. Carli PM, Sgro C, Parchin-Geneste N, Isambert N, Mugneret F, Girodon F, Maynadie M. Increased therapy-related leukemia secondary to breast cancer. Leukemia 2000; 14:1014–1017.

87. Chaplain G, Milan C, Sgro C, Carli PM, Bonithon-Kopp C. Increased risk of acute leukemia after adjuvant chemotherapy for breast cancer: a population-based study. J Clin Oncol 2000; 18:2836–2842.

88. Linassier C, Barin C, Calais G, Letortorec S, Bremond JL, Delain M, Petit A, Georget MT, Cartron G, Raban N, Benboubker L, Leloup R, Binet C, Lamagnere JP, Colombat P. Early secondary acute myelogenous leukemia in breast cancer patients after treatment with mitoxantrone, cyclophosphamide, fluorouracil and radiation therapy. Ann Oncol 2000; 11:1289–1294.

89. Yagita M, Ieki Y, Onishi R, Huang CL, Adachi M, Horiike S, Konaka Y, Taki T, Miyake M. Therapy-related leukemia and myelodysplasia following oral administration of etoposide for recurrent breast cancer. Int J Oncol 1998; 13:91–96.

90. Pedersen-Bjergaard J, Daugaard G, Hansen SW, Philip P, Larsen SO, Rorth M. Increased risk of myelodysplasia and leukaemia after etoposide, cisplatin, and bleomycin for germ-cell tumours. Lancet 1991; 338:359–363.

91. Schneider DT, Hilgenfeld E, Schwabe D, Behnisch W, Zoubek A, Wessalowski R, Gobel U. Acute myelogenous leukemia after treatment for malignant germ cell tumors in children. J Clin Oncol 1999; 17:3226–3233.

92. Kollmannsberger C, Kuzcyk M, Mayer F, Hartmann JT, Kanz L, Bokemeyer C. Late toxicity following curative treatment of testicular cancer. Semin Surg Oncol 1999; 17:275–281.

93. Rodriguez-Galindo C, Poquette CA, Marina NM, Head DR, Cain A, Meyer WH, Santana VM, Pappo AS. Hematologic abnormalities and acute myeloid leukemia in children and adolescents administered intensified chemotherapy for the Ewing sarcoma family of tumors. J Pediatr Hematol Oncol 2000; 22:321–329.

94. Pedersen-Bjergaard J, Andersen MK, Christiansen DH. Therapy-related acute my-eloid leukemia and myelodysplasia after high-dose chemotherapy and autologous stem cell transplantation. Blood 2000; 95:3273–3279.

95. Darrington DL, Vose JM, Anderson JR, Bierman PJ, Bishop MR, Chan WC, Morris ME, Reed EC, Sanger WG, Tarantolo SR, et al. Incidence and characterization of secondary myelodysplastic syndrome and acute myelogenous leukemia following high-dose chemoradiotherapy and autologous stem-cell transplantation for lymphoid malignancies. J Clin Oncol 1994; 12:2527–2534.

96. Bhatia S, Ramsay NK, Steinbuch M, Dusenbery KE, Shapiro RS, Weisdorf DJ, Robison LL, Miller JS, Neglia JP. Malignant neoplasms following bone marrow transplantation. Blood 1996; 87:3633–3639.

97. Stone RM, Neuberg D, Soiffer R, Takvorian T, Whelan M, Rabinowe SN, Aster JC, Leavitt P, Mauch P, Freedman AS, et al. Myelodysplastic syndrome as a late complication following autologous bone marrow transplantation for non-Hodgkin's lymphoma. J Clin Oncol 1994; 12:2535–2542.

98. Govindarajan R, Jagannath S, Flick JT, Vesole DH, Sawyer J, Barlogie B, Tricot G. Preceding standard therapy is the likely cause of MDS after autotransplants for multiple myeloma. Br J Haematol 1996; 95:349–353.

99. Milligan DW, Ruiz De Elvira MC, Kolb HJ, Goldstone AH, Meloni G, Rohatiner AZ, Colombat P, Schmitz N. Secondary leukaemia and myelodysplasia after auto-grafting for lymphoma: results from the EBMT. EBMT Lymphoma and Late Effects Working Parties. European Group for Blood and Marrow Transplantation. Br J Haematol 1999; 106:1020–1026.

100. Pedersen-Bjergaard J, Pedersen M, Myhre J, Geisler C. High risk of therapy-related leukemia after BEAM chemotherapy and autologous stem cell transplantation for previously treated lymphomas is mainly related to primary chemotherapy and not to the BEAM-transplantation procedure. Leukemia 1997; 11:1654–1660.

101. Miller JS, Arthur DC, Litz CE, Neglia JP, Miller WJ, Weisdorf DJ. Myelodysplastic syndrome after autologous bone marrow transplantation: an additional late complication of curative cancer therapy. Blood 1994; 83:3780–3786.

102. Krishnan A, Bhatia S, Slovak ML, Arber DA, Niland JC, Nademanee A, Fung H, Bhatia R, Kashyap A, Molina A, O'Donnell MR, Parker PA, Sniecinski I, Snyder DS, Spielberger R, Stein A, Forman SJ. Predictors of therapy-related leukemia and myelodysplasia following autologous transplantation for lymphoma: an assessment of risk factors. Blood 2000; 95:1588–1593.

103. Micallef IN, Lillington DM, Apostolidis J, Amess JA, Neat M, Matthews J, Clark T, Foran JM, Salam A, Lister TA, Rohatiner AZ. Therapy-related myelodysplasia and secondary acute myelogenous leukemia after high-dose therapy with autologous hematopoietic progenitor-cell support for lymphoid malignancies. J Clin Oncol 2000; 18:947–955.

104. Sobecks RM, Le Beau MM, Anastasi J, Williams SF. Myelodysplasia and acute leukemia following high-dose chemotherapy and autologous bone marrow or peripheral blood stem cell transplantation. Bone Marrow Transplant 1999; 23:1161–1165.

105. Legare RD, Gribben JG, Maragh M, Hermanowski-Vosatka A, Roach S, Tantravahi R, Nadler LM, Gilliland DG. Prediction of therapy-related acute myelogenous leu-

kemia (AML) and myelodysplastic syndrome (MDS) after autologous bone marrow transplant (ABMIT) for lymphoma. Am J Hematol 1997; 56:45–51.

106. Martinez-Climent JA, Comes AM, Vizcarra E, Benet I, Arbona C, Prosper F, Solano C, Garcia Clavel B, Marugan I, Lluch A, Garcia-Conde J. Chromosomal abnormalities in women with breast cancer after autologous stem cell transplantation are infrequent and may not predict development of therapy-related leukemia or myelodysplastic syndrome. Bone Marrow Transplant 2000; 25:1203–1208.

107. Takeyama K, Seto M, Uike N, Hamajima N, Ino T, Mikuni C, Kobayashi T, Maruta A, Muto Y, Maseki N, Sakamaki H, Saitoh H, Shimoyama M, Ueda R. Therapy-related leukemia and myelodysplastic syndrome: a large-scale Japanese study of clinical and cytogenetic features as well as prognostic factors. Int J Hematol 2000; 71:144–152.

108. Andersen MK, Larson RA, Mauritzson N, Schnittger S, Jhanwar SC, Pedersen-Bjergaard J. Balanced Chromosome Abnormalities inv(16) and t(15;17) in Therapy-related Myelodysplastic Syndromes and Acute Leukemia: Report from an International Workshop. Genes, Chromosomes and Cancer 2002; 33: in press.

109. Molldrem JJ, Caples M, Mavroudis D, Plante M, Young NS, Barrett AJ. Antithymocyte globulin for patients with myeloablative syndrome. Br J Haematol 1997; 99:699–705.

110. Vadhan-Raj S, Broxmeyer HE, Spitzer G, LeMaistre A, Hultman S, Ventura G, Tigaud JD, Cork MA, Trujillo JM, Gutterman JU, et al. Stimulation of nonclonal hematopoiesis and suppression of the neoplastic clone after treatment with recombinant human granulocyte-macrophage colony-stimulating factor in a patient with therapy-related myelodysplastic syndrome. Blood 1989; 74:1491–1498.

111. Gradishar WJ, Le Beau MM, O'Laughlin R, Vardiman JW, Larson RA. Clinical and cytogenetic responses to granulocyte-macrophage colony-stimulating factor in therapy-related myelodysplasia. Blood 1992; 80:2463–2470.

112. Bessho M, Itoh Y, Kataumi S, Kawai N, Matsuda A, Jinnai I, Saitoh M, Hirashima K, Minamihisamatsu M. A hematological remission by clonal hematopoiesis after treatment with recombinant human granulocyte-macrophage colony-stimulating factor and erythropoietin in a patient with therapy-related myelodysplastic syndrome. Leuk Res 1992; 16:123–131.

113. Kantarjian HM, Estey EH, Keating MJ. Treatment of therapy-related leukemia and myelodysplastic syndrome. Hematol Oncol Clin North Am 1993; 7:81–107.

114. Preisler HD, Early AP, Raza A, Vlahides G, Marinello MJ, Stein AM, Browman G. Therapy of secondary acute nonlymphocytic leukemia with cytarabine. N Engl J Med 1983; 308:21–23.

115. Vaughan WP, Karp JE, Burke PJ. Effective chemotherapy of acute myelocytic leukemia occurring after alkylating agent or radiation therapy for prior malignancy. J Clin Oncol 1983; 1:204–207.

116. Duane SF, Peterson BA, Bloomfield CD, Michels SD, Hurd DD. Response of therapy-associated acute nonlymphocytic leukemia to intensive induction chemotherapy. Med Pediatr Oncol 1985; 13:207–213.

117. Kantarjian HM, Keating MJ, Walters RS, Smith TL, Cork A, McCredie KB, Freireich EJ. Therapy-related leukemia and myelodysplastic syndrome: clinical, cytogenetic, and prognostic features. J Clin Oncol 1986; 4:1748–1757.

118. Larson RA, Wernli M, Le Beau MM, Daly KM, Pape LH, Rowley JD, Vardiman JW. Short remission durations in therapy-related leukemia despite cytogenetic complete responses to high-dose cytarabine. Blood 1988; 72:1333–1339.

119. Hoyle CF, de Bastos M, Wheatley K, Sherrington PD, Fischer PJ, Rees JK, Gray R, Hayhoe FG. AML associated with previous cytotoxic therapy, MDS or myeloproliferative disorders: results from the MRC's 9th AML trial. Br J Haematol 1989; 72:45–53.

120. De Witte T, Muus P, De Pauw B, Haanen C. Intensive antileukemic treatment of patients younger than 65 years with myelodysplastic syndromes and secondary acute myelogenous leukemia. Cancer 1990; 66:831–837.

121. Ballen KK, Antin JH. Treatment of therapy-related acute myelogenous leukemia and myelodysplastic syndromes. Hematol Oncol Clin North Am 1993; 7:477–493.

122. Fenaux P, Jouet JP, Bauters F, Lai JL, Lepelley P. Translocation t(9;11)(p21;q23) with acute myelomonocytic leukemia after chemotherapy for osteosarcoma: good response to antileukemic drugs. J Clin Oncol 1987; 5:1304–1305.

123. Samuels BL, Larson RA, Le Beau MM, Daly KM, Bitter MA, Vardiman JW, Barker CM, Rowley JD, Golomb HM. Specific chromosomal abnormalities in acute nonlymphocytic leukemia correlate with drug susceptibility in vivo. Leukemia 1988; 2:79–83.

124. Cortes J et al. Abnormalities in the long arm of chromosome 11 (11q) in patients with de novo and secondary acute myelogenous leukemias and myelodysplastic syndromes. Leukemia 1994; 8:2174–2178.

125. Gardin C et al. Intensive chemotherapy with idarubicin, cytosine arabinoside, and granulocyte colony-stimulating factor (G-CSF) in patients with secondary and therapy-related myelogenous leukemia. Leukemia 1997; 11:16–21.

126. Anderson JE et al. Stem cell transplantation for secondary acute myeloid leukemia: evaluation of transplantation as initial therapy or following induction chemotherapy. Blood 1997; 89:2578–2585.

127. Yakoub-Agha I et al. Allogenic bone marrow transplantation for therapy-related myelodysplastic syndrome and acute myeloid leukemia: a long-term study of 70 patients-report of the French society of bone marrow transplantation. J Clin Oncol 2000; 18:963–971.

128. Hale GA et al. Bone marrow transplantation for therapy-induced acute myeloid leukemia in children with previous lymphoid malignancies. Bone Marrow Transplant 1999; 24:735–739.

129. Cesaro S et al. Successful treatment of secondary acute myeloid leukemia relapsing after allogeneic bone marrow transplantation with donor lymphocyte infusion failed to prevent recurrence of primary disease: a case report. Bone Marrow Transplant 1999; 23:625–628.

130. Pedersen-Bjergaard J et al. Acute nonlymphocytic leukemia, preleukemia, and acute myeloproliferative syndrome secondary to treatment of other malignant diseases. II. Bone marrow cytology, cytogenetics, results of HLA typing, response to antileukemic chemotherapy, and survival of a total series of 55 patients. Cancer 1984; 54:452–462.

131. Bennett JM et al. Acute myeloid leukemia and other myelopathic disorders following treatment with alkylating agents. Hematol Pathol 1987; 1:99–104.

132. Fourth International Workshop on Chromosomes in Leukemia (1982). Secondary leukemias associated with neoplasia: treated and untreated. Cancer Genet Cytogenet 1984; 11:319–321.

133. Le Beau MM et al. Clinical and cytogenetic correlations in 63 patients with therapy-related myelodysplastic syndromes and acute nonlymphocytic leukemia: further evidence for characteristic abnormalities of chromosomes no. 5 and 7. J Clin Oncol 1986; 4:325–345.

134. Michels SD et al. Therapy-related acute myeloid leukemia and myelodysplastic syndrome: a clinical and morphologic study of 65 cases. Blood 1985; 65:1364–1372.

135. Iurlo A et al. Cytogenetic and clinical investigations in 76 cases with therapy-related leukemia and myelodysplastic syndrome. Cancer Genet Cytogenet 1989; 43:227–241.

136. Traweek ST et al. Clonal karyotypic hematopoietic cell abnormalities occurring after autologous bone marrow transplantation for Hodgkin's disease and non-Hodgkin's lymphoma. Blood 1994; 84:957–963.

137. Friedberg JW et al. Outcome in patients with myeloplastic syndrome after autologous bone marrow transplantation for non-Hodgkin's lymphoma. J Clin Oncol 1999; 17:3128–3135.

138. Wheeler C et al. Low incidence of post-transplant myelodysplasia/acute leukemia (MDS/AML) in NHL patients autotranspanted after cyclophosphamide, carmustine and etoposide (Abstract). Blood 1997; 90:385b.

139. Taylor PRA et al. Low incidence of myelodysplastic syndrome following transplantation using autologous non-cryopreserved bone marrow. Leukemia 1997; 11: 1650–1653.

140. Laughlin MJ et al. Secondary myelodysplasia and acute leukemia in breast cancer patients after autologous bone marrow transplant. J Clin Oncol 1998; 16:1008–1012.

141. Sargur M et al. Marrow transplantation for acute nonlymphocytic leukemia following therapy for Hodgkin's disease. J Clin Oncol 1987; 5:731–734.

142. Bunin NJ et al. Partially matched bone marrow transplantation in patients with myelodysplastic syndromes. J Clin Oncol 1988; 6:1851–1855.

143. Appelbaum FR et al. Bone marrow transplantation for patients with myelodysplasia. Pretreatment variables and outcome. Ann Intern Med 1990; 112:590–597.

144. Geller RB et al. Successful marrow transplantation for acute myelocytic leukemia following therapy for Hodgkin's disease. J Clin Oncol 1988; 6:1558–1561.

145. Longmore G et al. Bone marrow transplantation for myelodysplasia and secondary acute nonlymphoblastic leukemia. J Clin Oncol 1990; 8:1707–1714.

146. De Witte T et al. Allogeneic bone marrow transplantation for secondary leukaemia and myelodysplastic syndrome: a survey by the Leukaemia Working Party of the European Bone Marrow Transplantation Group (EBMTG). Br J Haematol 1990; 74:151–155.

# 8
# The Role of Apoptosis in the Myelodysplastic Syndromes

**Yataro Yoshida**
*Takeda General Hospital, Kyoto, Japan*

## I. INTRODUCTION

The myelodysplastic syndromes (MDS) are a heterogeneous group of clonal hematopoietic disorders with unfavorable prognosis due to complications of cytopenias or because of transformation into acute myeloid leukemia (AML) (1,2). Cells of all three hematopoietic lineages show quantitative and qualitative abnormalities. Morphological dysplasia, impaired differentiation, and defective cellular functions as well as genetic instability are the fundamental abnormalities shared by the MDS clone. Conceivably, these abnormalities represent different facets of the abnormal clone. The precise etiology of primary MDS remains unknown, but it is believed to result from transformation at the level of the pluripotent hematopoietic stem cells (1).

The paradox of peripheral cytopenias in the presence of normo- or hypercellular marrow has in the past been accounted for by ineffective hematopoiesis. Excessive apoptosis may, in fact, be the explanation (3). Further contributing to the complexity, the increased levels of apoptosis that occur in early stages of MDS may decline as MDS progress toward the leukemic stage (4). Apoptosis has been the subject of numerous studies and reviews (5,6) and the results of these studies have generally supported these hypotheses. The role of apoptosis in MDS is discussed in this chapter, with specific focus on the detection of apoptosis in clinical samples and the possible mechanisms leading to apoptosis in this group of enigmatic diseases.

## II. APOPTOSIS AND ITS DETECTION

Apoptosis is a metabolically active cellular process. Tissue and cell expansion or renewal results from cell elimination and proliferation. Physiological elimination of cells is due to apoptosis, where the cell triggers a genetic program that induces enzyme and antigen expression leading to its death. Apoptosis is characterized morphologically by chromatin condensation, DNA oligomeric changes, nuclear disintegration, and cell shrinkage followed by the formation of membrane-bound apoptotic bodies. In contrast to necrosis, apoptotic cells have specific low-molecular-weight oligomeric DNA fragmentation patterns and do not induce an inflammatory response, but apoptotic cells are targets of phagocytosis by adjacent macrophages. Apoptosis is governed by a number of genes whose protein products act as either inducers or repressors of apoptosis. Proapoptotic genes include *c-myc*, *p53*, *tumor necrosis-factor-α* (*TNF-α*) *receptor* (*TNFR*), and *fas*. Antiapoptotic genes include *bcl-2*, *bcl-x*, *c-abl*, and *ras*.

Most of these apoptosis-related genes have been identified with homologs between species indicating a highly conserved nature of apoptosis throughout evolution. Bcl-2 is the prototype member of a family of over a dozen proteins encoded by species from mammals to nematodes. The antiapoptotic members of this family are Bcl-2, Bcl-$X_L$, and Mcl-1, while the death-promoting, proapoptotic members of the family include Bax, Bcl-$X_S$, Bad, Bak, Bik, and Bid. The Bcl-2 family of proteins function as homodimers or heterodimers and it is the ratio of the anti- versus proapoptotic proteins that determines the cellular susceptibility to death signals. Thus, they act as gatekeepers for a variety of apoptotic signals.

The final execution step of apoptosis is caused by the activation of a family of cysteine proteases known as caspases, the effector molecules of apoptosis. Caspases are present as inactive proenzymes and, when activated, cleave and activate each other in a cascade-like fashion (caspase cascade). Through their cleavage of a number of intracellular cytoskelton, nuclear, and cytoplasmic proteins, most of the morphological and biochemical events associated with apoptosis ensue.

### A.  Morphological Methods

Light or electron microscopic examination can detect apoptosis-related morphological changes. However, these morphological methods are of limited value, except perhaps for studies of cultured cells. These methods detect apoptosis only after cells show fully developed apoptotic changes.

### B.  Biochemical Methods

Internucleosomal DNA fragmentation, resulting in ladder-like fragments, is visualized by conventional DNA electrophoresis and is the biochemical hallmark of apoptosis. As such, DNA laddering is frequently used as biochemical evidence of apoptosis in tissue culture, but is rarely seen in clinical samples. DNA laddering is likely to be seen only when substantial numbers of cells are apoptotic.

## C. In Situ Method

The free 3' DNA ends generated by the endogenous nuclease can be labeled by the use of exogenous DNA-modifying enzymes. There are two slightly different end-labeling methods: the TdT-mediated dUTP-biotin nick end labeling (TUNEL) method uses specific TdT-mediated binding of UTP to the 3'-OH ends, while the in situ end-labeling (ISEL) method uses *Escherichia coli* polymerase to incorporate biotinylated dUTP to the DNA ends. Both methods allow for fluorescent microscopic or immunohistochemical detection of the labeled deoxynucleotides (biotinylated, coupled to fluorescein or digoxygenin) that become incorporated into damaged DNA. The advantage of the in situ methods is the sensitivity in detecting cells in relatively early stages of apoptosis, while the major limitation is lack of specificity and difficulty in cellular identification.

## D. Flowcytometric Studies

Flowcytometric analysis allows for the simultaneous identification of cell types and apoptotic markers, including permeability of dyes, DNA hypodiploidy, expression of apoptosis-related protein, and membrane alteration as identified with annexin-V. One advantage is that certain events taking place early in apoptosis can be detected by flowcytometry. They include apoptotic membrane changes, altered expression of apoptosis-related protein, as well as altered mitochondrial membrane potential. Annexin-V binds to phosphatidylserine expressed on the outer membrane of apoptotic cells, and is conceivably another early marker of apoptosis. A second advantage of flowcytometry in apoptosis detection is the rapid evaluation of large numbers of cells. Furthermore, by combining suitable antibodies, flowcytometry allows for simultaneous identification of apoptotic cell types.

## E. General Cautions

Cellular heterogeneity of the bone marrow (BM), the rapid and silent nature of apoptotic processes, and instantaneous engulfment of apoptotic cells by neighboring cells, macrophages in particular, represent major obstacles hampering the clinical investigation. Regardless of the methods, extreme care is needed in minimizing damage to the samples, which are highly vulnerable to various manipulations. In addition, the heterogeneous nature of the disease itself should be taken into consideration.

## III. EVIDENCE FOR APOPTOSIS IN MDS

### A.  Morphological Findings

The initial report on apoptosis having a role in MDS emerged from electron microscopic observation of BM biopsy (7). The proportion of apoptotic cells was significantly higher in the BM of MDS patients than in that of the controls. Similar observations (Table 1) have been made in subsequent works (8,9). Cell types showing apoptotic morphology were myeloid and erythroid cells of varying maturational stages (7–9). Marrow stromal cells showed minimal or no apoptosis. Macrophages engulfing apoptotic cells were commonly seen.

As stated above, electron microscopic study is useful for detection of apoptosis only when cells show typically apoptotic morphology, notably in advanced stages of apoptosis. Despite this limitation, the results of these ultrastructural studies provide a strong argument that excessive intramedullarly apoptosis is associated with MDS. Strangely enough, no comparable light microscopic studies have been reported to date. In fact, apoptosis is not readily seen either in smears or in clot sections of marrow aspirates. However, apoptosis is evident following short-term incubation of the peripheral blood (PB) or BM of the MDS patients (10,11). In these experimental settings, predominant cell types showing apoptosis were neutrophils for PB, and neutrophils and erythroblasts for BM.

### B.  Biochemical Findings

Demonstration of the internucleosomal DNA fragmentation in gel electrophoresis is likewise difficult when it is applied to clinical samples (Table 2). Fragmentation is rarely seen in fresh BM samples, although it becomes visible following short-term incubation (10,12) or by the use of a sensitive radiolabeling method (13). The biochemical method requires a large number of cells to extract sufficient DNA for electrophoresis, and yet DNA laddering may be seen only when substantial numbers of these cells are apoptotic (12,13).

Using a single-step DNA extraction and gel electrophoresis, Tsoplou et al. showed DNA fragmentation in 18 of 53 BM samples from MDS patients (14). It was more commonly seen in "good"-prognosis MDS, subtypes classified as refractory anemia (RA) or refractory anemia with ringed sideroblasts (RARS), than in "poor"-prognosis MDS, subtypes classified as refractory anemia with excess blasts (RAEB), refractory anemia with excess blasts in transformation (RAEB-t), or chronic myelomonocytic leukemia (CMML). Patients with positive DNA laddering had increased marrow cellularity, longer overall survival, and longer period to transformation to AML.

**Table 1** Ultrastructural Studies of Apoptosis in MDS

| | Clark and Lampert [7] | Bogdanovic et al. [8] | Shetty et al. [9] | | |
|---|---|---|---|---|---|
| Samples | Biopsy | Marrow particle | Biopsy and aspirates | | |
| Cases | $N = 21^a$<br>15 RA, 3 RARS<br>3 RAEB, 2 CMML | $N = 30$<br>8 RA, 3 RARS, 14 RAEB<br>2 RAEB-t, 3 CMML | $N = 10$<br>7 RA, 3 RARS | | |
| Controls | $N = 10$ | $N = 12$ | $N = 4$ | | |
| Apoptosis | | | Biopsy[b] | Asp HDF | Asp LDF |
| MDS | 3.57 (0.61–43.6)/mm$^2$ | 3.13% | Score 4 | 27% | 4% |
| Controls | 0.19 (0–0.68)/mm$^2$ | 1.05% | Score 0 | 8.5% | 1.5% |
| Significance | Yes | Yes | | Yes | |
| Cell types | Myeloid and erythroid | Myeloid and erythroid, but not stromal cells | Myeloid and erythroid cells of all stages of maturation | | |
| Notes | No difference in FAB types | High apoptosis in RAEB, low in CMML and RAEB-t | High apoptosis in HDF | | |

[a] Some cases were studied consecutively.
[b] Score 4 represents an intermediate level of ISEL (in situ end labeling) positive cells while Score 0 represents <15% ISEL positive cells.

MDS, myelodysplastic syndromes; $N$, number; RA, refractory anemia; RARS, refractory anemia with ringed sideroblasts; RAEB, refractory anemia with excess blasts; RAEB-t, refractory anemia with excess blasts in transformation; CMML, chronic myelomonocytic leukemia; FAB, French-American-British classification system; Asp, aspirate; HDF, high-density fraction; LDF, low-density fraction.

**Table 2** Formation of DNA Ladder in MDS

|  | Raza et al. [12] | Tsoplou et al. [14] | Bouscary et al. [13] |
|---|---|---|---|
| Fresh or incubation | 4-hr incubation | Fresh | Fresh |
| Cases | N = 6 | N = 51[a] | N = 15 |
|  | 2 RA, 4 RAEB | 9 RA, 10 RARS, 11 RAEB | |
|  |  | 8 RAEB-t, 15 CMML | |
| Controls |  | N = 12 | |
| Positive ladder |  |  | |
| MDS | MDS 4/6 | MDS 18/53 | MDS 4/15 |
| Control | AML 0/3, Normal 0/2 | Normal 0/12 | Normal 0 |
| Notes |  | Positive in good-prognosis group | Radiolabeled method; positive cases |
|  |  | Correlates with BM cellularity and longer survival | > 45% TUNEL |

[a] Some cases were studied consecutively.

MDS, myelodysplastic syndromes; N, number; RA, refractory anemia; RARS, refractory anemia with ringed sideroblasts; RAEB, refractory anemia with excess blasts; RAEB-t, refractory anemia with excess blasts in transformation; CMML, chronic myelomonocytic leukemia; AML, acute myeloid leukemia; BM, bone marrow; TUNEL, TdT-mediated dUTP-biotin nick end-labeled.

## C. Findings from In Situ Labeling

Both TUNEL and ISEL have the advantage of histochemical detection of apoptosis. Sample sizes can be much less than those required for biochemical methods and cells in early apoptotic stages can be visualized, an advantage not found in conventional electrophoresis. Thus, many investigators have used these in situ methods (Table 3).

In all reports, the results were consistent in that apoptosis was significantly higher in cells from MDS patients than in those of the controls (12,13,15–20), although there was wide variation in the incidence of positive cells in both. For instance, some TUNEL studies resulted in a mean positive value of 39–56% for the MDS samples, which was significantly higher than the corresponding values of 12–16% for the control marrow (13,15). While a lower overall incidence of apoptosis in another similar study might have resulted from technical differences, a TUNEL positive cell value of 5.2% for MDS samples was also significantly higher than the 0.6% value for the control marrow (20).

Positive cells in the in situ methods were mostly myeloid and erythroid cells and occasionally megakaryocytes. Both immature and mature cells were positive. Two groups of investigators (12,17) reported that marrow stromal cells from MDS patients were also apoptotic. Within the MDS subtypes, apoptosis has been more pronounced in less advanced MDS than in advanced MDS (16,18), although the opposite view has been reported (12,20). As compared with MDS, apoptosis appeared to be low in secondary (post-MDS) AML (13) and de novo AML (12). This was further confirmed in the same patients sequentially examined during the progression of MDS to AML (18).

Of interest is the study by Hellstrom-Lindberg et al. (15) in which apoptosis of marrow biopsy samples of MDS patients was examined before and after cytokine treatment. The investigators found a significant reduction in apoptosis in patients who responded to the combined treatment of granulocyte CSF (G-CSF) and erythropoietin (EPO). Since nonresponding patients did not show such a reduction in apoptotic cells, it may be that the cytokine treatment acts through amelioration of ineffective hematopoiesis (15). Clinical and hematological parameters, including age, degree of cytopenias, and percentage of blasts and ringed sideroblasts, showed no correlation with apoptosis as evaluated by the TUNEL method (15). Finally, another study (13) showed a correlation of TUNEL data with a low Bournemouth score, further supporting the relationship of high apoptosis with good prognosis (14).

## D. Flowcytometric Findings

Flowcytometric analysis using double labeling, one color for cell identification and another for DNA analysis or various apoptotic markers, permits evaluation

**Table 3**  In Situ Detection of Apoptosis in MDS

| | Raza et al. [12] | Bouscary et al. [13] | Hellstrom-Lindberg et al. [15] |
|---|---|---|---|
| Method | ISEL | TUNEL | TUNEL |
| Samples | Biopsy | Aspirate | Biopsy |
| | $N = 50$ | $N = 23$ | $N = 27$ |
| Cases | 19 RA, 6 RARS, 17 RAEB | | 6 RA, 11 RARS |
| | 7 RAEB-t, 1 CMML | | 10 RAEB |
| Controls | $N = 20$ AML plus 2 normal BM | $N = 5$ | $N = 11$ |
| Apoptosis | | | |
| MDS | 26 high, 9 intermed., 10 low | $39 \pm 5.7\%$ | $56.3 \pm 3.8\%$ |
| Controls | AML-negative; normal-low | $12.6 \pm 2.5\%$ | $16.2 \pm 1.4\%$ |
| Significance | RAEB-t highest (sparing blast cells) | Yes | Yes |
| Cell types | Differentiated cells of all 3 lineages | Myeloid > erythroid | Immature and mature myeloid and erythroid |
| Notes | Stromal cells also positive | Correlates with low Bournemouth score | Subsequent decrease in apoptosis in responders to G-CSF and EPO |

| | Kitagawa et al. [16] | Parcharidou et al. [17] | Kurotaki et al. [18] |
|---|---|---|---|
| Method | TUNEL | ISEL | TUNEL |
| Samples | Biopsy and autopsy | Biopsy | Aspiration or biopsy |
| | $N = 17$ | $N = 21$ | $N = 37$ |
| Cases | 4 RA, 1 RARS, 4 RAEB | 4 RA, 1 RARS, 10 RAEB | 10 RA, 27 RAEB |
| | 5 RAEB-t, 3 CMML | 5 RAEB-t, 1 CMML | |
| Controls | $N = 18$ | | $N = 10$ |

| | | | |
|---|---|---|---|
| Apoptosis | | | |
| MDS | 17.2 ± 4.9% | 11 high, 5 intermed., 2 low, 3 absent | RA 9.5 ± 3%, RAEB 5.6 ± 3% |
| Control | 3.4 ± 1.5% | | 1.0 ± 0.6% |
| Significance | Yes | | Yes |
| Cell types | All 3 lineages | All 3 lineages | All 3 lineages |
| Notes | RA or RAEB > RAEB-t or CMML Positive cells expressed Fas | Stromal cells also positive | Decreased apoptosis when leukemia developed |

| | Fontenay-Roupie et al. [19] | Shimazaki et al. [20] |
|---|---|---|
| Method | TUNEL | TUNEL |
| Samples | Aspirate | Biopsy |
| Cases | N = 23[a] 4 RA, 9 RARS, 12 RAEB | N = 51 32 RA, 1 RARS, 7 RAEB, 8 RAEB-t, 3 CMML |
| Controls | N = 8 | N = 10 |
| Apoptosis | | |
| MDS | 12/23 cases > 30% | 5.2% |
| Control | 15% | 0.6% |
| Significance | | Yes |
| Cell types | Mostly myeloid lineage | All 3 lineages |
| Notes | | More apoptosis in high-risk MDS |

[a] Some cases studied consecutively.

MDS, myelodysplastic syndromes; N, number; RA, refractory anemia; RARS, refractory anemia with ringed sideroblasts; RAEB, refractory anemia with excess blasts; RAEB-t, refractory anemia with excess blasts in transformation; CMML, chronic myelomonocytic leukemia; AML, acute myeloid leukemia; BM, bone marrow; TUNEL, TdT-mediated dUTP-biotin nick end-labeling method; ISEL, in situ end labeling; G-CSF, granulocyte colony-stimulating factor; EPO, erythropoietin.

**Table 4** Flowcytometric Detection of Apoptosis in MDS Marrow CD34+ Cells

| | Rajapaksa et al. [21] | | Parker et al. [22] | |
| --- | --- | --- | --- | --- |
| Cases | N = 24 | | N = 59 | |
| | 10 RA, 6 RARS, 8 RAEB | | 36 early (RA, RARS, RAEB < 10% blasts) | |
| | | | 23 late (RAEB > 10% blasts, MDS-AML) | |
| Controls | N = 10 | | N = 20 normal BM plus 25 de novo AML | |
| Parameters examined | Sub-G1 | c-Myc/Bcl-2 | Annexin-V | Bax & Bad/Bcl-2 & Bcl-X |
| MDS | RA 9.1% | 1.6 | Early 56.5% | 2.47 |
| | | | Late 16% | 1.4 |
| Control | Normal 2.1% | 1.2 | Normal 18.5% | 1.89 |
| | AML 1.2% | 0.9 | | |
| Significance | Yes | | Yes | |
| Notes | Reduced c-Myc/Bcl-2 as MDS evolved toward AML | | No correlation between proapoptotic/antiapoptotic protein ratio and annexin-V positivity | |

MDS, myelodysplastic syndromes; CD, clusters of differentiation (cellular markers); N, number; RA, refractory anemia; RARS, refractory anemia with ringed sideroblasts; RAEB, refractory anemia with excess blasts; AML, acute myeloid leukemia; BM, bone marrow; Sub-G1, Sub-G1 stage of cell cycle; c-Myc, a proapoptotic protein; Bcl-2 & Bcl-X, antiapoptotic proteins; Bax & Bad, proapoptotic proteins.

of apoptosis in specific cell types. Subdiploid DNA (from sub-G1 stage of the cell cycle) or specific apoptotic membrane changes such as binding of annexin-V are examples of apoptotic markers. These apoptotic markers can also be examined by flowcytometry following initial purification of the cells, for instance, CD34+ and CD34− cells (Table 4).

By employing flowcytometric quantification of sub-G1 DNA as stained with propiodium iodide, Rajapaksa et al. (21) showed elevated levels of apoptosis in MDS patients. The proportion of CD34+ cells with sub-G1 DNA was higher in early stages of MDS than in advanced stages of MDS or AML or for normal individuals. In addition, altered oncoprotein expression has been shown in CD34+ cell populations from MDS patients, and the ratio of cell death-related (c-Myc) to cell survival-related (Bcl-2) oncoproteins has also been roughly correlated with the incidence of cells with apoptotic sub-G1 DNA content (21). The oncoprotein ratio was higher in RA than in RAEB or AML, indicating reduced c-Myc/Bcl-2 ratio as MDS progressed toward AML. Combined treatment with G-CSF and EPO was associated with decreased levels of apoptotic CD34+ marrow cells and may contribute to the enhanced hematopoiesis in vivo (21).

Flowcytometric detection of specific apoptotic membrane changes, by using annexin-V, which binds to exposed phosphatidylserine, has been used as an early marker of apoptosis. Parker et al. (22) reported that apoptotic CD34+ cells as assessed by annexin-V–FITC (fluorine isothiocyanate) binding was significantly increased in less advanced MDS than in advanced MDS or control marrow. A total of 20 of the 31 cases with less advanced MDS had more than 50% apoptotic CD34+ cells (22). The investigators also examined expression of proapoptotic (Bax and Bad) and antiapoptotic (Bcl-2 and Bcl-X) proteins of peamealized CD34+ cells, and showed significantly higher ratios of pro- versus antiapoptotic proteins occurring in early MDS as compared with advanced MDS (22). Although no correlation was found between the degree of apoptosis and the Bcl-2 family protein ratios, a total of 13 of the 16 early MDS samples examined had a ratio greater than 2 compared with only three of the 16 advanced cases.

## IV. THE KEY ISSUES ON THE ROLE OF APOPTOSIS IN MDS

The results listed in the foregoing section support the following key issues. First, excessive apoptosis occurs in MDS and apparently is more pronounced in early stages of MDS than in advanced stages. Second, apoptosis is decreased in de novo AML or leukemic transformation of MDS. Although there appears to be some difference in the incidence of apoptosis in MDS marrow, the difference depends largely on the sensitivity of the methods used.

Excessive apoptosis in early stages of MDS most likely represents ineffective hematopoiesis (3–6). In fact, increased levels of apoptosis have also been demonstrated in pathological conditions associated with ineffective hematopoiesis other than MDS, as reviewed elsewhere (23). Mechanisms leading to excessive apoptosis and ineffective hematopoiesis in each condition may not be the same. However, excessive apoptosis apparently is one of the cellular abnormalities of MDS (3,4).

Decline of apoptosis in parallel with the progression of MDS toward the leukemic stage is supported by the expression of specific oncoproteins relevant to cell survival and apoptosis. A recent histochemical study examined the expression of antiapoptotic *bcl-2* in immature myeloid blast cells from patients with MDS (24). Cell survival activity as assessed by *bcl-2* expression was higher in advanced MDS and AML than in early stages of MDS. The early myeloid precursors, predominantly myeloblasts, were examined in marrow biopsy sections following immunostaining, and when serial biopsies were studied, Bcl-2 was found to correlate with stages of the disease. The cell survival activity was lower in early MDS stages than in late stages of the disease, and increased level of activity was associated with disease progression over time to AML (24). The findings collectively support the hypothesis that MDS progression is related to accumulation of blast cells with increased *bcl-2* expression and decreased apoptosis. Conceivably, as the disease progresses, an immature hematopoietic cell population with decreased apoptosis may arise from a background of increased apoptosis in early MDS. Myeloblasts as well as undifferentiated blast cells have been reported to be negative in the ISEL study (12), which is in agreement with this hypothesis.

## V. POSSIBLE MECHANISMS LEADING TO INCREASED APOPTOSIS IN MDS

The various factors described below are not mutually exclusive. Rather they are interrelated (Fig. 1).

### A. Cytokines

Excessive apoptosis in MDS marrow cells may result from inhibitory cytokines. In particular, several studies suggested some roles for TNF-$\alpha$. Elevated levels of TNF-$\alpha$ in patients' serum (25–29), marrow plasma (30), and marrow biopsy samples (31,32) have been reported. Semiquantitative assessment of TNF-$\alpha$ in MDS BM has suggested positive correlation with high ISEL labeling (31) and elevated caspase 3-like activity (32). Results from another study showed that the production of TNF-$\alpha$ by phorbolester-stimulated PB mononuclear cells from MDS patients was increased in low-risk MDS cases (33). Up-regulation of TNF-$\alpha$ mRNA in the BM aspirates has also been shown (34,35). TNF-$\alpha$ protein and

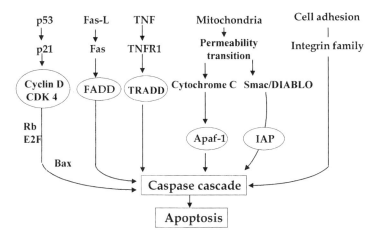

**Fig. 1** Possible lesions leading to apoptosis in MDS. p53 and p21, proapoptotic proteins; CDK 4, a cyclin-dependent kinase; Rb, retinoblastoma protein; E2F, transcription factor associated with Rb; Fas-L and Fas, ligand and the associated protein that induce an apoptotic signal; FADD, Fas-associated death domain protein; TNF, tumor necrosis factor; TNFR1, a receptor for TNF; TRADD, TNF receptor-associated death domain protein; Apaf-1, apoptotic protease activating factor-1; Smac, second mitochondria-derived activator of caspases; DIABLO, direct IAP-binding protein with lower binding constant; IAP, inhibitors of apoptosis.

soluble TNFR levels in the marrow plasma were significantly higher in early stages than in advanced stages of MDS (35). Addition of anti-TNF-α antibody to MDS BM cells significantly increased the numbers of hematopoietic colonies (35). Although altered levels of other cytokines such as interleukin-1-β (IL-1-β) and transforming growth factor-β (TGF-β) as well as Flt-3 ligand and Flt-3 receptor have been shown (34,36), the addition of anti-TGF-β antibody did not, however, have a positive effect on the ability to form hematopoietic colonies (35). Together, these results suggest that apoptosis in MDS may be mediated by TNF-α and that macrophages or other interstitial cells may be the most likely cellular source of TNF-α production. Raza et al. (37) postulated a dual role of TNF-α in the pathogenesis of MDS: TNF-α induces apoptosis in the maturing cells causing pancytopenia on the one hand, while on the other hand it stimulates the proliferation of the primitive progenitors, thus accounting for the hypercellular marrow.

## B.  Fas and Fas-ligand (Fas-L) System

Fas/Apo-1 (CD95) is a cell-surface protein that induces an apoptotic signal after binding to Fas-L or to a functional anti-Fas antibody. TNF-α induces Fas antigen

(38). Increased expression of *fas* in MDS BM cells has been shown by flowcytometry (13,19,35) and immunochemical studies (13,39). The cell types expressing *fas* included CD34+ cells (13) and myeloid and erythroid cells (13,39). Increased *fas* expression has been correlated to apoptosis in some studies (16,19), but not in all (39). Expression of *fas* showed no correlation with clinical parameters (13). Several groups examined mRNA levels of Fas and Fas-L, and found up-regulation of both mRNA levels (16,35). Kitagawa et al. (16) reported that *fas-L* is expressed not only in hematopoietic cells but also in macrophages, while *fas* expression is found in hematopoietic cells but not in macrophages. The investigators suggested that fas plays a role in inducing apoptosis in MDS BM cells and works in an autocrine (hematopoietic-hematopoietic cell interaction) and/or a paracrine fashion (hematopoietic-stromal cell interaction). Fas is functional as suggested by the use of Fas immunoglobulin, which resulted in improved hematopoietic colony formation by MDS cells (35). Finally, of interest is a recent report (40) of coculture of cell lysates of MDS BM cells with purified normal hematopoietic progenitor populations. The coculture showed suppression of the myeloid and erythroid colony growth; however, this suppression could be blocked by the addition of soluble recombinant fas Fc protein, which blocks the Fas/Fas-L system.

These results suggest that the Fas/Fas-L system may be functional and that defects in the CD95 pathway may contribute to the development of hematological malignancy by abrogating CD95-mediated growth control of activated cells. Expression of *fas* by CD34+ cells was negatively correlated with BM blast counts, suggesting that leukemic blasts lose *fas antigen* expression with progression of MDS (13). This is in accord with the hypothesis that leukemic cells evolving from MDS background are no longer susceptible to apoptosis, although it remains to be seen whether alteration in *fas* expression may be the sole reason for the leukemic progression of MDS. Alternatively, up-regulation of Fas-L on the "aberrant" blast cells from advanced MDS patients may be related to additional activation steps (35) but the mechanisms for blast protection from apoptosis remain unknown.

## C.  Cell Cycle Abnormalities

Certain tumor suppressor genes have been implicated in cell cycle control and apoptosis. Retinoblastoma protein (Rb) is hypophosphorylated in early G1, and is associated with the transcription factor E2F. With the progression in G1, Rb becomes phosphorylated by the cyclin-dependent kinase activity, leading to the release and transcriptional activity of E2F. E2F then activates genes necessary for G1/S transition of the cell cycle. Rb phosphorylation is regulated by cyclin D1. Although overexpression of *cyclin D1* is often found in cancers and lower *RB* expression is seen in some AML, altered expression of the *cyclin D1* or *RB* is rare in MDS (41).

Apoptosis and cell kinetics in MDS patients were examined following intravenous administration of iodo- and/or bromodeoxyuridine (42,43). Double labeling of marrow biopsy sections using ISEL and histochemical staining of the two thymine analogs indicated that 30–90% of S-phase cells in MDS were simultaneously apoptotic. More recently, it has been shown that such signal antonymy is a characteristic feature of MDS and is linked with altered expression of *E2F1* in some patients (44). As mentioned above, E2F is involved in G1/S transition. It remains to be seen whether overexpressed *E2F1* itself or untimely release of E2F1 is sufficient to induce cells to enter S phase, subsequently leading to apoptosis before completing S phase.

Another tumor suppressor gene *p53* maps chromosome 17p. The wild-type gene product may function as a negative regulator of the cell cycle and promote apoptosis. *p53* mutations in MDS are usually associated with loss of the wild-type allele (45). Nearly 70% of MDS or AML with 17p deletions harbor *p53* mutations. Such cases are characterized by dysgranulocytopoiesis, reduced marrow apoptosis, poor response to chemotherapy, and short survival (46). *p53* mutations are mostly seen in advanced stages of MDS (47). In contrast, high apoptosis has been shown in patients with AML and MDS with known *p53* overexpression. Orazi et al. reported that MDS patients with *p53* expression showed apoptosis in erythroid and myeloid cells of varying maturational stages and occasionally in megakaryocytes, but blast cells were spared (48). These findings indicate that disruption of p53-mediated apoptosis may partly explain disease progression of MDS.

TGF-β inhibitory effects on normal hematopoietic progenitors are mediated by many mechanisms including down-regulation of cyclin-dependent kinase 4 synthesis and gene expression of the cell cycle regulator P15$^{INK4b}$ as well as P15$^{INK4b}$ protein stability. Methylation of P15$^{INK4b}$ was detected in advanced MDS, frequently at AML transformation of MDS, but not at diagnosis when serially examined (49,50). These results indicate that leukemic cell proliferation might require an escape of regulation of the G1 phase of the cell cycle, and possibly escape from TGF-β inhibitory effect.

## D.  Caspase Activation

Studies of the apoptosis execution enzymes, caspases, are rather few. Ali et al. (51) reported a sequential activation of caspase-1 and caspase-3-like proteases during a 4-hr incubation of MDS BM cells. In the presence of a broad-spectrum caspase inhibitor, Z-VAD-FMK, apoptosis was attenuated. The same group also reported a correlation between TNF-α expression and high caspase-3-like activity in MDS BM cells. A more recent report by Bouscary et al. (52) showed that excess apoptosis was accompanied by increased caspase-3 activity in early stages of MDS. Caspase inhibitor Z-VAD-FMK dose-dependently reduced the number of annexin-V-positive cells in four of the nine evaluable cases with excessive apoptosis. However, in none of them did Z-VAD-FMK rescue hematopoiesis in vitro even though apoptosis was attenuated (52). The reasons remain unknown, but it may well be that a point of "no return" may exist along the apoptotic signaling cascade, after which cells are irreparably committed to die by as-yet-unknown mechanisms.

## E.  Bone Marrow Microenvironment

BM stroma from some MDS patients may induce apoptosis of normal hematopoietic progenitor cells. In four of the 11 patients with MDS subclassified as RA, Aizawa et al. (53) found that BM stroma cells failed to support the growth of normal progenitors in a coculture system. During the coculture, the normal progenitors underwent apoptosis. The expression of *fas* in hematopoietic cells was also induced by the MDS stroma. Recently, the same group established a stromal cell line LS801 from an MDS RA patient by introducing SV40-adenovirus vector containing *SV40* early gene (54). The LS801 stromal cell line also induced apoptosis of normal CD34+ cells and leukemic HL-60 and TF-1 cells. In this coculture, apoptosis was not attributable to Fas-L, TNF-$\alpha$, or IFN-$\gamma$, since their activity was not detectable in the conditioned medium of LS801 cells. Furthermore, when hematopoietic progenitors were kept separate from LS801 cells by a Millipore membrane to prevent their attachment, apoptosis was not seen, indicating direct cell-to-cell interaction is needed in the induction of apoptosis. It would be interesting to observe the fate of MDS cells in this coculture system.

## F.  Mitochondrial Abnormalities

Accumulating evidence implicates mitochondria in the execution of apoptotic pathway. At least three mitochondria-specific events have been defined in cells undergoing apoptosis: namely, loss of mitochondrial transmembrane potential, induction of mitochondrial permeability transition, and cytosolic translocation of apoptogenic factors, such as cytochrome C (Cyt C) and newly identified Smac/DIABLO (second mitochondria-derived activator of caspase/direct inhibitor of apoptotic proteins (IAP)-binding protein with lower binding constant) (55). The release of Cyt C can activate downstream events, such as processing of caspases. Smac/DIABLO is normally a mitochondrial protein, but when released into the cytoplasm, it promotes caspase-9 activation by binding to IAPs.

Abnormalities of mitochondrial metabolism have been postulated as the primary cause in acquired sideroblastic anemia (AISA). The mitochondrial respiratory chain is involved in mitochondrial iron uptake and supply of ferrous iron for heme synthesis. A heteroplasmic mutation of mitochondrial DNA may not only impair iron metabolism and heme synthesis but, through impaired mitochondrial energy production, also increase apoptosis (56). Such heteroplasmic mutation of mitochondrial DNA has also been shown in some cases of MDS.

## G. Oxidative Stress

TNF-$\alpha$ promotes apoptosis via intracellular oxygen free radical production and oxidation of DNA and proteins. Peddie et al. (29) postulated a role for intracellular oxygen free radical production, perhaps mediated by TNF-$\alpha$, in the pathogenesis of MDS. In line with this theory is the result from the addition of an antioxidant, $N$-acetylcysteine, to MDS BM culture, that is, reduction of TNF-$\alpha$ levels and apoptosis (57). The antioxidant treatment may play a role in guaranteeing MDS cell survival, and one of the mechanisms of action of amifostine may be similar antioxidant activity (58).

The expression of nitric oxide synthase (NOS) in MDS was examined in another study (59). Induction of NOS and production of the toxic metabolite NO is one of the TNF-$\alpha$–regulated effector mechanisms. Both the mRNA and protein level of inducible NOS (iNOS) were high in MDS but not detectable in control or AML BM. Double immunostaining method showed that iNOS was predominantly localized to BM macrophages. The investigators postulated that TNF-$\alpha$ up-regulation leads to iNOS production by macrophages as well as increased *fas* expression in MDS hematopoietic cells (59).

## VI. CONTROVERSIAL ISSUES

## A. Variability of the Data

A marked variation exists in the reported incidence of apoptosis in MDS. Electron microscopy (8) gave the lowest values whereas annexin-V assay (22) gave very high values (Table 1 and 4). Direct comparison of these extreme values is meaningless, since the former detects only cells with unequivocally apoptotic morphology in advanced stages of apoptosis, while the latter detects both early and intermediate apoptotic cells as well; probably, the former underestimates, while the latter overestimates apoptosis. Variability is also seen among studies using the TUNEL method (Table 3). Even considering that differences in patient selection and technical details (including differences in laboratory processing of cells) may be substantial, the variability is still confounding. This reflects the true difficulty in sensitively and specifically detecting cells dying as well as cells about to die via apoptosis. It is thus advisable to use more than two methods as well as a fair number of control samples.

## B. Is Apoptosis Observed Predominantly in Progenitor Cells or Maturing Cells?

Evidence for apoptosis in myelodysplastic maturing cells is derived from ultrastructural study (7–9) (Table 1), short-term incubation experiments (10,11), and in situ methods (12,13,17–20) (Table 3). Expression of *fas* has been shown not only in CD34+ cells, but also in myeloid and erythroid cells (13,39). Comparable degrees of TUNEL labeling have also been shown in both CD34+ and CD34− cells (14,60). In one study, apoptosis was detected in both CD34+ and CD34− cells in early MDS, but apoptosis was restricted to CD34+ cells in advanced MDS (14). In another study (9), ISEL labeling of high-density and low-density fractions of MDS BM cells showed that high-density fractions had significantly higher apoptotic rates than low-density fractions. Pelger-Huet-type neutrophils were typically apoptotic (9). These findings favor the view that apoptosis in MDS is not confined to progenitors, but seen in maturing cells as well.

By contrast, examination of apoptosis-related parameters, such as ratios of proapoptotic versus antiapoptotic proteins, annexin-V binding, and reactivity to the TUNEL method following separation of BM into CD34+ and CD34− cell fractions, showed that apoptosis was mainly seen in immature CD34+ progenitors (21,22). Apoptosis of CD34+ progenitor cells has also been reported in aplastic anemia, Fanconi anemia, and Blackfan-Diamond anemia (61–63), which are all associated with varying degrees of marrow hypoplasia. One would naturally assume that, if apoptosis is observed predominantly in progenitor cells in MDS, the BM would become hypocellular. Alternatively, the progenitor cells should have hyperproliferative activity to compensate for the apoptosis occurring within the progenitor cell population (37).

## C.  Is Apoptosis Central to MDS?

Excessive apoptosis has been suggested in certain conditions associated with ineffective hematopoiesis other than MDS (23). In this sense, apoptosis is clearly not specific to MDS. This brings up the critical question whether apoptosis is central to MDS or merely an effect but not a cause. Two possibilities may be raised to answer the question. First, increased apoptosis may represent a mechanism whereby the hematopoietic system allows elimination of unwanted cells. The marrow progenitors, when faced with the presence of chronic peripheral cytpopenias, are triggered, through a feedback increase of cytokines, to expand and provide more maturing cells. This concept deems apoptosis to be a response to peripheral cytopenias. However, this concept does not explain why peripheral cytopenias take place in MDS. An alternative hypothesis is that increased apoptosis may be a part of clonal abnormalities inherent to MDS (2–4,23). Conceivably, apoptosis is not merely an epiphenomenon in MDS, but is closely related to and caused by as-yet-unknown fundamental biological abnormalities of the MDS clone.

Very little is known about whether apoptotic MDS cells are clonal or not. The study by Bogdanovic et al. (8) found that apoptosis in patients with karyotypic abnormalities was not higher than in patients with normal karyotype, suggesting that discrete alterations in apoptosis are present even in the karyotypically normal clone. Lack of correlation of apoptosis to clonal cytogenetic abnormalities has also been shown with data of annexin-V binding (22). Novel techniques are needed to allow simultaneous detection of apoptosis, cytogenetics, and clonality at the single-cell level.

## D. Clinical Relevance of Apoptosis in MDS

As discussed above, most investigators support the thesis that apoptosis is more prominent in early stages of MDS than in advanced stages, and that apoptosis becomes less evident with the progression of MDS to AML. Except for these key issues, little is known of the clinical relevance of apoptosis.

If apoptosis is truly responsible for ineffective hematopoiesis in MDS, degrees of the cytopenias should most likely be related to apoptosis. Sporadic reports in line with this notion include serum levels of TNF-$\alpha$ showing correlation with the degree of anemia (26), TUNEL positivity correlating with low Bournemouth score (13), and apoptotic index correlating with leukopenia (8). Early stages of MDS have been associated with high apoptosis (14) and high TNF-$\alpha$ protein in marrow plasma (35), but not with the degree of peripheral cytopenias. Likewise, CD34+ cell apoptosis has not been related to cytopenias, marrow cellularity, or disease category (22). It has to be added, however, that apoptosis is a biological process that is not easy to evaluate in clinical samples. Given the difficulty of detecting apoptosis and limitations inherent to each of the methods of detection, a large-scale study involving apoptosis as one of the parameters is warranted although, in reality, would not be easy to carry out.

## E. Therapeutic Applications

Hematopoietic growth factors decrease apoptosis and improve blood counts (64). This is best illustrated by Hellstrom-Lindberg et al. (15), who found that the clinical effect of the combined therapy of G-CSF and EPO correlated with decreased levels of apoptosis in the BM of patients responding to the treatment. In addition, other compounds have been suggested to inhibit apoptosis. The phosphothiol-derivative amifostine has been suggested to generate trophic effect in MDS via its action as an antioxidant, or alternatively, through polyamine-like effects (58). Brief exposure of MDS BM cells to amifostine yielded a dose-dependent stimulation of hematopoietic progenitors and decreased apoptosis in CD34+ cells. Treatment with amifostine can promote multilineage hematopoietic stimulation in a proportion of MDS patients (58). In addition, amifostine combined with pentoxifylline, ciprofloxacin, and dexamethasone has shown some clinical efficacy (65,66). The efficacy of these combinations is presumed to occur through interference with the activity of TNF-$\alpha$.

Amifostine is an interesting novel treatment, but ongoing studies of amifostine either alone or in combination with other agents have to be completed before its role in MDS can be determined (67,68). Of importance, it must first be proven that apoptosis can be selectively modulated in a given tissue or cell type. Tissue-specific delivery of selective modulators of apoptosis must be considered to avoid the potential risks of tumor progression or of autoimmune disease.

## VII.  CONCLUSION AND FUTURE DIRECTIONS

Considerable progress has been made over the last decade in understanding the significance of apoptosis in MDS. A large body of evidence has shown that apoptosis is excessive in early stages of MDS and declines in advanced stages or in leukemic transformation of MDS. While apoptosis is a cell biological process conserved throughout evolution, our knowledge of apoptosis in mammalian cells and its genetic control and signaling is still sparse as compared with those in *Caenorhabdis* or *Drosophila*. Future studies should be directed: (1) to identify apoptotic signals, the accumulation of which either induces apoptosis or decreases the threshold of apoptotic induction; (2) to delineate causative lesions leading to abnormalities in apoptotic control in MDS; and (3) to develop more sensitive techniques for the detection of preapoptotic cells. The future thus lies in developing new insights into the biology of MDS and in establishing new therapeutic approaches.

## REFERENCES

1.  Bennett JM, Catovsky D, Daniel MT, Flandrin G, Galton DA, Gralnick HR, Sultan C. Proposals for the classification of the myelodysplastic syndromes. Br J Haematol 1982; 51:189–199.
2.  Yoshida Y, Stephenson J, Mufti GJ. Myelodysplastic syndromes: from morphology to molecular biology. Part I. Classification, natural history and cell biology of myelodysplasia. Int J Hematol 1993; 57:87–97.
3.  Yoshida Y. Hypothesis: apoptosis may be the mechanism responsible for the premature intramedullary cell death in the myelodysplastic syndrome. Leukemia 1993; 7: 144–146.
4.  Yoshida Y, Mufti GJ. Apoptosis and its significance in MDS: controversies revisited. Leuk Res 1999; 23:777–785.
5.  Greenberg PL. Apoptosis and its role in the myelodysplastic syndromes: implications for disease natural history and treatment. Leuk Res 1998; 22:1123–1136.
6.  Parker JE, Mufti GJ. Ineffective hematopoiesis and apoptosis in myelodysplastic syndromes. Br J Haematol 1998; 101:220–230.
7.  Clark DM, Lampert IA. Apoptosis is a common histopathological finding in myelo-

dysplasia: the correlate of ineffective hematopoiesis. Leuk Lymphoma 1990; 2:415–418.

8. Bogdanovic AD, Trpinac DP, Jancovic GM, Bumbasirevic VZ, Obradovic M, Colovic MD. Incidence and role of apoptosis in myelodysplastic syndrome: morphological and ultrastructural assessment. Leukemia 1997; 11:656–659.

9. Shetty V, Hussaini S, Broady-Robinson L, Allampallam K, Mundle S, Borok R, Broderick E, Mazzoran L, Zorat F, Raza A. Intramedullary apoptosis of hematopoietic cells in myelodysplastic syndrome patients can be massive: apoptotic cells recovered from high-density fraction of bone marrow aspirates. Blood 2000; 96:1388–1392.

10. Lepelley P, Campergue L, Grardel N, Preudhomme C, Cosson A, Fenaux P. Is apoptosis a massive process in myelodysplastic syndromes? Br J Haematol 1996; 95:368–371.

11. Hamada K, Takahashi I, Matsuoka M, Saita T, Mizobuchi N, Yorimitsu S, Takimoto H. Apoptosis of peripheral leukocytes in patients with myelodysplastic syndromes. Jpn J Clin Hematol 1998; 39:1079–1084 [Japanese].

12. Raza A, Gezer S, Mundle S, Gao XZ, Alvi S, Borok R, Rifkin S, Iftikhar A, Shetty V, Parcharidou A, Loew J, Marcus B, Khan Z, Chaney C, Showel J, Gregory S, Preisler H. Apoptosis in bone marrow biopsy samples involving stromal and hematopoietic cells in 50 patients with myelodysplastic syndromes. Blood 1995; 86:268–276.

13. Bouscary D, De Vos J, Guesnu M, Jondeau K, Viguier F, Melle J, Picard F, Dreyfus F, Fontenay-Roupie M. Fas/Apo-1 (CD95) expression and apoptosis in patients with myelodysplastic syndromes. Leukemia 1997; 11:839–845.

14. Tsoplou P, Kouraklis-Symeonidis A, Thanopoulou E, Zikos P, Orphanos V, Zoumbus NC. Apoptosis in patients with myelodysplastic syndromes: differential involvement of marrow cells in "good" versus "poor" prognosis patients and correlation with apoptosis-related genes. Leukemia 1999; 13:1554–1563.

15. Hellstrom-Lindberg E, Kanter-Lewensohn L, Ost A. Morphological changes and apoptosis in bone marrow from patients with myelodysplastic syndromes treated with granulocyte-CSF and erythropoietin. Leuk Res 1997; 21:415–425.

16. Kitagawa M, Yamaguchi S, Takahashi M, Tanizawa T, Hirokawa K, Kamiyama R. Localization of Fas and Fas ligand in bone marrow cells demonstrating myelodysplasia. Leukemia 1998; 12:486–492.

17. Parcharidou A, Raza A, Economopoulos T, Papageorgiou E, Anagnostou D, Papadaki T, Raptis S. Extensive apoptosis of bone marrow cells as evaluated by the in situ end-labelling (ISEL) technique may be the basis for ineffective haematopoiesis in patients with myelodysplastic syndromes. Eur J Haematol 1999; 62:19–26.

18. Kurotaki H, Tsushima Y, Nagai K, Yagihashi S. Apoptosis, bcl-2 expression and p53 accumulation in myelodysplastic syndrome, myelodysplastic-syndrome-derived acute myelogenous leukemia and de novo acute myelogenous leukemia. Acta Haematol 2000; 102:115–123.

19. Fontenay-Roupie M, Bouscary D, Guesnu M, Picard F, Melle J, Lacombe C, Gisselbrecht S, Mayeux P, Dreyfus F. Ineffective erythropoiesis in myelodysplastic syndromes: correlation with Fas expression but not with lack of erythropoietin receptor signal transduction. Br J Haematol 1999; 106:464–473.

20. Shimazaki K, Ohshima K, Suzumiya J, Kawasaki C, Kikuchi M. Evaluation of apoptosis as a prognostic factor in myelodysplastic syndromes. Br J Haematol 2000; 110:584–590.

21. Rajapaksa R, Ginzton N, Rott LS, Greenberg PL. Altered oncoprotein expression and apoptosis in myelodysplastic marrow cells. Blood 1996; 88:4275–4287.

22. Parker JE, Fishlock KL, Mijovic A, Czepulkowski B, Pagliuca A, Mufti GJ. "Low risk" myelodysplastic syndrome is associated with excessive apoptosis and an increased ratio of pro- versus anti-apoptotic bcl-2-related proteins. Br J Haematol 1998; 103:1075–1082.

23. Yoshida Y, Anzai N, Kawabata H. Apoptosis in myelodysplasia: a paradox or paradigm. Leuk Res 1995; 19:887–891.

24. Davis RE, Greenberg PL. Bcl-2 expression by myeloid precursors in myelodysplastic syndromes: relation to disease progression. Leuk Res 1998; 22:767–777.

25. Zoumbos N, Symeonidis A, Kourakli A, Katevas P, Matsouka P, Perraki M, Georgoulias V. Increased levels of soluble interleukin-2 receptors and tumor necrosis factor in serum of patients with myelodysplastic syndromes. Blood 1991; 77:413–414.

26. Verhoef GE, De Schouwer P, Ceuppens JL, Van Damme J, Goossens W, Boogaerts MA. Measurement of serum cytokine levels in patients with myelodysplastic syndromes. Leukemia 1992; 6:1268–1272.

27. Seipelt G, Ganser A, Duranceyk H, Maurer A, Ottmann OG, Hoelzer D. Induction of TNF-α in patients with myelodysplastic syndromes undergoing treatment with interleukin-3. Br J Haematol 1993; 84:749–751.

28. Stasi R, Brunetti M, Bussa S, Conforti M, Martin LS, La Pressa M, Bianchi M, Parma A, Pagano A. Serum levels of tumour necrosis factor-alpha predict response to recombinant human erythropoietin in patients with myelodysplastic syndrome. Clin Lab Haematol 1997; 19:197–201.

29. Peddie CM, Wolf CR, McLellan LI, Collins AR, Bowen DT. Oxidative DNA damage in CD34+ myelodysplastic cells is associated with intracellular redox changes and elevated plasma tumour necrosis factor-alpha concentration. Br J Haematol 1997; 99:625–631.

30. Gerusuk GM, Yamaguchi M, Beckman C, Kiener P, Anderson JE, Troutt AB, Loken MR, Deeg HJ. A role for fas, fas-ligand and TNF-α in the dysregulation of hematopoiesis in myelodysplastic syndrome (MDS). Blood 1996; 88:639a.

31. Dar S, Mundle S, Andric T, Qasi H, Shetty V, Reza S, Mativi Y, Allampallam K, Ali A, Venugopal P, Gezer S, Broady-Robinson L, Cartlidge J, Showel M, Hussaini S, Ragasa D, Ali I, Chaudhry A, Waggoner S, Lisak L, Huang RW, Raza A. Biological characteristics of myelodysplastic syndrome patients who demonstrated high versus no intramedullary apoptosis. Eur J Haematol 1999; 62:90–94.

32. Mundle SD, Reza S, Ali A, Mativi BY, Shetty V, Venugopal P, Gregory SA, Raza A. Correlation of tumor necrosis factor α (TNF-α) with high caspase 3-like activity in myelodysplastic syndromes. Cancer Lett 1999; 140:201–207.

33. Molnar L, Berki T, Hussain A, Nemeth P, Losonczy H. Detection of TNF α expression in the bone marrow and determination of TNF α production of peripheral blood mononuclear cells in myelodysplastic syndrome. Pathol Oncol Res 2000; 6:18–23.

34. Allampallam K, Shetty V, Hussaini S, Mazzoran L, Zorat F, Huang R, Raza A.

Measurement of mRNA expression for a variety of cytokines and its receptors in bone marrows of patients with myelodysplastic syndromes. Anticancer Res 1999; 19:5323–5328.

35. Gersuk GM, Beckham C, Loken MR, Kiener P, Anderson JE, Farrand A, Troutt AB, Ledbetter JA, Deeg HJ. A role for tumour necrosis factor-α, Fas and Fas-Ligand in marrow failure associated with myelodysplastic syndrome. Br J Hematol 1998; 103:176–188.

36. Shetty V, Mundle S, Alvi S, Showel M, Broady-Robinson L, Dar S, Borok R, Showel J, Gregory S, Rifkin S, Gezer S, Parcharidou A, Venugopal P, Shah R, Hernandez B, Klein M, Alston D, Robin E, Dominquez C, Raza A. Measurement of apoptosis, proliferation and three cytokines in 46 patients with myelodysplastic syndromes. Leuk Res 1996; 20:891–900.

37. Raza A, Mundle S, Shetty V, Alvi S, Chopra H, Span L, Parcharidou A, Dar S, Venugopal P, Borok R, Gezer S, Showel J, Loew J, Robin E, Rifkin S, Alston D, Hernandez B, Shah R, Kaiser H, Gregory S. Novel insights into the biology of myelodysplastic syndromes: excessive apoptosis and the role of cytokines. Int J Hematol 1996; 63:265–278.

38. Maciejewski J, Selleri C, Anderson S, Young NS. Fas antigen expression on CD34+ human marrow cells is induced by interferon γ and tumor necrosis factor α and potentiates cytokine-mediated hematopoietic suppression in vitro. Blood 1995; 85: 3183–3190.

39. Lepelley P, Grardel N, Erny O, Iaru T, Obein V, Cosson A, Fenaux P. Fas/APO-1 (CD95) expression in myelodysplastic syndromes. Leuk Lymphoma 1998; 30: 307–312.

40. Gupta P, Niehans GA, LeRoy SC, Gupta K, Morrison VA, SchulTz C, Knapp DJ, Kratzke RA. Fas ligand expression in the bone marrow in myelodysplastic syndromes correlates with FAB subtype and anemia, and predicts survival. Leukemia 1999; 13:44–53.

41. Preudhomme C, Vachee A, Lepelley P, Vanrumbeke M, Zandecki M, Quesnel B, Cosson A, Fenaux P. Inactivation of the retinoblastoma gene appears to be very uncommon in myelodysplastic syndromes. Br J Haematol 1994; 87:61–67.

42. Raza A, Mundle S, Iftikhar A, Gregory S, Marcus B, Khan Z, Alvi S, Shetty V, Dameron S, Wright V, Adler S, Loew LM, Shott S, Ali SN, Preisler H. Simultaneous assessment of cell kinetics and programmed cell death in bone marrow biopsies of myelodysplastics reveals extensive apoptosis as the probable basis for ineffective hematopoiesis. Am J Hematol 1995; 48:143–154.

43. Raza A, Alvi S, Broady-Robinson L, Showel M, Cartlidge J, Mundle SD, Shetty VT, Borok RZ, Dar SE, Chopra HK, Span L, Parcharidou A, Hines C, Gezer S, Venugopal P, Loew J, Showel J, Alston D, Hernandez B, Rifkin S, Robin E, Shah R, Gregory SA. Cell cycle kinetic studies in 68 patients with myelodysplastic syndromes following intravenous iodo- and/or bromodeoxyuridine. Exp Hematol 1997; 25:530–535.

44. Mundle SD, Mativi BY, Cartlidge JD, Dangerfield B, Broady-Robinson L, Li B, Shetty V, Venugopal P, Gregory SA, Preisler HD, Raza A. Signal antonymy unique to myelodysplastic marrows correlates with altered expression of E2F1. Br J Haematol 2000; 109:376–381.

45. Lai JL, Preudhomme C, Zandecki M, Flactif M, Vanrumbeke M, Lepelley P, Wattel E, Fenaux P. Myelodysplastic syndromes and acute myeloid leukemia with 17p deletions. An entity characterized by specific dysgranulopoiesis and a high incidence of P53 mutations. Leukemia 1995; 9:370–381.

46. Wattel E, Preudhomme C, Hecquet B, Vanrumbeke M, Quesnel B, Dervite I, Morel P, Fenaux P. p53 mutations are associated with resistance to chemotherapy and short survival in hematologic malignancies. Blood 1994; 84:3148–3157.

47. Sugimoto K, Hirano N, Toyoshima H, Chiba S, Mano H, Takaku F, Yazaki Y, Hirai H. Mutations of the p53 gene in myelodysplastic syndrome (MDS) and MDS-derived leukemia. Blood 1993; 81:3022–3026.

48. Orazi A, Kahsai M, John K, Neiman RS. p53 overexpression in myeloid leukemic disorders is associated with increased apoptosis of hematopoietic marrow cells and ineffective hematopoiesis. Mod Pathol 1996; 9:48–52.

49. Uchida T, Kinoshita T, Nagai H, Nakahara Y, Saito H, Hotta T, Murate T. Hypermethylation of the p15INK4B gene in myelodysplastic syndromes. Blood 1997; 90: 1403–1409.

50. Quesnel B, Guillerm G, Vereecque R, Wattel E, Preudhomme C, Bauters F, Vanrumbeke M, Fenaux P. Methylation of the p15INK5b gene in myelodysplastic syndromes is frequent and acquired during disease progression. Blood 1998; 91:2985–2990.

51. Ali A, Mundle SD, Ragasa D, Reza S, Shetty V, Mativi BY, Cartlidge JD, Azharuddin M, Qawi H, Dar S, Raza A. Sequential activation of caspase-1 and caspase-3-like proteases during apoptosis in myelodysplastic syndromes. J Hematother Stem Cell Res 1999; 8:343–356.

52. Bouscary D, Chen YL, Guesnu M, Picard F, Viguier F, Lacombe C, Dreyfus F, Fontenay-Roupie M. Activity of the caspase-3/CPP32 enzyme is increased in "early stage" myelodysplastic syndromes with excessive apoptosis, but caspase inhibition does not enhance colony formation in vitro. Exp Hematol 2000; 28:784–791.

53. Aizawa S, Nakano M, Iwase O, Yaguchi M, Hiramoto M, Hoshi H, Nabeshima R, Shima D, Handa H, Toyama K. Bone marrow stroma from refractory anemia of myelodysplastic syndrome is defective in its ability to support normal CD34-postive cell proliferation and differentiation in vitro. Leuk Res 1999; 23:239–246.

54. Aizawa S, Hiramoto M, Hoshi H, Toyama K, Shima D, Handa H. Establishment of stromal cell line from an MDS RA patient which induced an apoptotic change in hematopoietic and leukemic cells in vitro. Exp Hematol 2000; 28:148–155.

55. Brenner C, Kroemer G. Apoptosis. Mitochondria—the death signal integrators. Science 2000; 289:1150–1151.

56. Gattermann N. From sideroblastic anemia to the role of mitochondrial DNA mutations in myelodysplastic syndromes. Leuk Res 2000; 24:141–151.

57. Cortelezzi A, Cattaneo C, Sarina B, Cristiani S, Pomati M, Silvestris I, Motta M, Ibatici A, Gornati G, Volpe AD, Maiolo AT. Efficacy of N-acetylcysteine and all-trans retinoic acid in restoring in vitro effective hematopoiesis in myelodysplastic syndromes. Leuk Res 2000; 24:129–137.

58. List AF, Brasfield F, Heaton R, Glinsmann-Gibson B, Crook L, Taetle R, Capizzi R. Stimulation of hematopoiesis by amifostine in patients with myelodysplastic syndrome. Blood 1997; 90:3364–3369.

59. Kitagawa M, Takahashi M, Yamaguchi S, Inoue M, Ogawa S, Hirokawa K, Kamiyama R. Expression of inducible nitric oxide synthase (NOS) in bone marrow cells of myelodysplastic syndromes. Leukemia 1999; 13:699–703.

60. Mundle S, Venugopal P, Shetty V, Ali A, Chopra H, Handa H, Rose S, Mativi BY, Gregory SA, Preisler HD, Raza A. The relative extent and propensity of CD34+ vs. CD34− cells to undergo apoptosis in myelodysplastic marrows. Int J Hematol 1999; 69:152–159.

61. Philpott NJ, Scopes J, Marsh JC, Gordon-Smith EC, Gibson FM. Increased apoptosis in aplastic anemia bone marrow progenitor cells: possible pathophysiologic significance. Exp Hematol 1995; 23:1642–1648.

62. Koh PS, Hughes GC, Faulkner GR, Keeble WW, Bagby GC. The Fanconi anemia group C gene product modulates apoptotic responses to tumor necrosis factor-α and Fas ligand but does not suppress expression of receptors of the tumor necrosis factor receptor superfamily. Exp Hematol 1999; 27:1–8.

63. Perdahl EB, Naprstek BL, Wallace WC, Lipton JM. Erythroid failure in Diamond-Blackfan anemia is characterized by apoptosis. Blood 1994; 83:645–650.

64. Yoshida Y, Anzai N, Kawabata H. Apoptosis in normal and neoplastic hematopoiesis. Crit Rev Oncol Hematol 1996; 24:185–211.

65. Raza A, Qawi H, Lisak L, Andric T, Dar S, Andrews C, Venugopal P, Gezer S, Gregory S, Loew J, Robin E, Rifkin S, Hsu WT, Huang RW. Patients with myelodysplastic syndromes benefit from palliative therapy with amifostine, pentoxifylline, and ciprofloxacin with or without dexamethasone. Blood 2000; 95:1580–1587.

66. Novitzky N, Mohamed R, Finlayson J, du Toit C. Increased apoptosis of bone marrow cells and preserved proliferative capacity of selected progenitors predict for clinical response to anti-inflammatory therapy in myelodysplastic syndromes. Exp Hematol 2000; 28:941–949.

67. Hellstrom-Lindberg E. Treatment of adult myelodysplastic syndromes. Int J Hematol 1999; 70:141–154.

68. Cazzola M. Alternatives to conventional or myeloablative chemotherapy in myelodysplastic syndrome. Int J Hematol 2000; 72:134–138.

# 9

# Application of Single and Multiple Prognostic Factors in the Assessment of Patients with the Myelodysplastic Syndromes

**Carlo Aul and Aristoteles Giagounidis**
*St. Johannes Hospital, Duisburg, Germany*

**Ulrich Germing**
*Heinrich-Heine-Universität, Düsseldorf, Germany*

## I. INTRODUCTION

Myelodysplastic syndromes (MDS) are acquired hematopoietic stem cell disorders characterized by ineffective hematopoiesis, cellular dysfunction, and an increased risk of transformation into acute myeloid leukemia (AML). Increased apoptosis of myeloid cells is the central mechanism of ineffective hematopoiesis that leads to peripheral blood cytopenias. These disorders typically occur in older persons, although the proportion of younger adults diagnosed as having MDS appears to be rising in recent years. It has been estimated that the overall incidence of MDS in the human population is about 2–4/100,000/year (1). Incidence rates of 20–30/100,000/year in people over 70 demonstrate that MDS are among the most common hematological malignancies in this age group.

The diagnostic workup often starts from a chance finding on routine blood count. Anemia with normal or low reticulocyte counts is the most common finding, encountered in more than 90% of patients. The bone marrow smear yields evidence to confirm the diagnosis and is required for further subclassification of MDS. Although the World Health Organization (WHO) has recently published new proposals for morphological diagnosis (2), the French-American-British (FAB) classification (3) is still the gold standard for categorizing patients with

MDS; according to FAB criteria, five morphological subtypes are distinguished, including refractory anemia (RA), RA with ringed sideroblasts (RARS), RA with excess blasts (RAEB), RAEB in transformation (RAEB-t) and chronic myelo-monocytic leukemia (CMML).

One of the hallmarks of MDS is the heterogeneity, which is reflected not only by the variety of hematological manifestations, but also by the great differences in survival and AML incidence between individual patients. Whereas some patients succumb to complications of bone marrow failure or AML development within a few months of diagnosis, others show a relatively stable course and may survive for many years. Figure 1 shows the estimated overall survival of 1494 patients with MDS, diagnosed at the University of Düsseldorf over a period of almost 25 years and treated with supportive measures only. In good agreement with data from other centers, median survival of the entire patient population was about 2 years. Twenty percent of the patients exhibited a benign course of disease, surviving at least 5 years after diagnosis. Given the advanced age of most patients with the problem of attendant comorbidities, these patients should usually not receive active treatment for MDS. On the other hand, about the same proportion of patients is threatened by an aggressive course of disease that may be similar to that of de novo AML. The greatly reduced life expectancy of these patients often justifies the use of intensive therapeutic modalities such as AML-

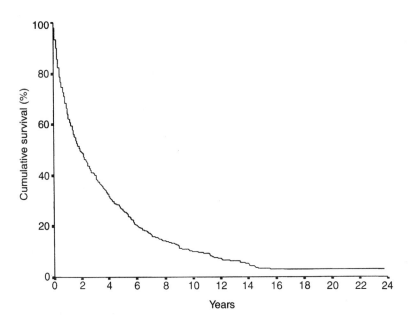

**Fig. 1**   Cumulative survival of 1494 primary MDS patients treated with supportive measures only. MDS, myelodysplastic syndromes.

type chemotherapy and autologous or allogeneic stem cell transplantation. Clearly, the marked differences in prognosis of MDS complicate therapeutic decisions.

The divergent life expectancies of newly diagnosed patients reflect the dynamic multistep pathogenesis of MDS. Pathogenesis is characterized by a series of genetic alterations affecting the myeloid progenitor cells in the bone marrow. Based on sequential morphological and cytogenetic bone marrow examinations, Tricot et al. (4) described three patterns of clonal evolution in MDS: (1) patients with an apparently stable disease with minimal or no increase in bone marrow blasts, (2) patients with an initially stable disease who, often upon occurrence of additional cytogenetic anomalies, abruptly progress to AML, and (3) patients with a gradual, but steady increase in bone marrow blasts that ultimately reach the diagnostic level of clinical AML.

Considering the marked heterogeneity of MDS, it was not surprising that many investigators tried to identify prognostic parameters for assigning patients to different risk groups. However, interpretation of therapeutic trials was largely hampered by nonuniform patient groups. A classic example is the outcome of treatment with low-dose cytosine arabinoside, which yielded response rates between 26 and 71% even in a large series of patients (5). It is likely that the wide range of treatment results is due to selection of patients with different risk factors. But now that new treatments such as immunomodulatory agents, intensive chemotherapy, or stem cell transplantation are becoming increasingly available, there is an urgent need for better and reliable risk stratification of MDS patients. This chapter summarizes our current knowledge of the prognostic parameters in MDS and discusses the clinical benefit of evaluating the survival probability and risk of AML development as based upon clinical, hematological, and cytogenetic factors.

Most of the studies reviewed reported results on adult patients with MDS. It is noteworthy, however, that in recent years increasing information has been compiled on pediatric cases of MDS, and this information has shown that prognostic factors in pediatric MDS appear to be different from those in adult MDS. This difference mainly results from the fact that most pediatric cases of MDS, which have been estimated to account for 1–3% of childhood malignancies, belong to the CMML subgroup whereas in adults, CMML accounts for only 10–15% of the patients. Further information on pediatric MDS is available in several excellent publications (6,7).

## II. PREREQUISITES FOR USING CLINICAL AND BIOLOGICAL VARIABLES AS RISK FACTORS

There are prerequisites for first identifying clinical parameters in risk evaluation of MDS. The parameters should be predictive of the patient's life expectancy.

In addition, large patient populations are usually required for identifying significant risk parameters. Reported patient series are often heterogeneous with regard to sample size, period of investigation, time of diagnosis, minimal diagnostic criteria of MDS, morphological subgroups, percentage of patients with secondary MDS, inclusion of treated patients, length of follow-up as well as application of statistical methods. This may explain why earlier studies failed to demonstrate significant differences between the survival curves of patients with and without abnormal karyotypes (8), whereas more recent investigations have clearly established the prognostic importance of cytogenetic analysis. Finally, for greatest selectivity and sensitivity in identifying risk factors, studies should be designed for the purpose of assessing the importance of these factors rather than subjecting completed studies to retrospective analysis.

The validity and utility of prognostic parameters should also be determined. First, to be widely applicable, prognostic parameters should be readily available to all practicing hematologists. For example, molecular genetic findings, despite their importance for understanding the varied natural course of MDS, are unlikely to be incorporated into risk analysis because such parameters are available only to specialists. Second, the independent statistical significance of the prognostic variable should be confirmed by multivariate analysis. For example, the prognostic value of the FAB classification diminishes, or gets lost, if the medullary blast cell count is included in the multivariate analysis. In addition, the prognostic value should also be confirmed by independent investigators in different patient series. Third, use of the prognostic parameter should be inexpensive. For example, magnetic resonance imaging of bone marrow is unlikely to become an integral part of the prognostic workup of newly diagnosed patients with MDS although it has been shown to provide valuable information for assessing overall survival and leukemia-free survival (9). Even the most significant variables such as chromosomal analysis are increasingly subjected to financial constraints. As an example, only 262 (18%) of 1494 patients recorded in the Düsseldorf bone marrow registry had been karyotyped despite the importance of MDS research at the University of Düsseldorf and the close cooperation between the university and the local hospitals and private practices. Furthermore, the cytogenetic evaluations were performed on patients who averaged 12 years younger than patients in whom no chromosome studies were performed. It is likely that the practicing clinicians did not perform a chromosomal analysis in elderly patients because they felt that their patients were too frail to obtain any therapeutic benefit from the result of karyotyping. Thus, without therapeutic benefit, almost any cost precludes the collection of the data and negates the utility of the prognostic parameter.

It is not clear whether there is a need for prognostic parameters that provide information on the patient's risk of transformation to acute leukemia. There are no studies demonstrating that MDS patients with transformation to acute leukemia die of causes different than those of patients whose medullary blast count remains below 30%. Mufti reported a study by Tricot in which the median survival of patients whose disease progressed to acute leukemia was not significantly different from that of patients whose disease did not transform (10). Complications due to peripheral blood cytopenias and functional defects of circulating blood elements were the leading causes of death in both patient groups. A similar conclusion regarding effects on median survival times is derived from our own data. Figure 2 shows the cumulative survival of 168 patients with RAEB-t who were treated with supportive care only. This morphological subgroup was chosen because RAEB-t patients carry the highest risk for disease progression to AML; in the entire group of patients, 65 cases of AML transformation were observed. The median survival for patients with or without AML development was almost identical, amounting to 7 and 5 months, respectively. Although transformation of MDS to AML may not directly impact survival, predicting the risk of AML transformation may be useful in evaluating new therapeutic treatments such as administration of hematopoietic growth factors (e.g., GM-CSF, granulocyte-monocyte colony-stimulating factor; G-CSF, granulocyte colony-stimulating fac-

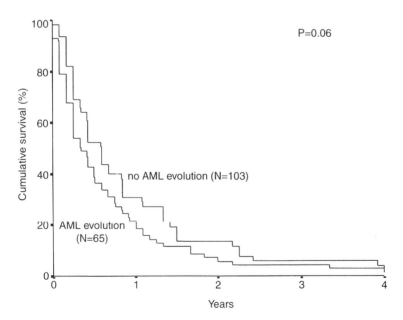

**Fig. 2** Cumulative survival rates of 168 RAEB-t patients treated with supportive measures only. The median survival for patients with or without AML development is not significantly different. N, number; P, probability of error; RAEB-t, refractory anemia with excess blasts in transformation; AML, acute myeloid leukemia.

tor; and interleukin 3), which potentially lower the risk of leukemic transformation (11,12).

Although a large number of prognostic factors have been described in the myelodysplastic syndromes (Table 1), only a few variables have gained practical acceptance. Since no single variable can identify precisely the clinical course and final outcome in the patient, scoring systems are used to enhance the predictive power by combining several features of the disease that have been proven through multivariate analysis to be of independent prognostic value. However, the clinical course of the individual patient may be wrongly predicted using these variables since scoring systems cannot yet anticipate clonal evolution in MDS.

Although prognostic factors were established to predict the natural course of MDS, several recent reports indicate that such factors are also helpful in pre-

**Table 1** Prognostic Factors in Myelodysplastic Syndromes

| | |
|---|---|
| Clinical parameters | DNA ploidy |
| Age | Hypodiploid marrow cells |
| Previous exposure to radiochemo-therapy | Molecular genetic findings |
| | *ras* and *fms* mutations |
| Laboratory features | *c-mpl* and *dcc* expression |
| Degree of peripheral blood cytopenias | *p53* mutations |
| Lactate dehydrogenase (LDH) activity | Abnormalities of CDK inhibitors |
| Serum deoxythymidine kinase (TK) | (e.g., *p15^{INK4B}*) |
| Soluble interleukin-2 receptor (SIL-2R) | Immunophenotyping |
| | CD13, CD33, and CD34 expression |
| Bone marrow morphology | Monoclonal antibody ratios |
| Blast cell percentage | Lymphoid markers |
| French-American-British (FAB) subtype | Fas/APO-1 (CD95) and Fas ligand expression |
| World Health Organization (WHO) subtype | Markers of cell proliferation (e.g., MIB-1) |
| Degree of hematopoietic dysplasia | P-170 glycoprotein expression |
| Cellularity | Bone marrow culturing |
| Myelofibrosis | Abortive myeloid cluster formation |
| Abnormal localization of immature precursors (ALIP) | Defective maturation within colonies |
| | Presence of clonogenic leukemic cells (CFU-L) |
| Chromosomal status | Long-term bone marrow cultures |
| Numerical abnormalities | |
| Structural abnormalities | |
| Karyotypic evolution | |
| Clonal status (NN, AA, AN) | |

AA, abnormal metaphases; AN, abnormal and normal metaphases; NN, normal metaphases, CDK, cyclin-dependent kinases; CD, marker proteins; CFU-L, colony-forming unit–leukocyte.

dicting the response to specific treatments. For example, cytogenetic abnormalities that are usually associated with an unfavorable clinical course are highly predictive of outcome after AML-type chemotherapy or allogeneic bone marrow transplantation (13,14). Hirst and Mufti reported that the rate of disease progression predicts the quality of remissions following intensive chemotherapy for MDS (15). Appelbaum and Anderson evaluated the relationship of the International Prognostic Scoring System (IPSS) risk categorization to the outcome of allogeneic bone marrow transplantation in 250 patients with MDS and found out that the IPSS score is closely correlated with the patients' disease-free survival and relapse rate after transplantation (16).

## III. CLINICAL PARAMETERS

In several studies (17–21), older age has been associated with poorer prognosis in MDS. Tricot et al. (17) reported that younger patients (<50 years) die less frequently of infectious and/or hemorrhagic complications than elderly patients (>70 years), while the percentage of patients transforming to AML was similar in both age groups. Sanz et al. (18) confirmed the prognostic value of age by univariate and multivariate analyses and incorporated this parameter in their scoring system. Considering age as an important parameter, it must also be realized that the vast majority of patients (>75%) are older than 60 years at diagnosis. Other authors have questioned the prognostic value of age, explaining the poorer life expectancy of older people by a higher incidence of deaths unrelated to MDS (22). A similar relationship was also shown for adverse prognosis and the male sex. Although survival was significantly shorter in men, Morel et al. found no difference in standard mortality ratios between male and female patients (22). A number of other clinical parameters, such as weight loss or presence of anemic symptoms, infections, and hemorrhages at diagnosis, have also been associated with an adverse prognosis in MDS (18,23).

Compared with primary MDS, secondary myelodysplastic syndromes, occurring after exposure of patients to chemotherapy and/or radiotherapy, show an unfavorable clinical course with a high rate of leukemic transformation. Therapy-induced MDS differ from primary MDS in several respects, including younger age of patients, more severe cytopenias, more pronounced bone marrow dysplasia ("trilineage MDS"), and a higher incidence of clonal karyotype anomalies (24). Also, reduced marrow cellularity, often combined with fibrosis (25–50% of cases), is common and increases the difficulty of obtaining adequate material for cytological evaluation. Furthermore, patients with secondary MDS usually present with an advanced stage of disease. In a study conducted at the M.D. Anderson Cancer Center (25), 73% of secondary MDS patients were classified as having RAEB or RAEB-t (the more advanced stages), whereas patients with primary

MDS usually show an even distribution between early and advanced stages. The poor prognosis of secondary MDS is largely explained by its association with unfavorable chromosome abnormalities such as deletions or monosomies of chromosomes 5 and/or 7 and complex aberrations (26). Thus, once cytogenetics are taken into consideration, there remains only a relatively small difference in survival between primary and secondary MDS patients.

## IV. LABORATORY FEATURES

Despite a close relationship between medullary blast cell percentage and peripheral blood cytopenias, hemoglobin levels and platelet counts are independent risk factors for predicting survival in MDS. Peripheral blood cytopenias reflect not only the extent of blast cell infiltration, but also the impaired maturation of hematopoietic progenitors in the bone marrow (dyshematopoiesis). The platelet count seems to be the most important prognostic factor among different cytopenias while the predictive value of neutrophil counts is less certain. Mufti et al. (27) hold that even mild granulocytopenia is of prognostic value and integrated a cut-off value of $2.5 \times 10^9/L$ in their scoring system (Bournemouth score). Other authors found that neutrophil counts become prognostic indicators only when falling below certain limits (0.5, 1.0, or $2.0 \times 10^9/L$) (8,18,28,29). In our own studies (30,31), we were unable to demonstrate shortened survival and increased risk of AML transformation among patients with reduced neutrophil counts; Figure 3 shows that in our population the survival probability for patients with a neutrophil count $\leq 2.5 \times 10^9/L$ or $>2.5 \times 10^9/L$ was almost identical. Mufti et al. and Kerkhofs et al. were the first to note that combinations of peripheral cytopenias (bi- and tricytopenia) carry a worse prognosis than isolated cytopenia (20,27).

The presence of circulating blast cells carries a poor prognosis, in terms of both survival and risk of leukemic transformation, and has been confirmed by numerous studies (8,18,30,32–34). In the Spanish series, patients with circulating blast cells had an actuarial median survival of only 6 months (18). Because the proportion of blast cells in the peripheral blood is a function of the blast cell content of the bone marrow, circulating blasts have no independent prognostic value when analyzed by multivariate analysis. It is noteworthy that the percentage of blast cells in the peripheral blood is a criterion of the FAB classification.

Besides peripheral blood findings, several other laboratory parameters have been evaluated for their prognostic value in MDS. Surprisingly, serum lactate dehydrogenase (LDH) activity has received little attention in the literature, although LDH levels have been identified as useful prognostic factors in a variety of other hematological malignancies (35,36). In two independent patient series we demonstrated that LDH activity is strongly correlated with survival (30,31).

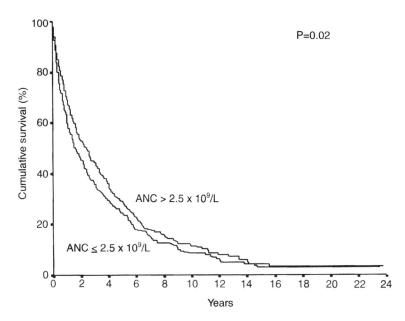

**Fig. 3**   Cumulative survival of 1306 primary MDS patients separated according to neutrophil count at the time of diagnosis. ANC, absolute neutrophil count; P, probability of error; MDS, myelodysplastic syndromes.

Median survival for patients with normal enzyme levels at diagnosis was 37 months, as compared with 11 months for patients with increased LDH activity (Fig. 4). By reflecting increased cell turnover, the elevated enzyme activity may represent a measure of ineffective hematopoiesis; however, there was no apparent correlation with the percentage of bone marrow blasts. In the CMML group, LDH activity was the only parameter besides the medullary blast cell count that was significantly related to the prognosis of patients (30). The independent prognostic value of LDH was confirmed by multivariate survival analysis. Furthermore, when cytogenetic data were included in the Cox regression model, the prognostic importance of LDH was maintained. Besides our group, Sanz et al. (18) and Maddox et al. (34) confirmed the prognostic value of LDH levels.

   Another interesting parameter that has only recently been incorporated into prognostic factor analysis is deoxythymidine kinase, a key enzyme of the salvage pathway for pyrimidine deoxyribonucleotide synthesis. Serum levels of deoxythymidine kinase (sTK) have been shown to provide prognostic information in AML, multiple myeloma, Hodgkin's disease, and non-Hodgkin's lymphomas (37). Studies in patients with AML have shown that serum TK is closely related to the degree of medullary blast cell infiltration and may thus serve as a measure

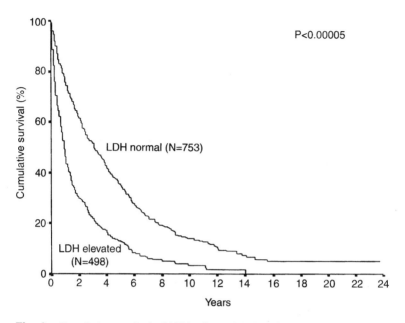

**Fig. 4** Cumulative survival of 1251 primary MDS patients separated according to serum lactate dehydrogenase (LDH) activity at the time of diagnosis. N, number; P, probability of error; MDS, myelodysplastic syndromes.

of leukemic cell burden (38). Investigations in MDS have shown that about 80% of patients present with increased enzyme levels (>5 U/μl) at the time of diagnosis. While there was no correlation between serum TK level and medullary blast cell count, TK activities tended to increase with progression of MDS. For patients with TK levels <10 U/μl, actuarial survival 2 years after diagnosis was 63%, as compared with 43% for those with enzyme values ≥10 U/μl (Fig. 5). The 5-year cumulative survival rates were 31 and 21%, respectively (39). Whereas Aul et al. found that sTK levels at diagnosis did not predict transformation to AML, Musto et al. reported a strong correlation between sTK and risk of AML development (40). In the Italian study, the independent prognostic value of sTk for predicting overall and leukemia-free survival was corroborated by multivariate analysis (40).

Several investigators have shown that plasma levels of soluble interleukin-2 receptor (sIL-2R) are increased in high-risk MDS (41,42). Ogata et al. have made a similar observation in a recent study of 80 MDS patients (43). These authors also noted that increased sIL-2R levels in low-risk MDS patients are predictive of an unfavorable clinical course. More specifically, 14 of 40 patients with RA or RARS presenting with elevated sIL-2R values developed significant

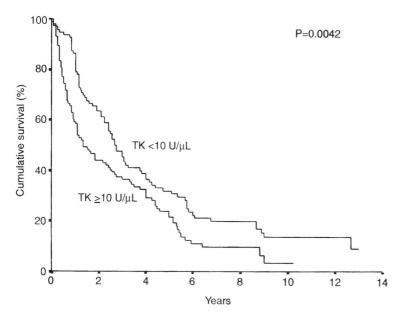

**Fig. 5** Cumulative survival of 212 primary MDS patients separated according to serum deoxythymidine kinase (TK) values at the time of diagnosis. P, probability of error; MDS, myelodysplastic syndromes.

complications (transfusion-dependent anemia, life-threatening infections, disease progression, or MDS-related death), whereas the clinical course of low-risk patients with low sIL-2R levels was uneventful.

## V.  BONE MARROW MORPHOLOGY

Cytological bone marrow (BM) smears are available in all cases of MDS and can therefore be used for prognostic purposes. Among quantitative parameters, the medullary blast cell count is by far the most important prognostic parameter. Whereas some authors found that distinction between cases with <5% and ≥5% blast cells in the bone marrow is sufficient for prognostic purposes, Sanz et al. (18) showed that the patients' life expectancy progressively shortens with increasing medullary blast cell percentage. Sanz et al. also demonstrated that RAEB is a heterogeneous disease that, by defining an extra cutoff point at 10% bone marrow blasts, can be separated into two subgroups with significantly different prognoses. Figures 6 and 7 show the estimated overall survival as well as the cumula-

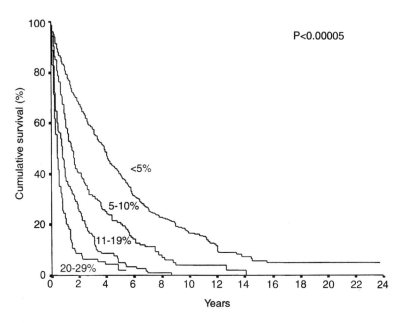

**Fig. 6** Cumulative survival of 1494 primary MDS patients treated with supportive care only and separated according to blast cell percentage in the bone marrow at the time of diagnosis. P, probability of error; MDS, myelodysplastic syndromes.

tive rates of AML transformation for 1494 primary MDS patients (treated with supportive care only) separated according to the bone marrow blast cell percentage at the time of diagnosis. As expected, the medullary blast cell burden is not only indicative of survival, but also possesses a strong predictive weight for the incidence of AML transformation. Cumulative risk of AML 2 years after diagnosis was 7% for patients with bone marrow blasts <5% and climbed up to 67% for the group with the highest blast cell percentage. Similarly, Iwabuchi et al. proposed a second cutoff value of 3% blast cells for patients with refractory anemia. These investigators found that patients with ≥3% blasts had a significantly worse prognosis than patients with <3% blasts in the bone marrow, but their results were based on an analysis of only 47 cases (45). Despite the observations of Iwabuchi et al. and Sanz et al., other researchers have not found a difference in survival when patients with 10–19% BM blasts were compared with those having 20–29% BM blasts (18,44).

The degree of bone marrow dysplasia has also been associated with an adverse prognosis in MDS. In Japanese patients, qualitative abnormalities of hematopoietic cells appeared to have higher prognostic significance than quantitative changes (33). Thiele et al. described a linkage of severe dyshematopoesis

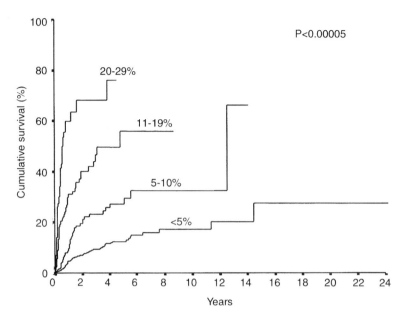

**Fig. 7** Cumulative risk of transformation to AML in 1494 primary MDS patients treated with supportive care only and separated according to blast cell percentage in the bone marrow at the time of diagnosis. P, probability of error; AML, acute myeloid leukemia; MDS, myelodysplastic syndromes.

to leukemic evolution of MDS (46). Whereas abnormalities of the erythroid series were of only minor importance, dysgranulopoiesis and dysmegakaryopoiesis had a strong prognostic weight. Varela et al. incorporated features of dyshematopoiesis into a new classification system in an attempt to improve the FAB classification that relies primarily on the percentage of blast cells in the bone marrow and peripheral blood (47), but little attention was given to this new classification system by practicing hematologists. In addition, there is a long-lasting debate on the prognostic importance of Auer rods in MDS. Contrary to previous assumptions, the presence of Auer rods does not indicate a rapidly progressive disorder, unless the bone marow blast count is increased (48). Furthermore, as only a minority of MDS patients (less than 3% in our series) have this morphological feature, this question of the significance of Auer rods is of academic interest only.

The increasing use of bone marrow biopsies has provided new possibilities for the prognostic evaluation of MDS patients and led to the definition of two additional variants of the syndrome (hypoplastic myelodysplasia and myelodysplasia with bone marrow fibrosis). Besides a precise assessment of bone marrow cellularity and myelofibrosis, histological specimens allow an investigation of the relationship between hematopoietic tissue and bony trabeculae. Krause et al., as cited in Boogaerts et al. (49), first described the presence of clusters (ALIPs, abnormal localization of immature precursors) of myeloid blast cells or promyelocytes aberrantly localized in the intertrabecular areas of the trephine sections. The prognostic impact of ALIPs was demonstrated by Tricot et al. (8) but the impact was confined to patients with RA and RARS. The survival time of ALIP-positive patients in the RA and RARS categories was significantly shorter than that of ALIP-negative cases (416 days vs. 1465 days). ALIP-positive patients also had an increased risk of AML transformation (44% vs. 5%). Boogaerts et al. confirmed the effects on survival, reporting a median survival of 28 months for ALIP-positive cases as compared with 65 months for ALIP-negative patients with RA/RARS (49). To clearly distinguish between true ALIPs and pseudoclusters of proerythroblasts and micromegakaryocytes in the bone marrow, Mangi and Mufti emphasized the importance of performing combined histopathological, cytochemical, and immunological studies (50). The size of the aggregates is also important because only patients with large blastic infiltrates were invariably characterized by short survival and early evolution to AML (51). Maschek et al. performed a multivariate analysis of several histological parameters in a large cohort of MDS cases and were able to corroborate the independent prognostic value of ALIPs (52).

Hyperfibrotic MDS was first described by Sultan et al. in a series of eight patients (53). Hyperfibrotic MDS, which is now considered a distinct MDS entity, is often associated with hyperplasia and marked dysplasia of megakaryopoiesis and must be distinguished from acute megakaryoblastic leukemia and myeloproliferative disorders with accompanying fibrosis. In fact, myelofibrosis occurs rarely in MDS. Maschek et al. observed a marked diffuse myelofibrosis in only 21 (3.7%) of 569 samples from patients with primary MDS (52). The median survival of these patients was markedly reduced in comparison with patients not having an increase in reticulin fibers (8 months vs. 18 months). In other series, marked myelofibrosis was also found to be associated with an unfavorable clinical course, the median survival ranging from 7 to 18 months (54,55). In some series, the negative prognostic influence of myelofibrosis on survival and AML transformation was confirmed by multivariate analysis (52,56). In the Hannover series, myelofibrosis had the strongest impact on prognosis in the otherwise good prognosis group of MDS patients presenting with <5% blast cells in the bone marrow (52). Ohyashiki et al. reported seven of 82 patients with primary MDS who developed severe myelofibrosis during the course of the disease had expired 1–9.5 months after the onset of myelofibrosis. Six of the seven patients had presented with chromosomal abnormalities, often complex aberrations, at the time of diagnosis of MDS (57).

Although not included in the original proposals of the FAB group, hypoplastic MDS is now accepted as separate entity, occurring in 8–19% of all MDS patients (29,58,59). Tuzuner et al. recently proposed criteria for the diagnosis of hypoplastic MDS, based upon the criteria being age-corrected or absolute bone marrow cellularity (60). Distinguishing hypoplastic MDS from aplastic anemia can be challenging, because trilineage dysplasia is sometimes difficult to assess and karyotypic abnormalities have also been discovered in patients with aplastic anemia (61). Irrespective of these challenges, bone marrow hypoplasia is not an adverse factor because patients with hypocellular MDS have similar prognosis to those with normocellular or hypercellular MDS (60). In the Hannover series of 352 patients, median survival was 22 months for hypoplastic MDS, 27 months for normocellular MDS, and 14 months for hypercellular MDS (58). Some authors reported that the incidence of leukemic transformation in hypoplastic MDS is slightly lower than in typical MDS (62). Others have claimed that certain karyotype abnormalities involving chromosomes 6 and 7 are associated with hypoplastic MDS (63,64).

## VI. FAB AND WHO CLASSIFICATION

The prognostic usefulness of the FAB classification has been demonstrated by numerous studies (8,18–23,27,29–33) and was the basis for its widespread acceptance among hematologists. In general, patients with RA and RARS survive significantly longer than patients with RAEB, RAEB-t, and CMML. However, despite its undisputed value, the FAB classification has certain limitations. These limitations result from the arbitrary demarcation of subgroups, overlapping features of patients in different FAB categories, overemphasis of morphological findings (e.g., Auer rods), and exclusion of other important prognostic variables such as peripheral blood cell counts and karyotype anomalies. A comparison between different studies shows that there is considerable heterogeneity in both survival (Table 2) and risk of AML transformation within defined FAB subgroups, particularly in patients with RARS and CMML.

We have previously proposed to distinguish two forms of sideroblastic anemia: (1) "pure" sideroblastic anemia (PSA), which shows only signs of dyserythropoiesis, and (2) refractory anemia with ringed sideroblasts (RARS), which is characterized not only by erythroid hyperplasia and ineffective erythropoiesis, but also by disturbed granulopoiesis and megakaryopoiesis. On retrospective analysis of 94 patients with sideroblastic anemia, we found that PSA and RARS differed considerably in terms of patient survival and incidence of AML (65). Almost identical results have now been obtained through a prospective study, with a 10 year follow-up period, of 232 new patients with acquired idiopathic

**Table 2** Natural History of Primary Myelodysplastic Syndromes: Median Survival of FAB Subgroups in 11 Studies Published Between 1985 and 1999

| Study (publication) | Patients ($n$) | Median survival (months) | | | | |
|---|---|---|---|---|---|---|
| | | RA | RARS | RAEB | RAEB-t | CMML |
| Mufti et al., 1985 (27) | 141 | 32 | 76 | 10.5 | 5 | 22 |
| Kerkhofs et al., 1987 (20) | 237 | 50 | >60 | 9 | 6 | >60 |
| Sanz et al., 1989 (18) | 370 | 26 | 34 | 9 | 5 | 12 |
| Goasguen et al., 1990 (154) | 503 | 32 | 45 | 19 | 11 | 15 |
| Morel et al., 1993 (74) | 408 | 51 | >84 | 18 | 15 | 21 |
| Maschek et al., 1994 (52) | 569 | 26.5 | 42 | 8.5 | 4.5 | 12.5 |
| Aul et al., 1992 (30) | 235 | 30 | 21 | 8 | 4 | 19 |
| Musilova et al., 1995 (77) | 240 | 57 | 35 | 10 | 4 | 32 |
| Oguma et al., 1995 (33) | 838 | 65 | 58 | 16 | 10 | 20 |
| Greenberg et al., 1997 (96) | 814 | 50 | 83 | 18 | 7 | 29 |
| Pfeilstöcker et al., 1999 (158) | 386 | 68 | 65 | 18 | 9 | 24 |

$n$, number; RA, refractory anemia; RARS, refractory anemia with ringed sideroblasts; RAEB, refractory anemia with excess blasts; RAEB-t, refractory anemia with excess blasts in transformation; CMML, chronic myelomonocytic leukemia; FAB, French-American-British classification system.

siderablastic anemia (AISA) (66). The Kaplan-Meier survival curves for the PSA and RARS patients from this prospective study show that the 5-year cumulative survival was 55 and 38%, respectively (Fig. 8). Predominant causes of death in the PSA group were infections and cardiovascular or cerebrovascular diseases, whereas in the RARS group nearly two-thirds of the deaths were attributable to complications of bone marrow failure, including transformation to AML for nine of the patients. The cumulative probability of leukemic progression 5 years after diagnosis was 0% for the PSA group and 15% for patients with RARS. Similar results were obtained in a study by Garand et al., who looked at the natural course of 84 patients with sideroblastic anemia (67). Patients with AISA-E (equivalent to our PSA group) survived significantly longer than patients with the myelodysplastic variant AISA-M (equivalent to our RARS group). Garand et al. also demonstrated a statistical difference in the risk of AML development between both patient groups. It thus appears that cytomorphological distinction between PSA and RARS provides valuable and reproducible prognostic information.

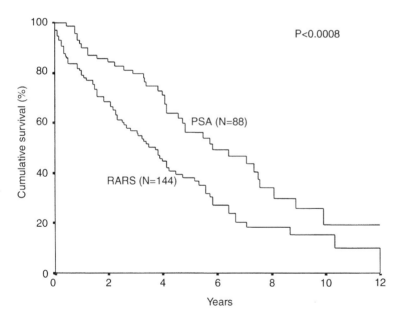

**Fig. 8** Cumulative survival of 232 patients with acquired idiopathic sideroblastic anemia. Patients with pure sideroblastic anemia (PSA) showing only signs of dyserythropoiesis have significantly better life expectancy than patients with refractory anemia with ringed sideroblasts (RARS) in whom the bone marrow smear also shows disturbed granulopoiesis and megakaryopoiesis. N, number; P, probability of error.

Chronic myelomonocytic leukemia, characterized by absolute monocytosis ($>1 \times 10^9$/L) in the peripheral blood, is also a heterogeneous disease. The considerable interstudy variation in survival among patients with CMML is in marked contrast to findings in RAEB and RAEB-t patients (see Table 2). Based on the presence or absence of increased peripheral leukocyte counts (cutoff level $13 \times 10^9$/L), the FAB Cooperative Group (68) later proposed to separate two subtypes of CMML (myelodysplastic and myeloproliferative variants). However, distinguishing between these two subtypes provides little prognostic information as their survival curves are almost identical (69).

By combining morphological, clinical, immunological, and cytogenetic methods, a WHO panel recently revised the FAB classification of myelodysplastic syndromes (2). By defining a medullary blast count of 20% as the dividing line between MDS and AML, the RAEB-t category was eliminated from the MDS classification. CMML was also not included in the revised classification. Refractory anemia (with or without ringed sideroblasts) was defined as a disorder involving the erythroid lineage only. As a new category, a group of patients with limited blast cell numbers ($<5$%) but with significant multilineage dysplasia was defined (refractory cytopenia with multilineage dysplasia). With regard to the distinctive morphological and clinical features, the 5q- syndrome was established as a separate category within MDS. Finally, the WHO panel proposed to categorize as ''myelodysplastic syndrome, unclassifiable'' MDS cases that did not fulfill the criteria of the other categories. At present, it is not clear whether the WHO classification will be of greater value than the FAB classification, thus supplanting the older system, for risk stratifying newly diagnosed MDS patients.

## VII. CHROMOSOMAL ANALYSIS

Cytogenetic investigations are increasingly used in the diagnostic workup of patients with myelodysplastic syndromes. Clonal karyotypic abnormalities are found in 32–76% of patients with primary MDS (70–80) and can be encountered in almost all cases of secondary MDS (81). Karyotype anomalies are probably late events in the pathogenesis of MDS, reflecting the progressive genomic instability of the premalignant clone. Abnormal clones are present in 30–50% of RA and RARS cases, whereas the incidence in patients with RAEB and RAEB-t varies between 60 and 90%. The frequency of cytogenetic anomalies in the CMML group is variable, ranging from 17 to 83% (82,83).

Although it has not been possible to identify genetic lesions specific to MDS, certain anomalies are clearly nonrandom changes. As compared with AML, which often shows reciprocal translocations and inversions, MDS are mainly affected by loss of chromosomal material. Out of 1663 MDS patients with cytogenetic defects reported by Johansson et al. (84), 22% presented with monosomies and 39% had structural abnormalities resulting in partial chromosomal loss. These findings have led to the hypothesis that loss of tumor suppressor genes or specific regulatory genes of hematopoietic cell proliferation and differentiation causes malignant transformation of stem cells in MDS (85).

The most common cytogenetic abnormalities in MDS are del(5q), monosomy 7/del(7q), and trisomy 8, which account for more than 60% of the cases with abnormal metaphases (80). Other recurrent anomalies are translocations involving 1q, rearrangements of 3q, trisomy 6, del(11q), del(12p), involvement of 12q, del(13q), del(17p), isochrome 17q, del(20q), trisomy 21, monosomy 21, and loss of sex chromosomes. Some defects are associated with characteristic hematological and morphological findings; for example, the 5q- syndrome, which was first described by Van den Berghe et al. (86), preferentially occurs in female patients and is associated with macrocytic anemia, normal or elevated platelet counts, erythroid hypoplasia, and presence of hypolobulated megakaryocytes in the bone marrow. Complex aberrations, often involving chromosomes 5 and 7, are three times as frequent in therapy-induced MDS as in primary MDS (26,81,87,88). Other unfavorable findings such as monosomy 7 also occur more frequently in secondary MDS than in primary MDS (89). In rare cases, rearrangements typical of AML, such as t(8;21), inv(16), or t(15;17), have been observed in MDS patients. However, such cases behave clinically like oligoblastic AML rather than preleukemia, and should be excluded from MDS (2).

As the frequency of chromosomal abnormalities generally increases with progression of MDS from RA and RARS to RAEB and RAEB-t (Table 3), it has for years been questioned whether karyotype constitutes an independent prognostic factor for survival and leukemic transformation. These uncertainties were partly due to methodological and statistical issues (e.g., analysis of insufficient numbers of metaphases, poor quality of banding pattern resolution, small patient samples, inclusion of treated patients, use of cytogenetic data obtained during the course rather than at diagnosis of MDS) or careless grouping of cytogenetic findings. For example, the generally negative influence of single defects on the natural course of MDS may be masked by including patients with del(5q), who often show a favorable prognosis. Recently, a number of studies have clearly shown that chromosomal analysis adds independent prognostic value to the medullary blast count and other conventional hematological parameters. Morel et al. (74), who performed a prognostic factor analysis in 408 cases of de novo MDS, found that patients with abnormal karyotype had shorter survival than patients with normal karyotype and that among patients with abnormal cytogenetics prognosis was poorer in patients with complex aberrations. The very poor prognosis of patients with complex cytogenetic abnormalities was confirmed in another

**Table 3** Percentage of Chromosomal Anomalies According to FAB Subtype: 2520 patients with Primary MDS from 12 Studies Published Between 1988 and 2000

| Study (publication) | Patients (n) | Entire group | RA | RARS | RAEB | CMML | RAEB-t |
|---|---|---|---|---|---|---|---|
| Billström et al., 1988 (70) | 111 | 44% | 52% | 31% | 53% | 10% | 0% |
| Yunis et al., 1988 (83) | 90 | 73% | 71% | 39% | 93% | 83% | 91% |
| Pierre et al., 1989 (71) | 247 | 45% | 33% | 39% | 69% | 40% | 57% |
| Suciu et al., 1990 (72) | 120 | 42% | 36% | 14% | 56% | 29% | 47% |
| Toyama et al., 1993 (73) | 401 | 50% | 41% | 75% | 64% | 40% | 50% |
| Bernasconi et al., 1994 (75) | 188 | 69% | 56% | 25% | 76% | 42% | 100% |
| White et al., 1994 (76) | 198 | 38% | 40% | 21% | 50% | 20% | 65% |
| Parlier et al., 1994 (79) | 104 | 55% | 63% | 50% | 56% | 44% | 70% |
| Werner et al., 1994 (82) | 66 | 56% | 68% | 0% | 71% | 17% | 62% |
| Musilova et al., 1995 (77) | 207 | 58% | 64% | 38% | 69% | 35% | 65% |
| Haase et al., 1995 (78) | 148 | 47% | 43% | 27% | 49% | 50% | 57% |
| Solé et al., 2000 (80) | 640 | 51% | 43% | 33% | 61% | 42% | 70% |

n, number; RA, refractory anemia; RARS, refractory anemia with ringed sideroblasts; RAEB, refractory anemia with excess blasts; CMML, chronic myelomonocytic leukemia; RAEB-t, refractory anemia with excess blasts in transformation; FAB, French-American-British classification system; MDS, myelodysplastic syndromes.

large study (73) and shown to be a consistent finding in all FAB subtypes. The survival of patients with complex cytogenetic abnormalities rarely exceeds a few months (90). For example, in our series of 262 untreated patients with primary MDS, patients with complex aberrations had a median survival of only 8 months, whereas it was 40 months for patients presenting with single or double defects (Fig. 9). Two years after diagnosis, the cumulative risk of AML transformation in these subgroups was 37 and 17%, respectively. In comparison, patients with normal chromosomes had a median survival of 55 months, and their actuarial risk of AML development 2 years after diagnosis was 13%. Verhoef et al. (91) also found significant differences in survival between patients with normal karyotype (median survival 30 months), single abnormalities (median survival 21 months), and complex aberrations (median survival 7 months). A number of other studies have shown that an isolated 5q- defect has a more favorable prognosis than any other karyotype in MDS, including a normal karyotype (92–94). Despite longer survival, patients with del(5q) have a comparably low risk of progression to AML (about 10%). The independent prognostic significance of chromosomal analysis in MDS has now been confirmed by multivariate analysis (74,95).

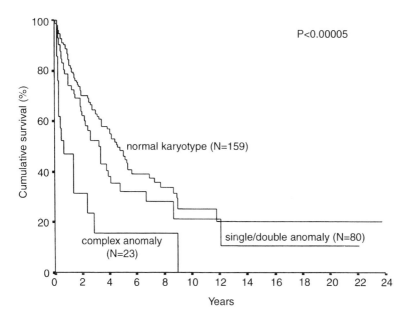

**Fig. 9** Cumulative survival of 262 untreated, primary MDS patients separated according to chromosomal status at the time of diagnosis. N, number; P, probability of error; MDS, myelodysplastic syndromes.

By evaluating 816 patients with primary MDS, the International MDS Risk Consensus Group was able to establish the importance of cytogenetic subgroups regarding survival and risk of evolution to AML (96). This study defined three subgroups with differing prognosis: (1) a favorable group including patients with normal karyotype, loss of the Y chromosome, del(5q), or del(20q); (2) an unfavorable group including patients with complex chromosomal defects (>3 anomalies), monosomy 7, or del(7q); and (3) an intermediate-risk group including other abnormalities such as trisomy 8 and double cytogenetic defects. Seventy percent of patients were segregated into the good-risk group, 16% into the poor-risk group, and 14% into the intermediate-risk group. The median survival times of patients in these three cytogenetic subgroups were 3.8, 0.8, and 2.4 years, respectively, and the times for 75% of the patients to remain free from disease transformation to AML were 5.6, 0.9, and 1.6 years (Fig. 10). In a recent study of 640 patients with de novo MDS, Solé et al. confirmed the prognostic usefulness of the IPSS cytogenetic subgroups (80). By univariate analysis, the investigators also identified additional subgroups with either excellent prognosis (12p deletions) or very poor prognosis (single 1q abnormalities). In addition, they showed that patients with trisomy 8, one of the most frequent defects in MDS, experienced short median survival (about 1 year) and a high risk of leukemic transformation (34% at 1 year after diagnosis), justifying exclusion of these cases from the intermediate-risk category established at the International MDS Risk Consensus Conference.

Acquisition of new karyotypic anomalies during the course of MDS (karyotypic evolution) has been shown to herald poor prognosis and is often associated with an abrupt shift to AML (4,97,98). The relevance of residual normal metaphases in a patient with cytogenetic defects is still a matter of debate. While patients with coexistence of abnormal and normal metaphases (AN) have been reported to have a longer survival and a lower risk of AML development than those patients in whom all metaphases are abnormal (AA), Kerkhofs et al. (20) reported that AN patients have a prognosis identical to AA patients, and Mecucci et al. (99) even claimed that patients with residual normal metaphases carry a worse prognosis than cases in which only aberrant metaphases are found.

Cellular DNA content, which can be measured easily by high-resolution flowcytometry, also appears to be a prognostic factor. In one study, it was demonstrated that the presence of hypodiploid marrow cells (correlating with loss of chromosomal material) is associated with shorter patient survival (100).

In summary, cytogenetics and related investigations are likely to play an increasing role in evaluating the prognosis in MDS patients. Newer techniques, such as fluorescence in situ hybridization using chromosome-specific DNA probes, offer a lower threshold of detection than traditional cytogenetic studies and will further expand the usefulness of chromosomal analysis as part of the diagnostic and prognostic workup in MDS.

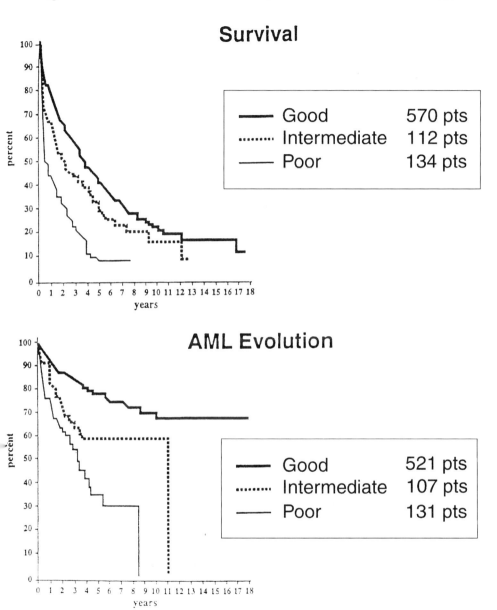

**Fig. 10** Cumulative survival (upper graph) and freedom from AML transformation (lower graph) of 816 patients with primary MDS according to cytogenetic risk categorization proposed by the International MDS Risk Consensus Conference. Good risk: normal karyotype, -Y, del(5q), or del(20q); poor risk: complex chromosomal abnormalities (≥3 anomalies, -7, or del(7q); intermediate risk: other cytogenetic defects. pts, patients; AML, acute myeloid leukemia; MDS, myelodysplastic syndromes. (From Ref. 96.)

## VIII.   MOLECULAR GENETIC FINDINGS

A number of proto-oncogene mutations have been described in patients with MDS. It has been suggested that mutations in the *ras* gene family are relevant to the pathogenesis of MDS and may be used as prognostic indicators. The *ras* genes code for GTP-binding proteins that participate in signal transduction from membrane receptors to the cell nucleus. Impaired GTPase activity of defective *ras* proteins leads to increased intracellular GTP levels, which confer a growth advantage upon affected cells. The incidence of *ras* mutations in patients with MDS is variable, ranging from 3 to 33% in different studies (101,102). Mutations of *ras* are particularly common in CMML and in MDS with accompanying monocytosis (103). Reviewing published data from 624 MDS patients, Parker and Mufti found an overall incidence of 16%, whereas 39% of samples from CMML patients scored positive (104). Mutations were preferentially reported in the neuroblastoma (N-*ras*) gene. Contrary to previous assumptions, *ras* mutations were found in both early and late stages of MDS development. Van Kamp et al. (101) performed a longitudinal analysis of point mutations of the N-*ras* proto-oncogene in patients with MDS who were followed for at least 2.5 years after diagnosis. In three of 90 patients tested, a mutation in codon 12 was found in the most recent blood smears. In all three cases the mutation was not detectable at diagnosis, but was acquired later during the course of MDS. In two of these patients, the mutational event was associated with rapid deterioration and transformation to AML. However, the third patient showed a protracted clinical course during a period of 5 years after acquisition of the mutation. These data indicate that activation of the N-*ras* gene in these three patients represents a secondary phenomenon associated with disease progression in some cases, but compatible with stable disease in others. Paquette et al. (105) retrospectively analyzed a large group of MDS patients to determine the effects of N-*ras* mutation on prognosis and risk of AML transformation. Of 220 evaluable patients, 20 (9%) had point mutations of N-*ras* involving codon 12. Individuals with N-*ras* mutations had a significantly shorter median survival than those who were N-*ras* negative (19 vs. 39 months). An increased risk of AML was also found in patients with N-*ras* mutations. These associations were independent of the percentage of bone marrow blasts and the presence of cytogenetic abnormalities. Whereas several more recent trials reported similar findings (106,107), other investigators found no correlation between *ras* mutations and adverse prognosis, in terms of both survival and transformation to AML (108,109). Thus, the prognostic value of *ras* mutations is still controversially discussed.

Mutations of *fms* and *c-mpl* may be relevant as well to prognosis. The *fms* proto-oncogene encodes the receptor for colony-stimulating factor 1 (alternatively known as macrophage colony-stimulating factor, M-CSF). Although relatively infrequent in MDS (110), *fms* mutations appear to have prognostic value.

Padua et al. (107) observed an increased frequency of transformation to AML in MDS patients harboring mutations of the *fms* proto-oncogene. Patients with oncogene mutations also had a significantly poorer survival compared with those without mutations (107). Bouscary et al. (111) reported overexpression of another oncogene, *c-mpl*, in 42% of patients with RAEB or RAEB-t and in 44% of patients with CMML, while no expression was found in patients with early-stage MDS. In patients with RAEB and RAEB-t, increased expression of *c-mpl* was associated with poor prognosis due to an increased risk of AML development. Forty-five percent of the *c-mpl*–positive patients evolved toward AML with a mean follow-up of 10.5 months, while 13% of the *c-mpl*–negative patients developed secondary leukemia with a mean follow-up of 21.1 months. However, the independent prognostic significance of these observations has not yet been demonstrated.

The *p53* tumor suppressor gene, which is located on the short arm of chromosome 17 (band 17p13), plays a key role in the regulation of the cell cycle. Mutations of *p53* have been reported in a wide range of human malignancies, including hematopoietic neoplasms (112). Mutant *p53* genes have been found in 0–25% of MDS patients, depending on the detection method and composition of the patient sample (113–117). Their presence is strongly correlated with complex chromosome changes including $-5/5q$-, $-7/7q$-, and 17p-. Therefore, it has been speculated that *p53* mutations reflect previous exposure to known or unknown carcinogens (117). Consistent with this assumption is the relatively high frequency of *p53* mutations in patients with therapy-related MDS (118). As expected, *p53* mutations have been shown by some investigators to predict short survival and an increased risk of AML transformation. In the study reported by Kaneko et al. (116), four of seven patients with *p53* mutations progressed to AML within 7 months after diagnosis of MDS, and the remaining three patients died within 7 months without developing AML. In addition, it appears that *p53* mutations indicate a poor response of patients to aggressive AML-type chemotherapy (119).

Miyake et al. (120) reported that expression of another tumor suppressor gene, *dcc* (deleted in colorectal carcinoma), was absent or extremely reduced in two of 24 MDS cases and in five of seven cases of overt leukemia that developed from MDS. It has therefore been suggested that inactivation of the *dcc* gene is related to AML transformation. However, these findings await confirmation by other investigators.

Recently, two groups of researchers have reported that the cyclin-dependent kinase (CDK) inhibitor gene $p15^{INK4B}$, which is involved in the regulation of the G1/S transition of the cell cycle, is frequently inactivated by methylation in advanced-stage MDS (121,122). Methylation of $p15^{INK4B}$ was observed in 20 (38%) of 53 MDS patients and was seen only in patients with a bone marrow blast count >10%. No correlation was found between karyotype and methylation status. On univariate analysis, patients with methylated $p15^{INK4B}$ had a median actuarial survival of 18 months as compared with 48 months in patients with the unmethylated CDK inhibitor gene. However, the prognostic significance of $p15^{INK4B}$ methylation was lost in multivariate analysis, owing to its strong correlation with the bone marrow blast percentage (121). These findings were confirmed in another study reported by Uchida et al. (122), who concluded that inactivation of genes by promoter hypermethylation may be late events in the MDS development.

In summary, a number of new molecular genetic findings with prognostic significance have been reported in the literature. However, such markers will rarely be available outside of research centers, which limits the clinical usefulness of the markers. For prognostic purposes, conventional hematological and cytogenetic parameters will instead be used.

## IX. IMMUNOPHENOTYPING

The role of immunophenotyping in the prognostic evaluation of patients with MDS has not been well established. Kristensen et al. reported that monoclonal antibody ratios (counts of cells with immature myeloid marker characteristics/ counts of cells with mature myeloid marker characteristics) are helpful for predicting prognosis in MDS (123). Several studies have shown that an increased percentage of cells having the marker CD34 (CD34+) or the presence of CD34+ cell aggregates in the bone marrow is associated with an adverse prognosis (124–126). However, Oriani et al. found no correlation between the results of CD34 immunostaining and FAB subtype. In addition, neither the percentage of CD34+ cells nor the number of CD34+ aggregates was correlated with the presence of ALIPs (126,127). Yet, using a cutoff level of 1% CD34+ cells in the bone marrow, patients with RAEB could be separated into two prognostic groups with significantly different survival times (127). The presence of circulating CD34+ cells was also found to be associated with an unfavorable prognosis. In the study of Sullivan et al. (128), 23 of 62 patients with newly diagnosed MDS had >1% CD34+ cells in the peripheral blood mononuclear cell fraction. The CD34 expression was preferentially observed in patients with advanced MDS and was correlated with shorter survival and higher rates of leukemic transformation. It is noteworthy that in this study the presence of circulating CD34+ cells was a better prognostic indicator than cytogenetics or CFU-GM (colony-forming unit–granulocyte/macrophage) colony growth. Up to now, however, the prognostic importance of CD34 expression has not been confirmed by multivariate analysis in a large patient population.

Recent findings suggest that apoptosis is an important pathophysiological mechanism in MDS, resulting in defective production of mature blood cells in the bone marrow (129). Researchers have tried to link apoptosis-related surface markers or oncoproteins to the natural course of MDS. Fas/APO-1 (CD95) is a cell surface molecule belonging to the tumor necrosis factor receptor family that induces apoptosis when bound by its ligand. Compared with a control population, Fas and Fas ligand expression are significantly increased in bone marrow cells from MDS patients (130,131). Examining a large number of MDS, AML-MDS (AML arising from MDS), and de novo AML bone marrow samples, Gupta et al. reported that Fas ligand expression predicts survival in MDS. Median survival of patients with Fas ligand expression on ≤12% bone marrow cells was 28 months as compared with 13 months for patients with >12% positive cells (132). However, the authors observed a strong correlation between Fas ligand expression and other hematological variables (FAB subtype, degree of anemia, transfusion requirements, percentage of abnormal metaphases upon cytogenetic analysis, Bournemouth score), suggesting that Fas ligand measurements provide no additional prognostic information to standard parameters. Recently, Shimazaki et al. (133) investigated the prognostic importance of medullary apoptosis and cell proliferation in 51 patients with various stages of MDS. Bone marrow biopsies were stained immunohistochemically for MIB-1 (marker for proliferating cells) and CD34 and apoptosis was visualized by detection of DNA fragmentation using TdT-incorporation of nucleotides on 3' ends of DNA. The results showed that the apoptotic rate was higher in MDS patients than in control subjects or in AML-MDS patients. The percentage of MIB-1-positive cells was higher in MDS and AML-MDS than in controls. Poor prognosis was indicated by high apoptotic rates, but was not significantly correlated with percentages of MIB-1 and CD34+ cells in the bone marrow (133).

Apart from its importance for predicting the response of patients to cytotoxic therapy, the multidrug resistance (*MDR-1*) gene product P-170 glycoprotein may serve as a prognostic marker in MDS. We investigated the predictive value of P-glycoprotein expression of bone marrow blast cells in 49 consecutive patients, most of them with advanced stages of MDS (134). Nineteen patients were found to be *MDR*-positive. P-glycoprotein expression was strongly correlated with CD34 positivity of blast cells, supporting previous findings that P-glycoprotein expression in MDS is associated with a stem cell phenotype (135,136). The median cumulative survival of patients with P-glycoprotein expression was 14 months as compared with 34 months in *MDR*-negative patients. Differences in AML incidence between both patients groups were not found in our study. In contrast, Sonneveld et al. reported that MDS patients with *MDR* expression have a high risk of leukemic transformation. During a median follow-up period of 8 months, 13 (81%) of 16 P-glycoprotein-positive patients developed AML, as compared with two (20%) of 10 P-glycoprotein-negative patients (136). Another multidrug-associated protein, MRP1, overexpression of which has been reported in human cell lines with non-P-170-glycoprotein-mediated multidrug resistance, was not found to be predictive of survival in a recent study of 56 patients with MDS (137).

## X.  BONE MARROW CULTURE STUDIES

Although MDS are typically associated with an increased bone marrow cellularity, the capacity to develop colony-forming units (CFU) of hematopoietic progenitor cells, including CFU-GM, CFU-E (erythrocyte), CFU-mega (megakaryocyte), CFU-GEMM (granulocyte, erythrocyte, monocyte, megakaryocyte), and BFU-E (burst-forming unit–erythroid), is low or even absent in the majority of patients. Most authors have reported on the colony growth of the progenitor cells CFU-GM. In about 50–90% of MDS patients, numbers of CFU-GM were found to be reduced (138–140). (Owing to variations in culture techniques, patient selection, and sample size, direct comparisons between different studies are often impossible.) Besides reduced colony growth, CFU-GM in MDS often show qualitative defects that are similar to those seen in AML (141,142). Further, Spitzer et al. (143) proposed to distinguish between "leukemic" and "nonleukemic" patterns of CFU-GM growth. Leukemic-type growth includes micro- or macrocluster formation with defective maturation of blasts within aggregates, single persisting blasts, or very low colony formation with <2 colonies/100,000 plated cells. Nonleukemic growth is characterized by persisting colony formation, even if moderately decreased in frequency.

In the literature, there are conflicting data as to the prognostic impact and value of this classification. While some authors found no difference in prognosis (144), others showed that a leukemic growth pattern predicted reduced survival and an increased risk of AML transformation (145–148). In a meta-analysis of 179 patients, median survival of patients with nonleukemic colony growth was 9–50 months as compared with only 5–10 months for patients with leukemic-type growth. The respective percentages of transformation to AML were 21–40% versus 50–80% (149). However, Tricot et al. emphasized that in vitro bone marrow cultures in individual patients are of limited prognostic value because of the large variability in colony growth and the broad overlap of in vitro culture findings between normal probands and MDS patients (8). Importantly, other studies demonstrated that there is a close correlation between in vitro bone marrow culture studies, proportion of medullary blast cells, and FAB subtype (150). Leukemic-type growth was much more common in patients with advanced-stage MDS than in patients belonging to good-prognosis FAB types. In addition, Gold et al. reported that abnormal marrow CFU-GM growth pattern correlated with abnormal marrow cytogenetic status (145). Finally, bone marrow culture studies are technically difficult, laborious, and costly, thus limiting their use as a routine prognostic tool in MDS.

In recent years, other cell biological assays have been applied to MDS patients. Long-term bone marrow cultures have been primarily used to examine the proliferative behavior of hematopoietic stem cells as well as to analyze the function of stromal cells in MDS. In some cases, these techniques have allowed detection of novel cytogenetic or molecular abnormalities that, owing to the small size of the hematopoietic clone, could not be demonstrated in conventional bone marrow specimens. It has been suggested that such findings have prognostic relevance (151). Other authors have tried to obtain prognostic information by assaying clonogenic leukemic cells (blast cell progenitors, also known as colony-forming unit–leukocyte, CFU-L) in MDS. In one study, circulating blast progenitors were identified in 74% of MDS samples. Large numbers of colonies were mainly found in patients with RAEB-t and evolving AML, demonstrating the adverse prognosis of circulating blast cell progenitors in MDS (152). Apart from its value for predicting the natural course of MDS, the CFU-L assay has also been successfully used to predict the response of patients to AML-type chemotherapy (152,153).

## XI. SCORING SYSTEMS

Considering the marked heterogeneity of MDS, it was not surprising that several authors devised scoring systems to assign patients to different risk groups. Initial scoring systems were based on relatively simple hematological parameters. Since then, the objective has been to improve upon the prognostic value of the FAB classification by combining several patient and disease characteristics that were shown by multivariate analysis to provide independent prognostic information, in particular, to incorporate cytogenetic findings into the risk analysis. Table 4 gives an overview on different scoring systems and the parameters on which these systems were based (18,27,30,47,74,79,96,154).

The first scoring system for risk evaluation of MDS patients was proposed in 1985 by the Bournemouth group (27). It was based on univariate analysis of conventional hematological parameters (bone marrow blast count >5%, hemoglobin concentration <10 g/dl, neutrophil count <2.5 × 10⁹/L, and platelet count <100 × 10⁹/L) in a cohort of 141 patients and it defined three risk groups, which differed significantly in both survival and rates of leukemic transformation. The predictive value of the Bournemouth score was confirmed in several independent studies (18,20,30,155–158). Later, the Bournemouth score was modified by adding leukocytosis as an unfavorable prognostic factor to allow its application to patients with CMML, who often present with neutrophilia rather than neutropenia (159). In addition, a number of investigators have proposed other modifications of the original Bournemouth score, employing different combinations and threshold values of hematological and clinical variables.

**Table 4** Comparison of Different Scoring Systems for Evaluating the Natural Course of Patients with Myelodysplastic Syndromes

| Prognostic variable | Scoring system (publication) | | | | | | | |
|---|---|---|---|---|---|---|---|---|
| | Bournemouth, 1985 (27) | FAB, 1985 (47) | Spanish, 1989 (18) | Simplified 3-D, 1990 (154) | Düsseldorf, 1992 (30) | Lille, 1993 (74) | Lausanne-Bournemouth, 1994 (79) | IPSS, 1997 (96) |
| Age | | | • | | | | | |
| Hemoglobin | • | | | • | • | | • | • |
| Neutrophils | • | • | | | | | | • |
| Platelets | • | • | • | • | • | • | • | • |
| LDH | | | | | • | | | |
| BM blasts | • | | • | • | • | • | • | • |
| Dyshematopoiesis | | • | | | | | | |
| Cytogenetics | | | | | | • | • | • |
| Maximum score | 4 | 15 | 5 | 3 | 4 | 4 | 2 | 3.5 |
| No. of risk groups | 3 | 3 | 3 | 3 | 3 | 3 | 3 | 4 |

FAB, French-American-British classification system; IPSS, International Prognostic Scoring System; LDH, serum lactate dehydrogenase; BM, bone marrow.

Other scoring systems were subsequently developed. Following review of 503 cases of patients with MDS, Goasguen et al. (154) published a simplified scoring system that used only bone marrow blast count, hemoglobin concentration, and platelet count as risk factors. Sanz et al. (18) published another score, as a result of multivariate analysis and validation on an independent series of patients, which employed bone marrow blast percentage, platelet count, and age as prognostic factors. By identifying additional cutoff values for the medullary blast cell proportion and peripheral platelet count, the Spanish group was able to separate patients with an increased medullary blast percentage (>5%) into three prognostically different risk groups with a median survival of 51 months (score 1), 15 months (score 2 or 3), and 4 months (score 4 or 5). However, the inclusion of age in the Sanz score has been critized by other authors who failed to demonstrate its prognostic impact in univariate and multivariate analyses (27,154). In addition, it was felt that the inclusion of age complicated clinical decision making, because patients who are less able to tolerate aggressive chemotherapy scored higher than younger patients (160).

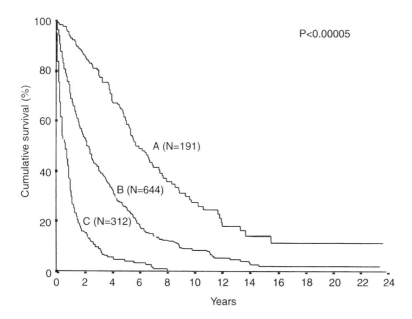

**Fig. 11**   Cumulative survival of 1147 untreated, primary MDS patients separated according to the Düsseldorf score, where A represents the low-risk group, B represents the intermediate-risk group, and C represents the high-risk group. Survival curves for risk groups A, B, and C are significantly different. N, number; P, probability of error; MDS, myelodysplastic syndromes.

**Table 5** International Prognostic Scoring System for Evaluating Prognosis in Patients with Myelodysplastic Syndromes

| Prognostic variable | Points | | | | |
|---|---|---|---|---|---|
| | 0 | 0.5 | 1 | 1.5 | 2.0 |
| Bone marrow blasts (%) | <5 | 5–10 | — | 11–20 | 21–30 |
| Number of cytopenias[a] | 0–1 | 2–3 | — | — | — |
| Cytogenetic category[b] | Good | Intermediate | Poor | — | — |

| Risk group | Score |
|---|---|
| Low | 0 |
| Intermediate-1 | 0.5–1.0 |
| Intermediate-2 | 1.5–2.0 |
| High | ≥2.5 |

[a] Cytopenias defined as platelets <100,000/μl; hemoglobin <10 g/dl; neutrophils <1500/μl.
[b] Good = normal karyotype, 5q-, 20q-, -Y; intermediate = other anomalies; poor = complex (≥3 abnormalities), chromosome 7 anomalies.
*Source*: Adapted from Ref. 96.

The Düsseldorf score is another simple scoring system that differs from the Bournemouth score by including lactate dehydrogenase (LDH) enzyme levels instead of neutrophil counts (30). Compared with the Bournemouth score, the Düsseldorf score was found to be advantageous in two respects. First, it was able to identify those patients with RA and RARS who, without showing an excess of bone marrow blasts at diagnosis, were bound for an unfavorable clinical course. Second, the inclusion of LDH levels provided for an accurate assessment of patients with CMML, whose prognosis is viewed too favorably when rated by the Bournemouth score. Another advantage of the Düsseldorf score is the identification of a true low-risk group (score 0) that is characterized by a 5-year survival probability of about 70%. The predictive value of the Düsseldorf score (Fig. 11) was confirmed in an independent sample of patients (31) and further validated by other investigators (158,161).

**Fig. 12** Cumulative survival (upper graph) and freedom from AML transformation (lower graph) of 816 primary MDS patients (untreated and minimally treated) separated according to classification in the International Prognostic Scoring System for myelodysplastic syndromes. Definition of subgroups is detailed in Table 5. pts, patients; AML, acute myeloid leukemia; MDS, myelodysplastic syndromes. (From Ref. 96.)

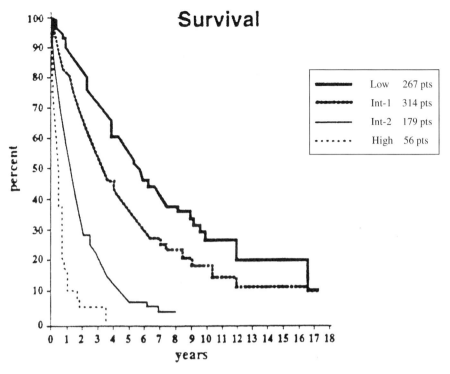

## Survival

| | Low | 267 pts |
| --- | --- | --- |
| | Int-1 | 314 pts |
| | Int-2 | 179 pts |
| | High | 56 pts |

percent

years

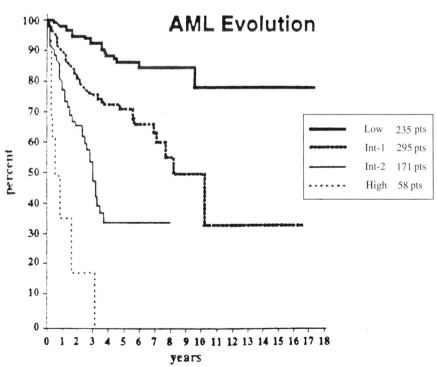

## AML Evolution

| | Low | 235 pts |
| --- | --- | --- |
| | Int-1 | 295 pts |
| | Int-2 | 171 pts |
| | High | 58 pts |

percent

years

Morel et al. (74) were the first to recognize the strong and independent prognostic value of chromosomal abnormalities in MDS. Based on the analysis of 408 cases with de novo MDS, they proposed a new scoring system that, besides bone marrow blast percentage and platelet count, incorporated cytogenetic data as a risk factor. Later, the International MDS Risk Analysis Workshop substantially advanced this prognostic categorization of patients with MDS. In this workshop, clinical, morphological, and cytogenetic data from 816 patients with primary MDS were retrospectively evaluated and subjected to univariate and multivariate risk analysis (96). (Patients who had previously been treated with short courses of low-dose oral chemotherapy or hematopoietic growth factors were included in this analysis. Patients with proliferative-type CMML, defined as patients with a white blood count $>12 \times 10^9$/L, were excluded from the analysis, because these patients were thought to represent myeloproliferative diseases rather than MDS. Cytopenias were defined as hemoglobin $<10$ g/dl, neutrophils $<1.8 \times 10^9$/L, and platelets $<100 \times 10^9$/L.) As a result of the multivariate analyses, age $>60$ years, gender (male sex), number of peripheral cytopenias, bone marrow blast count, and cytogenetics were shown to be the most important variables for disease outcome. In fact, 40% of the patients whose cases were reviewed at the Workshop had presented with cytogenetic anomalies, with del(5q) and trisomy 8 being the most common single abnormalities. Based on all of the parameters, a consensus scoring system was developed that distinguished four risk subgroups: low (score 0), intermediate-1 (score 0.5–1.0), intermediate-2 (score 1.5–2.0), and high (score $>2.5$) (Table 5). Figure 12 shows the cumulative overall survival and leukemia-free survival by subgroup. (Median survivals for the four risk groups were 5.7 years, 3.5 years, 1.2 years, and 0.4 years, respectively. The corresponding time intervals for 25% of the patients to undergo evolution to AML were 9.4 years, 3.3 years, 1.1 years, and 0.2 years, respectively.) When cytogenetics were omitted from the analysis, discrimination of clinical outcome was poorer, causing inaccurate risk assessment of a substantial proportion of intermediate-1 and intermediate-2 patients (162). Thus, the importance of a refined cytogenetic categorization of patients for risk assessment in MDS was convincingly shown by the Workshop.

As part of the consensus conference, the International Prognostic Scoring System (IPSS) was compared with other prognostic systems (FAB classification, Spanish score, Lille score) to determine the relative discriminatory abilities for assessing the natural course of MDS. In this analysis, the IPSS demonstrated greater discriminating power for both survival and AML evolution than the other scoring systems. Recently, the prognostic value of the IPSS has been confirmed in several independent patient series (80,163,164). In addition, direct comparison of different scoring systems performed by Pfeilstöcker et al. (158) showed that the IPSS carried the highest predictive value among all systems examined. It thus appears that the IPSS is an important tool for risk evaluation of newly diagnosed

MDS patients and will prove useful for design and analysis of therapeutic trials in these disorders.

## XII. CONCLUDING REMARKS

Since the identification of the MDS as a distinct entity of hematological diseases, considerable efforts have been made to define factors that are prognostically important. Now, to estimate disease progression and survival, the practicing clinician is not necessarily dependent on sophisticated laboratory and molecular investigations.

A good approach to help identify high-risk patients with MDS includes a combination of clinical, laboratory, morphological, and—if available—cytogenetic findings. Clinically speaking, patients over 60 years of age fare less well than younger patients. Concurrent infections and a poor health status also point toward a complicated clinical course. Further, treatment-related MDS are usually predictors of poor prognosis. Laboratory data such as peripheral blood cell findings, especially hemoglobin concentration and platelet count, may indicate a fairly good prognosis whereas increased LDH levels impact adversely on survival. Evidence of circulating blast cells in the peripheral blood and bone marrow morphology also help to identify patients with an aggressive clinical course. Further, the bone marrow blast count is a prominent prognostic feature, with patients having more than 10% blasts doing worse than those with a limited blast count. Patients with pure sideroblastic anemia have improved chances of survival than those with refractory anemia with ringed sideroblasts. The skilled morphologist might also predict the 5q- syndrome from the bone marrow morphology and therefore will identify another prognostically favorable subgroup. As for actual cytogenetic data, complex findings or monosomy 7 or del(7q) anomalies are associated with poor prognoses whereas patients with del(5q), del(20q), and -Y will do much better. If cytogenetic analysis is available, the IPSS score is a good approach to the prognostic evaluation of MDS patients.

It will be exciting to evaluate future developments. Additional molecular biological factors are still under investigation and there is yet a lack of predictors of therapeutic response in MDS. Certainly, large multicenter trials are needed to identify powerful determinants of clinical outcome after therapy.

## ACKNOWLEDGMENT

This publication was supported by the Bundesministerium für Bildung und Forschung (BMBF), Kompetenznetz, ''Akute und chronische Leukämien.''

## REFERENCES

1. Aul C, Gattermann N, Schneider W. Age-related incidence and other epidemiological aspects of myelodysplastic syndromes. Br J Haematol 1992; 82:358–367.
2. Harris NL, Jaffe ES, Diebold J, Flandrin G, Muller-Hermelink HK, Vardiman J, Lister TA, Bloomfield CD. World Health Organization classification of neoplastic diseases of the hematopoietic and lymphoid tissues: report of the Clinical Advisory Committee meeting—Airlie House, Virginia, November 1997. J Clin Oncol 1999; 17:3835–3849.
3. Bennett JM, Catovsky D, Daniel MT, Flandrin G, Galton DA, Gralnick HR, Sultan C. Proposals for the classification of the myelodysplastic syndromes. Br J Haematol 1982; 51:189–199.
4. Tricot G, Boogaerts MA, De Wolf-Peeters C, Van den Berghe, Verwilghen RL. The myelodysplastic syndromes: different evolution patterns based on sequential morphological and cytogenetic investigations. Br J Haematol 1985; 59:659–670.
5. Cazzola M, Anderson JE, Ganser A, Hellström-Lindberg E. A patient-oriented approach to treatment of myleodysplastic syndromes. Haematologica 1998; 83:910–935.
6. Passmore SJ, Hann IM, Stiller CA, Ramani P, Swansbury GJ, Gibbons B, Reeves BR, Chessels JM. Pediatric myelodysplasia: a study of 68 children and new prognostic scoring system. Blood 1995; 85:1742–1750.
7. Haas OA, Gadner H. Pathogenesis, biology, and management of myelodysplastic syndromes in children. Semin Hematol 1996; 33:225–235.
8. Tricot G, Vlietinck R, Boogaerts MA, Hendricks B, De Wolf-Peeters C, Van den Berghe H, Verwilghen RL. Prognostic factors in the myelodysplastic syndromes: importance of initial data on peripheral blood counts, bone marrow cytology, trephine biopsy and chromosomal analysis. Br J Haematol 1985; 60:19–32.
9. Takagi S, Tanaka O, Origasa H, Miura Y. Prognostic significance of magnetic resonance imaging of femoral marrow in patients with myelodysplastic syndromes. J Clin Oncol 1999; 17:277–283.
10. Mufti GJ. A guide to risk assessment in the primary myelodysplastic syndrome. Hematol Oncol Clin North Am 1992; 6:587–606.
11. Vadhan-Raj S, Keating M, LeMaistre A, Hittelman WN, McCredie K, Trujillo JM, Broxmeyer HE, Henney C, Gutterman JU. Effects of recombinant human granulocyte-macrophage colony-stimulating factor in patients with myelodysplastic syndromes. N Engl J Med 1987; 317:1545–1552.
12. Ganser A, Völkers B, Greher J, Ottmann OG, Walther F, Becher R, Bergmann L, Schulz G, Hoelzer D. Recombinant human granulocyte-macrophage colony-stimulating factor in patients with myelodysplastic syndromes—a phase I/II trial. Blood 1989; 73:31–37.
13. de Witte T, Suciu S, Peetermans M, Fenaux P, Strijckmans P, Hayat M, Jaksic B, Selleslag D, Zittoun R, Dardenne M, Solbu G, Zwierzina H, Muus P. Intensive chemotherapy for poor prognosis myelodysplasia (MDS) and secondary acute myeloid leukemia (sAML) following MDS of more than 6 months duration. A pilot

study by the Leukemia Cooperative Group of the European Organisation for Research and Treatment in Cancer (EORTC-LCG). Leukemia 1995; 9:1805–1811.

14. Nevill TJ, Fung HC, Shepherd JD, Horsman DE, Nantel SH, Klingemann HG, Forrest DL, Toze CL, Sutherland HJ, Hogge DE, Naiman SC, Le A, Brockington DA, Barnett MJ. Cytogenetic abnormalities in primary myelodysplastic syndrome are highly predictive of outcome after allogeneic bone marrow transplantation. Blood 1998; 92:1910–1917.

15. Hirst WJ, Mufti GJ. The rate of disease progression predicts the quality of remissions following intensive chemotherapy for myelodysplastic syndromes. Leuk Res 1994; 18:797–804.

16. Appelbaum FR, Anderson J. Allogeneic bone marrow transplantation for myelodysplastic syndrome: outcomes analysis according to IPSS score. Leukemia 1998; 12(suppl 1):S25–S29.

17. Tricot G, Vlietinck R, Verwilghen RL. Prognostic factors in the myelodysplastic syndromes: a review. Scand J Haematol 1986; 36(suppl 45):107–113.

18. Sanz GF, Sanz MA, Vallespi T, Canizo MC, Torrabadella M, Garcia S, Irriguible D, San Miguel JF. Two regression models and a scoring system for predicting survival and planning treatment in myelodysplastic syndromes: a multivariate analysis of prognostic factors in 370 patients. Blood 1989; 74:395–408.

19. Coiffier B, Adeleine P, Gentilhomme O, Felman P, Treille-Ritouet D, Byron PA. Myelodysplastic syndromes. A multiparametric study of prognostic factors in 336 patients. Cancer 1987; 60:3029–3032.

20. Kerkhofs H, Hermans J, Haak HL, Leeksma CH. Utility of the FAB classification for myelodysplastic syndromes: investigation of prognostic factors in 237 cases. Br J Haematol 1987; 65:73–81.

21. Cunningham I, MacCallum SJ, Nicholls MD, Byth K, Hewson JW, Arnold B, Motum PI, Mulligan SP, Crane GG. The myelodysplastic syndromes: an analysis of prognostic factors in 226 cases from a single institution. Br J Haematol 1995; 90: 602–606.

22. Morel P, Declercq C, Hebbar M, Bauters F, Fenaux P. Prognostic factors in myelodysplastic syndromes: critical analysis of the impact of age and gender and failure to identify a very-low-risk group using standard mortality ratio techniques. Br J Haematol 1996; 94:116–119.

23. Foucar K, Langdon RM, Armitage JO, Olson DB, Carroll TJ. Myelodysplastic syndromes. A clinical and pathologic analysis of 109 cases. Cancer 1985; 56:553 561.

24. Aul C, Gattermann N, Schneider W. Epidemiological and etiological aspects of myelodysplastic syndromes. Leuk Lymphoma 1995; 16:247–262.

25. Kantarjian HM, Estey EH, Keating MJ. Treatment of therapy-related leukemia and myelodysplastic syndrome. Hematol Oncol Clin North Am 1993; 7:81–107.

26. Estey EH. Prognosis and therapy of secondary myelodysplastic syndromes. Haematologica 1998; 83:543–549.

27. Mufti GJ, Stevens JR, Oscier DG, Hamblin TJ, Machin D. Myelodysplastic syndromes: a scoring system with prognostic significance. Br J Haematol 1985; 59: 425–433.

28. Heimpel H, Drings P, Mitrou P, Queisser W. Verlauf und prognostische Kriterien

bei Patienten mit "Präleukämie." Ergebnisse einer prospektiven Studie. [A prospective study on course and prognostic criteria in "preleukemia" (author's transl.).] Klin Wochenschr 1979; 57:21–29 [German].

29. Coiffier B, Adeleine P, Viala JJ, Bryon PA, Fière D, Gentilhomme O, Vuvan H. Dysmyelopoietic syndromes. A search for prognostic factors in 193 patients. Cancer 1983; 52:83–90.

30. Aul C, Gattermann N, Heyll A, Germing U, Derigs G, Schneider W. Primary myelodysplastic syndromes: analysis of prognostic factors in 235 patients and proposals for an improved scoring system. Leukemia 1992; 6:52–59.

31. Aul C, Gattermann N, Germing U, Runde V, Heyll A, Schneider W. Risk assessment in primary myelodysplastic syndromes: validation of the Düsseldorf score. Leukemia 1994; 8:1906–1913.

32. Morra E, Lazzarino M, Castello A, Inverardi D, Coci A, Alessandrino EP, Brusamolino E, Bernasconi P, Orlandi E, Bonfichi M, Merante S, Zei G, Bernasconi C. Risk assessment in myelodysplastic syndromes: value of clinical, hematologic and bone marrow histologic findings at presentation. Eur J Haematol 1990; 45:94–100.

33. Oguma S, Yoshida Y, Uchino H, Maekawa T, Nomura T, Mizoguchi H; Anemia Study Group of the Ministry of Health and Welfare. Clinical characteristics of Japanese patients with primary myelodysplastic syndromes: a co-operative study based on 838 cases. Leuk Res 1995; 19:219–225.

34. Maddox AM, Keating MJ, Smith TL, Speer J, Cork MA, Trujillo JM, McCredie KB, Freireich EJ. Prognostic factors for survival of 194 patients with low infiltrate leukemia. Leuk Res 1986; 10:995–1006.

35. Keating MJ, Smith TL, Gehan EA, McCredie KB, Bodey GP, Spitzer G, Hersh E, Gutterman J, Freireich EJ. Factors related to length of complete remission in adult acute leukemia. Cancer 1980; 45:2017–2029.

36. The International Non-Hodgkin's Lymphoma Prognostic Factors Project. A predictive model for aggressive non-Hodgkin's lymphoma. N Engl J Med 1993; 329: 987–994.

37. Luoni R, Ucci G, Riccardi A, Spriano P, Danova M, Cassano E, Molinari E, Ascari E. Serum thymidine kinase in hematologic malignancies. Haematologica 1988; 73: 31–35.

38. Hagberg H, Gronowitz S, Killander A, Källander C, Simonsson B, Sundström C, Oberg G. Serum thymidine kinase in acute leukaemia. Br J Cancer 1984; 49: 537–540.

39. Aul C, Gattermann N, Germing U, Winkelmann M, Heyll A, Runde V, Schneider W. Serum deoxythymidine kinase in myelodysplastic syndromes. Cancer 1994; 73: 322–327.

40. Musto P, Bodenizza C, Falcone A, D'Arena G, Scalzulli P, Perla G, Modoni S, Parlatore L, Valvano MR, Carotenuto M. Prognostic relevance of serum thymidine kinase in primary myelodysplastic syndromes: relationship to development of acute myeloid leukaemia. Br J Haematol 1995; 90:125–130.

41. Zwiezina H, Herold M, Schollenberger S, Geissler D, Schmalzl F. Detection of soluble IL-2 receptor in the serum of patients with myelodysplastic syndromes: induction under therapy with GM-CSF. Br J Haematol 1991; 79:438–443.

42. Yokose N, Ogata K, Ito T, An E, Tamura H, Dan K, Hamaguchi H, Sakamaki H, Onozawa Y, Nomura T. Elevated plasma soluble interleukin 2 receptor level correlated with defective natural killer and CD8+ T-cells in myelodysplastic syndromes. Leuk Res 1994; 18:777–782.

43. Ogata K, Yokose N, An E, Kamikubo K, Tamura H, Dan K, Sakamaki H, Onozawa Y, Hamaguchi H, Nomura T. Plasma soluble interleukin-2 receptor level in patients with primary myelodysplastic syndromes: a relationship with disease subtype and clinical outcome. Br J Haematol 1996; 93:45–52.

44. van der Weide M, Sizoo W, Nauta JJ, Krefft J, Langenhuijsen MM. Myelodysplastic syndromes: analysis of clinical and prognostic features in 96 patients. Eur J Haematol 1988; 41:115–122.

45. Iwabuchi A, Ohyashiki K, Ohyashiki JH, Kimura Y, Lin KY, Aizawa S, Nehashi Y, Miyazawa K, Yaguchi M, Toyama K. Percentages of bone marrow blasts and chromosomal changes in patients with refractory anaemia help to determine prognoses. Int J Hematol 1994; 60:207–213.

46. Thiele J, Vykoupil KF, Georgii A. Myeloid dysplasia (MD): a hematological disorder preceding acute and chronic myeloid leukemia. A morphological study on sequential core biopsies of the bone marrow in 27 patients. Virchows Arch A Pathol Anat Histol 1980; 389:343–367.

47. Varela BL, Chuang C, Woll JE, Bennett JM. Modifications in the classification of primary myelodysplastic syndromes: the addition of a scoring system. Hematol Oncol 1985; 3:55–63.

48. Seymour JF, Estey EH. The contribution of Auer rods to the classification and prognosis of myelodysplastic syndromes. Leuk Lymphoma 1995; 17:79–85.

49. Boogaerts MA, Verhoef GE, Demuynck H. Treatment and prognostic factors in myelodysplastic syndromes. Baillieres Clin Haematol 1996; 9:161–183.

50. Mangi MH, Mufti GJ. Primary myelodysplastic syndromes: diagnostic and prognostic significance of immunohistochemical assessment of bone marrow biopsies. Blood 1992; 79:198–205.

51. Lambertenghi-Deliliers G, Annaloro C, Oriani A, Soligo D, Pozzoli E, Polli EE. Prognostic relevance of histological findings on bone marrow biopsy in myelodysplastic syndromes. Ann Hematol 1993; 66:85–91.

52. Maschek H, Gutzmer R, Choritz H, Georgii A. Life expectancy in primary myelodysplastic syndromes: a prognostic score based upon histopathology from bone marrow biopsies of 569 patients. Eur J Haematol 1994; 53:280–287.

53 Sultan C, Sigaux F, Imbert M, Reyes F. Acute myelodysplasia with myelofibrosis: a report of eight cases. Br J Haematol 1981; 49:11–16.

54. Verhoef GEG, De Wolf-Peeters C, Ferrant A, Deprez S, Meeus P, Stul M, Zacheé P, Cassiman JJ, Van den Berghe H, Boogaerts MA. Myelodysplastic syndromes with bone marrow fibrosis: a myelodysplastic disorder with proliferative features. Ann Hematol 1991; 63:235–241.

55. Takahashi M, Koike T, Nagayama R, Fujiwara M, Koyama S, Ohnishi M, Nakamori Y, Soga N, Aoki S, Tatewaki W, Wada K, Moriyama Y, Shibata A. Myelodysplastic syndrome with myelofibrosis: myelodysplastic syndrome as a major primary disorder for acute myelofibrosis. Clin Lab Haematol 1991; 13:17–23.

56. Cassano E, Giordano M, Riccardi A, Coci A, Cazzola M. Myelodysplastic syn-

dromes: a multiparametric study of prognostic factors and a proposed scoring system. Haematologica 1990; 75:141–145.

57. Ohyashiki K, Sasao I, Ohyashiki JH, Murakami T, Iwabuchi A, Tauchi T, Saito M, Nakazawa S, Serizawa H, Ebihara Y, Toyama K. Clinical and cytogenetic characteristics of myelodysplastic syndromes developing myelofibrosis. Cancer 1991; 68:178–183.

58. Maschek H, Kaloutsi V, Rodriguez-Kaiser M, Werner M, Choritz H, Mainzer K, Dietzfelbinger M, Georgii A. Hypoplastic myelodysplastic syndromes: incidence, morphology, cytogenetics, and prognosis. Ann Hematol 1993; 66:117–122.

59. Yoshida Y, Oguma S, Uchino H, Maekawa T. Refractory myelodysplastic anaemias with hypocellular bone marrow. J Clin Pathol 1988; 41:763–767.

60. Tuzuner N, Cox C, Rowe JM, Watrous D, Bennett JM. Hypocellular myelodysplastic syndromes (MDS): new proposals. Br J Haematol 1995; 91:612–617.

61. Appelbaum FR, Barrall J, Storb R, Ramberg R, Doney K, Sale GE, Thomas ED. Clonal cytogenetic abnormalities in patients with otherwise typical aplastic anemia. Exp Hematol 1987; 15:1134–1139.

62. Kitagawa M, Kamiyama R, Takemura T, Kasuga T. Bone marrow analysis of the myelodysplastic syndromes: histological and immunohistochemical features related to the evolution of overt leukemia. Virchows Arch B Cell Pathol Incl Mol Pathol 1989; 57:47–53.

63. Moormeier JA, Rubin CM, Le Beau MM, Vardiman JW, Larson RA, Winter JN. Trisomy 6: a recurring cytogenetic abnormality associated with marrow hypoplasia. Blood 1991; 77:1397–1398.

64. de Planque MM, Kluin-Nelemans HC, van Krieken HJ, Kluin PM, Brand A, Beverstock GC, Willemze R, van Rood JJ. Evolution of acquired severe aplastic anaemia to myelodysplasia and subsequent leukaemia in adults. Br J Haematol 1988; 70: 55–62.

65. Gattermann N, Aul C, Schneider W. Two types of acquired idiopathic sideroblastic anaemia (AISA). Br J Haematol 1990; 74:45–52.

66. Germing U, Gattermann N, Aivado M, Hildebrandt B, Aul C. Two types of acquired idiopathic sideroblastic anaemia (AISA): a time-tested distinction. Br J Haematol 2000; 108:724–728.

67. Garand R, Gardais J, Bizet M, Bremond JL, Accard F, Callat MP, de Bouchony ET, Goasguen JE. Heterogeneity of acquired idiopathic sideroblastic anaemia (AISA). Leuk Res 1992; 16:463–468.

68. Bennett JM, Catovsky D, Daniel MT, Flandrin G, Galton DA, Gralnick HR, Sultan C, Cox C. The chronic myeloid leukemias: guidelines for distinguishing chronic granulocytic, atypical chronic myeloid, and chronic myelomonocytic leukaemia. Proposals by the French-American-British Cooperative Leukaemia Group. Br J Haematol 1994; 87:746–754.

69. Germing U, Gattermann N, Minning H, Heyll A, Aul C. Problems in the classification of CMML—dysplastic versus proliferative type. Leuk Res 1998; 22:871–878.

70. Billström R, Thiede T, Hansen S, Heim S, Kristoffersson U, Mandahl N, Mitelman F. Bone marrow karyotype and prognosis in primary myelodysplastic syndromes. Eur J Haematol 1988; 41:341–346.

71. Pierre RV, Catovsky D, Mufti GJ, Swansbury GJ, Mecucci C, Dewald GW, Ruutu T, Van den Berghe H, Rowley JD, Mitelman F, Reeves BR, Alimena G, Garson OM, Lawler SD, de la Chapelle A. Clinical-cytogenetic correlations in myelodysplasia (preleukemia). Cancer Genet Cytogenet 1989; 40:149–161.

72. Suciu S, Kuse R, Weh HJ, Hossfeld DK. Results of chromosome studies and their relation to morphology, course, and prognosis in 120 patients with de novo myelodysplastic syndrome. Cancer Genet Cytogenet 1990; 44:15–26.

73. Toyama K, Ohyashiki K, Yoshida Y, Abe T, Asano S, Hirai H, Hirashima K, Hotta T, Kuramoto A, Kuriya S, Miyazaki T, Kakishita E, Mizoguchi H, Okada M, Shrirakawa S, Takaku F, Tomonaga M, Uchino H, Yasunaga K, Nomura T. Clinical implications of chromosomal abnormalities in 401 patients with myelodysplastic syndromes: a multicentric study in Japan. Leukemia 1993; 7:499–508.

74. Morel P, Hebbar M, Lai JL, Duhamel A, Preudhomme C, Wattel E, Bauters F, Fenaux P. Cytogenetic analysis has strong independent prognostic value in de novo myelodysplastic syndromes and can be incorporated in a new scoring system: a report on 408 cases. Leukemia 1993; 7:1315–1323.

75. Bernasconi P, Alessandrino EP, Boni M, Bonfichi M, Morra E, Lazzarino M, Campagnoli C, Astori C. Karyotype in myelodysplastic syndromes: relations to morphology, clinical evolution, and survival. Am J Hematol 1994; 46:270–277.

76. White AD, Hoy TG, Jacobs A. Extended cytogenetic follow-up and clinical progress in patients with myelodysplastic syndromes. Leuk Lymphoma 1994; 12:401–412.

77. Musilova J, Michalova K, Zemanova Z, Neuwirthova R, Dohnalova A; Czechoslovak MDS Cooperative Group. Karyotype at diagnosis, subsequent leukemic transformation and survival in myelodysplastic syndrome (MDS). Leuk Res 1995; 19:303–308.

78. Haase D, Fonatsch C, Freund M, Wörmann B, Bodenstein H, Bartels H, Stollmann-Gibbels B, Lengfelder E. Cytogenetic findings in 179 patients with myelodysplastic syndromes. Ann Hematol 1995; 70:171–187.

79. Parlier V, van Melle G, Beris P, Schmidt PM, Tobler A, Haller E, Bellomo MJ. Hematological, clinical and cytogenetic analysis in 109 patients with primary myelodysplastic syndrome. Prognostic significance of morphology and chromosome findings. Cancer Genet Cytogenet 1994; 78:219–231.

80. Solé F, Espinet B, Sanz GF, Cervera J, Calasanz MJ, Luno E, Prieto F, Granada I, Hernandez JM, Cigudosa JC, Diez JL, Bureo E, Marques ML, Arranz F, Rios R, Martinez Climent JA, Vallespi T, Florensa L, Woessner S; Grupo Cooperative Espanol de Citogenetica Hematologica. Incidence, characterization and prognostic significance of chromosomal abnormalities in 640 patients with primary myelodysplastic syndromes. Br J Haematol 2000; 108:346–356.

81. Le Beau MM, Albain KS, Larson RA, Vardiman JW, Davis EM, Blough RR, Golomb HM, Rowley JD. Clinical and cytogenetic correlations in 63 patients with therapy-related myelodysplastic syndromes and acute nonlymphocytic leukemia: further evidence for characteristic abnormalities of chromosomes no. 5 and 7. J Clin Oncol 1986; 4:325–345.

82. Werner M, Nolte M, Maschek H, Kaloutsi H, Choritz H, Georgii A. Zytogenetik als Ergänzung zur Histopathologie am Beispiel des myelodysplastischen Syndroms.

[Cytogenics in addition to histopathology exemplified by myelodysplastic syndrome.] Pathologe 1994; 15:286–291 [German].

83. Yunis JJ, Lobell M, Arnesen MA, Oken MM, Mayer MG, Rydell RE, Brunning RD. Refined chromosome study helps define prognostic subgroups in most patients with primary myelodysplastic syndrome and acute myelogenous leukaemia. Br J Haematol 1988; 68:189–194.

84. Johansson B, Mertens F, Mitelman F. Cytogenetic deletion maps of hematologic neoplasms: circumstantial evidence for tumor suppressor loci. Genes Chromosomes Cancer 1993; 8:205–218.

85. Mittelman MM, Lessin LS. Oncogenes and growth factor genes in myelodysplasia. Hematol Pathol 1991; 5:37–41.

86. Van den Berghe H, Cassiman JJ, David G, Fryns JP, Michaux JL, Sokal G. Distinct haematological disorder with deletion of long arm of no. 5 chromosome. Nature 1974; 251:437–438.

87. Heim S. Cytogenetic findings in primary and secondary MDS. Leuk Res 1992; 16: 43–46.

88. Pedersen-Bjergaard J, Philip P, Larsen SO, Jensen G, Byrsting K. Chromosome aberrations and prognostic factors in therapy-related myelodysplasia and acute non-lymphocytic leukemia. Blood 1990; 76:1083–1091.

89. Kantarjian HM, Estey EH, Keating MJ. Treatment of therapy-related leukemia and myelodysplastic syndrome. Hematol Oncol Clin North Am 1993; 7:81–107.

90. Fenaux P, Morel P, Lai JL. Cytogenetics in myelodysplastic syndromes. Semin Hematol 1996; 33:127–138.

91. Verhoef G, De Wolf-Peeters C, Kerim S, Van De Broeck J, Mecucci C, Van den Berghe H, Boogaerts M. Update on the prognostic implication of morphology, histology, and karyotype in primary myelodysplastic syndromes. Hematol Pathol 1991; 5:163–175.

92. Van den Berghe H, Vermaelen K, Mecucci C, Barbieri D, Tricot G. The 5q- anomaly. Cancer Genet Cytogenet 1985; 17:189–255.

93. Mathew P, Tefferi A, Dewald GW, Goldberg SL, Su J, Hoagland HC, Noel P. The 5q- syndrome: a single-institution study of 43 consecutive patients. Blood 1993; 81:1040–1045.

94. Boultwood J, Lewis S, Wainscoat JS. The 5q- syndrome. Blood 1994; 84:3253–3260.

95. Sanz GF, Sanz MA. Prognostic factors in myelodysplastic syndromes. Leuk Res 1992; 16:77–86.

96. Greenberg P, Cox C, LeBeau MM, Fenaux P, Morel P, Sanz G, Sanz M, Vallespi T, Hamblin T, Oscier D, Ohyashiki K, Toyama K, Aul C, Mufti G, Bennett J. International scoring system for evaluating prognosis in myelodysplastic syndromes. Blood 1997; 89:2079–2088.

97. Second International Workshop on Chromosomes in Leukemia 1979. Chromosomes in preleukemia. Cancer Genet Cytogenet 1980; 2:108–113.

98. Benitez J, Carbonell F, Sanchez Fayos F, Heimpel H. Karyotypic evolution in patients with myelodysplastic syndromes. Cancer Genet Cytogenet 1985; 16:157–167.

99. Mecucci C, Van den Berghe H. Cytogenetics of myelodysplastic syndromes. Hematol Oncol Clin North Am 1992; 6:523–541.
100. Clark R, Peters S, Hoy T, Smith S, Whittaker K, Jacobs A. Prognostic importance of hypodiploid hemopoietic prescursors in myelodysplastic syndromes. N Engl J Med 1986; 314:1472–1475.
101. van Kamp H, de Pijper C, Verlaan-de Vries M, Bos JL, Leeksma CH, Kerkhofs H, Willemze R, Fibbe WE, Landegent JE. Longitudinal analysis of point mutations of N-ras proto-oncogene in patients with myelodysplasia using archived blood smears. Blood 1992; 79:1266–1270.
102. Yunis JJ, Boot AJ, Meyer MG, Bos JL. Mechanisms of ras mutation in myelodysplastic syndrome. Oncogene 1989; 4:609–614.
103. Bartram CR. Molecular genetic aspects of myelodysplastic syndromes. Hematol Oncol Clin North Am 1992; 6:557–570.
104. Parker J, Mufti GJ. Ras and myelodysplasia: lessons from the past decade. Semin Hematol 1996; 33:206–224.
105. Paquette RL, Landaw EM, Pierre RV, Kahan J, Lübbert M, Lazcano O, Isaac G, McCormick F, Koeffler HP. N-ras mutations are associated with poor prognosis and increased risk of leukemia in myelodysplastic syndrome. Blood 1993; 82:590–599.
106. Constantinidou M, Chalevelakis G, Economopoulos T, Koffa M, Liloglou T, Anastassiou C, Yalouris A, Spandidos DA, Raptis S. Codon 12 ras mutations in patients with myelodysplastic syndrome: incidence and prognostic value. Ann Hematol 1997; 74:11–14.
107. Padua RA, Guinn BA, Al-Sabah AI, Smith M, Taylor C, Pettersson T, Ridge S, Carter G, White D, Oscier D, Chevret S, West R. RAS, FMS and p53 mutations and poor clinical outcome in myelodysplasias: a 10-year follow-up. Leukemia 1998; 12:887–892.
108. Neubauer A, Greenberg P, Negrin R, Ginzton N, Liu E. Mutations in the ras proto-oncogenes in patients with myelodysplastic syndromes. Leukemia 1994; 8:638–641.
109. Lyons J, Janssen JW, Bartram C, Layton M, Mufti GJ. Mutation of Ki-ras and N-ras oncogenes in myelodysplastic syndromes. Blood 1988; 71:1707–1712.
110. Ridge SA, Worwood M, Oscier D, Jacobs A, Padua RA. FMS mutations in myelodysplastic, leukemic, and normal subjects. Proc Natl Acad Sci USA 1990; 87:1377–1380.
111. Bouscary D, Preudhomme C, Ribrag V, Melle J, Viguié F, Picard F, Guesnu M, Fenaux P, Gisselbrecht S, Dreyfus F. Prognostic value of *c-mpl* expression in myelodysplastic syndromes. Leukemia 1995; 9:783–788.
112. Harris CC, Hollstein M. Clinical implications of the *p53* tumor-suppressor gene. N Engl J Med 1993; 329:1318–1327.
113. Mori N, Wada M, Yokata J, Terada M, Okada M, Teramura M, Masuda M, Hoshino S, Motoji T, Oshimi K, Mizoguchi H. Mutations of the *p53* tumor suppressor gene in hematologic neoplasms. Br J Haematol 1992; 81:235–240.
114. Tsushita K, Hotta T, Ichikawa A, Saito H. Mutation of *p53* gene does not play a critical role in myelodysplastic syndrome and its transformation to acute leukemia. Br J Haematol 1992; 81:456–457.

115. Sugimoto K, Hirano N, Toyoshima H, Chiba S, Mano H, Takaku F, Yazaki Y, Hirai H. Mutations of the *p53* gene in myelodysplastic syndromes (MDS) and MDS-derived leukemia. Blood 1993; 81:3022–3026.

116. Kaneko H, Misawa S, Horiike S, Nakai H, Kashima K. TP53 mutations emerge at early phase of myelodysplastic syndrome and are associated with complex chromosomal abnormalities. Blood 1995; 85:2189–2193.

117. Jonveaux P, Fenaux P, Quiquandon I, Pignon JM, Lai JL, Loucheux-Lefebvre MH, Goosens M, Bauters F, Berger R. Mutations in the *p53* gene in myelodysplastic syndromes. Oncogene 1991; 6:2243–2247.

118. Orazi A, Cattoretti G, Heerema NA, Sozzi G, John K, Neiman RS. Frequent *p53* overexpression in therapy related myelodysplastic syndromes and acute myeloid leukemia: an immunohistochemical study of bone marrow biopsies. Mod Pathol 1993; 6:521–525.

119. Wattel E, Preudhomme C, Hecquet B, Vanrumbeke M, Quesnel B, Dervite I, Morel P, Fenaux P. *p53* mutations are associated with resistance to chemotherapy and short survival in hematologic malignancies. Blood 1994; 84:3148–3157.

120. Miyake K, Inokuchi K, Dan K, Nomura T. Expression of the *DCC* gene in myelodysplastic syndromes and overt leukemia. Leuk Res 1993; 17:785–788.

121. Quesnel B, Guillerm G, Vereecque R, Wattel E, Preudhomme C, Bauters F, Vanrumbeke M, Fenaux P. Methylation of the $p15^{INK4b}$ gene in myelodysplastic syndromes is frequent and acquired during disease progression. Blood 1998; 91:2985–2990.

122. Uchida T, Kinoshita T, Nagai H, Nakahara Y, Saito H, Hotta T, Murate T. Hypermethylation of the $p15^{INK4B}$ gene in myelodysplastic syndromes. Blood 1997; 90:1403–1409.

123. Kristensen JS, Hokland P. Monoclonal antibody ratios in malignant myeloid diseases: diagnostic and prognostic use in myelodysplastic syndromes. Br J Haematol 1990; 74:270–276.

124. Baur AS, Meugé-Moraw C, Schmidt PM, Partlier V, Jotterand M, Delacrétaz F. CD34/QBEND10 immunostaining in bone marrow biopsies: an additional parameter for the diagnosis and classification of myelodysplastic syndromes. Eur J Haematol 2000; 64:71–79.

125. Soligo D, Delia D, Oriani A, Cattoretti G, Orazi A, Bertolli V, Quirici N, Lambertenghi Deliliers G. Identification of CD34+ cells in normal and pathological bone marrow biopsies by QBEND10 monoclonal antibody. Leukemia 1991; 5:1026–1030.

126. Oriani A, Annaloro C, Soligo D, Pozzoli E, Cortelezzi A, Lambertenghi Deliliers G. Bone marrow histology and CD34 immunostaining in the prognostic evaluation of primary myelodysplastic syndromes. Br J Haematol 1996; 92:360–364.

127. Soligo DA, Oriani A, Annaloro C, Cortelezzi A, Calori R, Pozzoli E, Nosella D, Orazi A, Lambertenghi Deliliers G. CD34 immunohistochemistry of bone marrow biopsies: prognostic significance in primary myelodysplastic syndromes. Am J Hematol 1994; 46:9–17.

128. Sullivan SA, Marsden KA, Lowenthal RM, Jupe DM, Jones ME. Circulating CD34+ cells: an adverse prognostic factor in the myelodysplastic syndromes. Am J Hematol 1992; 39:96–101.

129. Kornblau SM. The role of apoptosis in the pathogenesis, prognosis, and therapy of hematologic malignancies (review). Leukemia 1998; 12(suppl 1):S41–S46.
130. Bouscary D, De Vos J, Guesnu M, Jondeau K, Viguier F, Melle J, Picard F, Dreyfus F, Fontenay-Roupie M. Fas/Apo-1 (CD95) expression and apoptosis in patients with myelodysplastic syndromes. Leukemia 1997; 11:839–845.
131. Kitagawa M, Yamaguchi S, Takahashi M, Tanizawa T, Hirokawa K, Kamiyama R. Localization of Fas and Fas ligand in bone marrow cells demonstrating myelodysplasia. Leukemia 1998; 12:486–492.
132. Gupta P, Niehans GA, LeRoy SC, Gupta K, Morrison VA, Schultz C, Knapp DJ, Kratzke RA. Fas ligand expression in the bone marrow in myelodysplastic syndromes correlates with FAB subtype and anemia, and predicts survival. Leukemia 1999; 13:44–53.
133. Shimazaki K, Ohshima K, Suzumiya J, Kawasaki C, Kikuchi M. Evaluation of apoptosis as a prognostic factor in myelodysplastic syndromes. Br J Haematol 2000; 110:584–590.
134. Runde V, Germing U, Aul C. Expression of CD34 and P-glycoprotein: prognostic significance in primary myelodysplastic syndromes. Int J Oncol 1995; 7:1–5.
135. List AF, Spier CM, Cline A, Doll DC, Garewal H, Morgan R, Sandberg AA. Expression of the multidrug resistance gene product (P-glycoprotein) in myelodysplasia is associated with a stem cell phenotype. Br J Haematol 1991; 78:28–34.
136. Sonneveld P, van Dongen JJ, Hagemeijer A, van Lom K, Nooter K, Schoester M, Adriaansen HJ, Tsuruo T, de Leeuw K. High expression of the multidrug resistance P-glycoprotein in high-risk myelodysplasia is associated with immature phenotype. Leukemia 1993; 7:963–969.
137. Poulain S, Lepelley P, Preudhomme C, Cambier N, Cornillon J, Wattel E, Cosson A, Fenaux P. Expression of the multidrug resistance-associated protein in myelodysplastic syndromes. Br J Haematol 2000; 110:591–598.
138. Partanen S, Juvonen E, Ruutu T. In vitro culture of haematopoietic progenitors in myelodysplastic syndromes. Scand J Haematol 1986; 36(suppl 45):98–101.
139. Greenberg L, Mara B. The preleukemic syndrome: correlation of in vitro parameters of granulopoiesis with clinical features. Am J Med 1979; 66:951–958.
140. Korthout M, De Bock R, van Bockstaele D, Peetermans M. Bone marrow cultures and prognosis in primary myelodysplastic syndromes. Leuk Res 1990; 14:85–89.
141. Raymakers R, De Witte T, Joziasse J, Van der Lely N, Boezeman J, Haanen C. In vitro growth pattern and differentiation predict for progression of myelodysplastic syndromes to acute nonlymphocytic leukemia. Br J Haematol 1991; 78:35–41.
142. Berthier R, Douady F, Metral J, Newton I, Schweitzer A, Hollard D. In vitro granulopoiesis in oligoblastic leukaemia: prognostic value, characterization and serial cloning of bone marrow colony and cluster forming cells in agar culture. Biomedicine 1979; 30:305–311.
143. Spitzer G, Verma DS, Dicke KA, Smith T, McCredie KB. Subgroups of oligoleukemia as identified by in vitro agar culture. Leuk Res 1979; 3:29–39.
144. May SJ, Smith SA, Jacobs A, Williams A, Bailey-Wood R. The myelodysplastic syndrome: analysis of laboratory characteristics in relation to the FAB classification. Br J Haematol 1985; 59:311–319.
145. Gold EJ, Conjalka M, Pelus LM, Jhanwar SC, Broxmeyer H, Middleton AB,

Clarkson BD, Moore MA. Marrow cytogenetic and cell-culture analyses of the myelodysplastic syndromes: insights to pathophysiology and prognosis. J Clin Oncol 1983; 1:627–634.

146. Tennant GB, Bowen DT, Jacobs A. Colony-cluster ratio and cluster number in cultures of circulating myeloid progenitors as indicators of high-risk myelodysplasia. Br J Haematol 1991; 77:296–300.

147. Coiffier B, Bryon PA, Fière D, Felman P, Gentilhomme O, Vu Van H, Viala JJ, Germain D. Agar culture of bone marrow cells in acute myeloid leukemia and dysmyelopoietic syndromes. Reevaluation of its prognostic value. Nouv Rev Fr Hematol 1982; 24:13–18.

148. Faille A, Dresch C, Poirier O, Balitrand N, Najean Y. Prognostic value of in vitro bone marrow culture in refractory anaemia with excess of myeloblasts. Scand J Haematol 1978; 20:280–286.

149. Greenberg PL. Biologic and clinical implications of marrow culture studies in the myelodysplastic syndromes. Semin Hematol 1996; 33:163–175.

150. Oscier DG, Worsley A, Darlow S, Figes A, Williams JD, Hamblin TJ. Correlation of bone marrow colony growth in the myelodysplastic syndromes with the FAB classification and the Bournemouth score. Leuk Res 1989; 13:833–839.

151. Kanamaru A, Tamura S. Application of long-term bone marrow cultures for studying the leukemic transformation of myelodysplastic syndromes. Leuk Lymphoma 1993; 11:345–352.

152. Aul C, Gattermann N, Schneider W. Comparison of in vitro growth characteristics of blast cell progenitors (CFU-L) in patients with myelodysplastic syndromes and acute myeloid leukemia. Blood 1992; 80:625–633.

153. Curtis JE, Messner HA, Hasselback R, Elhakim TM, McCulloch EA. Contributions of host- and disease-related attributes to the outcome of patients with acute myelogenous leukemia. J Clin Oncol 1984; 2:253–259.

154. Goasguen JE, Garand R, Bizet M, Bremond JL, Gardais J, Callat MP, Accard F, Chaperon J. Prognostic factors of myelodysplastic syndromes—a simplified 3-D scoring system. Leuk Res 1990; 14:255–262.

155. Maschek H, Gutzmer R, Choritz H, Georgi A. Comparison of scoring systems in primary myelodysplastic syndromes. Ann Hematol 1995; 70:301–308.

156. Rubio-Felix D, Giraldo P, Franco E, Gimeno J, Giralt M. Prognostic factors in myelodysplastic syndromes: analysis of five scoring systems. Hematol Oncol 1995; 13:139–152.

157. Balduini CL, Guarnone R, Pecci A, Centenara E, Invernizzi R, Ascari E. The myelodysplastic syndromes: predictive value of eight prognostic systems in 143 cases from a single institution. Haematologica 1999; 84:12–16.

158. Pfeilstöcker M, Reisner R, Nösslinger T, Grüner H, Nowotny H, Tüchler H, Schlögl E, Pittermann E, Heinz R. Cross-validation of prognostic scores in myelodysplastic syndromes on 386 patients from a single institution confirms importance of cytogenetics. Br J Haematol 1999; 106:455–463.

159. Worsley A, Oscier DG, Stevens J, Darlow S, Figes A, Mufti GJ, Hamblin TJ. Prognostic features of chronic myelomonocytic leukaemia: a modified Bournemouth score gives the best prediction of survival. Br J Haematol 1988; 68:17–21.

160. Sanz GF, Sanz MA, Greenberg PL. Prognostic factors and scoring systems in myelodysplastic syndromes. Haematologica 1998; 83:358–368.
161. Krieger O, Lutz D. Myelodysplastische syndrome. Onkol Forum 1993; 2:2–20.
162. Greenberg PL. Risk factors and their relationship to prognosis in myelodysplastic syndromes. Leuk Res 1998; 22(suppl 1):S3–S6.
163. Pérez-Rus G, del Toro J, Benitez J, Ballesteros M, Alvarez J, Prieto E, Cuesta P. Myelodysplastic syndromes: application of the International Prognostic Scoring System (IPSS). Leuk Res 1999; 23:S63.
164. Germing U, Hildebrandt B, Strupp C, Gattermann N, Aul C. Comparative study of the IPSS and Düsseldorf score for predicting the natural course of primary MDS. Leuk Res 1999; 23:S64.

# 10
# Response Criteria for Myelodysplastic Syndromes

**Bruce D. Cheson**
*National Cancer Institute, Bethesda, Maryland*

## I. INTRODUCTION

The term "myelodysplastic syndromes" (MDS) refers to a heterogeneous group of disorders characterized in most patients by peripheral cytopenias with a hypercellular bone marrow. In 1982, the French-American-British (FAB) group first published their classification scheme in an attempt at placing these diverse disorders into an organized framework to enable investigators to communicate with a common language. The FAB classification was modified in 1985, and, since that time, it has been the universally used categorization of these disorders (1,2). The morphological subtypes designated by the FAB committee included refractory anemia (RA), refractory anemia with ringed sideroblasts (RARS), refractory anemia with excess blasts (RAEB), refractory anemia with excess blasts in transformation (RAEB-T), and chronic myelomonocytic leukemia (CMML). Recently, a World Health Organization (WHO) steering committee proposed modifications of the FAB. The most controversial of these changes was a recommendation to decrease the number of blasts required to distinguish acute myeloid leukemia (AML) from MDS from 30% blasts to 20%. This alteration eliminated the category of RAEB-T, which had been added in the 1985 modification. In addition, the WHO committee created a category of MDS/MPD (myeloproliferative disorder) that included those patients with chronic myelomonocytic leukemia (CMML) (3). However, these recommendations have not yet been universally accepted. A major area of concern reflects the fact that the distinction between AML and MDS relates more to the clinical features and the pace of the disease than merely the number of blasts counted in the bone marrow. Moreover, lowering the percentage of blasts to be classified as AML would make it difficult to compare future data with past studies.

The prognosis of the various FAB subtypes ranges from a few months to several years. The likelihood of transformation to AML varies by FAB subtype (4–7): approximately 10–20% for RA or RARS, 20–30% for CMML, 40–50% for RAEB, and 60–75% for RAEB-T. As a result of bleeding and infection, the MDS are uniformly fatal even without progression to AML (8,9). The International Prognostic Scoring System (IPSS) was developed to create clinically meaningful prognostic groups even within FAB subtype. The IPSS uses bone marrow cytogenetics, percentage of bone marrow blasts, number of cytopenias, age, and sex to predict the likelihood of transformation to AML and the duration of survival. The IPSS distinguishes patients into four prognostic subgroups that are of relatively low risk of transformation and a better survival (IPSS low or intermediate-1), or a relatively high risk of transformation to AML with a poorer survival (IPSS intermediate-2 or high). These subgroups have been suggested to be useful for developing risk-based treatment options (10).

The MDS differ from many other hematological malignancies in their chronicity and the morbidity and mortality caused by chronic cytopenias, often without disease progression to AML (8). As such, alleviation of disease-related complications, measured by clinically meaningful hematological improvement, and enhanced quality of life (QOL) are important goals of therapy.

## II.  TREATMENT OF MDS

Over the decades, various strategies have been used to treat patients with MDS. In large part, the type of treatment has been determined by the MDS FAB subtype and, more recently, IPSS category, with differing goals of treatment (10). Bone marrow transplantation is the only curative therapy for patients with MDS, but it is successful in only a minority of patients (11–14). For patients with one of the more indolent subtypes (RA, RARS; IPSS low and intermediate-1), the goal of treatment is to improve the cytopenias and to delay the progression to a more aggressive subtype. Therefore, treatment is commonly of lower intensity, consisting of cytokines and biological response modifiers, and immunosuppressive therapy. The different agents have met with varying success in ameliorating cytopenias and treating infections; however, they have clearly failed in the ultimate goal of therapy, which is to prolong patient survival. Whether they maintain or improve their quality of life remains to be determined (10).

Other treatments that have been used in these patients include low doses of single agents or attenuated combinations of chemotherapy drugs (14). These therapies may be somewhat more intensive than the biological agents and may, therefore, be associated with greater toxicities, occasionally requiring inpatient administration (14).

For some patients, particularly those with RAEB or RAEB-T, "high intensity" therapies are often recommended. These may include multiagent chemotherapy regimens such as those used in patients with overt AML (15). In contrast to patients with lower-risk MDS, the goal of these treatments is to alter the natural history of the disease by achieving a meaningful clinical response (e.g., complete remission) that may translate into a prolongation of progression-free survival and, it is hoped, overall survival.

Treatment of MDS has been frustrating, not only because of the failure of any therapy short of transplantation to cure patients, but also because of the risk for significant treatment-related morbidity and mortality as a consequence of impaired bone marrow function. As a result, observation is still, unfortunately, an acceptable standard arm for randomized clinical trials. It has been extremely difficult to compare the results of various approaches in the phase II setting: treatment reports have tended to include relatively small numbers of heterogeneous patients, with substantial selection bias, and there have been marked differences in response criteria (16). Reviewing clinical trials from various international cooperative groups and cancer centers, the greatest problem has been with the inconsistent definition of the rather vague, but often used, term of "hematological improvement" (HI). HI has been used to indicate any level of response ranging from modest improvements in a single lineage to variable levels of improvement in multiple lineages in others (17–19). Given the various definitions and the fluctuations in counts that may be experienced by patients with MDS, HI is often difficult to interpret in single-arm trials.

## III. RESPONSE CRITERIA

The problems associated with differences in response definitions initially became apparent when attempts were made to assess the efficacy of low-dose cytarabine in MDS and AML (20,21): in the various studies significantly different response criteria were used, and when more standardized criteria were applied to the data, response rates were generally lower than had been reported. Another problem that may be encountered with increasing frequency relates to some of the newer classes of drugs that are more likely to be cytostatic than cytotoxic, or may induce

**Table 1**  Measurement of Response/Treatment Effect in MDS

ALTERING DISEASE NATURAL HISTORY

1. Complete remission (CR)

   Bone marrow evaluation: Repeat bone marrow showing less than 5% myeloblasts with normal maturation of all cell lines, with no evidence for dysplasia.[a] When erythroid precursors constitute less than 50% of bone marrow nucleated cells, the percentage of blasts is based on all nucleated cells; when there are 50% or more erythroid cells, the percentage blasts should be based on the nonerythroid cells.

   Peripheral blood evaluation (absolute values must last at least 2 months)[b]

   Hemoglobin greater than 11 g/dL (untransfused, patient not on erythropoietin)

   Neutrophils 1500/mm³ or more (not on a myeloid growth factor)

   Platelets 100,000/mm³ or more (not on a thrombopoetic agent)

   Blasts, 0%

   No dysplasia

2. Partial remission (PR) (absolute values must last at least 2 months):

   All the CR criteria (if abnormal before treatment), except:

   Bone marrow evaluation: Blasts decreased by 50% or more over pretreatment, or a less advanced MDS FAB classification than pretreatment. Cellularity and morphology are not relevant.

3. Stable disease

   Failure to achieve at least a PR, but with no evidence of progression for at least 2 months.

4. Failure

   Death during treatment or disease progression characterized by worsening of cytopenias, increase in the percentage bone marrow blasts, or progression to an MDS FAB subtype more advanced than pretreatment.

5. Relapse after CR or PR—one or more of the following:
   a) Return to pretreatment bone marrow blast percentage.
   b) Decrement of 50% or greater from maximum remission/response levels in granulocytes or platelets.
   c) Reduction in hemoglobin concentration by at least 2 g/dL or transfusion dependence.[c]

6. Disease progression
   a) For patients with less than 5% blasts: a 50% or more increase in blasts to more than 5% blasts.
   b) For patients with 5% to 10% blasts: a 50% or more increase to more than 10% blasts.
   c) For patients with 10% to 20% blasts: a 50% or more increase to more than 20% blasts.
   d) For patients with 20% to 30% blasts: a 50% or more increase to more than 30% blasts.
   e) One or more of the following: 50% or greater decrement from maximum remission/response levels in granulocytes or platelets, reduction in hemoglobin concentration by at least 2 g/dL, or transfusion dependence.[c]

7. Disease transformation
   Transformation to AML (30% or more blasts).

8. Survival and progression-free survival
   (See Table 2.)

CYTOGENETIC RESPONSE
(Requires 20 analyzable metaphases using conventional cytogenetic techniques.)
   Major: No detectable cytogenetic abnormality, if preexisting abnormality was present.
   Minor: 50% or more reduction in abnormal metaphases.
   Fluorescent in situ hybridization may be used as a supplement to follow a specifically defined cytogenetic abnormality.

**Table 1** Continued

QUALITY OF LIFE

Measured by an instrument such as the FACT Questionnaire.

    Clinically useful improvement in specific domains:

        Physical

        Functional

        Emotional

        Social

        Spiritual

HEMATOLOGIC IMPROVEMENT (HI)

(Improvements must last at least 2 months in the absence of ongoing cytotoxic therapy.)[b]

Hematologic improvement should be described by the number of individual, positively affected cell lines (eg, HI-E; HI-E + HI-N; HI-E + HI-P + HI-N).

1. Erythroid response (HI-E)

    Major response: For patients with pretreatment hemoglobin less than 11 g/dL, greater than 2 g/dL increase in hemoglobin; for RBC transfusion-dependent patients, transfusion independence.

    Minor response: For patients with pretreatment hemoglobin less than 11 g/dL, 1 to 2 g/dL increase in hemoglobin; for RBC transfusion-dependent patients, 50% decrease in transfusion requirements.

2. Platelet response (HI-P)

    Major response: For patients with a pretreatment platelet count less than 100,000/mm$^3$, an absolute increase of 30,000/mm$^3$ or more; for platelet transfusion-dependent patients, stabilization of platelet counts and platelet transfusion independence.

    Minor response: For patients with a pretreatment platelet count less than 100,000/mm$^3$, a 50% or more increase in platelet count with a net increase greater than 10,000/mm$^3$ but less than 30,000/mm$^3$.

3. Neutrophil response (HI-N)

Major response: For absolute neutrophil count (ANC) less than $1500/mm^3$ before therapy, at least a 100% increase, or an absolute increase of more than $500/mm^3$, whichever is greater.

Minor response: For ANC less than $1500/mm^3$ before therapy, ANC increase of at least 100%, but absolute increase less than $500/mm^3$.

4. Progression/relapse after HI: One or more of the following: a 50% or greater decrement from maximum response levels in granulocytes or platelets, a reduction in hemoglobin concentration by at least 2 g/dL, or transfusion dependence.§

For a designated response (CR, PR, HI), all relevant response criteria must be noted on at least 2 successive determinations at least 1 week apart after an appropriate period following therapy (eg, 1 month or longer).

[a] The presence of mild megaloblastoid changes may be permitted if they are thought to be consistent with treatment effect. However, persistence of pretreatment abnormalities (eg, pseudo-Pelger-Huet cells, ringed sideroblasts, dysplastic megakaryocytes) are not consistent with CR.

[b] In some circumstances, protocol therapy may require the initiation of further treatment (eg, consolidation, maintenance) before the 2-month period. Such patients can be included in the response category into which they fit at the time the therapy is started.

[c] In the absence of another explanation such as acute infection, gastrointestinal bleeding, hemolysis, and so on.

*Source*: Ref. 16.

cellular differentiation; therefore, time to disease progression may be a more relevant primary end point, rather than response rate (22). Thus, response criteria included in a clinical trial should be able to reflect the goals of the specific treatments.

In 1999 a group of international investigators with expertise in MDS standardized response criteria for clinical trials involving patients with MDS (16). These guidelines are presented in Table 1. Four levels of hematological response were recommended to distinguish those response categories for therapies that are palliative in intent (e.g., HI, QOL) from those for which a change in the natural history of the disease might be a realistic objective (complete remission, partial remission). A 2-month duration of response was required so that transient fluctuations in blood counts were not confused with actual responses.

Although disappearance of a cytogenetic abnormality appears to have prognostic significance in other hematological malignancies, such as chronic myelogenous leukemia (23,24), whether cytogenetic response correlates with outcome in MDS will require prospective evaluation in clinical trials.

Limited data also exist regarding the value of assessing QOL end points in MDS (25,26). In a study conducted by the Cancer and Leukemia Group B (CALGB) patients were randomized to either azacytidine or observation. Not only were response, toxicity, survival, and transformation important end points, but a QOL assessment was included in the study. Although there was no apparent survival advantage to the 5-azacytidine therapy, there did appear to be some improvement in patient QOL. The use of this criterion in appropriate clinical trials, employing instruments such as the WHO Performance Score or the FACT Questionnaire (26), may provide valuable insights into the patients' physical, functional, emotional, and social status.

The International Working Group also provided definitions of major end points such as disease-free survival, progression-free survival, and time to treatment failure (Table 2). Even if new therapies do not prolong survival, these parameters may be used to select the agents to study further. Without the standardization offered by the international guidelines, results can vary widely even using the same database, as has been observed and reported for non-Hodgkin's lymphoma (27).

Another major factor that needs to be considered when comparing studies and reporting results of trials is the distribution of patient risk groups. This point has become quite clear in patients with non-Hodgkin's lymphomas, where the International Prognostic Index (IPI) is now routinely used (28). Therefore, patients should be stratified not only on the basis of FAB subtype, but, perhaps more importantly, by IPSS risk group (29). Other stratification factors could include age and performance status, as recommended by the National Comprehensive Cancer Network (NCCN) Panel on MDS (10,29). Thus, when data are re-

**Table 2** Definitions of End Points for Clinical Trials in MDS

| End point | Response category | Definition | Point of measurement |
|---|---|---|---|
| Overall survival | All patients | Death from any cause | Entry onto trial |
| Event-free survival | All patients[a] | Failure or death from any cause | Entry onto trial |
| Progression-free survival | All patients | Disease progression or death from MDS | Entry onto trial |
| Disease-free survival | CR | Time to relapse | First documentation of response |
| Cause-specific death | All patients | Death related to MDS | Death |

[a] Under circumstances where presentation of EFS may be appropriate for responders only, this point should be clearly stated.
IPSS should be used as the primary stratification. Complete blood counts should be evaluated at least monthly, or more often if clinically indicated, to establish the durability of responses.
*Source*: Ref. 16.

ported, the various IPSS categories should be presented separately not only for response but for progression-free and overall survival.

## IV. CONCLUSIONS

A large number of new and unique agents that target biological or molecular pathways either are currently or will soon be in clinical trials in MDS. A critical problem is that few patients are entered onto these studies and, those who are have often received extensive prior therapy prior to the new investigational drugs, so they are less likely to respond.

In our search to identify new agents with promising activity, uniformly accepted response criteria would facilitate the interpretation of data and the ability to compare results among various studies. In addition, such criteria would provide a framework upon which to test scientific correlative studies of new biological and immunological insights into MDS. These considerations led to the new recommended guidelines for response in MDS (16).

It is unlikely any of the single agents will have a major impact on patient outcome. However, failure of a single agent to induce significant benefit may not be the fault of the drug, but rather be due to the manner in which it was tested: a clinical trial evaluating a suboptimal dose or schedule may lead to an erroneous impression that a compound is inactive. Similarly, while overly liberal response criteria can overestimate the activity of a new agent, overly restrictive criteria can lead to negative results with the premature discarding of potentially valuable agents. For example, antiangiogenic drugs are likely to be cytostatic and, therefore, may not induce traditional responses in phase II studies. Nevertheless, it is more likely that combinations of agents will be required to make a significant impact on patient outcome.

The goals of clinical research in MDS include prolonging survival of patients. Secondary end points of clinical importance include amelioration of cytopenias and improvement in QOL. In phase II trials, response rates may suggest activity of an agent; however, this end point is rarely sufficient for drug approval by regulatory agencies since increases in response rates have not necessarily translated into prolongation of time to treatment failure or survival. Therefore, phase III trials are generally required to demonstrate an improvement in efficacy.

The international guidelines are an attempt to provide uniformity to the design, conduct, and analysis of clinical trials in patients with MDS. They are currently required for all National Cancer Institute–sponsored trials in MDS. However, as with guidelines in other diseases, the need for modifications does not become apparent until they are applied prospectively in clinical trials (30–32). Moreover, revised criteria will likely be required as more is learned about the molecular biology and genetics of these disorders. Until that time, the standardized guidelines will, it is hoped, improve communication among investigators and improve interpretability of data and comparability among clinical trials.

## REFERENCES

1.  Bennett JM, Catovsky D, Daniel M-T, Flandrin G, Galton DAG, Gralnick H, Sultan C. Proposals for the classification of the myelodysplastic syndromes. Br J Haematol 1982; 51:189.
2.  Bennett JM, Catovsky D, Daniel MT, Flandrin G, Galton DAG, Gralnick HR, Sultan C. Proposed revised criteria for the classification of acute myeloid leukemia. A report of the French-American-British group. Ann Intern Med 1985; 103:626.
3.  Harris NL, Jaffe ES, Diebold J, Flandrin G, Muller-Harmelink HK, Vardiman J, Lister TA, Bloomfield CD. World Health Organization classification of neoplastic diseases of the hematopoietic and lymphoid tissues: report of the clinical advisory committee meeting—Airlie House, Virginia. J Clin Oncol 1999; 17:3835.
4.  Tricot G, Vlietinck R, Boogaerts MA, Hendrickx B, De Wolf-Peeters C, Van den Berghe H, Verwilghen RL. Prognostic factors in the myelodysplastic syndromes: importance of initial data on peripheral blood counts, bone marrow cytology, trephine biopsy and chromosome analysis. Br J Haematol 1985; 60:19.

5. Todd WM, Pierre RV. Preleukaemia: a long-term prospective study of 326 patients. Scand J Haematol 1986; 36:114.
6. Vallespí T, Torrabadella M, Julia A, Irriguible D, Jaen A, Acebedo G, Triginer J. Myelodysplastic syndromes: a study of 101 cases according to the FAB classification. Br J Haematol 1985; 61:81.
7. Kerkhofs H, Hermans J, Maak HL, Leeksma CH. Utility of the FAB classification for myelodysplastic syndromes: investigation of prognostic factors in 237 cases. Br J Haematol 1987; 65:83.
8. Weisdorf DJ, Oken MM, Johnson GJ, Rydell RE. Chronic myelodysplastic syndrome: short survival with or without evolution to acute leukaemia. Br J Haematol 1983; 55:691.
9. Kantarjian HM, Keating MJ, Walters RS, Smith TL, Cork A, McCredie KB, Freireich EJ. Therapy-related leukemia and myelodysplastic syndrome: clinical, cytogenetic, and prognostic features. J Clin Oncol 1986; 4:1748.
10. Greenberg P, Bishop M, Deeg J, Estey E, Erba H, Gore S, Nimer S, O'Donnell M, Stone R, Tallman M. NCCN Practice Guidelines for the Myelodysplastic Syndromes. Oncology 1998; 12:53.
11. De Witte T. New treatment approaches for myelodysplastic syndrome and secondary leukemias. Ann Oncol 1994; 5:401.
12. Anderson JE, Appelbaum FR, Schoch G, Gooley T, Anasetti C, Bensinger WI, Bryant E, Buckner CD, Chauncey T, Clift RA, Deeg HJ, Doney K, Flowers M, Hansen JA, Martin PJ, Matthews DC, Nash RA, Sanders JE, Shulman H, Sullivan KM, Witherspoon RP, Storb R. Allogeneic marrow transplantation for myelodysplastic syndrome with advanced disease morphology: a phase II study of busulfan, cyclophosphamide, and total-body irradiation and analysis of prognostic factors. J Clin Oncol 1996; 14:220.
13. De Witte T, Van Biezen A, Hermans J, Labopin M, Runde V, Or R, Meloni G, Mauri SB, Carella A, Apperly J, Gratwohl A, Laporte J-P. Autologous bone marrow transplantation for patients with myelodysplastic syndrome (MDS) or acute myeloid leukemia following MDS. Blood 1997; 90:3853.
14. Cheson BD. Standard and low-dose chemotherapy for the treatment of myelodysplastic syndromes. Leuk Res 1998; 22:s17.
15. Bernstein SH, Brunetta VL, Davey FR, Wurster-Hill D, Mayer RJ, Stone RM, Schiffer CA, Bloomfield CD. Acute myeloid leukemia-type chemotherapy for newly diagnosed patients with antecedent cytopenias having myelodysplastic syndrome as defined by French-American-British criteria: a Cancer and Leukemia Group B study. J Clin Oncol 1996; 14:2486.
16. Cheson BD, Bennett JM, Kantarjian H, Pinto A, Schiffer CA, Nimer SD, Lowenberg B, Beran M, de Witte TM, Stone RM, Mittelman M, Sanz GF, Wijermans PW, Gore S, Greenberg PL. Report of an international working group to standardize response criteria for myelodysplastic syndromes. Blood 2000; 96:3671.
17. Silverman LR, Demakos EP, Peterson B, Odchimar-Reissig R, Nelson D, Kornblith AB, Stone R, Holland JC, Powell BL, DeCastro C, Ellerton J, Larson RA, Schiffer CA, Holland JF. A randomized controlled trial of subcutaneous azacitidine (AZA C) in patients with the myelodysplastic syndrome (MDS): a study of the Cancer and Leukemia Group B (CALGB). Proc ASCO 1998; 17:14a.

18. Beran M, Kantarjian H, O'Brien S, Koller C, Al-Bitr M, Arbuck S, Pierce S, Abbruz-
    zese JL, Andreef M, Keating M, Freireich E, Estey E. Topotecan, a topoisomerase
    I inhibitor is active in the treatment of myelodysplastic syndrome and chronic myelo-
    monocytic leukemia. Blood 1996; 88:2473.

19. List AF, Holmes H, Vempaty H, Greenberg PL, Bennett JM. Phase II study of ami-
    fostine in patients with myelodysplastic syndromes (MDS): impact on hematopoie-
    sis. Proc ASCO 1999; 18:51a.

20. Cheson BD, Jasperse DM, Simon R, Friedman MA. A critical appraisal of low-dose
    cytosine arabinoside in patients with acute non-lymphocytic leukemia and myelo-
    dysplastic syndromes. J Clin Oncol 1986; 4:1857.

21. Cheson BD, Simon R. Low-dose ara-C in acute nonlymphocytic leukemia and myelo-
    dysplastic syndromes: a review of 20 years' experience. Semin Oncol 1987; 14:126.

22. Cheson BD, Zwiebel JA, Dancey J, Murgo A. Novel therapeutic agents for the treat-
    ment of myelodysplastic syndromes. Semin Oncol 2000; 27:560.

23. Kantarjian HM, Smith TL, O'Brien S, Beran M, Pierce S, Talpaz M. Prolonged
    survival in chronic myelogenous leukemia after cytogenetic response to interferon-
    alpha therapy. Ann Intern Med 1995; 122:254.

24. Cortes J, Talpaz M, O'Brien S, Rios MB, Majlis A, Keating M, Freireich EJ, Kantar-
    jian H. Suppression of cytogenetic clonal evolution with interferon alfa therapy in
    patients with Philadelphia chromosome-positive chronic myelogenous leukemia. J
    Clin Oncol 1998; 16:3279.

25. Kornblith A, Herndon II J, Silverman LR et al. The impact of 5-azacytidine on the
    quality of life of patients with the myelodysplastic syndrome (MDS) treated in a
    randomized phase III trial of the Cancer and Leukemia Group B (CALGB). Proc
    Am Soc Clin Oncol 1998; 17:49a.

26. Cella D. Quality of life outcomes: measurement and validation. Oncology (Hunting-
    ton) 1996; 10:233.

27. Grillo-López AJ, Cheson BD, Horning SJ, Peterson BA, Carter WD, Varns CL,
    Klippenstein DL, Shen CD. Response criteria for NHL: importance of "normal"
    lymph node size and correlations with response rates. Ann Oncol 2000; 11:399.

28. Shipp MA, Harrington DP, Anderson JR, Armitage JO, Bonadonna G, Brittinger
    G, Cabanillas F, Canellos GP, Coiffier B, Connors JM, Cowan RA, Crowther D,
    Dahlberg S, Engelhard M, Fisher RI, Gisselbrecht C, Horning SJ, Lepage E, Lister
    TA, Meerwaldt JH, Montserrat E, Nissen NI, Oken MM, Peterson BA, Tondini C,
    Velasquez WS, Yeap B. Development of a predictive model for aggressive
    lymphoma: the International Non-Hodgkin's Lymphoma Prognostic Factors Project.
    N Engl J Med 1993; 329:987.

29. Greenberg P, Cox C, LeBeau M, Fenaux P, Morel P, Sanz G, Sanz M, Vallespi T,
    Hamblin T, Oscier D, Ohyashiki K, Toyama K, Aul C, Mufti G, Bennett J. Interna-
    tional scoring system for evaluating prognosis in myelodysplastic syndromes. Blood
    1997; 89:2079.

30. Cheson BD, Cassileth PA, Head DR, Schiffer CA, Bennett JM, Bloomfield CD,
    Brunning R, Gale RP, Grever MR, Keating MJ, Sawitsky A, Stass S, Weinstein H,
    Woods WG. Report of the National Cancer Institute-sponsored workshop on defini-
    tions of diagnosis and response in acute myeloid leukemia. J Clin Oncol 1990; 8:
    813.

31. Cheson BD, Bennett JM, Rai KR, Grever MR, Kay NE, Schiffer CA, Oken MM, Keating MJ, Boldt DH, Kempin SJ, Foon KA. Guidelines for clinical protocols for chronic lymphocytic leukemia: report of the NCI-sponsored Working Group. Am J Hematol 1988; 29:152.

32. Cheson BD, Bennett JM, Grever M, Kay N, Keating MJ, O'Brien S, Rai KR. National Cancer Institute–Sponsored Working Group guidelines for chronic lymphocytic leukemia: revised guidelines for diagnosis and treatment. Blood 1996; 87:4990.

# 11

# Mechanisms of Drug Resistance in Myelodysplastic Syndromes and Acute Myeloid Leukemia

**Robert B. Geller and Alan F. List**
*University of Arizona College of Medicine,*
*Tucson, Arizona*

## I. INTRODUCTION

Resistance to chemotherapy remains the major obstacle to achieving durable, complete remissions in patients with myeloid malignancies. In many cases, patients respond to induction therapy, but the remission is of short duration and is associated with resistance to conventional antineoplastics at relapse. These resistant cells may be present at diagnosis or develop during treatment. In recent years, an important mechanism of pleiotropic drug resistance, multidrug resistance (MDR), as well as other mechanisms of resistance have been identified, and their role in clinical drug resistance in myelodysplastic syndromes (MDS) and adult acute myeloid leukemia (AML) explored (1,2). In particular, patients with MDS and secondary AML frequently express multidrug transporters that contribute to MDR (3–8). In this chapter, the prevalence and biological and clinical significance of MDR in AML and MDS will be discussed, as well as pharmacological approaches to overcome clinical MDR.

## II. MULTIDRUG RESISTANCE

### A. Drug Resistance Associated with Permeability Glycoprotein

Over the past two decades, we have witnessed the characterization of an important mechanism of drug resistance, termed "multidrug resistance" (MDR). MDR was first applied to describe the in vitro phenomenon in which tumor cells become cross-resistant to several structurally unrelated chemotherapeutic agents following exposure to a single cytotoxic drug (9). These drugs share few functional and structural similarities, with the exception of hydrophobicity and neutral or positive charge, and are generally naturally derived or semisynthetic xenobiotics, such as the anthracyclines, epipodophyllotoxins, taxanes, and vinca alkaloids (Table 1) (10).

One of the most important mechanisms of MDR in AML and MDS is mediated by the multidrug resistance gene-1 (*MDR1*), which encodes a transmembrane glycoprotein known as permeability glycoprotein (P-gp) (1,11,12). P-gp functions as an adenosine triphosphate (ATP)-dependent efflux pump, which is capable of extruding a wide variety of compounds, ranging from peptides and steroid hormones to antineoplastics (11).

## 1. Mechanism of Drug Resistance Associated with P-gp

In humans, two genes, *MDR1* and *MDR2*, encode for P-gp; both are located on chromosome 7 (12). Despite their homology, only the *MDR1* gene encodes the drug efflux protein that confers MDR. P-gp is a member of a superfamily of ATP-binding cassette (ABC) transporters, which now exceeds 50 members. The 170-kD P-gp consists of two structurally homologous halves, each containing six transmembrane domains, one ATP-binding site (Fig. 1), and the highly conserved "Walker A" and "Walker B" motif (12). Although initial studies suggested that phosphorylation of P-gp is essential for drug transport (13), mutational inactivation of the primary phosphorylation sites does not impair transport function

**Table 1**  Cytotoxic Drugs that Induce Multidrug Resistance and Are Transported by Permeability Glycoprotein

| | |
|---|---|
| Anthracyclines | Vinca alkaloids |
| Doxorubicin | Vincristine |
| Daunorubicin | Vinblastine |
| Idarubicin | Vinorelbine |
| Epirubicin | Other |
| Epipodophyllotoxins | Mitoxantrone |
| Etoposide | Dactinomycin |
| Teniposide | Trimetrexate |
| Taxanes | Mitomycin |
| Paclitaxel | Mithramycin |
| Docetaxel | |

*Source*: Adapted from Ref. 10.

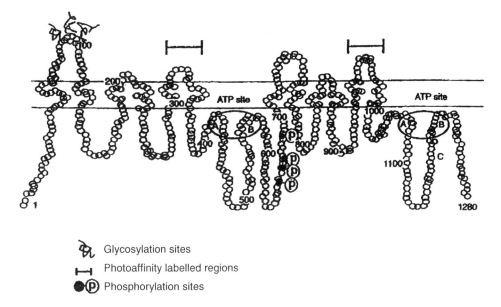

🐝 Glycosylation sites
⊢—⊣ Photoaffinity labelled regions
●ⓟ Phosphorylation sites

**Fig. 1** Schematic representation of MDR1 permeability glycoproteins. (From Ref. 12.)

(14,15). Surface glycosylation epitopes may contribute to routing and stability of the protein and offer sufficient antigenicity to serve as targets for monoclonal antibodies, such as MRK16, that recognize P-gp (16).

P-gp has a wide variety of substrates (Table 1), all of which are large hydrophobic and amphipathic molecules (10) that enter the cytosol via passive diffusion after intercalation into the cell membrane. Evidence suggests that P-gp acts as a flippase to capture extracellular substrates as they enter the cell membrane or cytosol (17,18) rather than functioning in a "classical" pump fashion by binding cytosolic substrates and extruding them across the membrane. The flippase mechanism appears to be highly conserved and is demonstrable in the prokaryote *Lactococcus lactis* through a homolog of P-gp that also has broad substrate specificity (19). Although the precise mechanism by which P-gp transports hydrophobic drugs is still not resolved, it is realized that this process is ATP-dependent. Transport from the inner lipid leaflet of the plasma membrane to the outer leaflet allows these drugs to be propelled from the plasma membrane by diffusion (20).

Several noncytotoxic agents, such as verapamil, quinidine, and cyclosporine A (CSA), inhibit P-gp-mediated drug export by competing with antineoplastic substrates for binding to P-gp (21). The efficient inhibition of P-gp-mediated drug efflux by these modulators may be derived from their superior passive diffusion into the cell, permitting the generation of high intracellular concentrations relative to the slow passive diffusion of most cytotoxic agents. According to Michaelis-Menten kinetics, these modulators have a P-gp-binding-affinity advantage when compared with the binding affinity of cytotoxic agents (22).

## 2. MDR1 Expression in MDS and AML

P-gp expression is evident in many solid tumors and in hematological malignancies (3), with tumors derived from tissues that naturally express P-gp demonstrating constitutive expression (1–3,23). Hematopoietic malignancies that frequently express P-gp include secondary and elderly AML, MDS, T-cell non-Hodgkin's lymphoma, and relapsed multiple myeloma (3–8,23–30). Although the fraction of leukemic cells that express P-gp may increase at relapse compared with the fraction at initial diagnosis, analysis of *MDR1* gene polymorphisms supports the notion that chemotherapy administered during induction selectively eradicates sensitive cell populations while fostering expansion of the P-gp-positive clone (5,31). Several recent studies have also demonstrated that P-gp expression in the leukemic blasts of patients with de novo AML (Table 2) and high-risk MDS varies directly with age and with cytogenetic pattern (4,6–8,31–40). This quanti-

**Table 2** Expression of MDR-1 or P-gp in De Novo Acute Myeloid Leukemia

| Study | No. of patients | Percent of patients with expression of multidrug resistance |
|---|---|---|
| Sato et al., 1990 [4] | 15 | 67 |
| Pirker et al., 1991 [7] | 63 | 71 |
| Marie et al., 1991 [6] | 35 | 19 |
| Zhou et al., 1992 [31] | 51 | 43 |
| Campos et al., 1992 [8] | 150 | 47 |
| te Boekhorst et al., 1993 [33] | 52 | 58 |
| Ino et al., 1994 [34] | 52 | 27 |
| Lamy et al., 1994 [35] | 51 | 53 |
| Leith et al., 1995 [36] | 171 | 75 |
| Leith et al., 1995 [37] | 193 | 72 |
| te Boekhorst et al., 1995 [38] | 38 | 74 |
| Guerci et al., 1995 [39] | 69 | 41 |
| van de Heuvel-Eibrink et al., 1997 [40] | 130 | 44 |

*Source*: Adapted from Ref. 32.

tative difference between studies is related, in part, to the analytical assays used for P-gp analysis (41–43).

## 3. Laboratory Analysis of P-gp Expression in Leukemia Samples

Since low levels of P-gp expression may be sufficient to confer chemotherapy resistance, assays designed to detect expression and function of P-gp in clinical samples must be highly sensitive. These assays should optimally distinguish the leukemia population from normal cells present within a clinical sample (36,44). This is particularly important in leukemia samples from peripheral blood and bone marrow aspirates as these samples contain a variable admixture of normal hematopoietic progenitors, lymphocytes, T cells, natural killer cells, and monocytes, all of which may express MDR1 and P-gp (42,43). Because of these challenges, highly sensitive and quantitative multiparametric flow cytometric assays have now been developed that permit simultaneous assessment of P-gp protein in the blast population and quantitative assessment of P-gp efflux. Such assays can be performed quickly, within 6–8 hr of procurement of a clinical specimen, so that P-gp expression and function may be used for appropriate clinical decisions.

To quantify P-gp on leukemic blasts in clinical samples, the sample should be labeled with P-gp-specific antibody that recognizes a distinct surface epitope of the protein (e.g., MRK-16 or MM4.17), an anti-CD34 antibody (i.e., the stem cell/progenitor antigen), and an anti-CD33 antibody (i.e., a myeloid-specific antigen), or with other antibodies that characterize a patient's leukemia antigenic phenotype (44–46). In studies by the Southwest Oncology Group (SWOG), biotinylated MRK-16 or MM4.17 antibody recognition is amplified using a highly sensitive avidin-phycoerythrin (PE)/Texas Red duochrome second-step reagent, which offers greater sensitivity than detection with a fluorescein isothiocyanate (FITC)-conjugated second-step reagent for discerning low levels of P-gp expression (34,36,44–46). The duochrome approach is highly specific since it allows for the accurate analysis of P-gp expression in a phenotypically gated myeloblast population. Functional activity of drug transport proteins can then be evaluated from flow cytometric measurements of the efflux by fluorescent drugs or dyes. To overcome the very weak intrinsic fluorescence of many of the chemotherapeutic agents, most clinical assays utilize a stronger fluorescent dye such as 3,3-diethyloxacarbocyanine iodide (DiOC$_2$) or rhodamine 123 (RHO 123), which are both P-gp substrates (36,44,46).

Functional efflux assays can be performed reproducibly on fresh or thawed cryopreserved specimens (36,45,46). For these efflux studies, the specimens are initially incubated in 37°C media containing the drug or dye to allow its uptake by passive diffusion. The blasts are then washed and incubated in dye-free media to allow efflux to occur. Parallel experiments are performed in the presence or absence of a P-gp modulator and changes in cellular fluorescence after efflux are measured. The physical characteristics of $DiOC_2$ and Rho 123 allow the cells to be costained with anti-CD34 and P-gp-specific antibodies. This allows examination of dye efflux in precisely defined blast populations. Thus, dye efflux in the blast population can be reliably distinguished from efflux from normal lymphocytes and myeloid cells that express P-gp. This distinction is particularly important in cases in which only a minor cell population displays efflux or the blast percentage is low (45,46).

Many groups have recently reported that P-gp expression and efflux are not always correlated in AML samples, making identification of patients who are candidates for treatment with P-gp modulators potentially difficult (36,46). Two disparate phenotypes have been observed in AML: first, samples that express P-gp but lack functional drug/dye efflux and, second, samples that demonstrate drug/dye efflux, but lack expression of P-gp. The latter cases implicate the presence of alternative drug efflux transporters and highlight the biological complexity of MDR (36,46). P-gp efflux capacity also varies inversely with progenitor maturity, resulting in loss of function with differentiation; this may explain the close linkage between P-gp function and the stem cell phenotype described in malignant myeloblasts and normal progenitors. Functional assays, therefore, have offered biological rationales for the reported discordance between P-gp expression and function and should facilitate proper interpretation of the results of clinical trials with MDR modulators.

## B. Other Forms of Drug Resistance

### 1. Alternative Mechanisms of Drug Resistance in Leukemia Cells

Although P-gp may confer clinical resistance to many antileukemia drugs, such as anthracyclines, epipodophyllotoxins, and amsacrine, other mechanisms of MDR are also demonstrable (47–51). The MDR protein (MRP) genes are a family of six transporter proteins that, like MDR1, are members of the ABC gene superfamily (52). The MRP genes encode multispecific organic anion transporters, with substrate specificity restricted to anionic amphophilic natural products or anion-conjugated (e.g., glutathione-, glucuronate-, sulfate-) neutral or positively charged molecules (53). While MPR1 is a multispecific drug transporter, MRP2 (alternatively known as c-MOAT) is implicated in cisplatin resistance and phosphatidylcholine transport. Gene transfection studies indicate that MRP2 also confers resistance to methotrexate, etoposide, doxorubicin, epirubicin, and mitoxantrone (54,55). MRP3, another organic transporter, displays higher avidity for glucuronate-conjugated substrates rather than the glutathione conjugates of

MRP1 and MRP2 (56). Attempts to generate stable overexpression of MRP3 by transfection have yielded only low levels of expression but these cells display resistance to etoposide and teniposide (57–59). MRP4 functions as a cellular efflux pump for several human immunodeficiency virus antivirals and may contribute to resistance to anticancer purine analogs (e.g., 6-mercaptopurine and thioguanine) (60). MRP5 overexpression yields low-level resistance to the thiopurines, but does not confer resistances to anthracyclines, vinca alkaloids, podophyllotoxins, or methotrexate (61). Both MRP4 and MRP5 are believed to function primarily as nucleoside analog transporters. Currently, both the physiological function and potential involvement of MRP6 in drug resistance remain unclear (62).

The *MRP1* gene is located on chromosome 16p13.1 and confers resistance to anion-conjugated anthracyclines and vinca alkaloids. MRP1 overexpression is demonstrable in a variety of untreated and refractory hematological malignancies including AML (47–51,63). The frequency of phenotypic detection of MRP1 in untreated AML approximates 30% (47), with a corresponding frequency that is at least equivalent or even slightly higher than in untreated cases at relapse (48,49). Coexpression of MRP1 and MRP2 with P-gp is frequently observed (47,64–66). Although the prognostic relevance of the MRP1 protein remains in question, functional assays suggest that the transporter may contribute to treatment failure, particularly when coexpressed with P-gp (67).

Recently, a subunit of the major vault protein (MVP) was identified in doxorubicin-resistant cell lines that lacked P-gp and MRP proteins and was designated LRP (lung resistance protein) (67,68). MVP has been implicated in the nuclear trafficking of cytotoxic agents by gene inactivation studies. In addition, several investigators have found significant expression of LRP in blast cells of patients with high-risk AML or advanced MDS and correlation of expression in some studies to treatment outcomes (68–70).

Another ABC-transmembrane transporter termed ''breast cancer resistance protein'' or mitoxantrone resistance (MXR) transporter was recently characterized (71–73). Similar to P-gp and MRP1, BCRP is associated with enhanced drug efflux, which is ATP dependent. However, this protein may also be involved in intracellular drug re-distribution and is unique in that it is a half-transporter. As a half-transporter, BCRP may require the formation of homodimers or heterodimers with another half-transporter to manifest export function. The changes in drug distribution are most notable for DNA-interactive drugs, where the protein facilitates drug redistribution from the nucleus to the cytoplasm in BCRP-transfected or drug-resistant cells. The exact mechanism for this redistribution is not known.

Diverse patterns of BCRP expression have been observed. Interestingly, BCRP has been shown to be highly expressed in the placenta and at lower levels in the liver, small intestine, colon, and ovary but its normal function in these tissues is unknown. When BCRP mRNA was examined in the blast cells from

21 patients with acute leukemia, BCRP mRNA varied considerably, with low or barely detectable expression in half of the samples, whereas seven samples had relatively high expression. High expression did not correlate with high expression of P-gp, suggesting that BCRP may cause resistance to certain antileukemia drugs in P-gp-negative cases (74). Thus far, BCRP has been associated with resistance to anthracenes, such as doxorubicin and mitoxantrone, and the topoisomerase inhibitor, topotecan, and cyclin-dependent kinase inhibitor, flavopiridol (74).

### 2. Laboratory Methods for Measuring Expression and Function of MRP and LRP

As with P-gp detection, it is preferable to detect MRP1 protein rather than MRP mRNA by reverse transcriptase or other molecular techniques, to distinguish normal and malignant cell expression. Given this, multicolor flow cytometric assays for detection of the MRP1 and LRP proteins have also been developed. MRP-1 is detected with the MRP-specific antibody MRPm6 and with a PE-labeled second-step reagent to optimize detection. LRP can similarly be detected using the monoclonal antibody LRP-56 (46). When compared with immunohistochemistry on cytospin preparations, the flow cytometry assays were found to be not only more rapid, but also more sensitive (74). However, despite the higher sensitivity of flow cytometry for LRP detection, only the results of immunocytochemical detection have consistently shown an adverse prognostic relationship to remission rate and duration in AML (75,76).

Another benefit to flow cytometric methods is that they also provide for drug/dye efflux measurements. P-gp, MRP, and LRP display specific patterns of drug/dye efflux and the patterns from primary human AML samples are similar to those established using cell-line models (46,77). P-gp, for instance, can transport $DiOC_2$ and Rho 123 and is inhibited by the modulators CSA and PSC 833 (78,79). Although intracellular drug redistribution is demonstrable in LRP-overexpressing cell lines and primary human AML samples, a specific inhibitor of LRP is not available. Therefore, flow cytometric screening assays to assess unique patterns of substrate transport are useful in detection of functional transport proteins that may contribute to MDR in clinical specimens (46).

### C. Prognostic Significance of Drug Resistance

### 1. Prognostic Significance of MDR Expression

The clinical significance of MDR1 expression in patients with MDS and AML varies based on the methodology applied. In some, but not all, studies evaluating MDR1 by either mRNA expression or P-gp immunodetection, overexpression of P-gp is associated with a lower probability of complete remission (Table 3) (4,6–8,31–34,37,80–103). The lack of agreement among studies relates, in part, to

**Table 3** Prognostic Significance of MDR1 in De Novo Acute Myeloid Leukemia

| Study | No. of patients | MDR1 expression[a] | | Negative correlation of expression and complete remission[b] | Negative correlation of expression to survival[b] |
|---|---|---|---|---|---|
| | | RNA | Protein | | |
| Sato et al., 1990 [4] | 36 | + | | Yes | Yes |
| Kuwazuru et al., 1990 [80] | 17 | | + | Yes | Yes |
| Pirker et al., 1991 [7] | 63 | + | | Yes | Yes |
| Marie et al., 1991 [6] | 23 | + | | Yes | — |
| Campos et al., 1992 [8] | 150 | | + | Yes | Yes |
| Zhou et al., 1992 [31] | 51 | + | + | Yes | Yes |
| Marie et al., 1993 [81] | 42 | + | + | Yes | — |
| te Boekhorst et al., 1993 [33] | 47 | | + | Yes | Yes |
| Ino et al., 1994 [34] | 52 | | + | No | No |
| Wood et al., 1994 [82] | 54 | | + | Yes | No |
| Hart et al., 1994 [83] | 36 | + | | Yes | Yes |
| Zochbauer et al., 1994 [84] | 52 | + | + | Yes | Yes |
| Del Poeta et al., 1996 [85] | 117 | | + | Yes | Yes |
| Guerci et al., 1995 [39] | 69 | | + | Yes | Yes |
| Stevers et al., 1995 [86] | 130 | | + | No | No |
| Zhou et al., 1995 [87] | 51 | + | | Yes | — |
| Schuurhuis et al., 1995 [64] | 17 | + | + | No | No |
| Del Poeta et al., 1994 [88] | 158 | | + | Yes | Yes |
| Nussler et al., 1994 [89] | 102 | | + | Yes | Yes |
| List et al., 1996 [90] | 21 | | + | Yes | Yes |
| Samdani et al., 1996 [91] | 96 | | + | Yes | Yes |
| Goasguen et al., 1996 [90] | 25 | | + | No | No |
| van de Heuvel-Eibrink et al., 1997 [40] | 120 | | + | Yes | Yes |
| Hunault et al., 1997 [93] | 110 | + | + | Yes | Yes |
| Del Poeta et al., 1997 [94] | 223 | | + | Yes | Yes |
| Martinez et al., 1997 [95] | 50 | | + | Yes | Yes |
| Filipits et al., 1997 [96] | 80 | | + | Yes | Yes |
| Lohri et al., 1997 [97] | 57 | + | | — | No |
| Leith et al., 1995 [37] | 352 | | + | Yes | Yes |
| Legrand et al., 1998 [98] | 53 | | + | Yes | — |
| Borg et al., 1998 [99] | 91 | | + | Yes | Yes |
| Kasimir-Bauer et al., 1998 [100] | 40 | | + | No | — |
| Senent et al., 1998 [101] | 82 | | + | Yes | No |
| Pallis et al., 1999 [102] | 47 | | + | Yes | Yes |
| Michieli et al., 1999 [103] | 96 | | + | Yes | Yes |

[a] "+" indicates that RNA or protein was measured in the study; an empty box indicates that there was no measurement of the RNA/protein.
[b] "—"indicates that correlations or outcomes were not reported.
*Source*: Adapted from Ref. 32.

the lack of standardization for the assays used for MDR1 detection. Furthermore, even with highly specific assays, it is uncertain whether low numbers of MDR1-expressing cells contribute to a poor outcome of treatment. In an attempt to evaluate the importance of varying numbers of MDR1-positive blasts, te Boekhorst et al. showed that even small numbers of these cells (1–5%) represent an increased risk of refractory disease (38). These data suggest that even small numbers of MDR1+ cells may be relevant and that assays with sufficient sensitivity to detect P-gp expression in small populations need to be standardized.

More recently, Leith et al. evaluated the clinical and biological relevance of MDR1 overexpression in 211 elderly patients, including 161 de novo and 50 secondary AML (44). All patients had detailed karyotyping performed as well as quantitation of expression of MDR1 and functional drug efflux. The frequency of patients with unfavorable cytogenetics was 32%, MDR2 protein expression was 71%, and functional drug efflux was 58%. In a univariate analysis, the presence of secondary AML, unfavorable cytogenetics, and MDR1 were each independently associated with lower rates of complete remission. In addition, poor response to therapy was strongly associated with unfavorable cytogenetics and MDR1 expression. These data confirm earlier reports that MDR1 expression is an independent prognostic variable for response in AML.

The expression of P-gp and MRP1 specifically in patients with MDS was evaluated in two studies (104,105). In one of these studies, List et al. evaluated P-gp expression in 45 bone marrow specimens, including 32 cases of MDS, seven cases of MDS that progressed to AML, and six cases of therapy-related hematological disorders (104). P-gp reactivity was not related to specific cytogenetic abnormalities. However, there was a strong correlation between P-gp expression and expression of CD34, suggesting that MDR in MDS may be closely linked to a stem cell phenotype. A second study, by Poulain et al., had differing results (105). Bone marrows from 56 patients with MDS, including 23 cases of MDS progression to AML, were evaluated. The results suggested that MRP1 expression correlated with disease stage; 28 of the 56 cases (50%) expressed MRP1, with expression being more frequent in those patients whose disease progressed to AML than in those whose disease did not progress from primary MDS (70% vs. 36%, $p = 0.02$). No correlation was observed between MDR1 expression and P-gp, LRP, or CD34 expression. Twenty-six patients were treated with intensive chemotherapy; MDR1 was not found to be predictive for response in this relatively small study.

## 2. Prognostic Significance of MRP and LRP Expression

Studies have been performed to evaluate the clinical significance of MRP and LRP expression in de novo AML (Table 4) (39,44,49,64,70,76,84,87,92,92,98–100,102,103,106–108). Virtually all of these analyses did not demonstrate a sig-

**Table 4**  Prognostic Significance of MRP1 and LRP in De Novo Acute Myeloid Leukemia

| Study | No. of patients | Expression[a] RNA | Protein | Negative correlation of expression and complete remission | Negative correlation of expression to survival[b] |
|---|---|---|---|---|---|
| MRP1 | | | | | |
| Hart et al., 1994 [83] | 36 | + | | No | — |
| Schuurhuis et al., 1995 [64] | 17 | + | | No | No |
| Schneider et al., 1995 [49] | 29 | + | | No | — |
| Zhou et al., 1995 [87] | 52 | + | | No | — |
| te Boekhorst et al., 1995 [38] | 35 | + | | No | No |
| Hunault et al., 1997 [93] | 110 | + | | No | No |
| Filipits et al., 1997 [96] | 80 | | + | No | No |
| Lohri et al., 1997 [97] | 57 | + | | No | No |
| Hart et al., 1997 [106] | 47 | + | | No | — |
| Leith et al., 1997 [44] | 352 | | + | No | No |
| Kasimir-Bauer et al., 1998 [100] | 40 | | + | No | — |
| Legrand et al., 1998 [98] | 53 | | + | No | — |
| Legrand et al., 1999 [106a] | 50 | | + | Yes | Yes |
| Borg et al., 1998 [99] | 91 | | + | No | No |
| LRP | | | | | |
| List et al., 1996 [70] | 21 | | + | Yes | Yes |
| Goasguen et al., 1996 [92] | 25 | | + | No | No |
| Leith et al., 1997 [44] | 352 | | + | No | No |
| Hart et al., 1997 [106] | 67 | + | | Yes | — |
| Pirker et al., 1997 [107] | 23 | | + | Yes | Yes |
| Filipits et al., 1998 [76] | 86 | | + | Yes | Yes |
| Borg et al., 1998 [99] | 91 | | + | Yes | Yes |
| Legrand et al., 1998 [108] | 53 | | + | No | — |
| Pallis et al., 1999 [102] | 47 | | + | No | — |
| Michieli et al., 1999 [103] | 96 | | + | No | No |

[a] "+" indicates that RNA or protein was measured in the study; an empty box indicates that there was no measurement of the RNA/protein.
[b] "—"indicates that correlations or outcomes were not reported.
*Source*: Adapted from Ref. 32.

nificant correlation between MRP1 and achieving complete remission while results evaluating LRP expression are more evenly divided. Interestingly, deletion of the MRP1 gene in AML patients harboring the inv(16) karyotype was associated with a favorable impact on disease-free survival and overall survival (109), which could, in part, explain why patients with this karyotype respond well to therapy.

Additional retrospective and prospective studies are currently underway using multicolor flow cytometry to assess the expression of P-gp, MRP, and LRP,

**Table 5**  P-gp, MRP, and LRP Expression Patterns in Acute Myeloid Leukemia According to Age and Disease Stage

| | Frequency of AML (% of patients)[a] | | |
| --- | --- | --- | --- |
| | Patient age at diagnosis | | |
| Protein | ≤55 years (N = 349) | >55 years (N = 203) | Recurrent or relapsed (N = 93) |
| P-gp | 37% | 73% | 46% |
| MRP | 10% | 10% | 33% |
| LRP | 44% | 56% | 81% |

[a] For each patient, more than one of the listed proteins may be expressed.
N, number of patients in group.
*Source*: Adapted from Ref. 46.

as well as to assess the drug/dye efflux for patients with AML. Preliminary studies indicate that the expression patterns of P-gp, MRP, and LRP are quite different based upon age and disease stage (Table 5) (46). In younger de novo AML patients, P-gp expression is relatively infrequent (37%), LRP expression was observed in 44% of cases, and MRP expression was relatively rare (10%). Expression of P-gp, but not MRP or LRP, increased with age. Interestingly, while the frequency of P-gp expression did not change significantly at relapse, LRP and MRP expression increased; these studies suggest that the MRP and LRP phenotypes may emerge more frequently at relapse, which is consistent with other reports (49,84,87). MRP1 and LRP have been, however, infrequently associated with clinical outcome using immunodetection methods (Table 4) while P-gp expression was often correlated (Table 3). LRP expression, measured by flow cytometry, in de novo AML, was also of no prognostic significance (Table 4).

Expression patterns of P-gp, LRP, and MRP in individual patient samples may be highly complex (46). The most frequent phenotype observed in younger AML patients is the lack of expression of each of the three major MDR proteins (33% of cases). For cases that expressed these proteins, the most common phenotypes are represented by LRP alone (22%), expression of P-gp alone (17%), and coexpression of P-gp and LRP (15%). Within an individual patient, these proteins may be expressed on the same or different blast populations, indicating clonal heterogeneity (46).

## III.  REVERSAL OF MULTIDRUG RESISTANCE

Since the initial recognition of MDR1 as a mechanism of drug resistance with independent prognostic relevance, attempts have been made to impede P-gp func-

**Table 6**   First-Generation P-gp Modulators

| | |
|---|---|
| Calcium channel blockers | Antibiotics |
|   Verapamil |   Cefoperazone |
|   Nifedipine |   Ceftriazone |
|   Bepridil |   Erythromycin |
|   Nicardipine | Cyclosporines |
| Other cardiovascular drugs |   Cyclosporine A |
|   Amiodarone | Phenothiazines |
|   Dipyramidole |   Trifluoperazine |
|   Quinidine |   Fluphenazine |
| Antimalarials | Hormones |
|   Quinine |   Tamoxifen |
|   Quinacrine |   Toremifene |
|   Cinchonine |   Progesterone |

*Source*: Adapted from Ref. 10.

tion using competitive inhibitors of antineoplastic transport across the cell membrane. Such agents include calcium channel blockers, calmodulin inhibitors, immunosuppressive agents, quinolones, indole alkaloids, detergents, steroids, and antiestrogens (Table 6) (10,110–113); several of these reversal agents share common chemical features, including lipophilicity, a benzene ring, and neutral or cationic charge. In vitro studies indicate that combinations of different modulators, such as verapamil and CSA, may result in synergistic P-gp inhibition. This observation suggests that the precise drug-binding site within the transport channel varies among reversing agents. Indeed, verapamil, CSA, PSC 833, and other reversing agents increase the intracellular retention of daunorubicin in AML cells that overexpress P-gp, but not in P-gp-negative cells (52,113–116). This pharmacological effect is associated with increased in vitro anthracycline cytotoxicity in clonogenic assays (117–121).

Despite the importance of these observations, few definitive clinical trials have been performed with effective MDR modulators. Several phase II/III studies in solid tumors included verapamil, quinidine, or trifluoroperazine with doxorubicin or epirubicin. Unfortunately, these studies provided limited information since appropriate serum levels for modulation of MDR could not be achieved (122,123). Other studies of cytotoxins combined with modulators included verapamil plus vinblastine or etoposide (124); high-dose verapamil or R-verapamil plus chemotherapy; diltiazem plus vincristine, tamoxifen, and vinblastine; and nifedepine plus etoposide (125–131). These trials have shown that reversing MDR is feasible, although clinical efficacy in patients with refractory solid tumors was limited.

For optimal modulation, it is necessary to achieve a steady-state plasma concentration that is one or two times greater than the concentration needed in vitro to overcome MDR in assays approximating physiological protein concentrations. For many of these modulators with chemical activities, this concentration exceeds that necessary for producing other pharmacological actions. In addition, variances in bioavailability, protein binding, and pharmacokinetics lead to unpredictable plasma concentrations that may cause unacceptable toxicity or inadequate target inhibition. At present, CSA and the cyclosporine D analog PSC 833 have undergone the most extensive testing (132–136) and can be administered at doses sufficient to achieve effective serum levels. However, the cyclosporines also alter drug and bilirubin elimination via inhibition of alternate ABC transporters in biliary canaliculi and within the renal tubuli. As a consequence of these changes in elimination, the cyclosporines may increase toxicity of anticancer drugs administered at standard doses. In addition, CD34+ hematopoietic progenitor cells are potentially harmed by combinations of myelotoxic drugs and modulators since these cells express P-gp (137). Fortunately, severe myelosuppression with inhibition of P-gp has not occurred.

In 1988, the first report of clinical reversal of drug resistance in patients with hematological malignancies was published (131). A myeloma patient refractory to VAD (vincristine, doxorubicin, and dexamethasone) was treated with VAD plus verapamil, with restoration of response. Based upon this experience, a larger group of patients with multiple myeloma or non-Hodgkin's lymphoma was treated with high doses of verapamil in an attempt to achieve effective plasma concentrations (121,131). The high plasma concentrations of verapamil required for P-gp inhibition led to cardiac arrthythmias in the majority of patients. In a subsequent study of verapamil combined with VAD, cardiac monitoring showed that most patients experienced electrocardiographic irregularities. Despite these problems, approximately half of the patients from the later study achieved a response. Subsequent studies of CSA or PSC 833 as MDR reversal agents combined with VAD demonstrated encouraging results (134,135,138).

Other investigations of drug resistance reversal have been undertaken. A refractory AML patient, having failed standard induction treatment, achieved a short remission when treated with daunorubicin and cytarabine in combination with CSA (139). Subsequent to this study, several phase I and II trials were initiated in AML patients who were either refractory to primary treatment or had relapsed after a previous response (136,140). In one study, 20 refractory or relapse patients were treated with mitoxantrone and etoposide in combination with CSA (136). The dose of the cytostatic agents was not reduced and, consequently, the toxicity of this regimen was considerable, related primarily to severe marrow hypoplasia and mucositis. Although the toxicity was regarded as unacceptable, a number of positive responses including complete remissions were noted. In a dose escalation study of CSA, 42 patients with either refractory or relapsed AML or blast-crisis chronic myeloid leukemia received sequential treatment with infusional daunorubicin and high-dose cytarabine combined with CSA; the dose of

CSA was increased until plasma levels sufficient to inhibit P-gp were reached (93). The toxicity of this regimen, which consisted primarily of myelosuppression, nausea, and hyperbilirubinemia, correlated with CSA dosage. More importantly, sequential analysis of specimens demonstrated that, for patients who initially achieved a complete remission with CSA treatment, this regimen successfully eliminated clones expressing MDR1 at relapse.

Quinine was the first modulator to complete phase III testing in patients with AML and advanced MDS (141). In a French cooperative group study, patients were randomized to receive an induction regimen containing mitoxantrone and cytarabine with placebo or quinine. A total of 131 patients were enrolled and P-gp analysis was successful in 91 of these patients. In the 42 patients who expressed P-gp, 52% of those patients who received quinine achieved complete remission compared with 18% who did not receive the quinine ($p = 0.02$). In addition, median survival was also significantly improved in the quinine group (13 months vs. 8 months, $p = 0.01$) and the quinine was well tolerated. Owing to the significant improvement in rate of complete remission and median survival seen at the interim analysis, the study was terminated early.

The Medical Research Council (MRC) conducted one of two trials on the benefit of P-gp inhibition by CSA in patients with high-risk AML. CSA was added to standard- versus timed-sequential ADE (Ara-C, daunorubicin, and etoposide) induction in patients with relapsed or refractory AML (142). Most patients enrolled in this study, unfortunately, received a CSA dosage (5 mg/kg/day) inadequate for P-gp blockade. As a consequence, no demonstrable clinical benefit was seen.

In a second trial that was conducted by SWOG, patients received treatment with CSA at 16 mg/kg/day, yielding mean blood concentrations exceeding 1600 ng/ml, sufficient for modulation of P-gp-mediated resistance in a surrogate biological assay (143). Patients with relapsed, refractory, or secondary AML received sequential treatment with high-dose cytarabine followed by continuous-infusion daunorubicin over 72 hr. Daunorubicin was given either without or with CSA, also as a 72-hr continuous infusion. Responding patients received one course of consolidation therapy, which included the same components assigned for induction. Among 226 patients evaluable for induction outcome, treatment with CSA significantly reduced the incidence of resistant disease (47% vs. 31%; $p = 0.0077$) and yielded a trend favoring improvement in the rate of complete remission (33% vs. 40%; $p = 0.14$). There was no significant difference in the frequency of induction deaths (12%). Estimated 2-year relapse-free survival was 34% for CSA-treated patients compared with 9% for the control cohort ($p = 0.035$) (Fig. 2). In addition, treatment with CSA significantly improved median survival in patients with P-gp positive leukemia by threefold (12 months vs. 4 months) and yielded a significant improvement in overall survival (Fig. 3), such that the overall survival of the CSA-treated cohort was 22% as compared

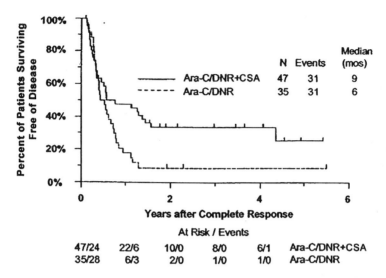

**Fig. 2** Kaplan-Meier estimate of relapse-free survival of patients achieving complete remission, according to assigned treatment. Tick marks indicate surviving patients in continuous complete remission. Ara-C, cytosine arabinoside; DNR, daunorubicin; CSA, cyclosporin A; N, number; mos, months. (From Ref. 116.)

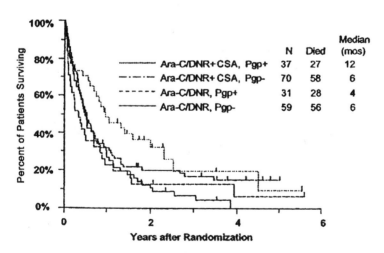

**Fig. 3** Kaplan-Meier estimate of overall survival by assigned treatment and permeability glycoprotein (P-gp) expression. Survival estimates include only patients evaluable for P-gp. Ara-C, cytosine arabinoside; DNR, daunorubicin; CSA, cyclosporine A; N, number; mos, months. (From Ref. 116.)

with 12% for the control cohort ($p = 0.046$). The administration of CSA delayed excretion of bilirubin and significantly increased steady-state blood concentrations of both daunorubicin and its metabolite daunorubicinol. Interestingly, the rate of complete remission increased and the frequency of resistance to induction therapy decreased with rising daunorubicin steady-state serum concentration in CSA-treated patients, whereas a similar relationship was not seen in the control group. An analogous impact on both relapse-free and overall survival was noted with CSA treatment, whereas survival inversely correlated with steady-state daunorubicin concentration in the control group. Thus, steady-state serum anthracycline concentration may be a critical determinant of treatment outcome when the anthracene is administered with an efflux modulator (such as CSA), whereas in the absence of the efflux modulator greater systemic daunorubicin exposure may only contribute to greater nonhematological toxicities.

Promising results of initial studies incorporating ''first-generation'' pharmacological inhibitors of P-gp (Table 6) fostered interest in the development of pharmacological modulators with greater potency and specificity (10). Among these ''second-generation'' inhibitors, PSC 833 has completed extensive testing in high-risk AML patients. PSC 833 is a cyclosporine D analog with 10-fold greater potency for P-gp inhibition than CSA. Although PSC 833 lacks intrinsic renal toxicity and immunosuppressive properties, both CSA and PSC 833 delay hepatic elimination of chemotherapeutics derived from natural products (134–136). Because of this pharmacokinetic interaction, considerable effort was invested during phase I testing to determine appropriate dosing of antineoplastic drugs in combination with PSC 833. For such targeted therapy to be successful, P-gp must be the dominant cellular resistance mechanism limiting the chemotherapeutic cytotoxicity and the modulated antineoplastic must display high P-gp binding affinity.

The development of more potent P-gp antagonists with greater target specificity held promise that such agents may yield more promising results with less toxicity. This was demonstrated in a trial in which infusional daunorubicin (34 mg/m$^2$ and 45 mg/m$^2$ daily) and cytarabine were combined with escalating dosages of PSC 833 (144). The results of this study demonstrated that PSC 833 (10 mg/kg/day) can be administered with conventional doses of infusional daunorubicin without increased nonhematological toxicity. Of equal importance, pharmacokinetic studies revealed that PSC 833 decreased daunorubicin elimination, thereby contributing to increased cytotoxin efficacy by increasing systemic exposure (two- to threefold) in two-thirds of the patients. Sequential analysis of *MDR1* gene expression in leukemia specimens from patients who had relapsed after study-induced remission demonstrated elimination of the *MDR1* gene message, suggesting effective modulation of P-gp-mediated MDR. Regardless of P-gp phenotype, LRP-positive cases had a lower probability of complete remission as compared with LRP-negative cases. LRP expression is an adverse biological feature that is not affected by P-gp antagonists.

Three additional feasibility studies were conducted to evaluate combinations of PSC 833 with conventional rapid infusion of chemotherapy during reinduction of poor-prognosis AML patients (145,146). These studies were designed as chemotherapy dose-escalation trials in combination with standard doses of PSC 833. Results indicate that rapid chemotherapy infusion is feasible, even in elderly patients, but requires 30–60% dose reduction in the targeted antineoplastic to accommodate elevations in peak ($C_{max}$) chemotherapy concentration and to minimize attendant toxicity.

Recently completed were four randomized trials evaluating the potential benefit of PSC 833 modulation of MDR in older patients with AML or in relapsed AML (Table 7) (146,147). Two of these trials, the Eastern Cooperative Oncology Group (ECOG) and the Cancer and Leukemia Group-B (CALGB) studies, were prematurely terminated owing to either lack of benefit or excessive toxicity in the PSC 833 treatment arm (146,147). In each of these studies, the targeted chemotherapy agents were administered by rapid infusion, necessitating dose reduction to accommodate mean changes in drug elimination. The other two trials, which are being conducted by the Dutch (P. Sonneveld, personal communication, 2000) and British [UK/(C301), 2000] study groups, are currently being evaluated, but preliminary results indicate that the principal end point of this study, i.e., an improvement in relapse-free survival, has not been reached.

There were several differences in study design between these four randomized trials with PSC 833 and the positive result with CSA modulation in the SWOG trial (143,146,147). These differences, besides the modulator used, include the sequential schedule of antineoplastic administration employed in the SWOG trial along with the 72-hr infusion of full-dose daunorubicin, and the administration of CSA during induction, and consolidation therapy. In contrast, the PSC 833 trials utilized rapid infusion of attenuated doses of the targeted antineoplastics, raising concerns that underdosing may have occurred in up to one-third of patients in whom a pharmacokinetic interaction was not anticipated. In addition, etoposide, which is a weak and inconsistent substrate for P-gp in cell-line models, was included in three of the PSC 833 studies (148,149). Preclinical investigations show that sensitization of MDR cells to anthracyclines or other xenobiotics by P-gp antagonists is both concentration- and time-dependent, and is optimized by prolonged concurrent exposure to the targeted antineoplastics (150). Extending the duration of daunorubicin infusion attenuates peak serum concentration ($C_{max}$) and limits anthracycline toxicity, permitting exploitation of a dose-response relationship with P-gp blockade. Therefore, both the schedule of antineoplastic drug administration and the selection of an antileukemia agent whose activity is limited by its affinity for P-gp may be important determinants of the success of modulator strategies in AML. (In addition, the possibility that

**Table 7** Phase III Trials for Investigation of PSC 833 in Acute Myeloid Leukemia

| Country/Institution and study code | No. of patients | Date of initiation | Criteria for eligibility | Treatment | End point | Outcome |
|---|---|---|---|---|---|---|
| USA/ECOG 2995 [146] | 127 | 1996 | Relapsed or refractory AML | MEC (induction and consolidation) | Complete remission | Premature closure due to efficacy |
| USA/CALGB 9720[147] | 126 | 1996 | ≥60 yrs | D-E-Ara-C (induction and consolidation) | Complete remission | Premature closure due to toxicity |
| Netherlands/HOVON MRC (C302) | 428 | 1995 | ≥60 yrs | DNR + Ara-C (induction) | Remission-free survival | Negative findings |
| UK/C301 | 256 | 1996 | Relapsed or refractory AML | MEC (induction) | Complete remission | Negative findings |

MEC, mitoxantrone and etoposide and cytarabine; D-E-Ara-C, daunorubicin and etoposide and cytarabine; DNR, daunorubicin.
*Source:* Adapted from Ref. 32.

CSA acts on a cellular target in addition to P-gp cannot be excluded when considering the results of these studies.) Results from the SWOG study have demonstrated that modulation of leukemia cell resistance should remain a therapeutic objective of future clinical studies (143).

Currently, other P-gp modulators are being evaluated. Some of these inhibitors, such as Vertex Pharmaceuticals' VX-710 and VX-853, inhibit both P-gp and MRP1 transport functions. The small molecule LY-335979 is a potent and selective inhibitor of P-gp that displays high binding affinity and does not alter anthracycline hepatic elimination. This agent has completed phase II testing and will enter phase III in AML within the ECOG.

Another approach to circumvention of MDR has included antisense oligonucleotides. These oligonucleotides are short sequences of DNA that form specific hydrogen bonds with complementary single-stranded mRNA sequences, allowing for regulation of specific gene expression (151). Motomura et al. evaluated the possibility of using antisense oligonucleotides against MDR1 mRNA to suppress overexpression of P-gp in AML blast cells and drug-resistant cell lines (152). In their analysis, incubation with these antisense oligonucleotides reduced the in vitro expression of P-gp in both AML blast cells and drug-resistant K562 cells. In addition, P-gp function of the treated blast cells was inhibited based upon the results of intracellular rhodamine and intracellular DNA studies. Importantly, the antisense-treated blast cells recovered their sensitivity to anthracyclines. These initial laboratory studies suggest that antisense oligonucleotides may merit clinical testing to overcome MDR in leukemia therapy.

At present, no other novel agents or approaches are available to overcome MRP-mediated resistance in AML as the few remaining modulators have significant adverse effects. Genistein is an effective reversal agent of MRP in vitro cell lines, but it cannot be safely administered to patients (153). The uricosuric probenecid may also reverse MRP1-mediated resistance in vitro, but it has the disadvantage of inhibiting platelet aggregation in patients who have thrombocytopenia and, therefore, would be difficult to administer in patients with hematological malignancies (154,155).

## IV. RESISTANCE TO Ara-C

Ara-C remains one of the most potent antileukemia drug available today and, combined with an anthracene, accounts for the principal components of remission-induction regimens for leukemia. Conventional induction regimens employ a relatively moderate dose of Ara-C, 100–200 mg/m$^2$, by continuous infusion for 7 days (156). However, dose escalation of Ara-C has been used successfully to overcome refractory disease in relapsing AML (1–3 g/m$^2$ every 12 hr daily for 3–5 days) and, more recently, higher dosages of Ara-C (1–3 g/m$^2$ every 12–

24 hr, once daily or every other day for 3–5 days) have been used during induction therapy and consolidation cycles (157–159). The CALGB has performed a randomized trial comparing varied doses of Ara-C during consolidation therapy in patients who had achieved a complete remission: results demonstrated significant survival and relapse-free survival advantages with high doses of Ara-C in younger (≤55 years) patients with selected good-risk cytogenetic abnormalities (160).

These prospective clinical trials have demonstrated that partial insensitivity to Ara-C may be overcome by saturating intracellular activation and degradation processes (161). Ara-C must be phosphorylated to Ara-CTP for incorporation into DNA, a reaction that is controlled by deoxycytidine kinase. This process may be negatively influenced by multiple factors, including a large pool of competing metabolites such as deoxycytidine, while catabolism occurs via the enzyme deoxycytidine deaminase. Similarly, despite saturating intracellular concentrations of cytarabine, rare mutations of the gene encoding deoxycytidine kinase may limit Ara-CTP generation and, therefore, cytotoxicity (162,163).

Because Ara-C has its greatest effect on rapidly dividing cells, stimulation of myeloblast division by administration of granulocyte colony-stimulating factor (G-CSF) or granulocyte-monocyte colony-stimulating factor (GM-CSF) may improve activity of Ara-C. Laboratory studies have shown that leukemia cell exposure to pharmacological doses of CSFs recruits dormant cells into cell cycle, allowing greater fractional kill by cytarabine. In an attempt to achieve a greater rate of complete remission in high-risk patients with AML, comparative clinical trials have been performed evaluating the role of administering either G-CSF or GM-CSF with induction therapy (Table 8) (164). In all studies except one, there were no adverse effects with the addition of either growth factor, although a clinical benefit was not observed. In the trial reported by Estey et al., administration of GM-CSF was associated with inferior survival but this was a dose escalation trial where patients were not uniformly treated (165).

## V. SUMMARY

AML and MDS represent clonal diseases, which are derived from transformation of an uncommitted stem cell. Drug resistance, which is essential for the survival of stem cells, is often seen in patients with these diagnoses and likely represents a conserved physiological function. Even though patients with AML and advanced MDS may present with disease sensitive to chemotherapy, the majority will relapse with more resistant disease.

Several different mechanisms of pharmacological drug resistance are recognized in these diseases. The most widely acknowledged mechanism involves expression of MDR1 that impacts the clinical efficacy of anthracyclines, epipodophyllotoxins, and amsacrine, which are often included as standard therapy for

**Table 8**  Controlled Trials of Growth Factors as Priming Therapy for Acute
Myeloid Leukemia

| Study | No. of patients | Cytokine/source and the comparative treatment | Day of growth factor infusion[a] | Leukemia stimulation |
|---|---|---|---|---|
| Buchner et al., 1997 | 75 | GM-CSF [yeast] vs. control | −2 | No |
| Rowe et al., 1998 | 245 | GM-CSF [yeast] vs. placebo | −2 | No |
| Ohno et al., 1994 | 58 | G-CSF vs. placebo | −2 | No |
| Estey et al., 1994 | 197 | G-CSF vs. control | −1 | Yes |
| Heil et al., 1995 | 80 | GM-CSF [*E. coli*] vs. placebo | −2 | No |
| Estey et al., 1992 | 232 | GM-CSF [*E. coli*] vs. control | −8 | No |
| Witz et al., 1998 | 229 | GM-CSF [*E. coli*] vs. placebo | +1 | No |
| Zittoun et al., 1996 | 51 | GM-CSF [*E. coli*] vs. control | −1 | No |
| Lowenberg et al., 1997 | 316 | GM-CSF [*E. coli*] vs. control | −1 | No |
| Peterson et al., 1996 | 174 | GM-CSF [*E. coli*] vs. placebo | −5 | No |
| Thomas et al., 1999 | 192 | GM-CSF [*E. coli*] vs. placebo | −2 | No |

[a] The day of growth factor infusion is relative to the day of chemotherapy completion (Day 0).
G-CSF, granulocyte colony-stimulating factor; GM-CSF, granulocyte monocyte colony-stimulating factor.
*Source*: Adapted from Ref. 172. This reference also lists the study publications cited in this table.

induction. Other mechanisms of multidrug resistance include MRP, LRP, and
BCRP, which are currently undergoing investigation as to their roles in myeloid
malignancies. Because of the importance of these mechanisms, the expression
and function of MDR, MRP, and LRP should be assessed in clinical trials. In
addition, approaches to reversing these mechanisms of resistance are just beginning to be evaluated and understood. Even though the results from initial trials
differ in their potential for improving patient outcome, continued evaluation and
experimentation to overcome these mechanisms of drug resistance will be critical
to improve overall survival for patients with AML or MDS.

## REFERENCES

1.  Goldstein LJ, Galski H, Fojo A, Willingham M, Lai SL, Gazdor A, Pirker R, Green
    A, Crist W, Brodeur GM, et al. Expression of a multidrug resistance gene in human
    cancers. J Natl Cancer Inst 1989; 81:116–124.
2.  Borst P. Genetic mechanisms of drug resistance. A review. Acta Oncol 1991; 30:
    87–105.
3.  Arceci RJ. Clinical significance of P-glycoprotein in multidrug resistance malig-
    nancies. Blood 1993; 81:2215–2222.

4. Sato H, Gottesmann MM, Goldstein LJ, Pastan I, Block AM, Sandberg AA, Preisler HD. Expression of the multidrug resistance gene in myeloid leukemias. Leuk
   Res 1990; 14:11–21.
5. Musto P, Melillo L, Lombardi G, Matera R, di Giorgio G, Carotenuto M. High
   risk of early resistant relapse for leukaemic patients with presence of multidrug
   resistance associated P-glycoprotein positive cells in complete remission. Br J
   Haematol 1991; 77:50–53.
6. Marie JP, Zittoun R, Sikic BI. Multidrug resistance (mdr1) gene expression in adult
   acute leukemias: correlations with treatment outcome and in vitro drug sensitivity.
   Blood 1991; 78:586–592.
7. Pirker R, Wallner J, Geissler K, Linkesch W, Haas OA, Bettelheim P, Hopfner M,
   Scherrer R, Valent P, Havelec L, et al. *MDR1* gene expression and treatment outcome in acute myeloid leukemia. J Natl Cancer Inst 1991; 83:708–712.
8. Campos L, Guyotat D, Archimbaud E, Calmard-Oriol P, Tsuruo T, Troncy J,
   Treille D, Fiere D. Clinical significance of multidrug resistance P-glycoprotein expression on acute nonlymphoblastic leukemia cells at diagnosis. Blood 1992; 79:
   473–476.
9. Biedler JL, Riehm H. Cellular resistance to actinomycin D in Chinese hamster cells
   in vitro: cross-resistance, radioautographic and cytogenetic studies. Cancer Res
   1970; 30:1174–1184.
10. Covelli A. Modulation of multidrug resistance (MDR) in hematological malignan-
    cies. Ann Oncol 1999; 10(suppl 6):53–59.
11. Kartner N, Riordan JR, Ling V. Cell surface P-glycoprotein associated with multi-
    drug resistance in mammalian cell lines. Science 1983; 221:1285–1288.
12. Hrycyna CA, Zhang S, Ramachandra M, et al. Functional and molecular character-
    ization of the human multidrug transporter. In: Gupta S, Tsuruo T, eds. Multidrug
    Resistance in Cancer Cells. Chichester, England: Wiley, 1996:29.
13. Germann UA. P-glycoprotein—a mediator of multidrug resistance in tumour cells.
    Eur J Cancer 1996; 32A:927–944.
14. Germann UA, Chambers TC, Ambudkar SV, Licht T, Cardarelli CO, Pastan I,
    Lottesman MM. Characterization of phosphorylation-defective mutants of hu-
    man P-glycoprotein expressed in mammalian cells. J Biol Chem 1996; 271:1708–
    1716.
15. Goodfellow HR, Sardini A, Ruetz S, Callaghan R, Gros P, McNaughton PA, Hig-
    gins CF. Protein kinase C-mediated phosphorylation does not regulate drug trans-
    port by the human multidrug resistance P-glycoprotein. J Biol Chem 1996; 271:
    13668–13674.
16. N-glycosylation and deletion mutants of the human MDR1 P-glycoprotein. J Biol
    Chem 1993; 268:7474–7481.
17. Sarkadi B. Fluorescent cellular indicators are extruded by the multidrug resistance
    protein. J Biol Chem 1993; 268:21493–21496.
18. Raviv Y, Pollard HB, Bruggeman EP, Pastan I, Gottesman MM. Photosensitized
    labeling of a functional multidrug transporter in living drug-resistant tumor cells.
    J Biol Chem 1990; 265:3975–3980.
19. Bolhuis H, van Veen HW, Molenaar D, Poolman B, Driessen AJM, Konings WN.
    Multidrug resistance in *Lactococcus lactis*: evidence for ATP-dependent drug ex-

trusion from the inner leaflet of the cytoplasmic membrane. EMBO J 1996; 15: 4239–4245.

20. Higgins CF, Gottesman MM. Is the multidrug transporter a flippase? Trends Biochem Sci 1992; 17:18–21.

21. Eytan GD, Regev R, Oren G, Assaraf YG. The role of passive transbilayer drug movement in multidrug resistance and its modulation. J Biol Chem 1996; 271: 12897–12902.

22. Smith AJ, de Vree JM, Ottenhoff R, Oude Elferink RP, Schinkel AH, Borst P. Hepatocyte-specific expression of the human MDR3 P-glycoprotein gene restores the biliary phosphatidylcholine excretion absent in Mdr2 ($-/-$) mice. Hepatology 1998; 28:530–536.

23. Pileri SA, Sabattini E, Falini B, Tazzari PL, Gherlinzoni F, Michieli MG, Damiani D, Zucchini L, Gobbi M, Tsuruo T, et al. Immunohistochemical detection of the multidrug transport protein P170 in human normal tissues and malignant lymphomas. Histopathology 1991; 19:131–140.

24. Nooter K, Herwijer H. Multidrug resistance (mdr) genes in human cancer. Br J Cancer 1991; 63:663–669.

25. Niehans GA, Jaszcz W, Brunetto V, Perri RT, Gajl-Peczalska K, Wick MR, Tsuruo T, Bloomfield CD. Immunohistochemical identification of P-glycoprotein in previously untreated, diffuse, large cell and immunoblastic lymphomas. Cancer Res 1992; 52:3768–3775.

26. Dalton WS, Grogan T, Rybski JA, Scheper RJ, Richter L, Kailey J, Broxterman HJ, Pinedo HM, Salmon SE. Immunohistochemical detection and quantitation of P-glycoprotein in multiple drug resistant human myeloma cells:association with level of drug resistance and drug accumulation. Blood 1989; 73:747–752.

27. Dan S, Esumi M, Sawada U, Hayashi N, Uchida T, Yamazaki T, Ashiya M, Satoh Y, Ohshim T, Horie T, et al. Expression of a multidrug resistance gene in human malignant lymphomas and related disorders. Leuk Res 1991; 15:1139–1143.

28. Rodriguez C, Commes T, Robert J, Rossi JF. Expression of P-glycoprotein and anionic glutathione S-transferase genes in non-Hodgkin's lymphoma. Leuk Res 1993; 17:149–156.

29. Yuen AR, Sikic BI. Multidrug resistance in lymphomas. J Clin Oncol 1994; 12: 2453–2459.

30. Fojo AT, Ueda K, Slamon DJ, Poplack DG, Gottesman MM, Pastan I. Expression of a multidrug-resistance gene in human tumors and tissues. Proc Natl Acad Sci USA 1987; 84:265–269.

31. Zhou DC, Marie JP, Suberville AM, Zittoun R. Relevance of mdr1 gene expression in acute myeloid leukemia and comparison of different diagnostic methods. Leukemia 1992; 6:879–885.

32. Sonneveld P, List AF. Chemotherapy resistance in acute myeloid leukemia. Baillieres Best Pract Res Clin Haematol 2001; 14:211–233.

33. te Boekhorst PAW, Leeuw K, Schoester M, et al. Predominance of functional multidrug resistance (MDR-1) phenotype in CD34+ leukemia cells. Blood 1993; 82: 3157–3162.

34. Ino T, Miyazaki H, Isogai M, Nomura T, Tsuzuki M, Tsuruo T, Ezaki K, Hirano M. Expression of P-glycoprotein in de novo acute myelogenous leukemia at initial

diagnosis; results of molecular and functional assays, and correlation with treatment outcome. Leukemia 1994; 8:1492–1497.

35. Lamy T, Goasguen JE, Mordelet E, Grulois I, Dauriac C, Drenou B, Chaperon J, Fauchet R, le Prise PY. P-glycoprotein (P-170) and CD34 expression in adult acute myeloid leukemia (AML). Leukemia 1994; 8:1879–1883.

36. Leith CP, Chen IM, Kopecky KJ, Appelbaum FR, Head DR, Godwin JE, Weick JK, Willman CL. Correlation of multidrug resistance (MDR1) protein expression with functional dye/drug efflux in acute myeloid leukemia by multiparameter flow cytometry: identification of discordant MDR−/fflux+ and MDR1+/efflux− cases. Blood 1995; 86:2329–2342.

37. Leith CP, Kopecky KJ, Chen IM, et al. MDR1 expression is highly predictive for achievement of complete remission (CR) in acute myeloid leukemia (AML) in the elderly:a Southwest Oncology Group study. Blood 1995 1; 86:286a (abstr).

38. te Boekhorst PA, Lowenberg B, van Kapel J, Nooter K, Sonneveld P. Multidrug resistant cells with high proliferative capacity determine response to therapy in acute myeloid leukemia. Leukemia 1995; 9:1025–1031.

39. Guerci A, Merlin JL, Missoum N, Feldmann L, Marchal S, Witz F, Rose C, Guerci O. Predictive value for treatment outcome in acute myeloid leukemia of cellular daunorubicin accumulation and P-glycoprotein expression simultaneously determined by flow cytometry. Blood 1995; 85:2147–2153.

40. van de Heuvel-Eibrink MM, van der Holt B, te Boekhorst PA, Pieters R, Schoester M, Lowenberg B, Sonneveld P. MDR 1 expression is an independent prognostic factor for response and survival in de novo acute myeloid leukemia. Br J Haematol 1997; 99:76–83.

41. Paietta E, Andersen J, Racevskis J, et al. Multidrug resistance gene (*mdr1*) transcript or CD34 antigen expression levels do not predict for complete remissions in de novo adult acute myeloid leukemia (AML): an Eastern Cooperative Oncology Group study. Blood 1994; 84:9771.

42. Klimecki WT, Futscher BW, Grogan TM, Dalton WS. P-glycoprotein expression and function in circulating blood cells from normal volunteers. Blood 1994; 83:2451–2458.

43. Chaudhary PM, Roninson IB. Expression and activity of P-glycoprotein, a multidrug efflux pump, in human hematopoietic stem cells. Cell 1994; 66:85 (abstr).

44. Leith CP, Kopecky KJ, Chen IM, et al. Development of a highly sensitive multiparameter flow cytometric assay correlating MDR1 expression and function; clinical application to acute myeloid leukemia. Adv Blood Disord 1997; 3:307–314.

45. Beck WT, Grogan TM, Willman CL, Cordon-Cardo C, Parham DM, Kuttesch JF, Andreeff M, Bates SE, Berard CW, Boyett JM, Brophy NA, Broxterman HJ, Chan HS, Dalton WS, Dietel M, Fojo AT, Gascoyne RD, Head D, Houghton PJ, Srivastava DK, Lehnert M, Leith CP, Paietta E, Pavelic ZP, Weinstein RI. Methods to detect P-glycoprotein-associated multidrug resistance in patients' tumors: consensus recommendations. Cancer Res 1996; 56:3010–3020.

46. Willman CL. The prognostic significance of the expression and function of multidrug resistance transporter proteins in acute myeloid leukemia: studies of the Southwest Oncology Group Leukemia Research Program. Semin Hematol 1997; 34(4 suppl 5):25–33.

47.  Burger H, Nooter K, Sonneveld P, Van Wingerden KE, Zaman GJ, Stoter G. High expression of the multidrug resistance-associated protein (MRP) in chronic and prolymphocytic leukaemia. Br J Haematol 1994; 88:348–356.
48.  Hart SM, Ganeshagru K, Hoffbrand AV, Prentice HG, Mehta AB. Expression of the multidrug resistance-associated protein (mrp) in acute leukemia. Leukemia 1999; 48:2163–2168.
49.  Schneider E, Cowan KH, Bader H, Toomey S, Schwartz GN, Karp JE, Burke PJ, Kaufmann SH. Increased expression of the multidrug resistance–associated protein gene in relapsed leukemia. Blood 1995; 85:186–193.
50.  Eijdems EW, Zaman GJ, de Haas M, Versantvoort CH, Flens MJ, Scheper RJ, Kamst E, Borst P, Baas F. Altered MRP is associated with multidrug resistance and reduced drug accumulation in human SW-1573 cells. Br J Cancer 1995; 72: 298–306.
51.  Muller M, Meijer C, Zaman GJ, Borst P, Scheper RJ, Mulder NH, de Vries EG, Jansen PL. Overexpression of the gene encoding the multidrug resistance–associated protein results in increased ATP-dependent glutathione S-conjugate transport. Proc Natl Acad Sci USA 1994; 91:13033–13037.
52.  Borst P, Evers R, Kool M, Wijnholds. A family of drug transporters: the multidrug resistance-associated proteins. J Natl Cancer Inst 2000; 92:1295–1302.
53.  Cui Y, Konig J, Buchholz JK, Spring H, Leier I, Keppler D. Drug resistance and ATP-dependent conjugate transport mediated by the apical multidrug resistance protein, MRP2, permanently expressed in human and canine cells. Mol Pharmacol 1999; 55:929–937.
54.  Ohga T, Koike K, Ono M, Makino Y, Itagaki Y, Tanimoto M, Kuwano M, Kohno K. Role of the human Y box-binding protein YB-1 in cellular sensitivity to the DNA-damaging agents cisplatin, mitomycin C, and ultraviolet light. Cancer Res 1996; 56:4224–4228.
55.  Versantvoort CH, Broxterman HJ, Bagrij T, Scheper RJ, Twentyman PR. Regulation by glutathione of drug transport in multi-drug resistant human lung tumor cell lines overexpressing multidrug resistance-associated protein. Br J Cancer 1995; 72:82–89.
56.  Hirohashi T, Suzuki H, Sugiyama Y. Characterization of the transport properties of cloned rat multidrug resistance-associated protein 3 (MRP3). J Biol Chem 1999; 274:15181–15185.
57.  Kool M, van Der Linden M, de Haas M, Scheffer GL, de Vree JM, Smith AJ, Jansen G, Peters GJ, Ponne N, Scheper RJ, Elferink RP, Baas F, Borst P. MRP3, an organic anion transporter able to transport anti-cancer drugs. Proc Natl Acad Sci USA 1999; 96:6914–6919.
58.  Ortiz DF, Li S, Iyer R, Zhang X, Novikoff P, Arias IM. MRP3, a new ATP-binding cassette protein localized to the canalicular domain of the hepatocyte. Am J Physiol 1999; 276:G1493–1500.
59.  Konig J, Rost D, Cui Y, Keppler D. Characterization of the human multidrug resistance protein isoform MRP3 localized to the basolateral hepatocyte membrane. Hepatology 1999; 29:1156–1163.
60.  Schuetz JD, Connelly MC, Sun D, Paibir SG, Flynn PM, Srinivas RV, Kumar A, Fridland A. MRP4: a previously unidentified factor in resistance to nucleoside-based antiviral drugs. Nat Med 1999; 5:1048–1051.

61. Wijnholds J, Mol CA, van Deemter L, de Haas M, Scheffer GL, Baas F, Beijnen JH, Scheper RJ, Hatse S, De Clercq E, Balzarini J, Borst P. Multidrug-resistance protein 5 is a multispecific organic anion transporter able to transport nucleotide analogs. Proc Natl Acad Sci USA 2000; 97:7476–7481.

62. Kool M, van der Linden M, de Haas M, Baas F, Borst P. Expression of human MRP6, a homologue of the multidrug resistance protein gene MRP1, in tissues and cancer cells. Cancer Res 1999; 59:175–182.

63. Slapak CA, Mizunuma N, Kufe DW. Expression of the multidrug resistance associated protein and P-glycoprotein in doxorubicin-selected human myeloid leukemia cells. Blood 1994; 84:3113–3121.

64. Schuurhuis GJ, Broxterman HJ, Ossenkoppele GJ, Baak JP, Eekman CA, Kuiper CM, Feller N, van Heijningen TH, Klumper E, Pieters R, et al. Functional multidrug resistance phenotype associated with combined overexpression of Pgp/ MDR1 and MRP together with 1-beta-D-arabinofuranosylcytosine sensitivity may predict clinical response in acute myeloid leukemia. Clin Cancer Res 1995; 1:81– 93.

65. Legrand O, Simonin G, Zittoun R, Maria JP. Comparison of MDR1, MRP and LRP expression with in vitro drug sensitivity in vivo response to treatment in fresh blast cells from adult acute myeloid leukemia patients. Blood 1997; 90:180a.

66. Van der Kolk DM, de Vries EG, Koning JA, van den Berg E, Müller M, Vellenga E. Activity and expression of the multidrug resistance proteins MRP1 and MRP2 in acute myeloid leukemia cells, tumor cell lines, and normal hematopoietic CD34+ peripheral blood cells. Clin Cancer Res 1998; 4:1727–1736.

67. Scheper RJ, Broxterman HJ, Scheffer GL, Kaaijk P, Dalton WS, van Heijningen TH, van Kalken CK, Slovak ML, de Vries EG, van der Valk P, et al. Overexpression of a M(r) 110,000 vesicular protein in non-P-glycoprotein mediated multidrug resistance. Cancer Res 1993; 53:1475–1479.

68. List AF, Spier CS, Abbaszadegan M, et al. Non-P-glycoprotein (Pgp) mediated multidrug resistance (MDR): identification of a novel drug resistance phenotype with prognostic relevance in acute myeloid leukemia. Blood 1993; 82:443a.

69. Scheffer GL, Wijngaard PL, Flens MJ, Izquierdo MA, Slovak ML, Pinedo HM, Meijer CJ, Clevers HC, Scheper RJ. The drug resistance-related protein LRP is the human major vault protein. Nat Med 1995; 1:578–582.

70. List AF, Spier CS, Grogan TM, Johnson C, Roe DJ, Greer JP, Wolff SN, Broxterman HJ, Scheffer GL, Scheper RJ, Dalton WS. Overexpression of the major vault transporter protein lung-resistance protein predicts treatment outcome in the acute myeloid leukemia. Blood 1996; 87:2464–2469.

71. Ross DD, Yang W, Abruzzo LV, et al. Atypical multidrug resistance: breast cancer resistance protein messenger RNA expression in mitoxantrone-selected cell lines. J Natl Cancer Inst 1999; 91:429.

72. Ross DD. Novel mechanisms of drug resistance in acute leukemia. Leukemia 2000; 14:467–473.

73. Ross DD, Doyle LA, Schiffer CA, Lee EJ, Grant CE, Cole SP, Deeley RG, Yang W, Tong Y. Expression of multidrug resistance-associated protein (MRP) mRNA transcripts in blast cells from acute myeloid leukemia (AML) patients. Leukemia 1996; 10:48–55.

74.  Ross DD, Karp JE, Chem TT, Doyle LA. Expression of breast cancer resistance protein in blast cells from patients with acute leukemia. Blood 2000; 96:365–368.

75.  Dorr R, Karanes C, Spier C, Grogan T, Greer J, Moore J, Weinberger B, Schiller G, Pearce T, Litchman M, Dalton W, Roe D, List AF. Phase I/II study of the P-glycoprotein modulator PSC 833 in patients with acute myeloid leukemia. J Clin Oncol 2001 19:1589–1599.

76.  Filipits M, Pohl G, Stranzl T, Suchomel RW, Scheper RJ, Jager U, Geissler K, Lechner K, Pirker R. Expression of the lung resistance protein predicts poor outcome in de novo acute myeloid leukemia. Blood 1998; 91:1508–1513.

77.  Minderman H, Vanhoefer U, Toth K, Yin MB, Minderman MD, Wrzosek C, Slovak ML, Rustum YM. DiOC2(3) is not a substrate for multidrug resistance protein (MRP)-mediated drug efflux. Cytometry 1996; 25:14–20.

78.  Zaman GJ, Lankelma J, van Tellingen O, Beijnen J, Dekker H, Paulusma C, Oude Elferink RP, Baas F, Borst P. Role of glutathione in the export of compounds from cells by the multidrug-resistance-associated protein. Proc Natl Acad Sci USA 1995; 92:7690–7694.

79.  Vanhoefer U, Cao S, Minderman H, Toth K, Skenderis BS 2nd, Slovak ML, Rustum YM. d,l-buthionine (S,R)-sulfoximine potentiates in vivo the therapeutic efficacy of doxorubicin against multidrug resistance protein expressing tumors. Clin Cancer Res 1996; 2:1961–1968.

80.  Kuwazuru Y, Hanada S, Furukawa T, Yoshimura A, Sumizawa T, Utsonomiya A, Ishibashi K, Saito T, Uozumi K, Maruyama M, et al. Expression of P-glycoprotein in adult T-cell leukemia cells. Blood 1990; 76:2065–2071.

81.  Marie JP, Bastie JN, Coloma F, Faussat Suberville AM, Delmer A, Rio B, Delmas-Marsalet B, Leroux G, Casassus P, Baumelou E, et al. Cyclosporin A as a modifier agent in the salvage treatment of acute leukemia (AL). Leukemia 1993; 7:821–824.

82.  Wood P, Burgess R, MacGregor A, Liu Yin JA. P-glycoprotein expression on acute myeloid leukemia blast cells at diagnosis predicts response to chemotherapy and survival. Br J Haematol 1994; 87:509–514.

83.  Hart, SM, Ganeshaguru K, Hoffbrand AV, Prentic HG, Mehta AB. Expression of the multidrug resistance-associated protein (MRP) in acute leukaemia. Leukemia 1994; 8:2163–2168.

84.  Zochbauer S, Gsur A, Bruner R, Kyrle PA, Lechner K, Pirker R. P-glycoprotein expression as a favorable prognostic factor in acute myeloid leukemia. Leukemia 1994; 8:974–977.

85.  Del Poeta G, Stasi R, Aronica G, Venditti A, Cox MC, Bruno A, Buccisano F, Masi M, Tribalto M, Amadori S, Papa G. Clinical relevance of P-glycoprotein expression in de novo acute myeloid leukemia. Blood 1996; 87:1997–2004.

86.  Stevers EL, Smith FO, Woods WG, Lee JW, Bleyer WA, Willman CL, Bernstein ID. Cell surface expression of the multidrug resistance P-glycoprotein (P-170) as detected by monoclonal antibody MRK-16 in pediatric acute myeloid leukemia fails to define a poor prognostic group: a report from the Childrens Cancer Group. Leukemia 1995; 9:2042–2048.

87.  Zhou DC, Zittoun R, Marie JP. Expression of multidrug resistance–associated pro-

tein (MRP) and multidrug resistance genes (*MDR1*) in acute myeloid leukemia. Leukemia 1995; 9:1661–1666.

88. Del Poeta G, Stasi R, Vendetti A, Suppo G, Aronica G, Bruno A, Masi M, Tabilio A, Papa G. Prognostic value of cell marker analysis in de novo acute myeloid leukemia. Leukemia 1994; 8:388–394.

89. Nussler V, Pelka-Fleischer R, Zwierzina H, Nerl C, Beckert B, Gullis E, Giesler F, Bock S, Bartl R, Petrides PE, et al. Clinical importance of P-glycoprotein–related resistance in leukemia and myelodysplastic syndromes—first experience with their reversal. Ann Hematol 1994; 69(suppl 1):S25–S29.

90. List AF, Karfanes C, Dorr R, et al. Modulation of anthracycline resistance in poor-risk acute myeloid leukemia (AML) with SDZ PSC 833: results of a phase I/II multicenter study. Blood 1996; 88:29a.

91. Samdani A, Vijapurkar U, Grimm MA, Spier CS, Grogan TM, Glinsmann-Gibson BJ, List AF. Cytogenetics and P-glycoprotein (PGP) are independent predictors of treatment outcome in acute myeloid leukemia (AML). Leukemia Res 1996; 20: 175–180.

92. Goasguen JE, Lamy T, Bergeron C, Ly Sunaram B, Mordelet E, Gorre G, Dossot JM, Le Gall E, Grosbois B, Le Prise PY, Fauchet R. Multifactorial drug resistance phenomenon in acute leukemias: impact of P170-MDR1, LRP56 protein, glutathi-one-transferases and metallothionein systems on clinical outcome. Leuk Lymphoma 1996; 23:567–576.

93. Hunault M, Zhou D, Delmer A, Ramond S, Viguie F, Cadiou M, Perrot JY, Levy V, Rio B, Cymbalista F, Zittoun R, Marie JP. Multidrug resistance gene expression in acute myeloid leukemia: major prognosis significance for in vivo drug resistance to induction chemotherapy. Ann Hematol 1997; 74:65–71.

94. Del Poeta G, Venditta A, Aronica G, Stasi R, Cox MC, Buccisano F, Bruno A, Tamburini A, Suppo G, Simone MD, Epicino AM, Del Moro B, Masi M, Papa G, Amadori S. P-glycoprotein expression in de novo acute myeloid leukemia. Leuk Lymphoma 1997; 27:257–274.

95. Martinez A, San Miguel JF, Valverde B, Barez A, Moro MJ, Garcia-Marcos MA, Perez-Simon JA, Vidriales B, Orfao A. Functional expression of MDR-1 in acute myeloid leukemia: correlation with the clinical-biological, immunophenotypical and prognostic disease characteristics. Ann Hematol 1997; 75:81–86.

96. Filipits M, Suchomel RW, Zochbauer M, Brunner R, Lechner K, Pirker R. Multi-drug resistance-associated protein in acute myeloid leukemia: no impact on treat-ment outcome. Clin Cancer Res 1997; 3:1419–1425.

97. Lohri A, van Hille B, Bacchi M, Fopp M, Joncourt F, Reuter J, Cerny T, Fey MF, Herrmann R. Five putative drug resistance parameters (MDR1/P-glycoprotein, MDR-associated protein, gluthathione-S-transferase, bcl-2 and topoisomerase IIalpha) in 57 newly diagnosed acute myeloid leukemias. Swiss Group for Clinical Cancer Research (SAKK). Eur J Haematol 1997; 59:206–215.

98. Legrand O, Simonin G, Perrot JY, et al. Pgp and MRP activities using calcein-AM are prognostic factors in adult acute myeloid leukemia patients. Blood 1998; 91:4480–4488.

99. Borg AG, Burgess R, Green LM, Scheper RJ, Liu Yin JA. Overexpression of lung-resistance protein and increased P-glycoprotein function in acute myeloid leukemia

cells predict a poor response to chemotherapy and reduced patient survival. Br J Haematol 1998; 103:1083–1091.

100. Kasimir-Bauer S, Ottinger H, Meusers P, Beelen G, Seeber S, Scheulen ME, et al. In acute myeloid leukemia, co-expression of at least two proteins, including P-glycoprotein, the multidrug resistance-related protein, bcl-2, mutant p53 and the heat-shock protein 27, is predictive of the response to induction chemotherapy. Exp Hematol 1998; 26:1111–1117.

101. Senent L, Jarque I, Martin G, Sempere A, Gonzalez-Garcia Y, Gomis F, Perez-Sirvent M, De La Rubia J, Sanz MA. P-glycoprotein expression and prognostic value in acute myeloid leukemia. Haematologica 1998; 83:783–787.

102. Pallis M, Turzanski J, Harrison G, Wheatley K, Langabeer S, Burnett AK, Russell NH. Use of standardized flow cytometric determinants of multidrug resistance to analyse response to remission induction chemotherapy in patients with acute myeloblastic leukaemia. Br J Haematol 1999; 104:307–312.

103. Michieli M, Damiani D, Ermacora A, Masolini P, Raspadori D, Visani G, Scheper RJ, Baccarani M. P-glycoprotein, lung resistance-related protein and multidrug resistance associated protein in de novo acute nonlymphocytic leukaemias: biological and clinical implications. Br J Haematol 1999; 104:328–335.

104. List AF, Spier CM, Cline A, Doll DC, Garewal H, Morgan R, Sandberg AA. Expression of the multidrug resistance gene product (P-glycoprotein) in myelodysplasia is associated with a stem cell phenotype. Br J Haematol 1991; 78:28–34.

105. Poulain S, Lepelley P, Preudhomme C, Cambier N, Cornillon J, Wattel E, Cosson A, Fenaux P. Expression of the multidrug resistance-associated protein in myelodysplastic syndromes. Br J Haematol 2000; 110:591–598.

106. Hart SM, Ganeshaguru K, Scheper RJ, Prentice HG, Hoffbrand AV, Mehta AB. Expression of the human major vault protein LRP in acute myeloid leukemia. Exp Hematol 1997; 25:1227–1232.

106a. Legrand O, Zittoun R, Marie JP. Role of MRP 1 in multidrug resistance in acute myeloid leukemia. Leukemia 1999; 13:578–584.

107. Pirker R, Pohl G, Stranzl T, et al. Expression of the lung resistance protein (LRP) predicts poor outcome in de novo acute myeloid leukemia. Blood 1997; 90:2519a.

108. Legrand O, Simonin G, Zittoun R, Marie JP. Lung resistance protein (LRP) gene expression in adult acute myeloid leukemia: a critical evaluation by three techniques. Leukemia 1998; 12:1367–1374.

109. Kuss BJ, Deeley RG, Cole SP, Willman CL, Kopecky KJ, Wolman SR, Eyre HJ, Lane SA, Nancarrow JK, Whitmore SA, et al. Deletion of gene for multidrug resistance in acute myeloid leukaemia with inversion in chromosome 16: prognostic implications. Lancet 1994; 343:1531–1534.

110. Lehnert M, Dalton WS, Roe D, Emerson S, Salmon SE. Synergistic inhibition by verapamil and quinine of P-glycoprotein-mediated multidrug resistance in a human myeloma cell line model. Blood 1991; 77:348–354.

111. Tsuruo T, Iida H, Tsukagoshi S, Sakurai Y. Potentiation of vincristine and adriamycin effects in human hemopoietic tumor cell lines by calcium channel antagonists and calmodulin inhibitors. Cancer Res 1983; 43:2267–2272.

112. Tsuruo T, Iida H, Kitatani Y, Yokota K, Tsukagoshi S, Sakurai Y. Effects of quini-

dine and related compounds on cytotoxicity and cellular accumulation of vincristine and adriamycin in drug-resistant tumor cells. Cancer Res 1984; 44:4303–4307.

113.  Berman E, McBride M. Comparative cellular pharmacology of daunorubicin and
      indarubicin in human multidrug-resistant leukemia cells. Blood 1992; 79:3267–
      3273.

114.  Nooter K, Sonneveld P, Oostrum R, Herwijer H, Hagenbeek T, Valerio D. Overex-
      pression of the mdr1 gene in blast cells from patients with acute myelocytic leuke-
      mia is associated with decreased anthracycline accumulation that can be restored
      by cyclosporin-A. Int J Cancer 1990; 45:263–268.

115.  Ross DD, Wooten PJ, Tong Y, Cornblatt B, Levy C, Sridhara R, Lee EJ, Schiffer
      CA. Synergistic reversal of multidrug-resistance phenotype in acute myeloid leuke-
      mia cells by cyclosporin A and cremjaphor EL. Blood 1994; 83:1337–1347.

116.  List AF, Kopecky KJ, Willman CL, Head DR, Persons DL, Slovak ML, Dorr R,
      Karanes C, Hynes HE, Dorosho JH, Shurafa M, Appelbaum FR. Benefit of
      cyclosporine modulation of drug resistance in patients with poor-risk acute myeloid
      leukemia: a Southwest Oncology Group study. Blood 2001; 98:3212–3220.

117.  Ross DD, Wooten PJ, Sridhara R, Ordónez JV, Lee EJ, Schiffer CA. Enhancement
      of daunorubicin accumulation, retention, and cytoxicity by verapamil or cyclospo-
      rin A in blast cells from patients with previously untreated acute myeloid leukemia.
      Blood 1993; 82:1288–1299.

118.  Solary E, Bidan JM, Calvo F, Chauffert B, Caillot D, Mugneret F, Gauville C,
      Tsuruo T, Carli PM, Guy H. P-glycoprotein expression and in vitro reversion of
      doxorubicin resistance by verapamil in clinical specimens from acute leukemia and
      myeloma. Leukemia 1991; 5:592–597.

119.  Marie JP, Helou C, Thevenin D, Delmer A, Zittoun R. In vitro effect of P-glycopro-
      tein (P-gp) modulators on drug sensitivity of leukemic progenitors (CFU-L) in
      acute myelogenous leukemia (AML). Exp Hematol 1992; 20:565–568.

120.  Visani G, Fogli M, Tosi P, Ottaviani E, Gamberi B, Cenacchi A, Manfroi S, Tura S.
      Comparative effects of racemic verapamil vs R-verapamil on normal and leukemic
      progenitors. Ann Hematol 1993; 66:273–276.

121.  Miller TP, Grogan TM, Dalton WS, Spier CM, Scheper RJ, Salmon SE. P-glyco-
      protein expression in malignant lymphoma and reversal of clinical drug resistance
      with chemotherapy plus high-dose verapamil. J Clin Oncol 1991; 9:17–24.

122.  Ozols RF, Cunnion RE, Klecker RW Jr, Hamilton TC, Ostchega Y, Parrillo JE,
      Young RC. Verapamil and adriamycin in the treatment of drug-resistant ovarian
      cancer patients. J Clin Oncol 1987; 5:641–647.

123.  Jones RD, Kerr DJ, Harnett AN, Rankin EM, Ray S, Kaye SB. A pilot study of
      quinidine and epirubicin in the treatment of advanced breast cancer. Br J Cancer
      1990; 62:133–135.

124.  Cairo MS, Siegel S, Anas N, Sender L. Clinical trial of continuous infusion vera-
      pamil, bolus vinblastine, and continuous infusion VP-16 in drug-resistant pediatric
      tumors. Cancer Res 1989; 49:1063–1066.

125.  Trump DL, Smith DC, Ellis PG, Rogers MP, Schold SC, Winer EP, Panella TJ,
      Jordon VC, Fine RL. High-dose oral tamoxifen, a potential multidrug-resistance-
      reversal agent: phase I trial in combination with vinblastine. J Natl Cancer Inst
      1992; 84:1811–1816.

126. Berg SL, Tolcher A, O'Shaughnessy JA, Denicoff AM, Noone M, Ognibene FP, Cowan KH, Balis FM. Effect of R-verapamil on the pharmacokinetics of paclitaxel in women with breast cancer. J Clin Oncol 1995; 13:2039–2042.

127. Motzer RJ, Lyn P, Fischer P, Lianes P, Ngo RL, Cordon-Cardo C, O'Brien JP. Phase I/II trial of dexverapamil plus vinblastine for patients with advanced renal cell carcinoma. J Clin Oncol 1995; 13:1958–1965.

128. Tolcher AW, Cowan KH, Solomon D, Ognibene F, Goldspiel B, Chang R, Noone MH, Denicoff AM, Barnes CS, Gossard MR, Fetsch PA, Berg SL, Balis FM, Venzon DJ, O'Shaughnessy JA. Phase I crossover study of paclitaxel with R-verapamil in patients with metastatic breast cancer. J Clin Oncol 1996; 14:1173–1184.

129. Mickisch GH, Noordizij MA, van der Gaast A, Gebreamlack P, Kohrmann KU, Mogler-Drautz E, Kupper H, Schroder FH. Dexverapamil to modulate vinblastine resistance in metastatic renal cell carcinoma. J Cancer Res Clin Oncol 1995; 121(suppl 3):R11–16.

130. Linn SC, van Kalken CK, van Tellingen O, van der Valk P, van Groeningen CJ, Kuiper CM Pinedo HM, Giaccone G. Clinical and pharmacologic study of multidrug resistance reversal with vinblastine and bepridil. J Clin Oncol 1994; 12:812–819.

131. Durie BG, Dalton WS. Reversal of drug-resistance in multiple myeloma with verapamil. Br J Haematol 1988; 68:203–206.

132. Sonneveld P, Durie BG, Lokhorst HM, Marie JP, Solbu G, Suciu S, Zittoun R, Lowenberg B, Nooter K. Modulation of multidrug-resistant multiple myeloma by cyclosporin. The Leukaemia Group of the EORTC and the HOVON. Lancet 1992; 340:255–259.

133. Lum BL, Kaubisch S, Yahanda AM, Adler KM, Jew L, Ehsan MN, Brophy NA, Halsey J, Gosland MP, Sikic BI. Alteration of etoposide pharmacokinetics and pharmacodynamics by cyclosporine in a phase I trial to modulate multidrug resistance. J Clin Oncol 1992; 10:1635–1642.

134. Sonneveld P, Marie JP, Huisman C, Vekhoff A, Schoester M, Faussat AM, van Kapel J, Groenewegen A, Charnick S, Zittoun R, Lowenberg B. Reversal of multidrug resistance by SDZ PSC 833, combined with VAD (vincristine, doxorubicin, dexamethasone) in refractory multiple myeloma. A phase I study. Leukemia 1996; 10:1741–1750.

135. Sonneveld P, Suciu S, Weijermans P et al. Cyclosporine A combined with VAD vs. VAD in patients with refractory multiple myeloma: an EORTC/HOVON randomized phase II study. Blood 1997; 90:356a.

136. Kornblau SM, Estey E, Madden T, Tran HT, Zhao S, Consoli U, Snell V, Sanchez-Williams G, Kantarjian H, Keating M, Newman RA, Andreeff M. Phase I study of mitoxantrone plus etoposide with multidrug blockade by SDZ PSC-833 in relapsed or refractory acute myelogenous leukemia. J Clin Oncol 1997; 15:1796–1802.

137. Drach D, Zhao S, Drach J, Mahadevia R, Gattringer C, Huber H, Andreeff M. Subpopulations of normal peripheral blood and bone marrow cells express a functional multidrug resistant phenotype. Blood 1992; 80:2729–2734.

138. Dalton WS, Grogan TM, Meltzer PS, Scheper RJ, Durie BG, Taylor CW, Miller TP, Salmon SE. Drug-resistance in multiple myeloma and non-Hodgkin's lymphoma: detection of P-glycoprotein and potential circumvention by addition of verapamil to chemotherapy. J Clin Oncol 1989; 7:415–424.

139. Sonneveld P, Nooter K. Reversal of drug-resistance by cyclosporin-A in a patient with acute myelocytic leukaemia. Br J Haematol 1990; 75:208–211.

140. Marie JP, Faussat-Suberville AM, Zhou D, Zittoun R. Daunorubicin uptake by leukemic cells: correlations with treatment outcome and mdr1 expression. Leukemia 1993; 7:825–831.

141. Wattel E, Solary E, Hecquet B, Caillot D, Ifrah N, Brion A, Mahe B, Milpied N, Janvier M, Guerci A, Rochant H, Cordonnier C, Dreyfus F, Buzyn A, Hoang-Ngoc L, Stoppa AM, Gratecos N, Sadoun A, Stamatoulas A, Tilly H, Brice P, Maloisel F, Lioure B, Desablens B, Fenaux P, et al. Quinine improves the results of intensive chemotherapy in myelodysplastic syndromes expression P glycoprotein: results of a randomized study. Br J Haematol 1998; 102:1015–1024.

142. Liu Tin JA, Wheatley K, Rees J, Burnett A. Comparison of two chemotherapy regimens with or without cyclosporine-A in relapsed/refractory acute myeloid leukemia: results of the U.K. Medical Research Council AML-R trial. Blood 1998; (suppl 1):231a.

143. List AF, Kopecky KJ, Willman CL, et al. Benefit of cyclosporine modulation of drug resistance in patients with poor-risk acute myeloid leukemia: a Southwest Oncology Group Study. Blood. In press.

144. Advani R, Saba HI, Tallman M, et al. Treatment of poor prognosis AML with PSC833 plus mitoxantrone, etoposide, cytarabine. Blood 1997; 90:356a.

145. Visani G, Milligan D, Leoni F, et al. A phase I dose-finding study of PSC 833, a novel MDR reversing agent, with mitoxantrone, etoposide and cytarabine in poor prognosis acute leukemia. Blood 1997; 90:356b.

146. Greenberg P, Avandi R, Tallman M, et al. Treatment for refractory/relapsed AML with PSC833 plus mitoxantrone, etoposide, cytarabine (PSC-MEC) vs. MEC: randomized phase II trial (E2995). Blood 1999; (suppl 1):383a.

147. Lee EJ, George SL, Caligiuri M, Szatrowski TP, Powell BL, Lemke S, Dodge RK. Smith R, Baer M, Schiffer CA. Parallel phase I studies of daunorubicin given with cytarabine and etoposide with or without the multidrug resistance modulator PSC-833 in previously untreated patients 60 years of age or older with acute myeloid leukemia: results of Cancer and Leukemia Group B study 9420. J Clin Oncol 1999; 17:2831–2839.

148. Politi PM, Arnold ST, Felsted RL, Sinha BK. P-glycoprotein-independent mechanism of resistance to VP-16 in multidrug-resistant tumor cell lines: pharmacokinetic and photoaffinity labeling studies. Mol Pharmacol 1990; 37:790–796.

149. Sehested M, Friche E, Jensen PB, Demant EJ. Relationship of VP-16 to the classical multidrug resistance phenotype. Cancer Res 1992; 52:2874–2879.

150. Cass CE, Janowska-Wieczorek A, Lynch MA, Sheinin H, Hindenburg AA, Beck WT. Effect of duration of exposure to verapamil on vincristine activity against multidrug-resistant human leukemic cell lines. Cancer Res 1989; 49:5798–5804.

151. Stein CA, Cheng YC. Antisense oligonucleotides as therapeutic agents—is the bullet really magical? Science 1993; 261:1004–1012.

152. Motomura S, Motoji T, Takanashi M, Wang YH, Shiozaki H, Sugawara I, Aikawa E, Tomida A, Tsuruo T, Kanda N, Mizoguchi H. Inhibition of P-glycoprotein and recovery of drug sensitivity of human acute leukemic blast cells by multidrug resistance gene (*mdr1*) antisense oligonucleotides. Blood 1998; 91:3163–3171.

153. Berger W, Elbling L, Hauptmann E, Micksche M. Expression of the multidrug resistance-associated protein (MRP) and chemoresistance of human non-small-cell lung cancer cells. Int J Cancer 1997; 73:84–93.

154. Packham MA, Rand ML, Perry DW, Ruben DH, Kinlough-Rathbone RL. Probenicid inhibits platelet responses to aggregating agents in vitro and has synergistic inhibitory effect with penicillin G. Thromb Haemost 1996; 76:239–244.

155. Weisman SM, Felsen D, Vaughan ED Jr. Indications and contraindications for the use of nonsteroidal antiinflammatory drugs in urology. Semin Urol 1985; 3:301–310.

156. Löwenberg B, Downing JR, Burnett A. Acute myeloid leukemia. Engl J Med 1999; 341:1051–1062.

157. Stone RM, Spriggs DR, Dhawan RK, Arthur KA, Mayer RJ, Kufe DW. A phase I study of intermittent continuous infusion high dose cytosine arabinoside for acute leukemia. Leukemia 1990; 4:843–847.

158. Bishop JF, Matthews JP, Young GA, Szer J, Gillett A, Joshua D, Bradstock K, Enno A, Wolf MM, Fox R, et al. A randomized study of high-dose cytarabine in induction in acute myeloid leukemia. Blood 1996; 87:1710–1717.

159. Geller RB, Burke PJ, Karp JE, Humphrey RL, Braine HG, Tucker RW, Fox MG, Zahurak M, Morrell L, Hall KL, et al. A two-step timed sequential treatment for acute myelocytic leukemia. Blood 1989; 74:1499–1506.

160. Mayer RJ, Davis RB, Schiffer CA, Berg DT, Powell BL, Schulman P, Omura GA, Moore JO, McIntyre OR, Frei E 3rd. Intensive postremission chemotherapy in adults with acute myeloid leukemia. Cancer and Leukemia Group B. N Engl J Med 1994; 331:896–903.

161. Grant S. Ara-C: Cellular and molecular pharmacology. Adv Cancer Res 1998; 72:197–233.

162. Stegmann AP, Honders MW, Hagemeijer A, Hoebee B, Willemze R, Landegent JE. In vitro-induced resistance to the deoxycytidine analogues cytarabine (AraC) and 5-aza-2′-deoxycytidine (DAC) in a rat model for acute myeloid leukemia is mediated by mutations in the deoxycytidine kinase (*dck*) gene. Ann Hematol 1995; 71:41–47.

163. Stegmann AP, Honders MW, Willemze R, Landegent JE. De novo induced mutations in the deoxycytidine kinase (*dck*) gene in rat leukemic clonal cell lines confer resistance to cytarabine (AraC) and 5-aza-2′-deoxycytidine (DAC). Leukemia 1995; 9:1032–1038.

164. Rowe JM. Concurrent use of growth factors and chemotherapy in acute leukemia (review). Curr Opin Hematol 2000; 7:197–202.

165. Estey E, Thall PF, Kantarjian H, O'Brien S, Koller CA, Beran M, Gutterman J, Deisseroth A, Keating M. Treatment of newly diagnosed acute myelogenous leukemia with granulocyte-macrophage colony-stimulating factor (GM-CSF) before and during continuous-infusion high-dose ara-C + daunorubicin: comparison to patients treated without CM-CSF. Blood 1992; 79:2246–2255.

# 12
# Myelodysplastic Syndrome and Juvenile Myelomonocytic Leukemia in Children

**Henrik Hasle**
*Skejby Hospital and Aarhus University, Aarhus, Denmark*

**Charlotte Niemeyer**
*Universitats-Kinderklinik, Freiburg, Germany*

## I. INTRODUCTION

Myelodysplastic syndrome (MDS) and juvenile myelomonocytic leukemia (JMML) in children have attained increasing attention in recent years. With this attention, it has become evident that there are significant differences between MDS in children and adults (Table 1). MDS and JMML are very rare in children, with a combined annual incidence of 3.6/million (1,2), the incidence being highest in infants. In contrast with that of children, the incidence in adults is greater and increases with age, with the incidence estimated between 35 and 120 per million per year (3). Refractory anemia with ringed sideroblasts, which constitutes 25% of the adult cases of MDS (4), is also extremely rare in children (5,6). Monosomy 7 is by far the most common cytogenetic abnormality in children whereas 5q-, observed frequently in adults, is very rare in children (7). Associated abnormalities occur much more often in children (in up to one-third) than in adults. Finally, the therapeutic possibilities are limited in adults and the therapy often has a palliative perspective whereas the aim in all children with MDS is cure.

**Table 1**  Differences Between Myelodysplastic Diseases in Children and Adults

| Parameter | Children | Adults |
|---|---|---|
| Incidence/million | 3.6 | >35 |
| Refractory anemia with ringed sideroblasts | <2% | 25% |
| Cytogenetic aberrations | 60% | 40% |
| −7/7q- | 30% | 10% |
| −5/5q- | 1–2% | 20% |
| Associated abnormalities | 30% | <5% |
| General aim of treatment | Curative | Palliative |

*Source*: Data from Ref. 1–7.

## A.  Historical Background of the Classification of Childhood MDS

The classification of childhood MDS has been inconsistent and confusing. Official guidelines have been lacking and even the most recent recommendations for the classification of childhood cancer do not mention MDS (8). This lack of a widespread accepted classification may have contributed to underdiagnosing MDS in children. Despite underdiagnosis, MDS and JMML remain uncommon in children, each disease constituting less than 5% of the hematological malignancies (Table 2). The rarity of MDS and the heterogeneous nature of the disease have further contributed to the difficulties in classifying childhood MDS.

A myriad of terms have been used over the last decades to designate MDS, reflecting the conceptual and diagnostic difficulties of the disorders. A case of presumably refractory anemia or refractory anemia with excess blasts was described as monocytic leukemia in the 1930s (9). One case that retrospectively may be classified as refractory anemia was described in 1958 as chronic monocytic leukemia (10). Most cases, however, were classified as acute myeloid leukemia (AML), despite a low number of blasts (11). The term "preleukemia" was introduced in pediatrics in the early 1970s (12–15) but the number of reported cases of childhood preleukemia remained extremely sparse; only 11 cases were identified in a review published in 1980 (16).

MDS in children has previously been lumped together with cases of transient pancytopenia preceding acute lymphocytic leukemia (pre-ALL) and collectively these were described as preleukemic states (17–19). However, these two conditions are distinct and should not be confused (20).

The French-American-British (FAB) group proposed in 1982 a classification scheme for MDS (21,22). This scheme was based upon a review of bone marrow smears from adults and was comprised of five subgroups: refractory anemia (RA), RA with ringed sideroblasts (RARS), RA with excess blasts (RAEB), RAEB in transformation (RAEB-t), and chronic myelomonocytic leukemia

**Table 2**  Incidence of Hematological Malignancies in Children 0–14 Years of Age: Combined Data from Denmark (1980–1991) and British Columbia (1982–1996)

| Disease type | Number of cases | Frequency (% of total) | Annual incidence per million children |
|---|---|---|---|
| ALL | 815 | 79 | 38.5 |
| AML[a] | 115 | 11 | 5.4 |
| MDS[a] | 38 | 4 | 1.8 |
| Myeloid leukemia of DS | 19 | 2 | 0.9 |
| JMML | 25 | 2 | 1.2 |
| CML | 13 | 1 | 0.6 |
| PV/ET | 3 | 0 | 0.1 |
| Unclassified | 3 | 0 | 0.1 |
| Total | 1031 | 100 | 48.7 |

[a] Excluding Down syndrome.
ALL, acute lymphocytic leukemia; AML, acute myeloid leukemia; MDS, myelodysplastic syndrome; DS, Down syndrome; JMML, juvenile myelomonocytic leukemia; CML, chronic myeloid leukemia; PV, polycythemia vera; ET, essential thrombocytemia.
*Source*: Data from Ref. 1 and 2.

(CMML). The FAB classification of AML was widely and rapidly accepted in pediatrics, whereas the FAB classification of MDS into the five named subgroups has slowly and partially been accepted among pediatricians. Since its introduction into pediatrics in the mid-1980s (23–25), the FAB classification system has been utilized by many researchers and clinicians, has prognostic impact (26,27), and has simplified communication in pediatric MDS. However, some investigators have experienced major problems in applying the FAB classification in a pediatric population (28) owing to specific diseases and morphological features in children and the frequent occurrence of associated anomalies.

## B.  Current Approach to the Classification of Childhood MDS

While the FAB classification has been generally accepted for adults with MDS, the classification of MDS in childhood has been the subject of some controversy. Some investigators have subdivided children with MDS either as having more adult-type MDS or as suffering from a disorder that is primarily observed in infancy and that has myeloproliferative features. In addition, other investigators have emphasized that MDS that develops in inherited bone marrow failure disorders is difficult to classify according to the FAB criteria. Also, hematological features of some nonclonal disorders, e.g., mitochondrial disorders, may be indistinguishable from true clonal MDS (29).

Recently, after a series of international meetings, consensus was reached on some of the difficult and controversial issues.

1. Nonclonal disorders with dysplastic morphological features should not be considered to be MDS.
2. The distinct disorder of young children, previously classified as CMML or juvenile chronic myeloid leukemia (JCML), is now termed "juvenile myelomonocytic leukemia" (JMML). This new terminology is utilized in the recent World Health Organization (WHO) classification on neoplastic diseases of the hematopoietic and lymphoid tissues (30). The WHO classification places JMML together with CMML and atypical chronic myeloid leukemia into a separate category of disorders that combine features of myeloproliferative and myelodysplastic syndromes.
3. Monosomy 7 is the most common acquired abnormality noted in hematopoietic cells of children with MDS (6). Some investigators considered monosomy 7 to represent a distinct hematological disorder described as monosomy 7 syndrome (26). However, monosomy 7 occurs in all FAB subtypes of myeloid neoplasia, and it has recently been shown that the morphological diagnosis along with the FAB subtype is the strongest predictor of length of survival (27). For these reasons, the concept of monosomy 7 being a distinct syndrome has been abandoned.
4. Clinical and biological features suggest that myeloid leukemia in children with Down syndrome (DS) is distinct from the disease in non-DS children (31). DS is often preceded by an MDS phase and, in some children, by a transient myeloproliferative disorder during the neonatal period. MDS, as well as AML, in DS is highly chemosensitive and carries an excellent prognosis when treated on modified AML protocols.

The classification of MDS in childhood has been greatly facilitated by the acknowledgment that JMML has primarily myeloproliferative features and that MDS in DS does not share the biological features of other types of MDS. Accordingly, this chapter is divided into three main parts: juvenile myelomonocytic leukemia, myeloid leukemia in DS, and MDS (both de novo and secondary MDS).

## II. JUVENILE MYELOMONOCYTIC LEUKEMIA

## A. History

JMML, the pediatric equivalent of what the FAB group termed CMML, has for historical reasons often been described together with chronic myeloid leukemia

(CML). The historical reasons for including JMML as a form of CML date back to the 1950s and early 1960s when several papers presented series of children with chronic leukemia and underscored the difference between CML in infants and in older children (32–36). A distinction was made between CML of the adult form and of the juvenile form, introducing the term "juvenile CML" (JCML) (36). Since that time, JCML has been the most widely used name in the British and American literature (37), although the French groups favored the term "chronic myelomonocytic leukemia" (38–40).

It was only around 1990 that JMML was included in the group of myelodysplastic syndromes (41–43). There has been some reluctance to accept the term "CMML" in children because of the obvious differences in disease presentations between children and adults. Attempting to avoid Babylonian confusion, the new unifying name—juvenile myelomonocytic leukemia—was proposed and has attained general international acceptance (44–46).

The criticism among hematologists of including CMML in the group of MDS (47) has similarly been raised among pediatricians. Whether JMML is classified as MDS or as a myeloproliferative disorder is a semantic question since JMML is a bridging disorder. Regardless of the heading used, the unique clinical features certainly justify that data on JMML patients be reported separately.

## B. Epidemiology

Incidence studies from Denmark and British Columbia (1,2) showed similar JMML incidences of 1.2/million children per year, corresponding to 2.4% of all hematological malignancies (Table 2) in accordance with earlier studies (35,36,40). However, a smaller study from England showed a very low incidence of JMML (48). Differences in classification practice may be important, but it is also possible that geographic differences in incidence exist.

The median age at presentation is 1.8 years; 35% are below 1 year of age at presentation, and only 4% are more than 5 years of age (49). JMML displays a male predominance with a male:female ratio of 2:1 (6,49).

Neurofibromatosis type 1 (NF1) is associated with more than a 200-fold increased risk of JMML (50). NF1 is known clinically in about 15% of the children with JMML and is relatively more common in children diagnosed after 5 years of age (49).

Associated abnormalities other than NF1 are found in 7% of the JMML cases (49). With the exception of Noonan syndrome, there is little consistency in the findings and no causal associations have been documented.

A JMML-like picture has been observed in several infants with Noonan syndrome (51–54). One study showed evidence of a monocytic proliferation in four of 40 neonates with Noonan syndrome (53). Most cases resolved spontaneously but AML occurred in one case (51). The only case that was tested showed polyclonal hematopoiesis (51). In vitro studies show excessive growth of granulo-cyte-macrophage colonies as in JMML, but the exact nature of this disorder remains unclear.

## C. Clinical and Laboratory Features

Marked hepatosplenomegaly may be the first sign leading the child to medical attention. Otherwise, patients present with pallor, fever, infection, bleeding, and cough, and a macular-papular skin rash is seen in 35% of the patients (49). Almost all patients show an increased white blood cell (WBC) count (Fig. 1) with absolute monocytosis, anemia, and thrombocytopenia. A WBC count greater than or equal to $50 \times 10^9$/L is found in 30% of the cases and only 7% have a WBC count greater than or equal to $100 \times 10^9$/L (49). Increased fetal hemoglobin (HbF) is a main characteristic of JMML with a notable exception for children having monosomy 7; almost all of these patients have normal HbF for the age (49). Diabetes insipidus has been reported as the presenting feature in a few cases with JMML and monosomy 7 (27).

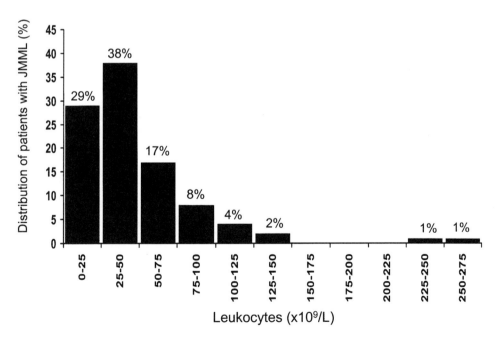

**Fig. 1** Distribution of white blood cells in patients with juvenile myelomonocytic leukemia (JMML). (Based on data from Ref. 49.)

## D.  Cytogenetics

Based on standard banding cytogenetics, 25–30% of children with JMML show monosomy 7 (mostly as the sole abnormality), 10% other aberrations (almost half of them with 7q-), and 60% a normal karyotype (7,49).

Data from the European Working Group on MDS in Childhood (EWOG-MDS) did not show any major clinical differences between JMML in patients with and without monosomy 7 (49). However, patients with monosomy 7 show some hematological characteristics; they present with lower WBC counts, higher percentages of monocytes in the blood, decreased myeloid:erythroid ratio in the bone marrow (BM), higher mean corpuscular volume, and normal or only moderately elevated HbF (49).

Monosomy 7 is seen at about the same frequency when JMML develops in NF1 as when it occurs in children without predisposing conditions (49).

## E.  Differential Diagnoses

International agreement has been attained on diagnostic criteria to help distinguish JMML from other disorders with myeloproliferative features (55) (Table 3). There remain, however, a number of diagnostic pitfalls that require attention.

**Table 3**   Diagnostic Guidelines for Juvenile Myelomonocytic Leukemia

| Clinical and laboratory findings | Observation |
| --- | --- |
| Suggestive clinical features | Hepatosplenomegaly |
| | Lymphadenopathy |
| | Pallor |
| | Skin rash |
| Laboratory criteria: | No Philadelphia chromosome and no *bcr-abl* rearrangement |
| Minimum criteria for tentative diagnosis (all 3 must be fulfilled) | |
| | Peripheral blood monocyte count $> 1 \times 10^9/L$ |
| | Blasts $< 20\%$ of bone marrow cells |
| Criteria for definite diagnosis (at least 2 must be fulfilled) | Hemoglobin F increased for age |
| | Myeloid precursors in peripheral blood smear |
| | White blood cell count $> 10 \times 10^9/L$ |
| | Clonal abnormality |
| | GM-CSF hypersensitivity of myeloid progenitors in vitro |

GM-CSF, granulocyte-monocyte colony-stimulating factor.
*Source*: Adapted from Ref. 55.

Infections, inborn errors of metabolism, and immunodeficiency may cause monocytosis and lead to an incorrect diagnosis of JMML, especially in infants; therefore, a period of observation is recommended in cases without clear-cut features.
Further, a few cases of viral infections mimicking JMML have been reported,
including Epstein-Barr virus (56), cytomegalovirus (57), herpes virus-6 (58), and
parvovirus (59). Immunodeficiencies such as leukocyte adhesion defect may also
mimic JMML (60).

## F.  Pathophysiology

JMML is a clonal disorder that arises from a pluripotent stem cell (61–65). Recently, new insights in the understanding of its pathogenesis were obtained and
could provide prospects for innovative rational therapy approaches.

   JMML mononuclear cells of both peripheral blood and bone marrow yield
excessive numbers of monocyte-macrophage colonies when cultured in semisolid
systems, even without the addition of exogenous growth factors (66–68). This
so-called "spontaneous proliferation" of JMML myeloid progenitors, a response
first observed over 20 years ago, can be prevented by prior depletion of adherent
cells. Several investigators suggested that the endogenous production of interleukin 1 (IL-1) (69), granulocyte-monocyte colony-stimulating factor (GM-CSF)
(70), or tumor necrosis factor $\alpha$ (TNF-$\alpha$) (71) by monocytes accounts for the
abundant growth of myeloid colonies. Supporting this position is the fact that
neutralizing antibodies and receptor antagonists to IL-1 (72), GM-CSF (73), and
TNF-$\alpha$ (71) have been shown to suppress colony formation. TNF-$\alpha$ appears to
act through GM-CSF by specifically modulating gene expression (74,75).

   Pure populations of JMML monocytes failed, however, to consistently
overproduce the above cytokines (73). Therefore, a primarily paracrine-based
growth mechanism driven by monocytes was felt to be unlikely. Instead, a hypersensitivity of JMML myeloid progenitors toward GM-CSF was shown to be the
most consistent observation (76). Indeed, GM-CSF hypersensitivity has become
the hallmark of the disease and an important diagnostic tool (Fig. 2) (45). GM-
CSF may be mandatory for survival of JMML cells; diphtheria toxin fused to
GM-CSF is toxic to JMML blasts (77), and treatment with a GM-CSF analog
that acts as a receptor antagonist induced apoptosis (78,79). While the importance
of GM-CSF in the pathophysiology of JMML is unchallenged, some investigators
reported an additional strong growth response toward stem cell factor (SCF) (80).

   The hypothesis that a specific defect in the GM-CSF signal transduction
pathway plays a major role in the pathogenesis of JMML led to studies at the
receptor and cytoplasmic signaling level. While GM-CSF receptor mutations
could not be demonstrated (81), abnormalities in the Ras signal transduction pathway downstream of the receptor became evident (Fig. 3). Members of the Ras
family of signaling proteins regulate cellular proliferation by cycling between

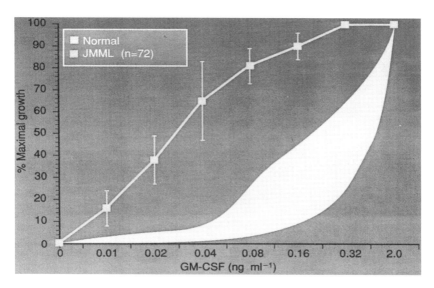

**Fig. 2** Dose-response curve for GM-CSF stimulated in vitro growth of GM-CFU in JMML (line) and normal bone marrow cells (white area). GM-CSF, granulocyte-monocyte colony-stimulating factor; GM-CFU, granulocyte-monocyte colony-forming units; JMML, juvenile myelomonocytic leukemia; n, number. (From Ref. 45.)

an active guanosin triphosphate (GTP-)-bound state (Ras-GTP) and an inactive guanosine diphosphate (Ras-GDP)-bound state. Ras activation is a crucial component of the proliferative response to growth factors. Point mutations of *ras* that cause high constitutive Ras-GTP levels (82) were noted in up to 25% of JMML patients (64,83,84). The conversion from Ras-GTP to the RAS-GDP is facilitated by GTP-ase-activating proteins (GAPs); GAPs therefore act as negative regulators of Ras function. Two GAPs, p120GAP (known as RasGAP) and neurofibromin, the protein encoded by the gene for NF1, regulate Ras in mammalian cells.

A link between NF1 and JMML has long been appreciated (85). About 15% of children with JMML carry the clinical diagnosis of NF1 (49). In addition, *NF1* mutations have been detected in JMML patients in the absence of the clinical diagnosis of NF1 (86,87), suggesting that JMML may be the presenting feature of NF1. The *NF1* gene functions as a tumor-suppressor gene, and loss of the normal *NF1* allele was noted in leukemic cells of NF1 patients (88,89). As expected, leukemic cells showed an elevated percentage of Ras in the GTP-bound state (90). *NF1* and *ras* mutations are mutually exclusive in JMML patients, indicating that one abnormality is sufficient to activate Ras.

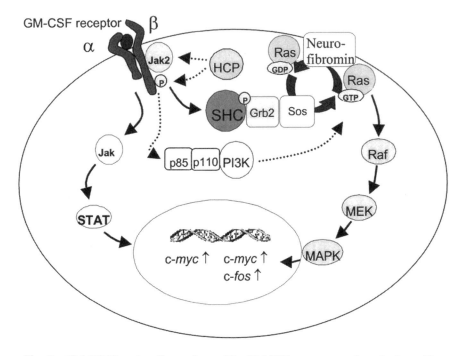

**Fig. 3** GM-CSF-Ras signaling pathway. The GM-CSF receptor consists of a low-affinity-binding α subunit with specificity and a high-affinity β subunit shared with other cytokines. Downstream signaling events include activation of the JAK/Stat pathway, the phosphatidylinositol 3-kinase/mitogen-activated kinase pathway, and the Ras/mitogen-activated kinase pathway. The latter is activated through adapter proteins like SHC and Grb2, and a guanine nucleotide exchange factor, such as Sos. Ras itself can activate Raf, and subsequently the phosphorylation cascade continues on to nuclear proteins.

The evidence that GM-CSF hypersensitivity in JMML is Ras-mediated is provided by experiments with homozygous mice lacking the *NF1* gene. Hematopoietic cells of these $NF1^{-/-}$ animals are hypersensitive to GM-CSF (90,91). Introduction of a neurofibromin-related functional GAP domain restored normal growth characteristics (92). The $NF1^{-/-}$ progenitor cells showed a constitutive activation of the Ras-Raf-MAP kinase signaling pathway and hyperactivation of MAP kinase after growth factor stimulation (93). By generating mice whose hematopoietic system was reconstituted with $NF1^{-/-}$ hematopoietic stem cells, it was demonstrated that loss of the *NF1* gene by itself is sufficient to produce the myeloproliferation associated with JMML (91).

The importance of hyperactive Ras in the pathogenesis of JMML suggests that novel therapeutics directed against components of the Ras signaling transduction cascade might ameliorate myeloproliferation. Posttranslational Ras processing initiated by farnesyltransferase is essential for the biological activity of Ras proteins. In vitro, the farnesyltransferase inhibitor L-744,832 inhibited growth of JMML progenitors (94) and partially blocked GM-CSF-induced MAP kinase activation in $NF1^{-/-}$ murine hematopoietic cells (95). However, the same inhibitor had no effect on the myeloproliferative disorder noted in irradiated mice reconstituted with $NF1^{-/-}$ progenitor cells (95). Future studies will have to clarify whether targeted disruption of Ras signaling has therapeutic efficacy in JMML.

## G.  Prognosis and Natural Course

A few cases of spontaneous remission (27) and long-term survival without therapy (40) have been reported. However, almost all patients will eventually progress if left untreated. Most often patients die from organ failure, especially respiratory failure, due to leukemic infiltrates. Blastic transformation is less frequent, with an older series showing blastic transformation in up to 25% of patients (40). A recent Japanese study showed blast count increasing, to more than 30% of the bone marrow cells, in eight of 78 patients, often with additional cytogenetic abnormalities (96). With the more widespread use of stem cell transplantation (SCT), very few patients will experience blastic transformation (49).

A poor prognosis is associated with low platelet count, elevated HbF, and age of 2 years or more (26,40,49). The EWOG-MDS data showed platelet count below $33 \times 10^9/L$ to be the strongest factor indicating a poor prognosis (49) (Fig. 4). The International Prognostic Scoring System (IPSS) for MDS (97) does not provide prognostic information for JMML (98).

## H.  Treatment of JMML

JMML is resistant to conventional-dose chemotherapy (49). Treatment with oral mercaptopurine and sequential cytarabine can give clinical and hematological responses in some patients (99). Isotretinoin, which effectively reduced spontaneous growth in vitro, has also been shown to induce durable responses (100). Nevertheless, allogeneic SCT is the only reported curative strategy for these children, curing about 30% of patients (101–106), but the rate of relapse is high, in the order of 40–50%. Most relapses occur early within the first year after SCT (Fig. 5). Less intensive schemes of graft-versus-host-disease (GvHD) prophylaxis seem to favor longer disease-free survival (105,106). Withdrawal of immunosuppression (107,108) or donor lymphocyte infusion (106) was successful in several children with recurrent disease, indicating a graft-versus-leukemia effect. Although the most effective preparative regimen is still unknown, some investigators reported that total-body irradiation might be associated with a higher relapse than busulfan-based regimens (Fig. 6) (105,106). The role of splenectomy prior to SCT is currently unknown because it has been common practice to remove large spleens prior to SCT (105). Recently a more favorable outcome for SCT

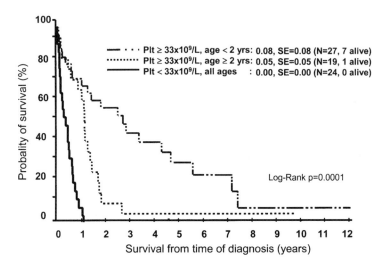

**Fig. 4** Probability of survival according to platelet count and age at diagnosis in patients with JMML not receiving stem cell transplantation. JMML, juvenile myelomonocytic leukemia; Plt, platelets; SE, standard error; N, number. (Based on data from Ref. 49.)

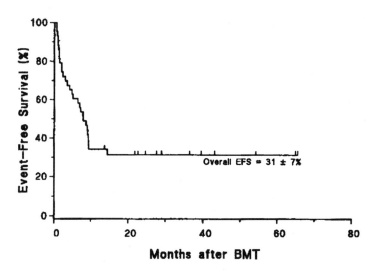

**Fig. 5** Probability of event-free survival for 43 children with JMML treated with allogeneic stem cell transplantation. (Hatch marks or changes in relative position on the graph represent data points.) JMML, juvenile myelomonocytic leukemia; BMT, bone marrow transplantation; EFS, event-free survival. (From Ref. 105.)

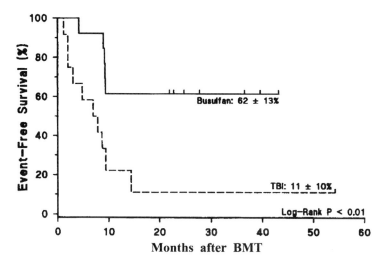

**Fig. 6** Impact of busulfan ($N = 13$) or total body irradiation (TBI) ($N = 12$) on the probability of event-free survival in children with juvenile myelomonocytic leukemia when given stem cell transplantation from HLA-identical siblings or 1-antigen-disparate donors. BMT, bone marrow transplantation; N, number. (From Ref. 105.)

in JMML has been reported with an event-free survival of about 60% for children transplanted from an HLA-matched sibling donor and 45% for children grafted from an HLA-compatible unrelated volunteer donor (109).

## III. MYELOID LEUKEMIA IN DOWN SYNDROME

While the risk of solid tumors is decreased for individuals with DS (110), these patients have a more than 50-fold increased risk of leukemia during the first 5 years of life and a 10-fold increased risk during years 5–29. After 30 years of age the risk of leukemia is close to that of non-DS individuals. The cumulated risk for leukemia by the age of 5 years is 2.1% and by 30 years 2.7%. Almost half the leukemias are myeloid and, furthermore, a myeloproliferative disorder indistinguishable from leukemia may occur in infants with DS.

### A. Transient Abnormal Myelopoiesis

Up to 10% of newborns with DS show anemia, thrombocytopenia, and increased WBC with circulating blasts. The clinical and morphological picture, which includes clonal abnormalities, may be indistinguishable from congenital leukemia;

the blast cells often have cell surface antigens characteristic of megakaryoblasts (111). (Similar features may occasionally be seen in a non-DS infant having trisomy 21 in the blast cells). The condition is referred to as transient abnormal myelopoiesis (TAM), transient leukemic reaction, or transient myeloproliferative disorder. Owing to the similarities with AML-M7, which is AML of megakaryo-blastic lineage, some have favored the name transient leukemia (111).

TAM involves selectively the trisomic cells in individuals with DS mosaic (112). Life-threatening complications may occur in a few patients, but spontaneous remission occurs in the majority within 3 months. No chemotherapy is indicated in TAM except in those with vital-organ involvement (113). AML develops 1–3 years later in about one-quarter of the children who have recovered from TAM (111). Risk factors for the subsequent AML development, however, are unknown (112). The mechanisms of the almost-uniform regression of TAM also remain unexplained.

The complexity of TAM and AML is illustrated by the report on a pair of identical twins with DS (114). Twin A had TAM with spontaneous regression and did not develop leukemia later on. Twin B had no hematological abnormalities in the newborn period but developed AML-M7 at 24 months of age.

## B. Myeloid Leukemia

DS is by far the most frequently encountered predisposing condition in children with a morphological diagnosis of MDS. DS is present in 25% of those diagnosed as RA, RAEB, or RAEB-t (1,2). JMML occurs in children at an incidence about half that of RA, RAEB, and RAEB-t (1), but only two cases of JMML associated with DS have been reported (115,116). The otherwise uncommon AML-M7 is frequently found in DS and is in most cases preceded by a history of MDS (117,118).

MDS and AML are differentiated on the basis of a blast count in the BM equal to or below 30% or greater than 30%, respectively. It has been common practice, however, to classify most cases of myeloid leukemia in DS as AML (31), although most patients present with less than 30% blasts in the BM (2). A complicating factor in the classification is that the BM in myeloid leukemia in DS children is often fibrotic and assessment of the blast count may be difficult. There are several distinctive features indicating biological differences between MDS/AML-M7 in children with DS versus those without DS. Furthermore, there seem to be no biological or therapeutic differences between MDS and AML in DS in contrast to that of non-DS children. In recognition of the unique biological features of AML and MDS in DS children, the disease may be best described by the term "myeloid leukemia of Down syndrome."

AML may occasionally occur in an older child or adult with DS. These cases have the common morphological and cytogenetic features of AML in non-

DS individuals. Such cases may represent ''normal'' AML occurring by chance in an individual with DS (119,120).

## C.  Clinical and Laboratory Features

The age distribution of myeloid leukemia in DS is very unusual (31,118,121,122) (Fig. 7). Of 307 patients, 150 (49%) were 1 year of age at diagnosis, 104 (34%) were 2 years of age, and only five (1.6%) were more than 4 years of age. Isolated thrombocytopenia is often the presenting feature. At diagnosis both platelet count and WBC are lower than in non-DS patients (31). The blast cells have morphological and antigen features of megakaryoblasts.

## D.  Cytogenetics

Numerical aberrations, mainly trisomy 8 and an extra chromosome 21 (tetrasomy 21), are the most common acquired cytogenetic abnormalities. Structural aberrations are uncommon, with the prognostically favorable cytogenetic abnormalities (t(8;21), t(15;17), inv(16)) occurring in 30% of the non-DS children with AML and being very uncommon in DS (31,118,123). The t(1;22) is the hallmark of

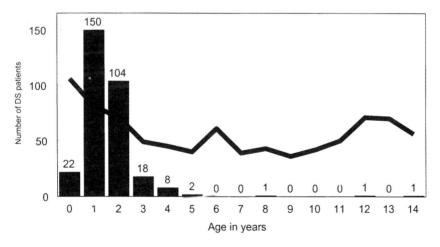

**Fig. 7**  Age distribution in 307 children with myeloid leukemia of Down syndrome (bars). Transient abnormal myelopoiesis of the newborn is excluded. Cumulated data from Japan ($N = 33$) (data from Ref. 121), Germany ($N = 38$) (data from Ref. 118), Scandinavia ($N = 69$) (G. Gustafsson, personal communication, 2000), UK ($N = 52$) (data from Ref. 122), and United States ($N = 115$) (data from Ref. 31). For comparison, the relative age distribution in 454 children with AML (line) is shown. (Data from Ref. 249.)

AML-M7 in infants. The translocation has not been associated with DS until a recent report on two DS patients aged 6 and 10 years with AML-M7 and t(1; 22) (124). Karyotype is not known to be a prognostic factor in DS.

The clonal cells in children with DS are myeloid progenitors with the potential for differentiation along the megakaryocytic and erythroid lineages (125); the granulocytic lineage is, in contrast to non-DS children, not involved in the leukemic process.

### E. Treatment

The prognosis of AML in DS was considered very poor before 1990. Since then, reports from the Nordic Society of Paediatric Haematology and Oncology (NO-PHO) (126) and the Pediatric Oncology Group (POG) (127) and later the Children's Cancer Group (CCG) (31) showed a surprisingly high survival rate when the DS patients received AML treatment (Fig. 8). DS was later shown to be the most important prognostic factor in AML (128). Several groups have reported long-term survival in DS patients well above 80% (118,121,127,128). DS patients treated on AML protocols have a significantly better outcome than those receiving minimal treatment (113); however, intensive timing of induction is associated with an increased mortality (31). DS children are at a low risk for relapse and,

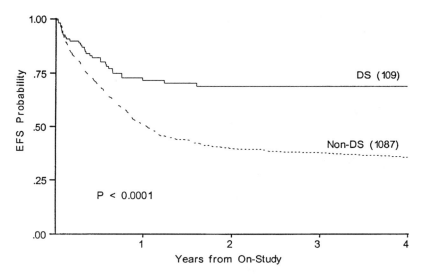

**Fig. 8**   Probability of event-free survival (EFS) in children with acute myeloid leukemia (AML) with and without Down syndrome (DS) treated according to the Children's Cancer Group (CCG) AML protocols (CCG 2861 and CCG 2891). P, probability (From Ref. 31.)

owing to the high risk for treatment-related toxicity, they benefit from less time-intensive therapy, allowing full count recovery prior to initiation of the next chemotherapeutic course (31). Long term survival has been reported in a few patients receiving only low-dose chemotherapy (111), but the results are inferior to those following intensive therapy and it is not recommended (113). SCT is associated with excess toxicity without therapeutic gain and is not indicated in the DS child in first remission (31,118). It is recommended to start therapy when the myeloid disorder is diagnosed and not wait until progression (113).

DS myeloblasts are 10-fold more sensitive to cytarabine in vitro than non-DS cells (129). The increased sensitivity of DS blasts may be related to the expression of chromosome 21 localized genes like cystathionine-$\beta$-synthetase and superoxide dismutase (129). An elevated cystathionine-$\beta$-synthetase activity may modulate cytarabine metabolism by decreasing levels of deoxycytidine triphosphate or decreasing generation of S-adenosyl-methionine and hypomethylation of the deoxycytidine kinase gene (129). Increased susceptibility of DS cells to undergo apoptosis may also contribute to the increased chemosensitivity.

It is remarkable that only the constitutional and not the acquired trisomy 21 is associated with a superior outcome (31). In vitro studies showed no increased transcript levels of cystathionine-$\beta$-synthetase in samples with acquired trisomy 21 (129). Further studies of the molecular mechanism of the increased sensitivity to chemotherapy in DS may lead to new approaches in the treatment of AML.

## IV.  MYELODYSPLASTIC SYNDROME

MDS can arise in an otherwise healthy child, when it may be named ''de novo'' or ''primary.'' It may also develop in a child with a known predisposing condition, when it is referred to as ''secondary.'' Secondary MDS is seen in patients (1) after chemo- or radiation therapy (named ''therapy-related MDS''), (2) with inherited bone marrow failure disorders, (3) with acquired aplastic anemia, and (4) with familial MDS. It is to be recognized, however, that children with so-called ''primary'' MDS may have an underlying, yet unknown, genetic defect predisposing them to MDS at young age. Therefore, the distinction between primary and secondary disease may become arbitrary. Instead, one might just specify whether the patient has a known predisposing condition.

### A.  Epidemiology

MDS represents 4% of all hematological malignancies in children (Table 2) corresponding to an annual incidence of MDS of 1.8/million children aged 0–14 years (1,2).

Constitutional abnormalities are present in about 30% of childhood MDS

(1,2,6,26,28). DS is by far the most common, seen in some 25% of those with a morphological diagnosis of RA, RAEB, or RAEB-t. MDS in DS is a unique entity and discussed separately above.

MDS has anecdotally been reported in a number of constitutional cytogenetic abnormalities other than trisomy 21, but only for trisomy 8 mosaicism is there solid evidence for an increased risk of MDS (130,131).

There are no clear data indicating that MDS occurring in patients with constitutional abnormalities other than DS and Fanconi anemia differ from MDS in other children. The patients should be included in series of MDS and the type and frequency of constitutional abnormalities should be reported. The outcome of patients with therapy-related MDS is poor and these patients should be reported separately.

## B.   Congenital Bone Marrow Failure

Fifty percent of Fanconi anemia patients develop MDS or AML before the age of 40 years (132). Cytogenetic analyses of the leukemia in Fanconi anemia show a high frequency of monosomy 7 and duplications of 1q (133,134). It is very difficult to diagnose RA in a patient with Fanconi anemia and the definition of clonality is problematic (134). The natural history and the therapy differ for MDS patients having Fanconi anemia versus those without (134). MDS and AML in patients with Fanconi anemia should be reported separately.

The survival of patients with severe congenital neutropenia (SCN) has significantly improved following the introduction of granulocyte colony-stimulating factor (G-CSF) treatment. Studies from the SCN International Register have shown a crude rate of MDS/AML development of 9% and an annual progression rate of 2% (135). Partial or complete loss of chromosome 7 is found in more than half the patients who develop MDS. Acquired mutations in the G-CSF receptor are found in most SCN patients with MDS/AML (136), but the role of the mutations in leukemogenesis remains to be examined. No cause-and-effect relationship between the development of MDS/AML and G-CSF therapy has been demonstrated and MDS/AML is not seen in cyclic or idiopathic neutropenia treated with G-CSF (135).

MDS may occur in as many as one-third of those with Shwachman-Diamond syndrome (137) and MDS and AML have occasionally been described in patients with Diamond-Blackfan anemia (2,27,138). No estimates of the relative risk are available but it is evident that the development of malignant myeloid disease in Diamond-Blackfan anemia is very rare. Indeed, not all bone marrow failure syndromes predispose to the development of MDS; e.g., patients with dyskeratosis congenita develop bone marrow failure in 95% of the cases but MDS has only been anecdotally documented (139).

## C. Acquired Aplastic Anemia

MDS develops in 10–15% of those patients with aplastic anemia not treated with SCT (140–142). Patients diagnosed as having nonsevere aplastic anemia may be overrepresented among those with development of clonal disease (143). MDS may occur sooner in children than in adults and is, in most cases, diagnosed within the first 3 years from presentation (141,142). Whether prolonged treatment with the combination of G-CSF and cyclosporine is associated with development of MDS is a controversial issue (141,144). Some of the more recent studies using shorter periods of G-CSF treatment have shown a lower incidence of MDS (145).

## D. Familial MDS

Familial occurrence of MDS, especially with −7/7q-, has been reported in a number of cases (41,146–149) and has been claimed to account for as many as one-third of the children with monosomy 7 (146). (There are no conspicuous clinical characteristics of the familial cases, except for higher age at presentation (6.4 vs. 2.7 years) (27,149).) In the EWOG-MDS series, 10% were familial cases (27). This frequency is in contrast to a population-based study (150) and a single-institution study (26), totaling 28 children with monosomy 7, who showed no relatives with MDS/AML. Familial MDS does also occur without −7/7q- (26,151). Some families show discordance for monosomy 7 (27); therefore, it is uncertain whether monosomy 7 per se increases the risk for familial cases. The inherited predisposing locus in familial MDS or AML with −7/7q- may not even be located on chromosome 7 (147). This is in accordance with the lack of leukemia cases among 183 people with constitutional aberrations of chromosome 7 (152) and the different parental origin of the remaining chromosome 7 in siblings with monosomy 7 (153).

## E. Therapy-Related MDS

The use of chemotherapy may cause therapy-related MDS (154–158). The risk is significantly increased 2–10 years after the treatment for the primary malignant disease and peaks 4–5 years following the leukemogenic therapy. There seem to be two different types of therapy-related malignant transformation (159,160). One is related to treatment with alkylating agents, leading to MDS after a latency period of 3–5 years, and is cytogenetically characterized by deletions or loss of whole chromosomes. The other type is associated with the use of epipodophyllotoxins, with acquired translocations involving chromosome band 11q23 often presenting as frank AML 1–3 years after treatment of the primary malignancy (155). Ongoing studies on polymorphic variation may identify individuals with a high genetic susceptibility to leukemia (161).

Therapy-related MDS constitutes less than 5% of the patients in series of MDS and JMML (1,2); however, MDS secondary to treatment of malignancies was found in 13% in a large series from Japan (162). New intensive-treatment protocols may lead to an increased risk of therapy-related diseases (163).

## F. Pathophysiology

Various studies have shown that MDS is a clonal disease, either arising in a progenitor cell restricted to myelopoiesis, erythropoiesis, and megakaryopoiesis, or initiating in a more immature cell involving the lymphoid series (164–166). The initiating events of MDS remain obscure in children as in adults. Because MDS is heterogeneous, different mechanisms of initiation and progression of the disease are likely to exist. Some form of genetic damage in a pluripotent hematopoietic progenitor cell may give rise to genetic instability, with subsequent development of numerous molecular and cellular abnormalities (167). Thus, it is not surprising that congenital disorders with DNA repair defects, like Fanconi anemia, are predisposing conditions for MDS. An estimated 30–50% of children with MDS have a known constitutional disorder and it is likely that most children with MDS have a congenital abnormality predisposing them to the initiating genetic change. It is further hypothesized that subsequent changes, e.g., mutations in proto-oncogenes like *ras*, *p53*, or *WT1*, and karyotypic changes like monosomy 7, are part of a final common pathway of disease progression (149,168–171). There is currently too little insight in the pathophysiology of MDS to answer the questions of whether and possibly how disease mechanisms of MDS in the elderly and in children differ.

## G. Clinical and Laboratory Features

The presenting feature of MDS is, in almost all cases, that of pancytopenia, although single-lineage cytopenia may occasionally be the presenting characteristic. In a few cases, the cytopenia has been an incidental finding during a routine workup, and in a few other cases, the cytopenia has been identified during evaluation of the patient for possible sibling bone marrow donor. Not all children with RA have anemia, but macrocytosis is a characteristic finding and frequently HbF is slightly elevated (172). Elevated WBC ($>20 \times 10^9$/L), in contrast, and marked hepatomegaly are strongly suggestive of AML.

In general, patients with RA or low-grade RAEB only require infrequent transfusions and severe infections are rarely observed. The condition may smolder with stable cytopenia for months or even years but will eventually progress in virtually all patients.

## H.  Bone Marrow Features

The bone marrow (BM) is usually normo- or hypercellular, although decreased cell content has been observed in up to 50% of the cases of childhood RA (172). The BM displays characteristic dysplastic features with megaloblastic erythropoiesis, bizarre small or unusual large megakaryocytes, dysgranulopoiesis, and often an increased percentage of myeloblasts. Characteristic dysplastic features were described by the FAB group but the description leaves room for personal interpretation and the degree of dysplasia is not included in the classification. As a result, dysplasia has been scored as mild, moderate, and marked, but without quantification or definitions of the dysplasia (173). Definitions of dysplasia have since been established by the pathology board of EWOG-MDS and the quantitative and qualitative dysplastic scoring system has been used in a prospective study (174,175). Such detailed morphological evaluations may prove to be an adjuvant tool in the diagnosis of MDS. The degree of dysplasia has prognostic relevance in adults with RA (176) but whether the dysplastic score has prognostic significance in children is not yet known.

## I.  Cytogenetics

An abnormal karyotype is found in 60–70% of the children with MDS (5–7,177). The numerical abnormalities dominate, with only 10% showing a translocation, a derivative, or a deletion as the sole abnormality. Structural abnormalities are frequently part of a complex karyotype with numerical abnormalities. This is in contrast to AML where structural abnormalities are by far the most frequent findings (178,179).

Monosomy 7 is the most common cytogenetic abnormality in childhood MDS, observed in approximately 30% of the cases (5,7,26,177). Trisomy 8 and trisomy 21 are, after monosomy 7, the most common numerical abnormalities. Constitutional trisomy 21 is usually clinically obvious when present, whereas constitutional trisomy 8 mosaicism may remain unrecognized (130) and should be tested when trisomy 8 is found in the BM.

There are only very few data on the prognostic value of cytogenetic abnormalities in children. Monosomy 7 is associated with a poor prognosis in childhood AML (178,180–182) and MDS in adults (97), but is not an unfavorable feature in childhood MDS (27).

AML-specific translocations, e.g., t(8;21)(q22;q22), t(15;17)(q22;q12), or inv(16)(p13;q22), may occur in cases with a low blast cell count (183–185). The response to therapy is favorable in such cases and these cases should be considered and treated as AML (183). Analyses utilizing polymerase chain reaction techniques are recommended to search for these abnormalities.

## J.  Differential Diagnosis

There are no established minimal diagnostic criteria for childhood MDS. The main diagnostic problems in the clinic are to differentiate MDS from AML and aplastic anemia.

### 1.  Separating MDS from AML

AML is the major differential diagnosis of MDS. There are, however, significant differences in cytogenetics and in response to therapy between MDS and AML (5,44,186), with MDS being meant for the biological entity resistant to chemotherapy. The fundamental biological differences between MDS and AML make the morphologically based classification a surrogate marker for the distinction between biological entities. The cutoff between RAEB-t and AML in the FAB system was set at 30% blasts in the BM (21) but, recently, the WHO eliminated RAEB-t and defined AML by a blast count exceeding 20% (30). This decision was primarily based on treatment considerations in adults and whether the proposal for reclassifying MDS may be useful in pediatrics remains untested. Until supportive data are presented, we suggest adherence to the 30% cutoff recognizing, however, that biological features, like those represented by chromosomal abnormalities, may be more important in distinguishing chemotherapy-resistant MDS from chemosensitive AML. In fact, MDS progressing to greater than 20% blasts will maintain the characteristic biological features and has little in common with de novo AML and t(8;21), t(15;17) or inv(16). To distinguish AML derived from MDS from true de novo AML, the term ''MDS-related AML'' (MDR-AML) has been suggested for the former (167).

The clinical course and the response to therapy in AML-M6 (187,188) (erthroid subtype of AML), AML-M7 (189), and AML with monosomy 7 (27,181,190) may be more similar to MDS than to the other types of AML, and biologically they may fit better into the classification of MDS. On the other hand, cases with a low blast cell count and AML-specific translocations may fit better into a classification of AML (183–185).

In borderline cases with BM blasts slightly less than 30% and no cytogenetic clues, the BM examination should be repeated after 2 weeks. At least 400 BM cells should be counted to decrease sample error. If the blast count of the BM is more than 30% in the second examination, the case should be regarded as AML.

### 2.  Acute Megakaryoblastic Leukemia

The FAB recommendation of distinguishing AML from MDS by a myeloblast cutoff level of 30% has been extended to the criteria for diagnosing AML-M7 (189,191–193). This practice has not always been followed; e.g., a review of 116 cases showed that about 50% of the cases had blasts less than 30% despite the statement "diagnosed as AML-M7 defined by the criteria of FAB" (194). In fact, the morphological features of M7 blasts are highly variable, including lymphoid-appearing (191). Nonetheless, megakaryoblasts can be characterized by the surface markers CD61 (GP IIIa), CD42b (GP Ib), CD41a (GP IIb/IIIa), and factor VIII–associated antigen. Cytochemical staining with myeloperoxidase (MPO) and Sudan black B is negative (195).

AML-M7 often occurs in infants and is associated with t(1;22)(p13:q13) in one-third of the cases (192,193). Complex numeric abnormalities are also frequently observed (189). The prognosis is inferior to other AML types (31,189,192,193). AML-M7 is frequently associated with DS and the clinical and biological features suggest that such cases represent a separate disorder (see above).

AML-M7 may be particularly difficult to distinguish from RAEB or RAEB-t. AML-M7 is often accompanied by marrow fibrosis, rendering it difficult to obtain an adequate aspirate; assessment of the blast count from a BM biopsy may be helpful. The presence of t(1;22)(p13;q13) may provide an additional diagnostic marker for AML-M7 (192,193).

It is at present unclear how to classify patients with extensive BM fibrosis and increased number of megakaryoblasts as shown by immunophenotype but with a total number of BM blasts below 30%. The clinical features, response to therapy, and cytogenetic findings in AML-M7 are, regardless of the blast count, in most cases closer-related to MDS than AML. We suggest that pediatric cases with organomegaly and ≤30% BM blasts be classified and treated as AML-M7 irrespective of BM blast count. In contrast, cases without organomegaly but with ≤30% BM blasts should be classified and treated as MDS. The latter condition is quite rare but may be seen in an older child.

### 3. Refractory Anemia Versus Aplastic Anemia

In adults with MDS, a hypoplastic variant has been observed in about 15% of all cases (196,197) but in these cases, cell content increases with progression of MDS. Similarly, earlier studies in children and adolescents showed decreased BM cellularity in 16% of the patients (41,43,173,198–200); however, the studies included only a few RA cases. A study on childhood RA showed decreased cell content in 17 of 34 patients (201). MDS also develops in 10–15% of those patients with aplastic anemia not treated with SCT (140–142). Most cases of MDS in children have been diagnosed within the first 3 years from presentation with aplastic anemia (141,142). The fast progression to MDS raises the question whether the patients had MDS from the beginning.

Hypoplastic MDS may be difficult to discriminate from aplastic anemia. However, careful sequential morphological studies, including BM biopsies, will almost always establish a distinction between the two entities (202–204). BM fibrosis, dilution, and sampling variation make it difficult to assess the cellularity from an aspirate; therefore, a trephine biopsy is essential for the evaluation of a child with suspected aplastic anemia or MDS. Clonal hematopoiesis is strongly suggestive of MDS, but may occasionally be seen in aplastic anemia (205,206). Cytogenetics may fail and fluorescence in situ hybridization (FISH) or human androgen receptor gene (HUMARA) assay may be useful to establish clonality. Point mutations of the N-*ras* oncogene are frequent in MDS but have not been observed in aplastic anemia (207). Overexpression of p53 is suggestive of MDS (208).

### 4. Other Differential Diagnoses

There are no definitive minimal diagnostic criteria for MDS (209). It may be very difficult to confirm a diagnosis of MDS in children, especially in infants when the blast cell count is low and there is no clonal marker. In cases with consistent hematological abnormalities over time, RA is a diagnosis of exclusion when infectious diseases like parvovirus (210–212) and human immunodeficiency virus (213), vitamin $B_{12}$ deficiency (214), drug therapy (215), rheumatoid arthritis (216), metabolic disorders (217), and other causes of cytopenia and dysplasia (216,218,219) have been ruled out.

### K. Prognosis and Natural Course

MDS and MDR-AML may develop at different rates (Fig. 9) (220). The percentage of blast cells in the BM may increase abruptly (curve A in Fig. 9) after a set of transforming events; this disease type is best described as MDR-AML. Other cases show a constant rate of progression, and the 20% or 30% threshold is passed only after a period of months or years (curve B in Fig. 9). Although any case above the threshold is conventionally defined as AML, cases consistent with curve B are better described as persistent MDS.

Children with RA can show a long and stable clinical course without treatment. In a series of 51 children with primary RA, the median time to progression to RAEB was 47 months (172). Both RA and RAEB patients with monosomy 7 may show stable disease without treatment for several years (27). SCT in the stable phase is associated with a favorable outcome. This is in contrast to MDS with $-7/7q-$ in adults, which is associated with a very poor prognosis (97) even when treated with SCT (221). Progression may occur rapidly without any preceding symptoms for both children and adults. Once progression has occurred, the outcome is very poor (222,223). Therefore, early transplantation is recommended.

Spontaneous regression of MDS has occasionally been reported in the literature (27,224–228). It has been suggested that spontaneous remission occurs

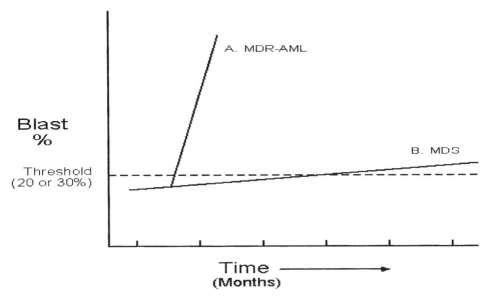

**Fig. 9** Myelodysplastic syndromes (MDS) as compared with MDS-related acute myeloid leukemia (MDR-AML): different rates of blast cell development. In A, the percentage of cells in the bone marrow increases suddenly; this disease type is best described as MDR-AML. In B, the rate remains constant, and the threshold is passed after months. Although any case above the threshold is conventionally defined as AML, cases consistent with curve B are better described as persistent MDS. (Adapted from Ref. 220.)

when MDS is a polyclonal expression of a multiorgan disease (51). However, most reported cases with spontaneous cytogenetic remission had clonal hematopoiesis and no signs of associated systemic disease. The frequency of spontaneous remission is unknown, but it is estimated to occur in less than 5% of the cases.

A large series of patients with chromosome 7 abnormalities were studied (27). Those with monosomy 7 as the sole abnormality had greater survival than those with complex abnormalities involving chromosome 7 (27).

The International Prognostic Scoring System for MDS weighted data on BM blasts count, cytopenia, and cytogenetics and separated patients into four prognostic groups (97). Preliminary data on childhood MDS showed that two-to-three-lineage cytopenia and a blast count >5% of the BM cells correlated with poor survival, whereas the cytogenetic groups did not provide prognostic information (98).

A pediatric prognostic scoring system proposed by the British group (26) assigned one point each for HbF > 10%, platelets <40 × 10⁹/L, and two or more cytogenetic abnormalities. A significantly higher survival was found in children with MDS and a score of 0. Application of the scoring system in other series has been hampered by HbF being evaluable in only a minority of the MDS patients.

## L.  Treatment of MDS

Allogeneic SCT is a curative treatment option and has emerged as the therapy of choice for all forms of MDS in childhood. A variety of other therapy strategies, such as hematopoietic growth factors, differentiating agents, hypomethylating agents, low-dose cytotoxic drugs, or other experimental agents, have been implemented in adults and in the elderly who do not qualify for SCT. Because none of these approaches has been shown to prolong survival, it is felt that they are generally not indicated in children and adolescents.

Results of SCT in pediatric MDS are often included in larger series of adult patients (229–232). There are only few reports specifically addressing the question of SCT in MDS of children (233–239). To summarize the results of these published MDS patient series, the probability of disease-free survival (DFS) for children transplanted with stem cells from an HLA-matched family donor (MFD) is about 0.50. Children receiving a graft from an HLA-matched unrelated donor (MUD) suffer a higher transplant-related mortality (TRM) and have a DFS of approximately 0.35. The European Group for Blood and Marrow Transplantation (EBMT) recently reported the results of an analysis of a large number of MDS patients less than 20 years of age transplanted between 1983 and 1998 (240). For the 163 patients receiving a MFD transplant, the 3-year actuarial probability of DFS, TRM, and relapse was 0.45, 0.30, and 0.36, respectively. MUD transplants had been performed in 84 patients, with probabilities of 0.36, 0.45, and 0.35 for DFS, TRM, and relapse, respectively.

Stage of disease as indicated by FAB type has a significant effect on relapse and outcome following SCT (222,232,240,241). In RA, the relapse rate is low provided the conditioning regimen is myeloablative (230,232). SCT early in the course of the disease has therefore been recommended for all children and adolescents with MDS. In children with RA and absence of profound cytopenia, postponement of SCT with a watch-and-wait strategy may be justified specifically in the presence of a normal karyotype.

For patients with advanced MDS, the potential benefit of AML-type induction chemotherapy prior to SCT to reduce relapse and improve DFS remains a contentious issue. In the absence of a prospective randomized study, opposing conclusions regarding the benefit of such intensive therapy have been suggested. In a recent analysis of EWOG-MDS on 53 children with primary advanced MDS, there was no benefit of intensive AML-type therapy preceding SCT (242). In this study of primary advanced MDS, outcome after SCT was not dependent on the percentage of blasts prior to SCT. Considering the significant morbidity and mortality of induction chemotherapy and a complete remission rate of only about 50% (186), AML-type therapy prior to SCT may not be warranted for most children with MDS. Conventional intensive chemotherapy without SCT is unlikely to eradicate the primitive pluripotent cells involved in MDS, rendering this therapy noncurative (186,243).

Children with MDS secondary to chemo- or radiation therapy generally have an extremely poor survival. Although remission can often be achieved with AML-type therapy, only very few patients remain disease-free and even SCT has only been reported to offer cure in about 20–30% of the patients (239,244–246). The incidence of severe or moderately severe treatment-related toxicity is increased (229,246) while the risk of relapse may be similar to that observed for patients with primary MDS (240).

Only a few cases of SCT in MDS arising from congenital bone marrow failure disorders or acquired aplastic anemia have been published and these publications have indicated a poor outcome for this heterogeneous group of patients. Early SCT before neoplastic transformation (247) or during less advanced MDS (248) may be associated with improved survival. Future cooperative studies like those of EWOG-MDS or the EBMT are needed to provide further information on the appropriate timing, conditioning regimen, and GvHD prophylaxis for the different subtypes of MDS in childhood.

## V. PERSPECTIVES

Significant progress has been made in the concept and treatment of JMML and MDS in childhood. We still need to improve the diagnostic precision, evaluate the role of any nonmyeloablative therapy, and further improve the results of SCT. Understanding the biological mechanisms of MDS and JMML is essential for further advancements. Clinical progress is possible only through the enrollment of patients in prospective cooperative studies like those of the EWOG-MDS and the North American Children's Oncology Group.

## REFERENCES

1. Hasle H, Kerndrup G, Jacobsen BB. Childhood myelodysplastic syndrome in Denmark: incidence and predisposing conditions. Leukemia 1995; 9:1569–1572.
2. Hasle H, Wadsworth LD, Massing BG, McBride M, Schultz KR. A population-based study of childhood myelodysplastic syndrome in British Columbia, Canada. Br J Haematol 1999; 106:1027–1032.
3. Aul C, Bowen DT, Yoshida Y. Pathogenesis, etiology and epidemiology of myelodysplastic syndromes. Haematologica 1998; 83:71–86.

4. Third MIC Cooperative Study Group. Recommendations for a morphologic, immunologic, and cytogenetic (MIC) working classification of the primary and therapy-related myelodysplastic disorders. Report of the workshop held in Scottsdale, Arizona, USA, on February 23–25, 1987. Cancer Genet Cytogenet 1988; 32:1–10.

5. Hasle H. Myelodysplastic syndromes in childhood—classification, epidemiology, and treatment. Leuk Lymphoma 1994; 13:11–26.

6. Luna-Fineman S, Shannon KM, Atwater SK, Davis J, Masterson M, Ortega J, Sanders J, Steinherz P, Weinberg V, Lange BJ. Myelodysplastic and myeloproliferative disorders of childhood: a study of 167 patients. Blood 1999; 93:459–466.

7. Harbott J, Haas OA, Kerndrup G, Michalová K, Sainati L, Slater R, Biondi A, Fenu S, Hasle H, Kühne T, Mann G, Stary J, van Wering ER, Baumann I, Nöllke P, Rogge T, Zimmermann M, Niemeyer C. Cytogenetic evaluation of children with MDS and JMML. Results of the European working group of childhood MDS (EWOG-MDS). Leukemia 2000; 14:961.

8. Kramárová E, Stiller CA. The international classification of childhood cancer. Int J Cancer 1996; 68:759–765.

9. Court D, Edward DG. Monocytic leukaemia in childhood. Arch Dis Child 1939; 14:231–244.

10. Pearson HA, Diamond LK. Chronic monocytic leukemia in childhood. J Pediatr 1958; 53:259–270.

11. Shuster S, Jones JH, Kilpatrick GS. Leukaemia and foetal haemoglobin: a case study. Br Med J 1960; 2:1556–1558.

12. Humbert JR, Hathaway WE, Robinson A, Peakman DC, Githens JH. Pre-leukemia in children with a missing bone marrow C chromosome and a myeloproliferative disorder. Br J Haematol 1971; 21:705–716.

13. Heimpel H, Kleihauer E, Olischlager A, Queisser W. [Functional disorders of the hematopoietic system in the preleukemic phase. Acute undifferentiated leukemia.] Med Klin 1972; 67:1004–1011 [German].

14. Lascari AD. Leukemia in childhood. In: Preleukemia. Springfield, IL: Charles C Thomas, 1973:97–110.

15. Smith WB, Ablin A, Goodman JR, Brecher G. Atypical megakaryocytes in preleukemic phase of acute myeloid leukemia. Blood 1973; 42:535–540.

16. Kleihauer E. The preleukemic syndromes (hematopoietic dysplasia) in childhood. Eur J Pediatr 1980; 133:5–10.

17. Bernard J, Schaison G. Transitory bone marrow failure. A series of 13 preleukemic cases in children. Am J Pediatr Hematol Oncol 1980; 2:141–144.

18. Pizzi E, Mauri A, Locasciulli A, Jankovic M, Zurlo MG, Carnelli V. [Preleukemic states in infancy: discussion of 3 cases.] Minerva Pediatr 1980; 32:831–836 [Italian].

19. Wegelius R. Bone marrow dysfunctions preceding acute leukemia in children: a clinical study. Leuk Res 1992; 16:71–76.

20. Hasle H, Heim S, Schroeder H, Schmiegelow K, Østergaard E, Kerndrup G. Transient pancytopenia preceding acute lymphoblastic leukemia (pre-ALL). Leukemia 1995; 9:605–608.

21. Bennett JM, Catovsky D, Daniel MT, Flandrin G, Galton DAG, Gralnick HR, Sultan C. Proposals for the classification of the myelodysplastic syndromes. Br J Haematol 1982; 51:189–199.

22. Bennett JM, Catovsky D, Daniel MT, Flandrin G, Galton DA, Gralnick HR, Sultan C. Proposed revised criteria for the classification of acute myeloid leukemia. A report of the French-American-British Cooperative Group. Ann Intern Med 1985; 103:620–625.

23. Cantù-Rajnoldi A, Porcelli P, Cattoretti G, Ferrari M, Romitti L, Adamoli L, Masera G. Myelodysplastic syndromes in children: Observation on five cases. Eur Paediatr Haematol Oncol 1984; 1:71–75.

24. Foucar K, Langdon RM 2nd, Armitage JO, Olson DB, Carroll TJ Jr. Myelodysplastic syndromes. A clinical and pathologic analysis of 109 cases. Cancer 1985; 56: 553–561.

25. van Wering ER, Kamps WA, Vossen JM, van der List-Nuver CJ, Theunissen PM. Myelodysplastic syndromes in childhood: three case reports. Br J Haematol 1985; 60:137–142.

26. Passmore SJ, Hann IM, Stiller CA, Ramani P, Swansbury GJ, Gibbons B, Reeves BR, Chessells JM. Pediatric myelodysplasia: A study of 68 children and a new prognostic scoring system. Blood 1995; 85:1742–1750.

27. Hasle H, Aricò M, Basso G, Biondi A, Cantù-Rajnoldi A, Creutzig U, Fenu S, Fonatsch C, Haas OA, Harbott J, Kardos G, Kerndrup G, Mann G, Niemeyer CM, Ptoszkova H, Ritter J, Slater R, Stary J, Stollmann-Gibbels B, Testi AM, van Wering ER, Zimmermann M, for the European Working Group on MDS in Childhood (EWOG-MDS). Myelodysplastic syndrome, juvenile myelomonocytic leukemia, and acute myeloid leukemia associated with complete or partial monosomy 7. Leukemia 1999; 13:376–385.

28. Bader-Meunier B, Mielot F, Tchernia G, Buisine J, Delsol G, Duchayne E, Lemerle S, Leverger G, de Lumley L, Manel AM, Nathanson M, Plantaz D, Robert A, Schaison G, Sommelet D, Vilmer E. Myelodysplastic syndrome in childhood: report of 49 patients from a French multicentre study. French Society of Paediatric Haematology and Immunology. Br J Haematol 1996; 92:344–350.

29. Bader-Meunier B, Rötig A, Mielot F, Lavergne JM, Croisille L, Rustin P, Landrieu P, Dommergues JP, Munnich A, Tchernia G. Refractory anaemia and mitochondrial cytopathy in childhood. Br J Haematol 1994; 87:381–385.

30. Harris NL, Jaffe ES, Diebold J, Flandrin G, Muller-Hermelink HK, Vardiman J, Lister TA, Bloomfield CD. The World Health Organization classification of neoplastic diseases of the hematopoietic and lymphoid tissues. Report of the Clinical Advisory Committee meeting—Airlie House, Virginia, November 1997. J Clin Oncol 1999; 17:3835–3849.

31. Lange BJ, Kobrinsky N, Barnard DR, Arthur DC, Buckley JD, Howells WB, Gold S, Sanders J, Neudorf S, Smith FO, Woods WG. Distinctive demography, biology, and outcome of acute myeloid leukemia and myelodysplastic syndrome in children with Down syndrome: Children's Cancer Group Studies 2861 and 2891. Blood 1998; 91:608–615.

32. Cooke JV. Chronic myelogenous leukemia in children. J Pediatr 1953; 42:537–550.

33. Barrett O, Conrad M, Crosby WH. Chronic granulocytic leukemia in childhood. Am J Med Sci 1960; 250:587–592.

34. Vahlquist B, Vuille JC. Chronic granulocytic leukemia in childhood. Acta Paediatr Scand 1960; 49:795–809.

35. Bernard J, Seligmann M, Acar J. [Chronic myeloid leukemia in children. A study of 20 cases.] Arch Fr Pediatr 1962; 19:881–894 [French].

36. Hardisty RM, Speed DE, Till M. Granulocytic leukaemia in childhood. Br J Haematol 1964; 10:551–566.

37. Freedman MH, Estrov Z, Chan HSL. Juvenile chronic myelogenous leukemia. Am J Pediatr Hematol Oncol 1988; 10:261–267.

38. Bernard J, Seligmann M. Les leucémies myélomonocytaires du nourrisson. Nouv Rev Fr Hematol 1968; 8:759–762 [French].

39. Weisgerber C, Schaison G, Chavelet F, Seligmann M, Bernard J. [Myelomonocytic leukemia in children. Study of 28 cases.] Arch Fr Pediatr 1972; 29:11–30 [French].

40. Castro-Malaspina H, Schaison G, Passe S, Pasquier A, Berger R, Bayle-Weisgerber C, Miller D, Seligmann M, Bernard J. Subacute and chronic myelomonocytic leukemia in children (juvenile CML). Clinical and hematologic observations, and identification of prognostic factors. Cancer 1984; 54:675–686.

41. Brandwein JM, Horsman DE, Eaves AC, Eaves CJ, Massing BG, Wadsworth LD, Rogers PC, Kalousek DK. Childhood myelodysplasia: suggested classification as myelodysplastic syndromes based on laboratory and clinical findings. Am J Pediatr Hematol Oncol 1990; 12:63–70.

42. Chessells JM. Myelodysplasia. Baillières Clin Haematol 1991; 4:459–482.

43. Hasle H, Jacobsen BB, Pedersen NT. Myelodysplastic syndromes in childhood: a population based study of nine cases. Br J Haematol 1992; 81:495–498.

44. Haas OA, Gadner H. Pathogenesis, biology, and management of myelodysplastic syndromes in children. Semin Hematol 1996; 33:225–235.

45. Emanuel PD, Shannon KM, Castleberry RP. Juvenile myelomonocytic leukemia: molecular understanding and prospects for therapy. Mol Med Today 1996; 2:468–475.

46. Aricò M, Biondi A, Pui CH. Juvenile myelomonocytic leukemia. Blood 1997; 90:479–488.

47. Michaux JL, Martiat P. Chronic myelomonocytic leukaemia (CMML)—a myelodysplastic or myeloproliferative syndrome? Leuk Lymphoma 1993; 9:35–41.

48. Jackson GH, Carey PJ, Cant AJ, Bown NP, Reid MM. Myelodysplastic syndromes in children. Br J Haematol 1993; 84:185–186.

49. Niemeyer CM, AricòM, Basso G, Cantù Rajnoldi A, Creutzig U, Haas OA, Harbott J, Hasle H, Kerndrup G, Locatelli F, Mann G, Stollmann-Gibbels B, van't Veer Korthof ET, van Wering ER, Zimmermann M. Chronic myelomonocytic leukemia in childhood: a retrospective analysis of 110 cases. European Working Group on Myelodysplastic Syndromes in Childhood (EWOG-MDS). Blood 1997; 89:3534–3543.

50. Stiller CA, Chessells JM, Fitchett M. Neurofibromatosis and childhood leukaemia/lymphoma: a population based UKCCSG study. Br J Cancer 1994; 70:969–972.

51. Bader-Meunier B, Tchernia G, Mielot F, Fontaine JL, Thomas C, Lyonnet S, La-

vergne JM, Dommergues JP. Occurrence of myeloproliferative disorder in patients with Noonan syndrome. J Pediatr 1997; 130:885–889.

52. Fukuda M, Horibe K, Miyajima Y, Matsumoto K, Nagashima M. Spontaneous remission of juvenile chronic myelomonocytic leukemia in an infant with Noonan syndrome. J Pediatr Hematol Oncol 1997; 19:177–179.

53. Choong K, Freedman MH, Chitayat D, Kelly EN, Taylor G, Zipursky A. Juvenile myelomonocytic leukemia and Noonan syndrome. J Pediatr Hematol Oncol 1999; 21:523–527.

54. Wieland R, Rössler J, Doell C, Niemeyer C, Havers W. Mild course of congenital juvenile myelomonocytic leukemia in an infant with Noonan syndrome. Leukemia 2000; 14:965.

55. Niemeyer CM, Fenu S, Hasle H, Mann G, Stary J, van Wering ER. Differentiating juvenile myelomonocytic leukemia from infectious disease. Blood 1998; 91:365–367.

56. Herrod HG, Dow LW, Sullivan JL. Persistent Epstein-Barr virus infection mimicking juvenile chronic myelogenous leukemia: immunologic and hematologic studies. Blood 1983; 61:1098–1104.

57. Kirby MA, Weitzman S, Freedman MH. Juvenile chronic myelogenous leukemia: differentiation from infantile cytomegalovirus infection. Am J Pediatr Hematol Oncol 1990; 12:292–296.

58. Lorenzana A, Lyons H, Sawaf H, Higgins M, Carrigan D, Emanuel PD. Human herpes virus-6 (HHV-6) infection in an infant mimicking juvenile chronic myelogenous leukemia. J Pediatr Hematol Oncol 1997; 19:370.

59. Yetgin S, Cetin M, Yenicesu I, Ozaltin F, Uckan D. Acute parvovirus B19 infection mimicking juvenile myelomonocytic leukemia. Eur J Haematol 2000; 65:276–278.

60. Kuijpers TW, Van Lier RA, Hamann D, de Boer M, Thung LY, Weening RS, Verhoeven AJ, Roos D. Leukocyte adhesion deficiency type 1 (LAD-1)/variant. A novel immunodeficiency syndrome characterized by dysfunctional beta2 integrins. J Clin Invest 1997; 100:1725–1733.

61. Busque L, Gilliland DG, Prchal JT, Sieff CA, Weinstein HJ, Sokol JM, Belickova M, Wayne AS, Zuckerman KS, Sokol L, Castleberry RP, Emanuel PD. Clonality in juvenile chronic myelogenous leukemia. Blood 1995; 85:21–30.

62. Lapidot T, Grunberger T, Vormoor J, Estrov Z, Kollet O, Bunin N, Zaizov R, Williams DE, Freedman MH. Identification of human juvenile chronic myelogenous leukemia stem cells capable of initiating the disease in primary and secondary SCID mice. Blood 1996; 88:2655–2664.

63. Nakazawa T, Koike K, Agematsu K, Itoh S, Hagimoto R, Kitazawa Y, Higuchi T, Sawai N, Matsui H, Komiyama A. Cytogenetic clonality analysis in monosomy 7 associated with juvenile myelomonocytic leukemia: clonality in B and NK cells, but not in T cells. Leuk Res 1998; 22:887–892.

64. Flotho C, Valcamonica S, Mach-Pascual S, Schmahl G, Corral L, Ritterbach J, Hasle H, Arico M, Biondi A, Niemeyer CM. RAS mutations and clonality analysis in children with juvenile myelomonocytic leukemia (JMML). Leukemia 1999; 13: 32–37.

65. Cooper LJN, Shannon KM, Loken MR, Weaver M, Stephens K, Sievers EL. Evi-

dence that juvenile myelomonocytic leukemia can arise from a pluripotential stem cell. Blood 2000; 96:2310–2313.

66. Altman AJ, Palmer CG, Baehner RL. Juvenile ''chronic granulocytic'' leukemia: a panmyelopathy with prominent monocytic involvement and circulating monocyte colony-forming cells. Blood 1974; 43:341–350.

67. Barak Y, Levin S, Vogel R, Cohen IJ, Wallach B, Nir E, Zaizov R. Juvenile and adult types of chronic granulocytic leukemia of childhood: growth patterns and characteristics of granulocyte-macrophage colony forming cells. Am J Hematol 1981; 10:269–275.

68. Estrov Z, Zimmerman B, Grunberger T, Chao J, Teshima IE, Chan HS, Freedman MH. Characterization of malignant peripheral blood cells of juvenile chronic myelogenous leukemia. Cancer Res 1986; 46:6456–6461.

69. Bagby GC Jr, Dinarello CA, Neerhout RC, Ridgway D, McCall E. Interleukin 1-dependent paracrine granulopoiesis in chronic granulocytic leukemia of the juvenile type. J Clin Invest 1988; 82:1430–1436.

70. Gualtieri RJ, Emanuel PD, Zuckerman KS, Martin G, Clark SC, Shadduck RK, Dracker RA, Akabutu J, Nitschke R, Hetherington ML, et al. Granulocyte-macrophage colony-stimulating factor is an endogenous regulator of cell proliferation in juvenile chronic myelogenous leukemia. Blood 1989; 74:2360–2367.

71. Freedman MH, Cohen A, Grunberger T, Bunin N, Luddy RE, Saunders EF, Shahidi N, Lau A, Estrov Z. Central role of tumour necrosis factor, GM-CSF, and interleukin 1 in the pathogenesis of juvenile chronic myelogenous leukaemia. Br J Haematol 1992; 80:40–48.

72. Schiro R, Longoni D, Rossi V, Maglia O, Doni A, Arsura M, Carrara G, Masera G, Vannier E, Dinarello CA, et al. Suppression of juvenile chronic myelogenous leukemia colony growth by interleukin-1 receptor antagonist. Blood 1994; 83:460–465.

73. Emanuel PD, Bates LJ, Zhu SW, Castleberry RP, Gualtieri RJ, Zuckerman KS. The role of monocyte-derived hemopoietic growth factors in the regulation of myeloproliferation in juvenile chronic myelogenous leukemia. Exp Hematol 1991; 19:1017–1024.

74. Iversen PO, Sioud M. Modulation of granulocyte-macrophage colony-stimulating factor gene expression by a tumor necrosis factor specific ribozyme in juvenile myelomonocytic leukemic cells. Blood 1998; 92:4263–4268.

75. Kochetkova M, Iversen PO, Lopez AF, Shannon MF. Deoxyribonucleic acid triplex formation inhibits granulocyte macrophage colony-stimulating factor gene expression and suppresses growth in juvenile myelomonocytic leukemic cells. J Clin Invest 1997; 99:3000–3008.

76. Emanuel PD, Bates LJ, Castleberry RP, Gualtieri RJ, Zuckerman KS. Selective hypersensitivity to granulocyte-macrophage colony-stimulating factor by juvenile chronic myeloid leukemia hematopoietic progenitors. Blood 1991; 77:925–929.

77. Frankel AE, Lilly M, Kreitman R, Hogge D, Beran M, Freedman MH, Emanuel PD, McLain C, Hall P, Tagge E, Berger M, Eaves C. Diphtheria toxin fused to granulocyte-macrophage colony-stimulating factor is toxic to blasts from patients with juvenile myelomonocytic leukemia and chronic myelomonocytic leukemia. Blood 1998; 92:4279–4286.

78. Iversen PO, Rodwell RL, Pitcher L, Taylor KM, Lopez AF. Inhibition of proliferation and induction of apoptosis in juvenile myelomonocytic leukemic cells by the granulocyte-macrophage colony-stimulating factor analogue E21R. Blood 1996; 88:2634–2639.

79. Iversen PO, Lewis ID, Turczynowicz S, Hasle H, Niemeyer C, Schmiegelow K, Bastiras S, Biondi A, Hughes TP, Lopez AF. Inhibition of granulocyte-macrophage colony-stimulating factor prevents dissemination and induces remission of human juvenile myelomonocytic leukemia in engrafted immunodeficient mice. Blood 1997; 90:4910–4917.

80. Sawai N, Koike K, Ito S, Okumura N, Kamijo T, Shiohara M, Amano Y, Tsuji K, Nakahata T, Oda M. Aberrant growth of granulocyte-macrophage progenitors in juvenile chronic myelogenous leukemia in serum-free culture. Exp Hematol 1996; 24:116–122.

81. Freeburn RW, Gale RE, Wagner HM, Linch DC. Analysis of the coding sequence for the GM-CSF receptor alpha and beta chains in patients with juvenile chronic myeloid leukemia (JCML). Exp Hematol 1997; 25:306–311.

82. Barbacid M. Ras oncogenes: their role in neoplasia (review). Eur J Clin Invest 1990; 20:225–235.

83. Miyauchi J, Asada M, Sasaki M, Tsunematsu Y, Kojima S, Mizutani S. Mutations of the N-*ras* gene in juvenile chronic myelogenous leukemia. Blood 1994; 83: 2248–2254.

84. Kalra R, Paderanga DC, Olson K, Shannon KM. Genetic analysis is consistent with the hypothesis that NF1 limits myeloid cell growth through p21ras. Blood 1994; 84:3435–3439.

85. Bader JL, Miller RW. Neurofibromatosis and childhood leukemia. J Pediatr 1978; 92:925–929.

86. Side LE, Emanuel PD, Taylor B, Franklin J, Thompson P, Castleberry RP, Shannon KM. Mutations of the NF1 gene in children with juvenile myelomonocytic leukemia without clinical evidence of neurofibromatosis, type 1. Blood 1998; 92:267–272.

87. Watanabe I, Horiuchi T, Hatta N, Matsumoto M, Koike K, Kojima S, Ohga S, Fujita S. Analysis of neurofibromatosis type 1 gene mutation in juvenile chronic myelogenous leukemia. Acta Haematol 1998; 100:22–25.

88. Shannon KM, O'Connell P, Martin GA, Paderanga D, Olson K, Dinndorf P, McCormick F. Loss of the normal NF1 allele from the bone marrow of children with type 1 neurofibromatosis and malignant myeloid disorders. N Engl J Med 1994; 330:597–601.

89. Side L, Taylor B, Cayouette M, Conner E, Thompson P, Luce M, Shannon K. Homozygous inactivation of the NF1 gene in bone marrow cells from children with neurofibromatosis type 1 and malignant myeloid disorders. N Engl J Med 1997; 336:1713–1720.

90. Bollag G, Clapp DW, Shih S, Adler F, Zhang YY, Thompson P, Lange BJ, Freedman MH, McCormick F, Jacks T, Shannon K. Loss of NF1 results in activation of the Ras signaling pathway and leads to aberrant growth in haematopoietic cells. Nat Genet 1996; 12:144–148.

91. Largaespada DA, Brannan CI, Jenkins NA, Copeland NG. Nf1 deficiency causes

Ras-mediated granulocyte/macrophage colony stimulating factor hypersensitivity and chronic myeloid leukaemia. Nat Genet 1996; 12:137–143.

92. Hiatt KK, Ingram DA, Zhang Y, Bollag G, Clapp DW. Neurofibromin GTPase-activating protein-related domains restore normal growth in Nf1 −/− cells. J Biol Chem 2001; 276:7240–7245.

93. Zhang YY, Vik TA, Ryder JW, Srour EF, Jacks T, Shannon K, Clapp DW. Nf1 regulates hematopoietic progenitor cell growth and ras signaling in response to multiple cytokines. J Exp Med 1998; 187:1893–1902.

94. Emanuel PD, Snyder RC, Wiley T, Gopurala B, Castleberry RP. Inhibition of juvenile myelomonocytic leukemia cell growth in vitro by farnesyltransferase inhibitors. Blood 2000; 95:639–645.

95. Mahgoub N, Taylor BR, Gratiot M, Kohl NE, Gibbs JB, Jacks T, Shannon KM. In vitro and in vivo effects of a farnesyltransferase inhibitor on Nf1-deficient hematopoietic cells. Blood 1999; 94:2469–2476.

96. Okamura J, Ohara A, Kigasawa H, Asami K, Mabuchi O, Yabe M, Manabe A, Kojima S, Tsuchida M, Hayashi Y, Ikuta K, Koike K, Akiyama Y, Hara J, Ikushima S, Nakahata T. The blastic transformation of juvenile myelomonocytic leukemia. Leukemia 2000; 14:967.

97. Greenberg P, Cox C, Le Beau MM, Fenaux P, Morel P, Sanz G, Sanz M, Vallespi T, Hamblin T, Oscier D, Ohyashiki K, Toyama K, Aul C, Mufti G, Bennett J. International scoring system for evaluating prognosis in myelodysplastic syndromes. Blood 1997; 89:2079–2088.

98. Hasle H, Fenu S, Kardos G, Kerndrup G, Mann G, Rogge T, Schultz KR, Stary J, Wadsworth LD, van Wering ER, Harbott J, Nöllke P, Niemeyer CM. International prognostic scoring system for childhood MDS and JMML. Leukemia 2000; 14: 968.

99. Lilleyman JS, Harrison JF, Black JA. Treatment of juvenile chronic myeloid leukemia with sequential subcutaneous cytarabine and oral mercaptopurine. Blood 1977; 49:559–562.

100. Castleberry RP, Emanuel PD, Zuckerman KS, Cohn S, Strauss L, Byrd RL, Homans A, Chaffee S, Nitschke R, Gualtieri RJ. A pilot study of isotretinoin in the treatment of juvenile chronic myelogenous leukemia. N Engl J Med 1994; 331: 1680–1684.

101. Sanders JE, Buckner CD, Thomas ED, Fleischer R, Sullivan KM, Appelbaum FA, Storb R. Allogeneic marrow transplantation for children with juvenile chronic myelogenous leukemia. Blood 1988; 71:1144–1146.

102. Bunin NJ, Casper JT, Lawton C, Murray K, Camitta BM, Greenwood M, Geil J, Ash RC. Allogeneic marrow transplantation using T cell depletion for patients with juvenile chronic myelogenous leukemia without HLA-identical siblings. Bone Marrow Transplant 1992; 9:119–122.

103. Donadieu J, Stephan JL, Blanche S, Cavazzana-Calvo M, Baruchel A, Herbelin C, Benkerrou M, Thomas C, Girault D, Fischer A. Treatment of juvenile chronic myelomonocytic leukemia by allogeneic bone marrow transplantation. Bone Marrow Transplant 1994; 13:777–782.

104. Lutz P, Zix-Kieffer I, Souillet G, Bertrand Y, Dhooge C, Rubie C, Mazingue F, Marguerite F, Machinaud-Lacroix F, Rialland X, Plouvier E, Behar C, Vilmer E,

Philippe N, Otten J. Juvenile myelomonocytic leukemia: analyses of treatment results in the EORTC Children's Leukemia Cooperative Group (CLCG). Bone Marrow Transplant 1996; 18:1111–1116.

105. Locatelli F, Niemeyer C, Angelucci E, Bender-Götze C, Burdach S, Ebell W, Friedrich W, Hasle H, Hermann J, Jacobsen N, Klingebiel T, Kremens B, Mann G, Pession A, Peters C, Schmid HJ, Stary J, Suttorp M, Uderzo C, van't Veer-Korthof ET, Vossen J, Zecca M, Zimmermann M. Allogeneic bone marrow transplantation for chronic myelomonocytic leukemia in childhood: a report from the European Working Group on Myelodysplastic Syndrome in Childhood. J Clin Oncol 1997; 15:566–573.

106. Matthes-Martin S, Mann G, Peters C, Lion T, Fritsch G, Haas OA, Pötschger U, Gadner H. Allogeneic bone marrow transplantation for juvenile myelomonocytic leukaemia: a single centre experience and review of the literature. Bone Marrow Transplant 2000; 26:377–382.

107. Orchard PJ, Miller JS, McGlennen R, Davies SM, Ramsay NK. Graft-versus-leukemia is sufficient to induce remission in juvenile myelomonocytic leukemia. Bone Marrow Transplant 1998; 22:201–203.

108. MacMillan ML, Davies SM, Orchard PJ, Ramsay NK, Wagner JE. Haemopoietic cell transplantation in children with juvenile myelomonocytic leukaemia. Br J Haematol 1998; 103:552–558.

109. Locatelli F, Zecca M, Duffner U, Bender-Götze C, Dini G, Ebell W, Hoogerbrugge PM, Klingebiel T, Kremens B, Messina C, Nöllke P, Nürnberger W, Pession A, Peters C, Souliet G, Stary J, Uderzo C, Zimmermann M, Zintl F. Busulfan, cyclophosphamide and melphalan as pretransplant conditioning regimen for children with MDS and JMML. Interim analysis of the EWOG-MDS/EBMT prospective study. Leukemia 2000; 14:971.

110. Hasle H, Clemmensen IH, Mikkelsen M. Risks of leukaemia and solid tumours in individuals with Down's syndrome. Lancet 2000; 355:165–169.

111. Zipursky A, Brown E, Christensen H, Sutherland R, Doyle J. Leukemia and/or myeloproliferative syndrome in neonates with Down syndrome. Semin Perinatol 1997; 21:97–101.

112. Homans AC, Verissimo AM, Vlacha V. Transient abnormal myelopoiesis of infancy associated with trisomy 21. Am J Pediatr Hematol Oncol 1993; 15:392–399.

113. Lange B. The management of neoplastic disorders of haematopoiesis in children with Down's syndrome. Br J Haematol 2000; 110:512–524.

114. Miller RW, Shurin SB. Neonatal myeloproliferative disorder in Down syndrome: transient or preleukemic? Proc ASPHO 1994; 3:24–24.

115. Matzke E, Winkler K, Grosch-Worner I, Marsmann G, Landbeck G, Fischer K, Poschmann A. [Juvenile chronic myeloid leukemia (JCML) case history and follow up studies on 9 patients.] Klin Pädiatr 1980; 192:157–168 [German].

116. Crombet O, Svarch E. Down syndrome and juvenile myelomonocytic leukemia. Pediatr Hematol Oncol 1999; 16:181–182.

117. Zipursky A, Thorner P, De Harven E, Christensen H, Doyle J. Myelodysplasia and acute megakaryoblastic leukemia in Down's syndrome. Leuk Res 1994; 18:163–171.

118. Creutzig U, Ritter J, Vormoor J, Ludwig WD, Niemeyer C, Reinisch I, Stollmann-Gibbels B, Zimmermann M, Harbott J. Myelodysplasia and acute myelogenous leukemia in Down's syndrome. A report of 40 children of the AML-BFM Study Group. Leukemia 1996; 10:1677–1686.

119. Sato A, Imaizumi M, Koizumi Y, Obara Y, Nakai H, Noro T, Saito T, Saisho T, Yoshinari M, Cui Y, Suzuki H, Funato T, Iinuma K. Acute myelogenous leukaemia with t(8;21) translocation of normal cell origin in mosaic Down's syndrome with isochromosome 21q. Br J Haematol 1997; 96:614–616.

120. Litz CE, Davies S, Brunning RD, Kueck B, Parkin JL, Gajl Peczalska K, Arthur DC. Acute leukemia and the transient myeloproliferative disorder associated with Down syndrome: morphologic, immunophenotypic and cytogenetic manifestations. Leukemia 1995; 9:1432–1439.

121. Kojima S, Sako M, Kato K, Hosoi G, Sato T, Ohara A, Koike K, Okimoto Y, Nishimura S, Akiyama Y, Yoshikawa T, Ishii E, Okamura J, Yazaki M, Hayashi Y, Eguchi M, Tsukimoto I, Ueda K. An effective chemotherapeutic regimen for acute myeloid leukemia and myelodysplastic syndrome in children with Down's syndrome. Leukemia 2000; 14:786–791.

122. Craze JL, Harrison G, Wheatley K, Hann IM, Chessells JM. Improved outcome of acute myeloid leukaemia in Down's syndrome. Arch Dis Child 1999; 81:32–37.

123. Teigler-Schlegel A, Baumann I, Creutzig U, Niemeyer C, Harbott J. Acquired chromosome aberrations in children with Down syndrome and myelodysplastic syndrome or acute myeloid leukemia. Leukemia 2000; 14:966.

124. Trejo RM, Aguilera RP, Nieto S, Kofman S. A t(1;22)(p13;q13) in four children with acute megakaryoblastic leukemia (M7), two with Down syndrome. Cancer Genet Cytogenet 2000; 120:160–162.

125. Zipursky A, Wang H, Brown EJ, Squire J. Interphase cytogenetic analysis of in vivo differentiation in the myelodysplasia of Down syndrome. Blood 1994; 84:2278–2282.

126. Slørdahl SH, Smeland EB, Holte H, Grønn M, Lie SO, Seip M. Leukemic blasts with markers of four cell lineages in Down's syndrome (''megakaryoblastic leukemia''). Med Pediatr Oncol 1993; 21:254–258.

127. Ravindranath Y, Abella E, Krischer JP, Wiley J, Inoue S, Harris M, Chauvenet A, Alvarado CS, Dubowy R, Ritchey AK, Land V, Steuber CP, Weinstein H. Acute myeloid leukemia (AML) in Down's syndrome is highly responsive to chemotherapy: experience on Pediatric Oncology Group AML Study 8498. Blood 1992; 80:2210–2214.

128. Lie SO, Jonmundsson G, Mellander L, Siimes MA, Yssing M, Gustafsson G. A population-based study of 272 children with acute myeloid leukaemia treated on two consecutive protocols with different intensity: best outcome in girls, infants, and children with Down's syndrome. Nordic Society of Paediatric Haematology and Oncology (NOPHO). Br J Haematol 1996; 94:82–88.

129. Taub JW, Huang X, Matherly LH, Stout ML, Buck SA, Massey GV, Becton DL, Chang MN, Weinstein HJ, Ravindranath Y. Expression of chromosome 21-localized genes in acute myeloid leukemia: differences between Down syndrome and

non-Down syndrome blast cells and relationship to in vitro sensitivity to cytosine arabinoside and daunorubicin. Blood 1999; 94:1393–1400.

130. Hasle H, Clausen N, Pedersen B, Bendix-Hansen K. Myelodysplastic syndrome in a child with constitutional trisomy 8 mosaicism and normal phenotype. Cancer Genet Cytogenet 1995; 79:79–81.

131. Brady AF, Waters CS, Pocha MJ, Brueton LA. Chronic myelomonocytic leukaemia in a child with constitutional partial trisomy 8 mosaicism. Clin Genet 2000; 58: 142–146.

132. Butturini A, Gale RP, Verlander PC, Adler-Brecher B, Gillio AP, Auerbach AD. Hematologic abnormalities in Fanconi anemia: an International Fanconi Anemia Registry study. Blood 1994; 84:1650–1655.

133. Auerbach AD, Allen RG. Leukemia and preleukemia in Fanconi anemia patients. A review of the literature and report of the International Fanconi Anemia Registry. Cancer Genet Cytogenet 1991; 51:1–12.

134. Maarek O, Jonveaux P, Le Coniat M, Derre J, Berger R. Fanconi anemia and bone marrow clonal chromosome abnormalities. Leukemia 1996; 10:1700–1704.

135. Freedman MH, Bonilla MA, Fier C, Bolyard AA, Scarlata D, Boxer LA, Brown S, Cham B, Kannourakis G, Kinsey SE, Mori PG, Cottle T, Welte K, Dale DC. Myelodysplasia syndrome and acute myeloid leukemia in patients with congenital neutropenia receiving G-CSF therapy. Blood 2000; 96:429–436.

136. Tidow N, Pilz C, Teichmann B, Muller-Brechlin A, Germeshausen M, Kasper B, Rauprich P, Sykora KW, Welte K. Clinical relevance of point mutations in the cytoplasmic domain of the granulocyte colony-stimulating factor receptor gene in patients with severe congenital neutropenia. Blood 1997; 89:2369–2375.

137. Smith OP, Hann IM, Chessells JM, Reeves BR, Milla P. Haematological abnormalities in Shwachman-Diamond syndrome. Br J Haematol 1996; 94:279–284.

138. van Dijken PJ, Verwijs W. Diamond-Blackfan anemia and malignancy. A case report and a review of the literature. Cancer 1995; 76:517–520.

139. Dokal I. Dyskeratosis congenita in all its forms. Br J Haematol 2000; 110:768–779.

140. Socie G, Henry-Amar M, Bacigalupo A, Hows J, Tichelli A, Ljungman P, McCann SR, Frickhofen N, Van't Veer-Korthof E, Gluckman E. Malignant tumors occurring after treatment of aplastic anemia. European Bone Marrow Transplantation-Severe Aplastic Anaemia Working Party. N Engl J Med 1993; 329:1152–1157.

141. Ohara A, Kojima S, Hamajima N, Tsuchida M, Imashuku S, Ohta S, Sasaki H, Okamura J, Sugita K, Kigasawa H, Kiriyama Y, Akatsuka J, Tsukimoto I. Myelodysplastic syndrome and acute myelogenous leukemia as a late clonal complication in children with acquired aplastic anemia. Blood 1997; 90:1009–1013.

142. Führer M, Rampf U, Burdach S, Dörffel W, Ebell W, Friedrich W, Haas R, Klingebiel T, Niemeyer C, Ritter J, Sörensen J, Stollmann-Gibbels B, Walther JU, Zeidler C, Bender-Götze C. Immunosuppresive therapy and bone marrow transplantation for aplastic anemia in children: results of the study SAA 94. Blood 1998; 92:156a.

143. Führer M, Burdach S, Ebell W, Gadner H, Haas R, Harbott J, Janka-Schaub G, Klingebiel T, Kremens B, Niemeyer C, Rampf U, Reiter A, Ritter J, Schulz A,

Walther U, Zeidler C, Bender-Götze C. Relapse and clonal disease in children with aplastic anemia (AA) after immunosuppressive therapy (IST): the SAA 94 experience. German/Austrian Pediatric Aplastic Anemia Working Group. Klin Pädiatr 1998; 210:173–179.

144. Locasciulli A, Arcese W, Locatelli F, Di Bona E, Bacigalupo A. Treatment of aplastic anaemia with granulocyte-colony stimulating factor and risk of malignancy. Italian Aplastic Anaemia Study Group. Lancet 2001; 357:43–44.

145. Kojima S, Hibi S, Kosaka Y, Yamamoto M, Tsuchida M, Mugishima H, Sugita K, Yabe H, Ohara A, Tsukimoto I. Immunosuppressive therapy using antithymocyte globulin, cyclosporine, and danazol with or without human granulocyte colony-stimulating factor in children with acquired aplastic anemia. Blood 2000; 96:2049–2054.

146. Carroll WL, Morgan R, Glader BE. Childhood bone marrow monosomy 7 syndrome: a familial disorder? J Pediatr 1985; 107:578–580.

147. Shannon KM, Turhan AG, Chang SS, Bowcock AM, Rogers PC, Carroll WL, Cowan MJ, Glader BE, Eaves CJ, Eaves AC, Kan YW. Familial bone marrow monosomy 7. Evidence that the predisposing locus is not on the long arm of chromosome 7. J Clin Invest 1989; 84:984–989.

148. Gilchrist DM, Friedman JM, Rogers PC, Creighton SP. Myelodysplasia and leukemia syndrome with monosomy 7: a genetic perspective. Am J Med Genet 1990; 35:437–441.

149. Luna-Fineman S, Shannon KM, Lange BJ. Childhood monosomy 7: epidemiology, biology, and mechanistic implications. Blood 1995; 85:1985–1999.

150. Hasle H, Olsen JH. Cancer in relatives of children with myelodysplastic syndrome, acute and chronic myeloid leukaemia. Br J Haematol 1997; 97:127–131.

151. Mijovic A, Antunovic P, Pagliuca A, Mufti GJ. Familial myelodysplastic syndromes: a key to understanding leukaemogenesis? Leuk Res 1997; 21(suppl 1):S6.

152. Hasle H, Olsen JH, Hansen J, Friedrich U, Tommerup N. Occurrence of cancer in a cohort of 183 persons with constitutional chromosome 7 abnormalities. Cancer Genet Cytogenet 1998; 105:39–42.

153. Minelli A, Maserati E, Giudici G, Tosi S, Olivieri C, Bonvini L, De Filippi P, Biondi A, Lo Curto F, Pasquali F, Danesino C. Familial partial monosomy 7 and myelodysplasia: different parental origin of the monosomy 7 suggests action of a mutator gene. Cancer Genet Cytogenet 2001; 124:147–151.

154. Pui CH, Hancock ML, Raimondi SC, Head DR, Thompson E, Wilimas J, Kun LE, Bowman LC, Crist WM, Pratt CB. Myeloid neoplasia in children treated for solid tumours. Lancet 1990; 336:417–421.

155. Pui CH, Ribeiro RC, Hancock ML, Rivera GK, Evans WE, Raimondi SC, Head DR, Behm FG, Mahmoud MH, Sandlund JT, Crist WM. Acute myeloid leukemia in children treated with epipodophyllotoxins for acute lymphoblastic leukemia. N Engl J Med 1991; 325:1682–1687.

156. Rubin CM, Arthur DC, Woods WG, Lange BJ, Nowell PC, Rowley JD, Nachman J, Bostrom B, Baum ES, Suarez CR, Shah NR, Morgan E, Maurer HS, McKenzie S, Larson RA, Le Beau MM. Therapy-related myelodysplastic syndrome and acute myeloid leukemia in children: correlation between chromosomal abnormalities and prior therapy. Blood 1991; 78:2982–2988.

157. Hayani A, Mahoney DH Jr, Taylor LD. Therapy-related myelodysplastic syndrome in children with medulloblastoma following MOPP chemotherapy. J Neurooncol 1992; 14:57–62.

158. Levine EG, Bloomfield CD. Leukemias and myelodysplastic syndromes secondary to drug, radiation, and environmental exposure. Semin Oncol 1992; 19:47–84.

159. Pedersen-Bjergaard J, Philip P, Larsen SO, Andersson M, Daugaard G, Ersboll J, Hansen SW, Hou-Jensen K, Nielsen D, Sigsgaard TC, et al. Therapy-related myelodysplasia and acute myeloid leukemia. Cytogenetic characteristics of 115 consecutive cases and risk in seven cohorts of patients treated intensively for malignant diseases in the Copenhagen series. Leukemia 1993; 7:1975–1986.

160. Pedersen-Bjergaard J, Rowley JD. The balanced and the unbalanced chromosome aberrations of acute myeloid leukemia may develop in different ways and may contribute differently to malignant transformation. Blood 1994; 83:2780–2786.

161. Davies SM. Therapy-related leukemia: is the risk life-long and can we identify patients at greatest risk? J Pediatr Hematol Oncol 2000; 22:302–305.

162. Sasaki H, Manabe A, Kojima S, Tsuchida M, Hayashi Y, Ikuta K, Okamura J, Koike K, Ohara A, Ishii E, Komada Y, Hibi S, Nakahata T. Myelodysplastic syndromes in childhood: a retrospective study in Japan. Leukemia 2000; 14:968.

163. Rodriguez-Galindo C, Poquette CA, Marina NM, Head DR, Cain A, Meyer WH, Santana VM, Pappo AS. Hematologic abnormalities and acute myeloid leukemia in children and adolescents administered intensified chemotherapy for the Ewing sarcoma family of tumors. J Pediatr Hematol Oncol 2000; 22:321–329.

164. Tefferi A, Thibodeau SN, Solberg LA Jr. Clonal studies in the myelodysplastic syndrome using X-linked restriction fragment length polymorphisms. Blood 1990; 75:1770–1773.

165. van Lom K, Hagemeijer A, Smith EME, Hahlen K, Groeneveld K, Löwenberg B. Cytogenetic clonality analysis in myelodysplastic syndrome: monosomy 7 can be demonstrated in the myeloid and in the lymphoid lineage. Leukemia 1995; 9:1818–1821.

166. Busque L, Gilliland DG. X-inactivation analysis in the 1990s: promise and potential problems. Leukemia 1998; 12:128–135.

167. Head DR. Revised classification of acute myeloid leukemia. Leukemia 1996; 10:1826–1831.

168. Neubauer A, Shannon K, Liu E. Mutations of the ras proto-oncogenes in childhood monosomy 7. Blood 1991; 77:594–598.

169. Paquette RL, Landaw EM, Pierre RV, Kahan J, Lübbert M, Lazcano O, Isaac G, McCormick F, Koeffler HP. N-ras mutations are associated with poor prognosis and increased risk of leukemia in myelodysplastic syndrome. Blood 1993; 82:590–599.

170. Misawa S, Horiike S, Kaneko H, Sasai Y, Ueda Y, Nakao M, Yokota S, Taniwaki M, Fujii H, Nakagawa H, Tsuda S, Kashima K. Significance of chromosomal alterations and mutations of the N-RAS and TP53 genes in relation to leukemogenesis of acute myeloid leukemia. Leuk Res 1998; 22:631–637.

171. Tamaki H, Ogawa H, Ohyashiki K, Ohyashiki JH, Iwama H, Inoue K, Soma T, Oka Y, Tatekawa T, Oji Y, Tsuboi A, Kim EH, Kawakami M, Fuchigami K, Tomonaga M, Toyama K, Aozasa K, Kishimoto T, Sugiyama H. The Wilms' tumor gene

WT1 is a good marker for diagnosis of disease progression of myelodysplastic syndromes. Leukemia 1999; 13:393–399.

172. Kardos G, Baumann I, Fenu S, Harbott J, Hasle H, Kerndrup G, Mann G, Niemeyer C, Rogge T, Schmitt-Gräff A, Schultz KR, Sianati L, Slater R, Stary J, Wadsworth LD, van Wering ER, Zimmermann M. Refractory anemia in childhood: a study of the European working group of MDS in childhood (EWOG-MDS). Leukemia 2000; 14:967.

173. Creutzig U, Cantù-Rajnoldi A, Ritter J, Romitti L, Odenwald E, Conter V, Riehm H, Masera G. Myelodysplastic syndromes in childhood. Report of 21 patients from Italy and West Germany. Am J Pediatr Hematol Oncol 1987; 9:324–330.

174. Cantù-Rajnoldi A, Baumann I, Fenu S, Kerndrup G, van Wering ER. Proposals of the EWOG-MDS pathology board for the evaluation of dysplastic findings on bone marrow aspirates. Leuk Res 1999; 23(suppl 1):S52.

175. Rogge T, Niemeyer CM. Myelodysplastic syndromes in childhood. Onkologie 2000; 23:18–24.

176. Rosati S, Anastasi J, Vardiman J. Recurring diagnostic problems in the pathology of the myelodysplastic syndromes. Semin Hematol 1996; 33:111–126.

177. Groupe Francais de Cytogénétique Hématologique. Forty-four cases of childhood myelodysplasia with cytogenetics, documented by the Groupe Francais de Cytogénétique Hématologique. Leukemia 1997; 11:1478–1485.

178. Grimwade D, Walker H, Oliver F, Wheatley K, Harrison C, Harrison G, Rees J, Hann I, Stevens R, Burnett A, Goldstone A. The importance of diagnostic cytogenetics on outcome in AML: analysis of 1,612 patients entered into the MRC AML 10 trial. The Medical Research Council Adult and Children's Leukaemia Working Parties. Blood 1998; 92:2322–2333.

179. Martinez-Climent JA, García-Conde J. Chromosome rearrangements in childhood acute myeloid leukemias and myelodysplastic syndromes. J Pediatr Hematol Oncol 1999; 21:91–102.

180. Leverger G, Bernheim A, Daniel MT, Flandrin G, Schaison G, Berger R. Cytogenetic study of 130 childhood acute nonlymphocytic leukemias. Med Pediatr Oncol 1988; 16:227–232.

181. Kalwinsky DK, Raimondi SC, Schell MJ, Mirro J Jr, Santana VM, Behm F, Dahl GV, Williams D. Prognostic importance of cytogenetic subgroups in de novo pediatric acute nonlymphocytic leukemia. J Clin Oncol 1990; 8:75–83.

182. Woods WG, Kobrinsky N, Buckley JD, Lee JW, Sanders J, Neudorf S, Gold S, Barnard DR, DeSwarte J, Dusenbery K, Kalousek D, Arthur DC, Lange BJ. Timed-sequential induction therapy improves postremission outcome in acute myeloid leukemia: a report from the Children's Cancer Group. Blood 1996; 87:4979–4989.

183. Chan GCF, Wang WC, Raimondi SC, Behm FG, Krance RA, Chen G, Freiberg A, Ingram L, Butler D, Head DR. Myelodysplastic syndrome in children: differentiation from acute myeloid leukemia with a low blast count. Leukemia 1997; 11: 206–211.

184. Xue Y, Yu F, Zhou Z, Guo Y, Xie X, Lin B. Translocation (8;21) in oligoblastic leukemia: is this a true myelodysplastic syndrome? Leuk Res 1994; 18:761–765.

185. Taj AS, Ross FM, Vickers M, Choudhury DN, Harvey JF, Barber JCK, Barton C,

Smith AG. t(8;21) myelodysplasia, an early presentation of M2 AML. Br J Haematol 1995; 89:890–892.

186. Hasle H, Kerndrup G, Yssing M, Clausen N, ⊆stergaard E, Jacobsen N, Jacobsen BB. Intensive chemotherapy in childhood myelodysplastic syndrome. A comparison with results in acute myeloid leukemia. Leukemia 1996; 10:1269–1273.

187. Malkin D, Freedman MH. Childhood erythroleukemia: review of clinical and biological features. Am J Pediatr Hematol Oncol 1989; 11:348–359.

188. Michiels JJ. Erythroleukemia and myelodysplastic syndromes: an historical appraisal and a personal view. Leuk Lymphoma 1993; 9:27–34.

189. Ribeiro RC, Oliveira MS, Fairclough D, Hurwitz CA, Mirro J, Behm FG, Head D, Silva ML, Raimondi SC, Crist WM, et al. Acute megakaryoblastic leukemia in children and adolescents: a retrospective analysis of 24 cases. Leuk Lymphoma 1993; 10:299–306.

190. Woods WG, Nesbit ME, Buckley J, Lampkin BC, McCreadie S, Kim TH, Piomelli S, Kersey JH, Feig S, Bernstein I, Hammond D, the Children's Cancer Study Group. Correlation of chromosome abnormalities with patient characteristics, histologic subtype, and induction success in children with acute nonlymphocytic leukemia. J Clin Oncol 1985; 3:3–11.

191. Bennett JM, Catovsky D, Daniel MT, Flandrin G, Galton DA, Gralnick HR, Sultan C. Criteria for the diagnosis of acute leukemia of megakaryocyte lineage (M7). A report of the French-American-British Cooperative Group. Ann Intern Med 1985; 103:460–462.

192. Carroll A, Civin C, Schneider N, Dahl G, Pappo A, Bowman P, Emami A, Gross S, Alvarado C, Phillips C, Krischer J, Crist W, Head D, Gresik M, Ravindranath Y, Weinstein H. The t(1;22)(p13;q13) is nonrandom and restricted to infants with acute megakaryoblastic leukemia: a Pediatric Oncology Group study. Blood 1991; 78:748–752.

193. Lion T, Haas OA, Harbott J, Bannier E, Ritterbach J, Jankovic M, Fink FM, Stojimirovic A, Hermann J, Riehm HJ, Lampert F, Ritter J, Koch H, Gadner H. The translocation t(1;22)(p13;q13) is a nonrandom marker specifically associated with acute megakaryocytic leukemia in young children. Blood 1992; 79:3325–3330.

194. Lu G, Altman AJ, Benn PA. Review of the cytogenetic changes in acute megakaryoblastic leukemia: one disease or several? Cancer Genet Cytogenet 1993; 67:81–89.

195. Imamura M, Kobayashi M, Kobayashi S, Yoshida K, Mikuni C, Ishikawa Y, Matsumoto S, Sakamaki S, Niitsu Y, Hinoda Y, et al. Failure of combination therapy with recombinant granulocyte colony-stimulating factor and erythropoietin in myelodysplastic syndromes. Ann Hematol 1994; 68:163–166.

196. Bartl R, Frisch B, Baumgart R. Morphologic classification of the myelodysplastic syndromes (MDS): combined utilization of bone marrow aspirates and trephine biopsies. Leuk Res 1992; 16:15–33.

197. Mangi MH, Mufti GJ. Primary myelodysplatic syndromes: diagnostic and prognostic significance of immunohistochemical assessment of bone marrow biopsies. Blood 1992; 79:198–205.

198. Nair R, Athale UA, Iyer RS, Nair CN, Pai SK, Kurkure PA, Kadam PR, Advani

SH. Childhood myelodysplastic syndromes: clinical features, cytogenetics and prognosis. Indian J Pediatr 1992; 59:443–448.

199. Tuncer MA, Pagliuca A, Hicsönmez G, Yetgin S, Ozsoylu S, Mufti GJ. Primary myelodysplastic syndrome in children: the clinical experience in 33 cases. Br J Haematol 1992; 82:347–353.

200. Mansoor AM, Bharadwaj TP, Sethuraman S, Chandy M, Pushpa V, Kamada N, Murthy PB. Analysis of karyotype, SCE, and point mutation of RAS oncogene in Indian MDS patients. Cancer Genet Cytogenet 1993; 65:12–20.

201. Kardos G, Baumann I, Fenu S, Harbott J, Hasle H, Kerndrup G, Mann G, Niemeyer C, Rogge T, Schmitt-Gräff A, Sianati L, Slater R, Stary J, van Wering ER, Zimmermann M. Refractory anemia in childhood: a study of the European working group of MDS in childhood (EWOG-MDS). Blood 1998; 92:629a.

202. Fohlmeister I, Fischer R, Mödder B, Rister M, Schaefer HE. Aplastic anemia and the hypocellular myelodysplastic syndrome: histomorphological diagnostic, and prognostic features. J Clin Pathol 1985; 38:1218–1224.

203. Elghetany MT, Hudnall SD, Gardner FH. Peripheral blood picture in primary hypocellular refractory anemia and idiopathic acquired aplastic anemia: an additional tool for differential diagnosis. Haematologica 1997; 82:21–24.

204. Baumann I, Führer M, Bender-Götze C, Rogge T, Niemeyer CM. Histopathological features of hypoplastic myelodysplastic syndrome and comparison with severe aplastic anemia in childhood. Leuk Res 1999; 23(suppl 1):S41.

205. Appelbaum FR, Barrall J, Storb R, Ramberg R, Doney K, Sale GE, Thomas ED. Clonal cytogenetic abnormalities in patients with otherwise typical aplastic anemia. Exp Hematol 1987; 15:1134–1139.

206. Mikhailova N, Sessarego M, Fugazza G, Caimo A, De Filippi S, van Lint MT, Bregante S, Valeriani A, Mordini N, Lamparelli T, Gualandi F, Occhini D, Bacigalupo A. Cytogenetic abnormalities in patients with severe aplastic anemia. Haematologica 1996; 81:418–422.

207. Shinohara K, Yujiri T, Kamei S, Ayame H, Tanaka M, Ando S, Tajiri M. Absence of point mutation of N-ras oncogene in bone marrow cells with aplastic anemia. Int J Cell Cloning 1992; 10:94–98.

208. Elghetany MT, Vyas S, Yuoh G. Significance of p53 overexpression in bone marrow biopsies from patients with bone marrow failure: aplastic anemia, hypocellular refractory anemia, and hypercellular refractory anemia. Ann Hematol 1998; 77: 261–264.

209. Öst A, Reizenstein P. Minimal diagnostic criteria for the myelodysplastic syndrome. Leuk Res 1992; 16:9–11.

210. Hasle H, Kerndrup G, Jacobsen BB, Heegaard ED, Hornsleth A, Lillevang ST. Chronic parvovirus infection mimicking myelodysplastic syndrome in a child with subclinical immunodeficiency. Am J Pediatr Hematol Oncol 1994; 16:329–333.

211. Rinn R, Chow WSW, Pinkerton PH. Transient acquired myelodysplasia associated with parvovirus B19 infection in a patient with congenital spherocytosis. Am J Hematol 1995; 50:71–72.

212. Yarali, N, Duru F, Sipahi T, Kara A, Tezic T. Parvovirus B19 infection reminiscent of myelodysplastic syndrome in three children with chronic hemolytic anemia. Pediatr Hematol Oncol 2000; 17:475–482.

213. Sandhaus LM, Scudder R. Hematologic and bone marrow abnormalities in pediatric patients with human immunodeficiency virus (HIV) infection. Pediatr Pathol 1989; 9:277–288.

214. Wollman MR, Penchansky L, Shekhter-Levin S. Transient 7q- in association with megaloblastic anemia due to dietary folate and vitamin B12 deficiency. J Pediatr Hematol Oncol 1996; 18:162–165.

215. Brichard B, Vermylen C, Scheiff JM, Ninane J, Cornu G. Haematological disturbances during long-term valproate therapy. Eur J Pediatr 1994; 153:378–380.

216. Yetgin S, Ozen S, Saatci U, Bakkaloglu A, Besbas N, Kirel B. Myelodysplastic features in juvenile rheumatoid arthritis. Am J Hematol 1997; 54:166–169.

217. Hinson DD, Rogers ZR, Hoffman GF, Schachtele M, Fingerhut R, Kohlschutter A, Kelley RI, Gibson KM. Hematological abnormalities and cholestatic liver disease in two patients with mevalonate kinase deficiency. Am J Med Genet 1998; 78:408–412.

218. Clatch RJ, Krigman HR, Peters MG, Zutter MM. Dysplastic haemopoiesis following orthotopic liver transplantation: comparison with similar changes in HIV infection and primary myelodysplasia. Br J Haematol 1994; 88:685–692.

219. Hirose M, Taguchi Y, Makimoto A, Yamada T, Okamoto T, Kuroda Y. New variant of congenital dyserythropoietic anemia with trilineage myelodysplasia. Acta Haematol 1995; 94:102–104.

220. Head D. Subclassification of myelodysplastic syndrome in children. J Pediatr Hematol Oncol 2001; (in press).

221. Nevill TJ, Fung HC, Shepherd JD, Horsman DE, Nantel SH, Klingemann HG, Forrest DL, Toze CL, Sutherland HJ, Hogge DE, Naiman SC, Le A, Brockington DA, Barnett MJ. Cytogenetic abnormalities in primary myelodysplastic syndrome are highly predictive of outcome after allogeneic bone marrow transplantation. Blood 1998; 92:1910–1917.

222. Anderson JE, Appelbaum FR, Schoch G, Gooley T, Anasetti C, Bensinger WI, Bryant E, Buckner CD, Chauncey TR, Clift RA, Doney K, Flowers M, Hansen JA, Martin PJ, Matthews DC, Sanders JE, Shulman H, Sullivan KM, Witherspoon RP, Storb R. Allogeneic marrow transplantation for refractory anemia: a comparison of two preparative regimens and analysis of prognostic factors. Blood 1996; 87:51–58.

223. Anderson JE, Gooley TA, Schoch G, Anasetti C, Bensinger WI, Clift RA, Hansen JA, Sanders JE, Storb R, Appelbaum FR. Stem cell transplantation for secondary acute mycloid leukemia: evaluation of transplantation as initial therapy or following induction chemotherapy. Blood 1997; 89:2578–2585.

224. Stollmann B, Fonatsch C, Havers W. Persistent Epstein-Barr virus infection associated with monosomy 7 or chromosome 3 abnormality in childhood myeloproliferative disorders. Br J Haematol 1985; 60:183–196.

225. Scheurlen W, Borkhardt A, Ritterbach J, Huppertz HI. Spontaneous hematological remission in a boy with myelodysplastic syndrome and monosomy 7. Leukemia 1994; 8:1435–1438.

226. Benaim E, Hvizdala EV, Papenhausen P, Moscinski LC. Spontaneous remission in monosomy 7 myelodysplastic syndrome. Br J Haematol 1995; 89:947–948.

227. Renneboog B, Hansen V, Heimann P, De Mulder A, Jannsen F, Ferster A. Sponta-

neous remission in a patient with therapy-related myelodysplastic syndrome (t-MDS) with monosomy 7. Br J Haematol 1996; 92:696–698.

228.  Mantadakis E, Shannon KM, Singer DA, Finkelstein J, Chan KW, Hilden JM, Sandler ES. Transient monosomy 7: a case series in children and review of the literature. Cancer 1999; 85:2655–2661.

229.  Longmore G, Guinan EC, Weinstein HJ, Gelber RD, Rappeport JM, Antin JH. Bone marrow transplantation for myelodysplasia and secondary acute nonlymphoblastic leukemia. J Clin Oncol 1990; 8:1707–1714.

230.  Anderson JE, Appelbaum FR, Fisher LD, Schoch G, Shulman H, Anasetti C, Bensinger WI, Bryant E, Buckner CD, Doney K, Martin PJ, Sanders JE, Sullivan KM, Thomas ED, Witherspoon RP, Hansen JA, Storb R. Allogeneic bone marrow transplantation for 93 patients with myelodysplastic syndrome. Blood 1993; 82:677–681.

231.  Anderson JE, Anasetti C, Appelbaum FR, Schoch G, Gooley TA, Hansen JA, Buckner CD, Sanders JE, Sullivan KM, Storb R. Unrelated donor marrow transplantation for myelodysplasia (MDS) and MDS-related acute myeloid leukaemia. Br J Haematol 1996; 93:59–67.

232.  Sutton L, Chastang C, Ribaud P, Jouet JP, Kuentz M, Attal M, Reiffers J, Tigaud JM, Rio B, Dauriac C, Legros M, Dreyfus F, Lioure B, Troussard X, Milpied N, Witz F, Oriol P, Cahn JY, Michallet M, Gluckman E, Ifrah N, Pico JL, Vilmer E, Leblond V. Factors influencing outcome in de novo myelodysplastic syndromes treated by allogeneic bone marrow transplantation: a long-term study of 71 patients Societe Francaise de Greffe de Moelle. Blood 1996; 88:358–365.

233.  Guinan EC, Tarbell NJ, Tantravahi R, Weinstein HJ. Bone marrow transplantation for children with myelodysplastic syndromes. Blood 1989; 73:619–622.

234.  Uderzo C, Locasciulli A, Cantù-Rajnoldi A, Mozzana R, Lambertenghi-Deliliers G, Masera G. Allogeneic bone marrow transplantation for myelodysplastic syndromes of childhood: report of three children with refractory anemia with excess of blasts in transformation and review of the literature. Med Pediatr Oncol 1993; 21:43–48.

235.  Locatelli F, Pession A, Bonetti F, Maserati E, Prete L, Pedrazzoli P, Zecca M, Prete A, Paolucci P, Cazzola M. Busulfan, cyclophosphamide and melphalan as conditioning regimen for bone marrow transplantation in children with myelodysplastic syndromes. Leukemia 1994; 8:844–849.

236.  Nichols K, Parsons SK, Guinan E. Long term follow-up of 12 pediatric patients with primary myelodysplastic syndrome treated with HLA-identical sibling donor bone marrow transplantation. Blood 1996; 87:4020–4022.

237.  Locatelli F, Zecca M, Niemeyer C, Angelucci E, Arcese G, Bender-Götze C, Bonetti F, Burdach S, Dini G, Ebell W, Friedrich W, Hasle H, Hermann J, Jacobsen N, Klingebiel T, Kremens B, Mann G, Miniero R, Pession A, Peters C, Paolucci P, Rossetti F, Schmid HJ, Stary J, Suttorp M, Uderzo C, van't Veer Korthof ET, Vossen J, Zimmermann M. Role of allogeneic bone marrow transplantation for the treatment of myelodysplastic syndromes in childhood. The European Working Group on Childhood Myelodysplastic Syndrome (EWOG-MDS) and the Austria-Germany-Italy (AGI) Bone Marrow Transplantation Registry. Bone Marrow Transplant 1996; 18(suppl 2):63–68.

238. Rubie H, Attal M, Demur C, Brousset P, Duchayne E, Rigal-Huguet F, Dastugue N, Robert A. Intensified conditioning regimen with busulfan followed by allogeneic BMT in children with myelodysplastic syndromes. Bone Marrow Transplant 1994; 13:759–762.

239. Leahey A, Friedman DL, Bunin NJ. Bone marrow transplantation in pediatric patients with therapy-related myelodysplasia and leukemia. Bone Marrow Transplant 1999; 23:21–25.

240. de Witte T, Hermans J, Vossen J, Bacigalupo A, Meloni G, Jacobsen N, Ruutu T, Ljungman P, Gratwohl A, Runde V, Niederwieser D, van Biezen A, Devergie A, Cornelissen J, Jouet JP, Arnold R, Apperley J. Haematopoietic stem cell transplantation for patients with myelodysplastic syndromes and secondary acute myeloid leukaemias: a report on behalf of the Chronic Leukaemia Working Party of the European Group for Blood and Marrow Transplantation (EBMT). Br J Haematol 2000; 110:620–630.

241. Anderson JE, Appelbaum FR, Schoch G, Gooley T, Anasetti C, Bensinger WI, Bryant E, Buckner CD, Chauncey T, Clift RA, Deeg HJ, Doney K, Flowers M, Hansen JA, Martin PJ, Matthews DC, Nash RA, Sanders JE, Shulmann H, Sullivan KM, Witherspoon RP, Storb R. Allogeneic marrow transplantation for myelodysplastic syndrome with advanced disease morphology: a phase II study of busulfan, cyclophosphamide, and total-body irradiation and analysis of prognostic factors. J Clin Oncol 1996; 14:220–226.

242. Niemeyer CM, Duffner U, Bender-Götze C, Ebell W, Hasle H, Klingebiel T, Kremens B, Nürnberger W, Vossen J, Zecca M, Zintl F, Locatelli F. AML-Type intensive chemotherapy prior to stem cell transplantation (SCT) does not improve survival in children and adolescents with primary myelodysplastic syndromes (MDS). Blood 2000; 96:521a.

243. Creutzig U, Bender-Götze C, Ritter J, Zimmermann M, Stollmann-Gibbels B, Körholz D, Niemeyer C. The role of intensive AML-specific therapy in treatment of children with RAEB and RAEB-t. Leukemia 1998; 12:652–659.

244. Sandler ES, Friedman DJ, Mustafa MM, Winick NJ, Bowman WP, Buchanan GR. Treatment of children with epipodophyllotoxin-induced secondary acute myeloid leukemia. Cancer 1997; 79:1049–1054.

245. Ballen KK, Gilliland DG, Guinan EC, Hsieh CC, Parsons SK, Rimm IJ, Ferrara JL, Bierer BE, Weinstein HJ, Antin JH. Bone marrow transplantation for therapy-related myelodysplasia: comparison with primary myelodysplasia. Bone Marrow Transplant 1997; 20:737–743.

246. Yakoub-Agha I, de La Salmoniere P, Ribaud P, Sutton L, Wattel E, Kuentz M, Jouet JP, Marit G, Milpied N, Deconinck E, Gratecos N, Leporrier M, Chabbert I, Caillot D, Damaj G, Dauriac C, Dreyfus F, Francois S, Molina L, Tanguy ML, Chevret S, Gluckman E. Allogeneic bone marrow transplantation for therapy-related myelodysplastic syndrome and acute myeloid leukemia: a long-term study of 70 patients-report of the French society of bone marrow transplantation. J Clin Oncol 2000; 18:963–971.

247. Zeidler C, Welte K, Barak Y, Barriga F, Bolyard AA, Boxer L, Cornu G, Cowan MJ, Dale DC, Flood T, Freedman M, Gadner H, Mandel H, O'Reilly RJ, Ramenghi U, Reiter A, Skinner R, Vermylen C, Levine JE. Stem cell transplantation in pa-

tients with severe congenital neutropenia without evidence of leukemic transformation. Blood 2000; 95:1195–1198.

248. Faber J, Lauener R, Wick F, Betts D, Filgueira L, Seger RA, Gungor T. Shwachman-Diamond syndrome: early bone marrow transplantation in a high risk patient and new clues to pathogenesis. Eur J Pediatr 1999; 158:995–1000.

249. Gurney JG, Severson RK, Davis S, Robison LL. Incidence of cancer in children in the United States. Sex-, race, and 1-year age-specific rates by histologic type. Cancer 1995; 75:2186–2195.

# 13
# Treatment of Anemia in Myelodysplastic Syndromes

**David T. Bowen**
*University of Dundee and Ninewells Hospital, Dundee, Scotland*

**Eva Hellström-Lindberg**
*Karolinska Institute and Huddinge University Hospital, Stockholm, Sweden*

## I. INTRODUCTION

Anemia is the major clinical problem for patients with myelodysplastic syndromes (MDS). Eighty percent of these patients are anemic at presentation and the majority require red cell transfusion at some stage of the disease. For most patients, supportive care with red cell transfusion is currently the most appropriate management strategy but with an increased understanding of the different mechanisms of anemia in this heterogeneous group of diseases, interventional therapy will increasingly be available for patient subgroups determined by biological criteria.

## II. MECHANISMS OF ANEMIA IN MDS

While the anemia of MDS can often be multifactorial, there are two broad pathological processes that impair red cell production and that are considered to be the major contributors to anemia:

Ineffective erythropoiesis
Hypoproliferative erythropoiesis

Ineffective erythropoiesis is more commonly seen when there are <10% blasts in refractory anemia (RA), refractory anemia with ringed sideroblasts (RARS), and refractory anemia with excess blasts (RAEB), while patients with >10% blasts have more hypoproliferative erythropoiesis, although these processes are not mutually exclusive. These two broad models can be described in more detail using a variety of in vivo and in vitro assays and the mechanisms for impairment of erythrocyte production are becoming increasingly understood. However, this increased understanding reveals a considerable heterogeneity of pathological processes, even within subtypes grouped according to the French-American-British (FAB) system, and the identification of common mechanisms remains elusive.

## A. Ineffective Erythropoiesis

### 1. Morphology

Studies of the mechanisms of anemia have evolved from the initial morphological observations, which were later used by the FAB group to define the entity of MDS (1). RA is typically characterized by erythroid hyperplasia, with nuclear abnormalities such as megaloblastoid change and nuclear irregularity. Bone marrow from patients with RARS tends to show less nuclear irregularity, an increase in proerythroblasts, and the classical iron deposition in mitochondria demonstrated upon staining with Perl's reagent. RAEB also shows nuclear dysplasia with less pronounced erythroid hyperplasia as blast cells increase.

### 2. Iron Studies Including Mitochondria

Erythrokinetic studies indicate that ineffective erythropoiesis is most prominent in patients with RA/RARS (2). Serum transferrin receptor (TfR) concentration is increased in RARS patients but is probably not a good marker of ineffectiveness (3). The recent identification of mitochondrial DNA mutations in patients with RARS indicates a failure of reduction of iron for utilization by ferrochelatase and subsequent incorporation into heme (4). A direct relationship with this defect and ineffective erythropoiesis has not yet been established although a loss of mitochondrial membrane potential correlates with other markers of apoptosis in RARS bone marrow (5).

### 3. In Vitro Erythroid Progenitor Growth: The Battle of Proliferation Versus Survival Versus Differentiation

Committed erythroid progenitor growth is reduced in most patients with MDS (6). Residual nonclonal erythroid progenitors can be identified in some patients (7). MDS bone marrow is relatively deficient in erythroid (compared to myeloid) clonogenicity as demonstrated both by replating of blast colonies (8) and by early commitment to the lineage of cells having the CD34+ surface receptor (9). Taken together with a lack of maturation from burst-forming units–erythrocytes (BFU-E) to colony-forming units–erythrocytes (CFU-E) (10), this suggests that the defect arises most often in a relatively primitive erythroid progenitor and possibly even at the stem cell level (11). A greater proportion of erythroid precursor cells from patients with RA/RARS are in $S/G_2M$ phases of the cell cycle (compared with normal marrow cells) but it is as yet unclear whether this represents an increased proliferation of the precursor compartment or prolonged S-phase (12,13).

The poor erythroid progenitor growth in MDS can be partially augmented in a proportion of patients by a variety of survival-augmentation (antiapoptotic) strategies. These include increased concentrations of early-acting hematopoietic growth factors such as stem cell factor (14) and granulocyte colony-stimulating factor (G-CSF) (15), antioxidants (e.g., amifostine) (16), glucocorticoids (17), and caspase inhibitors (11).

## 4. Apoptosis as the Mediator of Ineffective Erythropoiesis

The paradox of a morphologically expanded bone marrow erythron with peripheral anemia is explained by an increased rate of intramedullary erythroid cell death, most likely by augmented apoptosis (18–20). In retrospect, many of the techniques used above to describe ineffective erythropoiesis have also demonstrated augmented cell death (by apoptosis). More recently, direct demonstration of cellular apoptosis has become possible although this is a complex process and each technique identifies a different stage of the apoptotic pathway.

It is unclear within which hierarchical differentiation compartment the apoptosis in MDS is most prominent and this has important ramifications for directing antiapoptotic therapy. Apoptosis and DNA fragmentation can clearly be demonstrated in MDS bone marrow CD34+ cells (21,22) as well is in the erythroid precursors (5,18). A greater susceptibility to Fas-induced cell death promoted by increased caspase activity has been shown in mononuclear cells from RARS bone marrow, and caspase inhibition of CD34+ cells may enhance erythroid colony growth in RARS but not in normal bone marrow (11,23).

An interesting paradox is the observation that CD34+ cells from some patients with MDS are resistant to Fas-induced apoptosis following incubation with tumor necrosis factor (TNF)-$\alpha$ (24). This may explain the property of clonal expansion in the face of augmented apoptosis within the more mature compartment.

## 5. Intracellular Pathways and Erythroid Differentiation

Erythroid differentiation requires activation of the erythropoietin (EPO) receptor followed by appropriate activation of the JAK-STAT pathway. This process is linked to an increased expression of the transcription factor GATA-1, which is necessary for erythroid differentiation. While there is no evidence for abnormalities in the EPO receptor in MDS, studies have shown severely reduced STAT5 activation and GATA-1 expression in myelodysplastic bone marrow (25). However, this may not be a primary defect of only the abnormal clone. Down-regulation of GATA-1 has been demonstrated to be a caspase-mediated event in normal bone marrow and a study in MDS failed to show a correlation between erythroid colony growth and level of STAT5 activation, suggesting instead that erythroid deficiency was propagated by the Fas-caspase pathway (26,27).

## 6. What Is the Mechanism of Induction of Ineffective Erythropoiesis?

The primary defects responsible for ineffective erythropoiesis may be intrinsic, extrinsic or a combination of both.

*a. Intrinsic.* There have been no systematic studies of early erythropoiesis capable of defining the relationship between specific intrinsic genomic/gene expression defects and ineffective erythropoiesis. Mutations within the N-*ras* gene occur in approximately 10–20% patients with MDS and mutant N-*ras* transfection into human cord blood progenitor cells reproduces some of the erythropoietic defects seen in MDS (28). The significance of *ras* mutation in the pathogenesis of MDS, however, remains unclear.

*b. Extrinsic.* Recently there has been an increasing recognition of the role of extrinsic hematopoietic inhibitory factors such as TNF-α/interleukin-1β, although most in vitro studies have concentrated on the effects of these inhibitory cytokines on CD34+ cells and myeloid (not erythroid) progenitors (29). Clinically, however, the most impressive responses to immunosuppressive therapy are seen in the erythroid lineage (vide infra).

## B. Hypoproliferative Erythropoiesis

Hypoproliferative erythropoiesis is the more common erythropoietic defect in MDS, occurring when blasts exceed 10% of the bone marrow cells, and is much less studied than ineffective erythropoiesis. Morphologically, hypoproliferative erythropoiesis manifests as a reduced percentage of marrow erythroid precursors and nuclear and cytoplasmic morphological abnormalities are less striking. An almost-total red cell aplasia can occasionally be seen in both early and advanced MDS, but mechanisms probably differ in these groups. The occasional response to immunosuppression in RA suggests an overlap with pure red cell aplasia (30).

In contrast to RA and RARS, erythrokinetic studies indicate that patients with an excess of blasts/chronic myelomonocytic leukemia have predominantly a hypoproliferative erythroid defect (2). Poor progenitor growth does not allow further distinction between the processes of ineffective or hypoproliferative erythropoiesis.

Hypoproliferative erythropoiesis could occur in several ways:

Intrinsic failure of erythroid differentiation at a very early progenitor level
Extrinsic autoimmune suppression of a primitive erythroid progenitor
Progression of ineffective erythropoiesis to "burnout"
"Steal" of myeloid differentiation (with blast cell proliferation) from erythroid cells within the multipotential progenitor compartment

## C. Effective Erythroid Output: Reticulocytes in MDS

Effective erythroid output is best represented by reticulocyte analysis; an increased proportion of immature reticulocytes is a key feature of ineffective red cell production in MDS. This change is proportional to the erythropoietin drive and may represent "shift" reticulocytes (3). Other reticulocyte abnormalities in anemic MDS patients include an increased reticulocyte cell volume and reduced reticulocyte hemoglobin concentration (31).

## D. Additional Contributors to Anemia in MDS

Peripheral red cell destruction/loss may also produce anemia in MDS. Red cell loss may result from bleeding associated with thrombocytopenia and/or platelet functional defects. Red cell life span is shortened in some MDS patients and this may be due to hemolysis (often with a positive direct antiglobulin test) (32) or hypersplenism. Many diverse red cell abnormalities are also described in MDS although their clinical significance is less clear (33–35). Finally, many patients with long-standing transfusion therapy show progressively increasing transfusion need, but the mechanism is poorly understood.

## E. Myelodysplasia Subtypes with Preferential Erythroid Lineage Involvement

### 1. Pure (Dyserythropoietic) Sideroblastic Anemia

RARS patient can be divided into two groups on the basis of single-lineage (erythroid) versus multilineage dysplasia and degree of nonerythroid lineage cytopenias. Pure sideroblastic anemia (PSA) has a better prognosis (77% vs. 56% 3-year survival) with no cases of leukemic transformation in a recently reported study (36). However, myeloid colony growth may also be severely reduced in typical PSA patients indicating a stem cell origin also of this form of MDS (11).

## 2. 5q- Syndrome

The 5q- syndrome occurs predominantly in elderly women and is characterized by anemia, frequent thrombocytosis, and an isolated deletion of the long arm (or part thereof) of chromosome 5. The recent observation that the karyotypic defect is present in precursors of myeloid and lymphoid lineages as well as erythroid poses some fundamental mechanistic questions as to why the clinical picture predominates in the erythroid lineage (37).

## III. THERAPEUTIC APPROACHES

An improvement in the cytopenias associated with MDS may be achieved by three different (but often concurrent) pathophysiological routes:

> Expand effective erythropoiesis at the expense of the ineffective clone
> Convert ineffective to effective erythropoiesis within the MDS clone
> Eliminate the MDS clone to allow reconstitution with polyclonal hematopoiesis

While chemotherapy and stem cell transplantation can clearly achieve route 3, whether either of routes 1 and 2 is achieved with use of other effective therapeutic modalities is unclear.

A considerable problem when reviewing therapeutic studies in MDS is the extensive variation in clinical response criteria used by different study groups. It is important to distinguish responses that are merely "biological" (often transient and/or incomplete) and those that are meaningful to the patient. This has recently been partially addressed by the publication of suggested standardized response criteria to treatments for MDS; treatments are divided into those with modalities potentially causing change in the natural course of the disease and those aimed at improvement of peripheral blood values (38). Importantly, quality of life has been included as a response parameter.

## A. Symptoms of Anemia: What Needs Treating?

The impact of blood cytopenias upon quality of life has only recently begun to be studied in MDS, and preliminary information is available only in abstract and overview form (39,40). The most common symptoms of anemia that impair the quality of life of MDS patients are fatigue and exertional dyspnea (40). In a predominantly elderly, patient population (30), anemia will exacerbate comorbid conditions such as angina, chronic hypoxia (obstructive airways disease), peripheral vascular disease, and, most likely, dementia-like conditions. However, the contribution of anemia to comorbidity in elderly patients with chronic anemia and transfusion need has received limited attention. Similarly no study has systematically addressed the question of target levels for erythrocyte transfusion to maintain an outpatient life without increasing comorbidity. Thus, the response to our question (what needs treating?) is that any decision about target hemoglobin levels should be a result of a thorough discussion between the doctor and the patient. The treatment goal, whether the treatment consists of transfusion therapy, EPO, or other proerythrogenic therapies, should aim at the best possible quality of life and may be adjusted based on close observation of comorbid conditions.

## B. Supportive Care

### 1. The Concept

Supportive care remains the most appropriate management for many patients with good-prognosis MDS and for those with poor-prognosis disease whose age or performance status precludes them from receiving more intensive forms of therapy. The term "supportive care for the treatment of anemia" as currently used describes the replacement of red cells by cellular products with the intention of symptomatic control. Supportive care is the standard of care against which other forms of treatment should be compared. High-quality evidence for the effectiveness of supportive care in terms of outcome measures such as quality of life and survival is, however, lacking and has not been systematically studied. Supportive care could also potentially include any treatment that improves anemia but does not eradicate the MDS clone.

### 2. Red Cell Transfusion

At presentation the majority of cases of MDS will have a hemoglobin concentration $< 10$ g/dL. Chronic anemia, though seldom life-threatening, can lead to significant morbidity and is therefore important in relation to quality of life and to comorbid disease. Red cell transfusion should be considered in any patient symptomatic of anemia. Patients with MDS may, however, compensate well for their anemia and the need to introduce red cell transfusion will vary between individuals. It is of considerable importance to consider transfusing the patient on symptomatic grounds, preferably before symptoms develop and not just based upon the hemoglobin concentration. Indeed, recent studies have demonstrated that the incremental increase of hemoglobin concentration from 11 to 12 g/dl was associated with the largest improvement in quality of life (41). The frequency of red cell transfusion is variable, from as often as once every 1–2 weeks to more infrequently (every 6–12 weeks). For patients with short transfusion intervals, bleeding and hemolysis should be considered but most frequently the high transfusion requirement reflects profound erythroid failure (severe reticulocytopenia) with or without peripheral consumptive processes such as hypersplenism.

The risks associated with red cell transfusion are considerable, and many remain as yet unknown. Increasing recognition of transfusion-transmitted infection drives the search for alternative strategies for the management of anemia. Recent infectious agents considered or proven to be associated with red cell transfusion include hepatitis C, TT virus, and new-variant Creutzfeldt-Jakob disease. Although those transmitted infections with long incubation times appear of little relevance to the majority of MDS patients whose life expectancy is <6 years, there is a group of long-term transfused patients for whom this is a major issue. Red cell alloimmunization is common and increases with increasing numbers of units transfused and, despite this, reactions to red cell transfusion are equally frequent in patients without red cell alloantibodies (42). The practicalities and expense of obtaining compatible blood for alloimmunized patients are nevertheless significant. In countries practicing universal leukodepletion of red cell products, the risks of red cell alloimmunization have now fallen, but the many rare and potentially fatal complications of transfusion such as posttransfusion purpura and transfusion-associated graft-versus-host disease remain.

## 3. Iron Chelation Therapy

Patients with myelodysplasia may develop iron overload either as a result of repeated red cell transfusions or through excessive absorption of food iron by some patients with sideroblastic anemia. A limited study has demonstrated subclinical organ toxicity in multitransfused patients (43). However, there have been no larger studies on this subject or studies to distinguish the clinical consequences of iron loading specifically in MDS patients or other patient groups with similar median age.

Iron chelation therapy may be considered for patients with iron overload. Desferoxamine, administered as regular subcutaneous infusions, can reduce serum ferritin and liver iron concentration in MDS patients (44). Observational studies have also suggested that desferoxamine therapy may be associated with improved marrow function and reduced transfusion requirements (45,46). In some countries, Sweden for example, desferoxamine is often given as long-term infusion via an indwelling intravenous catheter (e.g., Portacath) with comparable results as subcutaneous infusions (E. Hellström-Lindberg, personal observation). There are also observational studies, which include MDS patients, of the effect of an orally active iron chelator, deferiprone, on iron excretion. Although this drug promotes increased urinary iron excretion, there remain questions as to its safety (agranulocytosis and possible hepatotoxicity) and efficacy (47).

Recommendations for iron chelation treatment in myelodysplasia are based on limited data and on a comparison with the effects of iron overload and its treatment in other transfusion-dependent conditions. It is difficult to recommend which group of MDS patients should be offered iron chelation therapy as the investment of time and discomfort associated with regular subcutaneous infusions of desferoxamine has to be weighed against the likelihood of net benefit in reducing the complications of iron overload. The rate of iron loading and the total iron load should be assessed from the transfusion history and on increments in serum ferritin levels and liver enzyme tests. Other factors to consider when contemplating iron chelation therapy include the likely prognosis of the myelodysplasia or any other preexisting disease; in practice, the MDS patients most likely to benefit are those with sideroblastic anemia, 5q- syndrome, or other forms of RA with minimal cytopenia in other lineages. Iron chelation should be considered by the time that a patient has received 5 g iron (approximately 25 units of red cells). Addition of vitamin C at 100–200 mg daily taken about 1 hr prior to desferoxamine infusion increases the proportional iron excretion but should not be started until approximately 4 weeks after desferoxamine therapy is initiated. The use of twice-daily subcutaneous bolus injections of desferoxamine (48) may be considered where infusions are not tolerated, but there is even less information about their potential value in myelodysplasia than for the subcutaneous infusions.

## C. Interventional Therapies

The aim of interventional therapy is to improve quality of life benchmarked against either the baseline untreated state or against best supportive care in the form of red cell transfusions. These interventional therapies have the potential to produce sustained increases in hemoglobin concentration and to thus avoid the up-and-down lifestyle accepted by so many regularly transfused patients and their physicians.

### 1. Hematopoietic Growth Factors

*a. EPO Alone.* The therapeutic efficacy of recombinant EPO in the treatment of anemia is now well established for selected patients with MDS. Cohort studies have clearly demonstrated responses and a randomized placebo-controlled study has confirmed the superior response rate of EPO over placebo (49) (Table 1).

There are two meta-analyses covering trials of EPO alone until late 1994, including 205 patients from 17 trials (50) and 115 patients from 10 trials (51), respectively. The overall response rates (using a 100% reduction of transfusion need as minimal response criteria) are 16% and 23.5%, respectively. Positive predictors of response in the larger meta-analysis were non-RARS FAB subtype, pretreatment serum EPO levels of less than 200 U/L, and the lack of need for transfusion. Patients with RARS responded less well to EPO therapy alone, with

**Table 1**   Larger Studies of Therapy with EPO Alone or EPO in Combination with G-CSF

| Author/year | Study type | Number of patients | Treatment | Inclusion criteria | Erythroid response | Parameters giving favorable outcomes/comments |
|---|---|---|---|---|---|---|
| Hellström-Lindberg, 1995 (50) | Meta-analysis | 205 | EPO | Various, all studies prior to 1995 | 16% overall (8% for RARS) | sEPO < 200 U/L No transfusion for RA/RAEB needed |
| Rose et al., 1995 (116) | Phase II | 116 | EPO | Hb < 80 g/L sEPO < 500 U/L | 28% (18% for transfusion-dependent patients)[a] | sEPO < 100 U/L RA |
| Italian Cooperative Study Group, 1998 (49) | Phase III | 87 | EPO/placebo | Hb < 90 g/L Blasts < 10% | 37% versus 11%[a] (p = 0.007) | Response significant in RA and in non-transfused patients |
| Negrin et al., 1996 (58) | Phase II | 55 | EPO + G−CSF | Hb < 100 g/L | 48%,[a] median duration of 10 months | sEPO |
| Hellström-Lindberg et al., 1998 (56) | Phase II | 71 | EPO + G−CSF | Hb < 100 g/L | 38%,[b] duration of 24 months | sEPO, transfusion need |
| Remacha et al., 1999 (57) | Phase II | 32 | EPO + G−CSF | Hb < 100 g/L sEPO < 250 U/L | 50%[a] | Predictive model (see Fig. 1) |
| Mantovani et al., 2000 (59) | Phase II | 33 | EPO + G−CSF | Blasts < 20% | 61% (12-week duration) 80% (36-week duration) | 50% response after 2 years |

[a] Response in transfusion-dependent patients was defined as >50% reduction in transfusion need.
[b] Response in transfusion-dependent patients was defined as elimination of transfusion need.
EPO, erythropoietin; G-CSF, granulocyte colony-stimulating factor; Hb, hemoglobin; sEPO, serum EPO; RA, refractory anemia; RARS, RA with ringed sideroblasts; RAEB, RA with excess blasts; P, probability.

**Table 2** Response Rates to EPO Based upon FAB Subtype, Pretreatment Serum
EPO Concentration, and Transfusion Need

| | Response rate by predictor | | | |
| --- | --- | --- | --- | --- |
| | No transfusion need | | Transfusion need | |
| FAB subtype | sEPO < 200 U/L | sEPO > 200 U/L | sEPO < 200 U/L | sEPO > 200 U/L |
| All subtypes other than RARS | 8/14 (57%) | 4/8 (50%) | 5/24 (21%) | 7/71 (10%) |
| RARS | 3/9 (33%) | 0/4 (0%) | 2/23 (9%) | 0/26 (0%) |

EPO, erythropoietin; sEPO, serum EPO; FAB, French-American-British classification system; MDS,
myelodysplastic syndromes; RARS, refractory anemia with ringed sideroblasts.
*Source*: Adapted from Ref. 50.

an overall response rate of 8% (Table 2) (50). The smaller study identified only
RAEB FAB subtype as a negative predictor. In the only double-blind, randomized, placebo-controlled study of EPO treatment in MDS, an overall benefit for
EPO over placebo ($p = 0.007$) was shown for MDS patients with <10% bone
marrow myeloblasts. However, analysis of patient subgroups demonstrated a significant effect of treatment only in nontransfused patients and in patients with
RA. Again, basal serum EPO levels of less than 200 U/L predicted for response
(49). Taking these studies together, it is likely that patients having RARS and a
transfusion need will respond poorly to EPO as monotherapy. Other parameters
predictive of response in smaller studies include low serum lactate dehydrogenase
(52) and serum TNF-α concentration (53), the presence of measurable blood
BFU-E (54), and relatively well-preserved effective erythropoiesis as measured
by erythrokinetics (55).

EPO therapy is generally well tolerated with the most common side effects
being flu-like symptoms and occasional splenic pain and enlargement.

*b. EPO Combined with G-CSF.* The synergistic effect of the combination of G-CSF plus EPO has now been demonstrated in vivo by three groups
(56–58). This effect was most pronounced in patients with RARS, who showed
the best response rate to the combination (~50%). Moreover, compared with
EPO treatment alone, the combination showed an effect also in patients with a
moderate (<2 units per month) transfusion need. The combination therapy was
well tolerated. A recent study, with different response criteria, demonstrated an
increased response rate with prolonged treatment in 33 patients (61% were responders at 12 weeks and 80% were responders at 36 weeks) (59). Seven responses developed between week 12 and 36 of which three were in patients with
RARS.

Using pretreatment serum EPO as a ternary variable ($<100$, 100–500, or $>500$ U/L) and a transfusion requirement ($<2$ or $\geq2$ U/month) of red blood cells (RBC) as a binary variable, a predictive model for response was developed from the data of 98 patients treated in two multicenter studies (60). Three groups of responders were identified (Fig. 1) with predicted response rates of 74%, 23%, and 7% (high-, intermediate-, and low-response groups, respectively). The model has since been independently validated in a small retrospective study (57) and, prospectively, in a Scandinavian phase IV study, which is still not finally reported (39). In the latter, the model showed a significant predictive value ($p = 0.004$), with 61% of the patients responding in the best predictive group.

The available data allow recommendation for a trial of G-CSF and EPO therapy for individual patients with symptomatic anemia who fulfill the criteria for the high, and possibly intermediate, response group of the predictive model. This combination therapy should be considered as the initial treatment, especially for patients with RARS and transfusion need since this subgroup of patients usually has a low response rate to EPO alone. Other patients may start with EPO

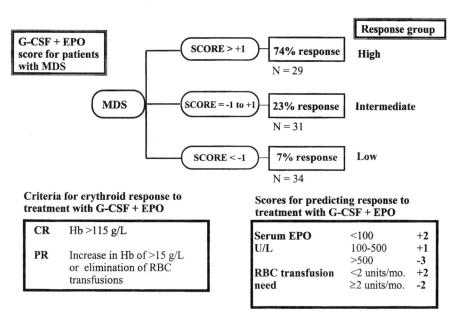

**Fig. 1** Logisitic regression-based predictive model for response rates to therapy with EPO plus G-CSF based upon pretreatment serum EPO concentration and transfusion need. EPO, erythropoietin; G-CSF, granulocyte colony-stimulating factor; MDS, myelodysplastic syndrome; N, number; RBC, red blood cells; Hb, hemoglobin; CR, complete remission; PR, partial remission. (Adapted from Ref. 60.)

as monotherapy and, if a response to EPO alone is not observed after 8 weeks, the patient can then be treated with the combination. Recent data suggest that prolonged treatment may be required to achieve a response.

    *c.  Dosing Schedule for EPO Alone or in Combination with G-CSF.*  Recommended dosing schedules for EPO are 50,000–70,000 U/week in 3–5 divided doses for a minimum of 6 weeks. It is likely that the number of doses per week could be reduced but such studies have still not been undertaken in MDS. In responders, the dose may often, but not always, be reduced to 20,000–40,000 U/week in 2–3 divided doses. For nonresponders, G-CSF should be added at a dose to normalize (and at least double) the neutrophil count if it is less than $1.5 \times 10^9$/L or double the neutrophil count if it is more than $1.5 \times 10^9$/L. While existing data indicate that treatment should be stopped at 10–12 weeks in the absence of response, emerging evidence suggests that a more prolonged therapeutic trial may be required to definitively exclude slow responders (59). As for all other patients on EPO treatment, functional iron deficiency has to be considered, although this has not been extensively studied as a cause for nonresponse to EPO in MDS.

    *d.  Durability of Response to EPO Alone or in Combination with G-CSF.* There are only limited data confirming the durability of therapy with EPO alone. One small study suggests that one-third of responders were able to either sustain the initial response or sustain response at reintroduction of EPO following recurrence of their anemia while off therapy. Responses at reintroduction could also be maintained on lower doses of EPO than that used at induction. Patients who lost their response did so for largely predictable reasons, including MDS transformation to acute myeloid leukemia and the development of a new malignancy (61).

    Maintenance therapy with the EPO/G-CSF combination suggests that the median response duration for these patients is at least 24 months (56,59). Thirty percent of patients maintained a response at 5 years (56), the majority of whom had RARS (56,59). A higher rate of sustained responses (50%) has also recently been reported at 1 and 2 years of combined EPO and G-CSF therapy (59).

    *e.  Pharmacoeconomics of EPO Therapy.*  Despite the clear efficacy of EPO for selected MDS patients, there is considerable variability in prescription between countries resulting from the complex pharmacoeconomic debate and (as yet) from the lack of data demonstrating clear outcome benefits on such parameters as survival, quality of life, and comorbidity (62). The detailed pharmacoeconomic equation is complex and will vary from center to center and country to country. Examples of this are (1) the difference in charges for red cells between Scotland (centrally held budget) and the rest of the United Kingdom (paid for locally) and (2) different funding sources for outpatient therapy (central national budget in Sweden vs. departmental local budgets in the United Kingdom). The denominators within these models are constantly changing; for example, the cost of red cells in the United Kingdom has nearly doubled with the advent of universal leukodepletion. Comparing countries, the cost for red cell transfusions is at least three times higher in the United States than in Europe. Limited pharmacoeconomic models have already been developed and some suggest that EPO therapy of cancer can be considered to be cost effective as presently delivered (63) or given ''lower rHuEPO [erythropoietin] dosages and higher numbers of transfused units of PRBCs [packed red blood cells]'' (64). Pharmacoeconomic models expressing the conflicting view can also be found in the literature (65).

*f. Mechanism of Action of EPO Alone or in Combination with G-CSF.* A response to EPO and G-CSF combination therapy is associated with reduction of bone marrow apoptosis, reduced but more effective bone marrow erythropoiesis, and, in RARS, reduced number of ringed sideroblasts (19). The mechanism of these effects remains uncertain. It is clear, however, that EPO prevents erythroid progenitors from undergoing apoptosis and promotes erythroid differentiation by initiating intracellular events (66); these events, in part, include activation of the STAT5 transcription factor and expression of antiapoptotic genes, such as *bcl-xl*, and genes associated with erythroid differentiation (e.g., GATA-1) (67,68). Signaling via the G-CSF receptor induces erythroid differentiation in vitro, even in the absence of the EPO receptor or STAT5 activity, and this may explain some of the synergy between G-CSF and EPO therapy in MDS patients in whom STAT5 activation is often compromised (69). However, why myelodysplastic erythroid precursors fail to respond adequately to relatively normal or moderately elevated serum EPO levels but may respond at supranormal concentrations remains to be elucidated.

*g. Parameters of Early Erythroid Response.* In addition to clear identification of parameters predictive of high rates of response to growth factor therapy, early identification of that response is highly desirable. It is, perhaps, even more desirable to identify nonresponders as early as possible to avoid unnecessary patient inconvenience, toxicity [e.g., thrombocytopenia (56)], and cost. The use of algorithms, which utilize baseline serum EPO plus incremental increases in TfR and hemoglobin concentration, to identify early response to EPO therapy in hematological malignancies is well established (70), although obtaining rapid EPO/TfR assay results is not usually practical. For MDS, an increase in serum TfR of $<18\%$ at 2 weeks predicted for nonresponse to EPO in the recent randomized study of EPO therapy (49). For responding patients, identification of *early* reticulocytosis through, for example, an increase in Sysmex R-2000 high-fluorescent reticulocytes has been little studied in MDS, although one small study showed early reticulocytosis as a better early indicator of response than increasing serum TfR (71).

*h. EPO plus GM-CSF or Other Agents.* Several smaller cohort studies have indicated that response rates to the combination of EPO and granulocyte-macrophage colony-stimulating factor (GM-CSF) are comparable to those with EPO and G-CSF (72–74). However, the only randomized study of GM-CSF combined with either placebo or EPO showed low response rates (<10% in each arm) and little difference between both arms of the study (75). Also, given that GM-CSF has more side effects than G-CSF, there is little evidence to recommend GM-CSF therapy in combination with EPO.

Small studies have also examined EPO combined with other agents, including growth factors such as interleukin-3, 13-*cis* retinoic acid, cyclosporine A, all-*trans* retinoic acid (ATRA), or vitamin D, but none appear superior to EPO alone or in combination with G-CSF.

## 2. Coenzymes/Hematopoietic Vitamins

In the diagnostic phase, careful exclusion of vitamin $B_{12}$ or folate deficiency is clearly essential before considering therapy. Therapeutic trials of pyridoxine, thiamine, hydroxocobalamin, and folic acid have shown, however, that these co-enzymes and vitamins are not generally useful for treating anemia. One exception is rare cases of acquired RARS with hypochromic microcytic indices (which probably represent late-onset inherited sideroblastic anemia); these cases may respond to pharmacological doses of pyridoxal phosphate (50 mg three times per day) (76).

## 3. Differentiating Agents

*a. Vitamins.* Various analogs of vitamin A and vitamin D have been shown to induce differentiation in in vitro models of MDS (77). However, despite initial optimism (78), randomized studies have confirmed that 13-*cis* retinoic acid therapy is not superior to placebo (79). In addition, response rates to ATRA are low and are associated with significant toxicity (80). The active metabolite of vitamin D, 1,25-dihydroxycholecalciferol, is too toxic for meaningful responses to be observed (81) and results with the potent analog EB1089 have been disappointing. Thus, the currently available agents have no role in the management of MDS.

*b. Interferons.* Both α- and γ-interferons induce hematological responses in a small proportion of patients, although with often-intolerable side effects. Erythroid responses are rarely sustained and not usually clinically meaningful (82–86).

*c. Chemical Inducers.* Small therapeutic studies of the widely used in vitro polar planar erythroid differentiating agent hexamethylene bisacetamide (HMBA) show limited erythropoietic benefit at the expense of significant toxicity

(87,88). Analogs of HMBA are potent erythroid differentiating agents that inhibit histone deacetylase and may be promising compounds for therapeutic study in MDS (89).

Sodium phenylbutyrate is another potent in vitro differentiating agent whose effect is mediated, at least in part, by histone deacetylase inhibition. Phenylbutyrate demonstrates in vitro antiproliferative and differentiation effects on primary myeloid cells from acute myeloid leukemia and MDS patients (90) but clinical studies have been disappointing.

Heme infusion (as heme arginate) was initially promising but has not been pursued (91).

## 4. Immune Modulation

Anecdotal responses have been reported with corticosteroids (92,93), but evidence for their efficacy is sparse. Two groups have demonstrated the efficacy of antilymphocyte/antithymocyte globulin (ALG or ATG) in raising the blood counts in a proportion of patients with MDS (94,95). Responses have primarily been observed in patients with RA, with considerably lower response in RAEB and lower still in RARS. ATG/ALG seems to be more effective in hypoplastic MDS and in patients with a paroxysmal nocturnal hemoglobinuria (PNH) clone (96) or with the human leukocyte antigen HLA DR15 (97), but these immune modulators may also induce significant improvements in other patients with low-risk MDS. Clinical trials with these agents are ongoing and the results are encouraging, especially since this treatment is capable of inducing durable red cell transfusion independence besides reducing transfusion need. Similar responses have been observed with cyclosporine A (although not usually durable), with higher response rates also observed in hypocellular MDS (98,99). Immunosuppressive therapy is discussed in greater detail in Chapter 14.

## 5. Antiapoptotic Therapy

The antiapoptotic therapy approach involves targeted inhibition of likely pro-apoptotic pathways. Most attention has been directed toward inhibition of TNF-$\alpha$ production or function or of downstream intracellular actions of TNF-$\alpha$, such as the induction of oxidative stress. The agents most associated with this approach for the treatment of MDS are amifostine and pentoxifylline. Other agents such as G-CSF (100) and EPO (19) also inhibit apoptosis and could be considered in this category.

The radioprotective antioxidant-aminothiol amifostine (WR 1065) was initially shown to stimulate in vitro hematopoietic clonogenic growth from both normal and MDS bone marrow (16,101). The first and largest therapeutic study of amifostine in MDS patients was encouraging, with hematopoietic stimulatory effects (single or multilineage) observed in 83% of the patients (15 of 18) (16).

Of the red cell transfusion–dependent patients, five of 15 had at least a 50% reduction in red cell transfusions during the study period and bone marrow from eight of the 15 evaluable patients showed improved BFU-E growth. [Response rates were lower in the expanded cohort reported in abstract form (102).] Responses to amifostine may be schedule dependent as only minor responses were seen with a continuous therapeutic schedule (103) in contrast to the 3-weekly-courses in the original study. However, evidence for a clinically meaningful effect on erythropoiesis, such as that obtained by EPO alone, EPO plus G-CSF, or ATG in RA patients, has not been reported.

Although amifostine has a multitude of potential therapeutic mechanisms, the hematopoietic stimulatory effect of both amifostine and reduced glutathione is consistent with other studies, suggesting a role for oxidative stress in the apoptotic induction of MDS cells (22,104). Occasional responders to amifostine showed karyotypic evidence of expansion of residual nonclonal hematopoiesis. A reduction in ringed sideroblasts was seen in responding RARS patients, which may represent the augmentation by amifostine of iron incorporation into heme within the abnormal clone. Although all therapeutic effects of amifostine are largely transient, these findings have produced a new avenue for therapeutic targets.

Pentoxifylline also inhibits TNF synthesis but is of doubtful efficacy as a single agent or in combination with ciprofloxacin, which reduces the hepatic metabolism and increases the bioavailability of pentoxifylline (105). A combination of pentoxifylline, ciprofloxacin, and dexamethasone (106) with or without amifostine (107) is associated with minor erythroid responses but the combinations are not clearly superior to each agent alone. The most active agent of this combination is likely to be dexamethasone but additive effects of two or more of these four drugs are also possible. An interesting observation of one of these studies (107), increasingly observed in other studies (59), was the slow rate of response with some patients showing initial response at 12 months.

Early results from clinical studies of thalidomide show that this agent can produce erythroid as well as multilineage responses in low-risk MDS patients. Thalidomide has several mechanisms of action including inhibition of macrophage TNF-$\alpha$ production, antiangiogenesis, and immunomodulation from helper T-cell $T_H2$ to $T_H1$ responses.

## 6. Chemotherapy: Eliminating the Ineffective Clone

The greatest body of published experience is with low-dose, subcutaneous cytosine arabinoside (Ara-C), which was initially thought to act as a differentiating agent but now is accepted to be primarily cytotoxic. Erythroid responses occur in the context of multilineage reconstitution of nonclonal hematopoiesis in approximately 30% of the patients (108). Hematological responses may be more frequent in patients with a hypocellular marrow, normal platelet count, and fewer than two chromosomal abnormalities (109) and also in those with the 5q- chromosomal abnormality (110). Some of these responses are durable but at the expense of significant hematological toxicity (108).

There is preliminary evidence that single-agent oral melphalan can induce complete hematological responses and thus provide transfusion independence in high-risk MDS, particularly for those with hypocellular marrows and normal cytogenetics (111,112). The mechanism of action is most likely cytotoxicity although release of hematopoietic suppression, as suggested by an increase in medium/high fluorescent reticulocytes observed as early as 1 week of treatment, may represent a component (D. Bowen, personal experience). Caution against the use of melphalan in younger patients is suggested owing to emergence of chemoresistant relapses with therapy-related karyotypes (113).

Two demethylating agents, 5-azacytidine and its analog 5-aza-2-deoxycytidine (decitabine), have been used in the treatment of MDS. Hematological responses have been observed in approximately 50% of the patients with MDS in all subgroups as defined by the International Prognostic Scoring System (IPSS) (114,115). 5-Azacytidine may be associated with less myelosuppression and this agent eliminated red cell transfusion dependence, while also augmenting erythroid colony growth in 82% of the patients in one study (114). The complete remission rate was, however, low. Decitabine showed promising results in a large phase II trial, with more complete remissions, especially in high-risk patients, but with responses usually following a more pronounced myelosuppression (115). Whether the effects of these agents reflect a cytotoxic mechanism of action or a genuine demethylation-induced differentiation remains unclear. However, since hypermethylation has been described as a potential mechanism behind loss of cell cycle control in MDS, these agents have the potential of adding to the therapeutic arsenal for MDS.

## IV. CLOSING COMMENTS

An outline of management recommendations for the treatment of anemia in MDS patients is presented in Figure 2. To improve treatment for patients with MDS, better tools will be required to define the underlying pathogenetic mechanisms in individual patients. It is clear that the anemia of MDS may have several different causes, each of which may show varying responses to different treatment options. Before any treatment for MDS is planned, it is important to estimate the overall prognosis including IPSS score, age, performance status, and comorbidity. In addition, therapy may be directed by more specific parameters such as bone marrow cellularity, the presence of a PNH clone, and serum EPO assays. New biological information may be helpful in developing new treatment modalities. In the meantime, carefully designed clinical trials incorporating standardized re-

---

**Recommendations for Management of Anemia in Myelodysplastic Syndromes**

- Red cell transfusions should be considered in all symptomatic anemic patients.

- Iron chelation therapy should be considered in regularly transfused patients after 25 red cell units, provided the estimated prognosis of survival is sufficent.

- Anemic patients with serum erythropietin ≤500 U/L and red cell transfusion requirement of <2 U/month should be considered for a trial of recombinant erthropoietin therapy at 50,000-70,000 U/week. Addition of G-CSF should be considered for non-responders at 8 weeks.

- Refractory anemia patients with hypocellular marrows should be considered for immunosuppressive therapy.

---

**Fig. 2** Summary of recommendations for management of anemia in patients with myelo-dysplastic syndromes.

sponse criteria should allow statistically sound predictive models to be developed that will, in turn, allow better selection of patients for existing therapeutic options.

## REFERENCES

1. Bennett JM, Catovsky D, Daniel MT, Flandrin G, Galton DA, Gralnick HR, Sultan C. Proposals for the classification of the myelodysplastic syndromes. Br J Haematol 1982; 51:189–199.
2. Cazzola M, Barosi G, Berzuini C, Dacco M, Orlandi E, Stefanelli M, Ascari E. Quantitative evaluation of erythropoietic activity in dysmyelopoietic syndromes. Br J Haematol 1982; 50:55–62.
3. Bowen DT, Culligan D, Beguin Y, Kendall R, Willis N. Estimation of effective and total erythropoiesis in myelodysplasia using serum transferrin receptor and erythropoietin concentrations, with automated reticulocyte parameters. Leukemia 1994; 8:151–155.
4. Ali FM, May A, Jones BM, Jacobs A. Enrichment of erythroblasts from human

bone marrow using complement-mediated lysis: measure of ferritin. Br J Haematol 1983; 53:227–235.

5.  Matthes TW, Meyer G, Samii K, Beris P. Increased apoptosis in acquired sideroblastic anaemia. Br J Haematol 2000; 111:843–852.

6.  May SJ, Smith SA, Jacobs A, Williams A, Bailey-Wood R. The myelodysplastic syndrome—analysis of laboratory characteristics in relation to the FAB classification. Br J Haematol 1985; 59:311–319.

7.  Asano H, Ohashi H, Ichihara M, Kinoshita T, Murate T, Kobayashi M, Saito H, Hotta T. Evidence for nonclonal hematopoietic progenitor cell populations in bone marrow of patients with myelodysplastic syndromes. Blood 1994; 84:588–594.

8.  Backx B, Broeders L, Touw I, Lowenberg B. Blast colony-forming cells in myelodysplastic syndrome: decreased potential to generate erythroid precursors. Leukemia 1993; 7:75–79.

9.  Sawada K, Sato N, Notoya A, Tarumi T, Hirayama S, Takano H, Koizumi K, Yasukouchi T, Yamaguchi M, Koike T. Proliferation and differentiation of myelodysplastic CD34+ cells: phenotypic subpopulations of marrow CD34+ cells. Blood 1995; 85:194–202.

10. Merchav S, Nielsen OJ, Rosenbaum H, Sharon R, Brenner B, Tatarsky I, Sciaglla P, Wieczorek L. In vitro studies of erythropoietin-dependent regulation of erythropoiesis in myelodysplastic syndromes. Leukemia 1990; 4:771–774.

11. Hellstrom-Lindberg E, Schmidt-Mende J, Forsblom AM, Christensson B, Fadeel B, Zhivotovsky B. Apoptosis in refractory anaemia with ringed sideroblasts is initiated at the stem cell level and associated with increased activation of caspases. Br J Haematol 2001; 112:714–726.

12. Dormer P, Schalhorn A, Wilmanns W, Hershko C. Erythroid and myeloid maturation patterns related to progenitor assessment in the myelodysplastic syndromes. Br J Haematol 1987; 67:61–66.

13. Jensen IM, Hokland M, Hokland P. A quantitative evaluation of erythropoiesis in myelodysplastic syndromes using multiparameter flow cytometry. Leuk Res 1993; 17:839–846.

14. Backx B, Broeders L, Lowenberg B. Kit ligand improves in vitro erythropoiesis in myelodysplastic syndrome. Blood 1992; 80:1213–1217.

15. Schmidt-Mende J, Tehranchi J, Forsblom AM, Joseph B, Christensson B, Fadeel B, Zhivotovsky B, Hellstrom-Lindberg E. Granulocyte-colony stimulating factor inhibits Fas-trigered apoptosis in bone marrow cells isolated from patients with refractory anaemia with ringed sideroblasts. Leukemia 2001; 15:742–751.

16. List AF, Brasfield F, Heaton R, Glinsmann-Gibson B, Crook L, Taetle R, Capizzi R. Stimulation of hematopoiesis by amifostine in patients with myelodysplastic syndrome. Blood 1997; 90:3364–3369.

17. Koeffler HP, Cline MJ, Golde DW. Erythropoiesis in preleukemia. Blood 1978; 51:1013–1019.

18. Raza A, Gezer S, Mundle S, Gao XZ, Alvi S, Borok R, Rifkin S, Iftikhar A, Shetty V, Parcharidou A, et al. Apoptosis in bone marrow biopsy samples involving stromal and hematopoietic cells in 50 patients with myelodysplastic syndromes. Blood 1995; 86:268–276.

19. Hellstrom-Lindberg E, Kanter-Lewensohn L, Ost A. Morphological changes and apoptosis in bone marrow from patients with myelodysplastic syndromes treated with granulocyte-CSF and erythropoietin. Leuk Res 1997; 21:415–425.

20. Lepelley P, Campergue L, Grardel N, Preudhomme C, Cosson A, Fenaux P. Is apoptosis a massive process in myelodysplastic syndromes? Br J Haematol 1996; 95:368–371.

21. Parker JE, Mufti GJ, Rasool F, Mijovic A, Devereux S, Pagliuca A. The role of apoptosis, proliferation, and the Bcl-2-related proteins in the myelodysplastic syndromes and acute myeloid leukemia secondary to MDS. Blood 2000; 96:3932–3938.

22. Peddie CM, Wolf CR, McLellan LI, Collins AR, Bowen DT. Oxidative DNA damage in CD34+ myelodysplastic cells is associated with intracellular redox changes and elevated plasma tumour necrosis factor-alpha concentration. Br J Haematol 1997; 99:625–631.

23. Boudard D, Sordet O, Vasselon C, Revol V, Bertheas MF, Freyssenet D, Viallet A, Piselli S, Guyotat D, Campos L. Expression and activity of caspases 1 and 3 in myelodysplastic syndromes. Leukemia 2000; 14:2045–2051.

24. Horikawa K, Nakakuma H, Kawaguchi T, Iwamoto N, Nagakura S, Kagimoto T, Takatsuki K. Apoptosis resistance of blood cells from patients with paroxysmal nocturnal hemoglobinuria, aplastic anemia, and myelodysplastic syndrome. Blood 1997; 90:2716–2722.

25. Hoefsloot LH, van Amelsvoort MP, Broeders LC, van der Plas DC, van Lom K, Hoogerbrugge H, Touw IP, Lowenberg B. Erythropoietin-induced activation of STAT5 is impaired in the myelodysplastic syndrome. Blood 1997; 89:1690–1700.

26. De Maria R, Zeuner A, Eramo A, Domenichelli C, Bonci D, Grignani F, Srinivasula SM, Alnemri ES, Testa U, Peschle C. Negative regulation of erythropoiesis by caspase-mediated cleavage of GATA-1. Nature 1999; 401:489–493.

27. Fontenay-Roupie M, Bouscary D, Guesnu M, Picard F, Melle J, Lacombe C, Gisselbrecht S, Mayeux P, Dreyfus F. Ineffective erythropoiesis in myelodysplastic syndromes: correlation with Fas expression but not with lack of erythropoietin receptor signal transduction. Br J Haematol 1999; 106:464–473.

28. Darley RL, Hoy TG, Baines P, Padua RA, Burnett AK. Mutant N-RAS induces erythroid lineage dysplasia in human CD34+ cells. J Exp Med 1997; 185:1337–1347.

29. Molldrem JJ, Jiang YZ, Stetler-Stevenson M, Mavroudis D, Hensel N, Barrett AJ. Haematological response of patients with myelodysplastic syndrome to antithymocyte globulin is associated with a loss of lymphocyte-mediated inhibition of CFU-GM and alterations in T-cell receptor V-beta profiles. Br J Haematol 1998; 102: 1314–1322.

30. Williamson PJ, Oscier DG, Bell AJ, Hamblin TJ. Red cell aplasia in myelodysplastic syndrome. J Clin Pathol 1991; 44:431–432.

31. Bowen D, Williams K, Phillips I, Cavill I. Cytometric analysis and maturation characteristics of reticulocytes from myelodysplastic patients. Clin Lab Haematol 1996; 18:155–160.

32. Sokol RJ, Hewitt S, Booker DJ. Erythrocyte autoantibodies, autoimmune haemolysis, and myelodysplastic syndromes. J Clin Pathol 1989; 42:1088–1091.

33. Higgs DR, Wood WG, Barton C, Weatherall DJ. Clinical features and molecular analysis of acquired hemoglobin H disease. Am J Med 1983; 75:181–191.

34. Lintula R. Red cell enzymes in myelodysplastic syndromes: a review. Scand J Haematol 1986; 45(suppl):56–59.

35. Chalevelakis G, Karaoulis S, Yalouris AG, Economopoulos T, Tountas N, Raptis S. Globin chain synthesis in myelodysplastic syndromes. J Clin Pathol 1991; 44: 134–138.

36. Germing U, Gattermann N, Aivado M, Hildebrandt B, Aul C. Two types of acquired idiopathic sideroblastic anaemia (AISA): a time-tested distinction. Br J Haematol 2000; 108:724–728.

37. Nilsson L, Astrand-Grundstrom I, Arvidsson I, Jacobsson B, Hellström-Lindberg E, Hast R, Jacobsen, SE. Isolation and characterization of hematopoietic progenitor/stem cells in 5q-deleted myelodysplastic syndromes: evidence for involvement at the hematopoietic stem cell level. Blood 2000; 96:2012–2021.

38. Cheson BD, Bennett JM, Kantarjian H, Pinto A, Schiffer CA, Nimer SD, Lowenberg B, Beran M, de Witte TM, Stone RM, Mittelman M, Sanz GF, Wijermans PW, Gore S, Greenberg PL. Report of an international working group to standardize response criteria for myelodysplastic syndromes. Blood 2000; 96:3671–3674.

39. Hellström-Lindberg E, Ahlgren T, Dahl I, Dybedal I, Grimfors G, Gulbrandsen N, et al. A final decision model for treating the anemia of myelodysplastic syndromes (MDS) with EPO + G-CSF. Blood 2000; 96(suppl 1):546a.

40. Thomas ML, Zhang, J, Greenberg P. Quality of life in individuals with myelodysplastic syndromes (MDS): a descriptive study. Blood 1999; 94(suppl 1):662a.

41. Demetri GD, Kris M, Wade J, Degos L, Cella D. Quality-of-life benefit in chemotherapy patients treated with epoetin alfa is independent of disease response or tumor type: results from a prospective community oncology study. Procrit Study Group. J Clin Oncol 1998; 16:3412–3425.

42. Fluit CR, Kunst VA, Drenthe-Schonk AM. Incidence of red cell antibodies after multiple blood transfusion. Transfusion 1990; 30:532–535.

43. Schafer AI, Cheron RG, Dluhy R, Cooper B, Gleason RE, Soeldner JS, Bunn HF. Clinical consequences of acquired transfusional iron overload in adults. N Engl J Med 1981; 304:319–324.

44. Jensen PD, Jensen FT, Christensen T, Ellegaard J. Evaluation of transfusional iron overload before and during iron chelation by magnetic resonance imaging of the liver and determination of serum ferritin in adult non-thalassaemic patients. Br J Haematol 1995; 89:880–889.

45. Haines ME, Wainscoat JS. Relapsing sideroblastic anaemia. Br J Haematol 1991; 78:285–286.

46. Jensen PD, Heickendorff L, Pedersen B, Bendix-Hansen K, Jensen FT, Christensen T, Boesen AM, Ellegaard. The effect of iron chelation on haemopoiesis in MDS patients with transfusional iron overload. Br J Haematol 1996; 94:288–299.

47. Pippard MJ, Weatherall DJ. Oral iron chelation therapy for thalassaemia: an uncertain scene. Br J Haematol 2000; 111:2–5.

48. Franchini M, Gandini G, de Gironcoli M, Vassanelli A, Borgna-Pignatti C, Aprili G. Safety and efficacy of subcutaneous bolus injection of deferoxamine in adult patients with iron overload. Blood 2000; 95:2776–2779.

49. Anonymous. A randomized double-blind placebo-controlled study with subcutaneous recombinant human erythropoietin in patients with low-risk myelodysplastic syndromes. Italian Cooperative Study Group for rHuEpo in Myelodysplastic Syndromes. Br J Haematol 1998; 103:1070–1074.

50. Hellstrom-Lindberg E. Efficacy of erythropoietin in the myelodysplastic syndromes: a meta-analysis of 205 patients from 17 studies. Br J Haematol 1995; 89: 67–71.

51. Rodriguez JN, Dieguez JC, Muniz R, Martino ML, Fernandez-Jurado A, Amian A, Canavate M, Prados D. [Human recombinant erythropoietin in the treatment of myelodysplastic syndromes anemia. Meta-analytic study.] Sangre (Barc.) 1994; 39: 435–439 [Spanish].

52. Di Raimondo F, Longo G, Cacciola E Jr, Milone G, Palumbo GA, Cacciola RR, Alessi M, Giustolisi R. A good response rate to recombinant erythropoietin alone may be expected in selected myelodysplastic patients. A preliminary clinical study. Eur J Haematol 1996; 56:7–11.

53. Musto P, Matera R, Minervini MM, Checchia-de Ambrosio C, Bodenizza C, Falcone A, Carotenuto M. Low serum levels of tumor necrosis factor and interleukin-1-beta in myelodysplastic syndromes responsive to recombinant erythropoietin. Haematologica 1994; 79:265–268.

54. Bowen D, Culligan D, Jacobs A. The treatment of anaemia in the myelodysplastic syndromes with recombinant human erythropoietin. Br J Haematol 1991; 77:419–423.

55. Verhoef GE, Zachee P, Ferrant A, Demuynck H, Selleslag D, Van Hove L, Deckers F, Boogaerts MA. Recombinant human erythropoietin for the treatment of anemia in the myelodysplastic syndromes: a clinical and erythrokinetic assessment. Ann Hematol 1992; 64:16–21.

56. Hellström-Lindberg E, Ahlgren T, Beguin Y, Carlsson M, Carneskog J, Dahl IM, Dybedal I, Grimfors G, Kanter-Lewensohn L, Linder O, Luthman M, Lofvenberg E, Nilsson-Ehle H, Samuelsson J, Tangen JM, Winqvist I, Oberg G, Osterborg A, Ost A. Treatment of anemia in myelodysplastic syndromes with granulocyte colony-stimulating factor plus erythropoietin: results from a randomized phase II study and long-term follow-up of 71 patients. Blood 1998; 92:68–75.

57. Remacha AF, Arrizabalaga B, Villegas A, Manteiga R, Calvo T, Julia A, Fernandez Fuertes I, Gonzalez FA, Font L, Junca J, del Arco A, Malcorra JJ, Equiza EP, de Mendiguren BP, Romero M. Erythropoietin plus granulocyte colony-stimulating factor in the treatment of myelodysplastic syndromes. Identification of a subgroup of responders. The Spanish Erythropathology Group. Haematologica 1999; 84: 1058–1064.

58. Negrin RS, Stein R, Doherty K, Cornwell J, Vardiman J, Krantz S, Greenberg PL. Maintenance treatment of the anemia of myelodysplastic syndromes with recombinant human granulocyte colony-stimulating factor and erythropoietin: evidence for in vivo synergy. Blood 1996; 87:4076–4081.

59. Mantovani L, Lentini G, Hentschel B, Wickramanayake PD, Loeffler M, Diehl V, Tesch H. Treatment of anaemia in myelodysplastic syndromes with prolonged administration of recombinant human granulocyte colony-stimulating factor and erythropoietin. Br J Haematol 2000; 109:367–375.

60. Hellström-Lindberg E, Negrin R, Stein R, Krantz S, Lindberg G, Vardiman J, Ost A, Greenberg P. Erythroid response to treatment with G-CSF plus erythropoietin for the anaemia of patients with myelodysplastic syndromes: proposal for a predictive model. Br J Haematol 1997; 99:344–351.

61. Hast R, Wallvik J, Folin A, Bernell P, Stenke L. Long-term follow-up of 18 patients with myelodysplastic syndromes responding to recombinant erythropoietin treatment. Leuk Res 2001; 25:13–18.

62. Bowen DT, Hellström-Lindberg E. Best supportive care for the anaemia of myelodysplasia: inclusion of recombinant erythropoietin therapy? Leuk Res 2001; 25: 19–21.

63. Cremieux PY, Finkelstein SN, Berndt ER, Crawford J, Slavin MB. Cost effectiveness, quality-adjusted life-years and supportive care. Recombinant human erythropoietin as a treatment of cancer-associated anaemia. Pharmacoeconomics 1999; 16: 459–472.

64. Sheffield RE, Sullivan SD, Saltiel E, Nishimura L. Cost comparison of recombinant human erythropoietin and blood transfusion in cancer chemotherapy-induced anemia. Ann Pharmacother 1997; 31:15–22.

65. Barosi G, Marchetti M, Liberato NL. Cost-effectiveness of recombinant human erythropoietin in the prevention of chemotherapy-induced anaemia. Br J Cancer 1998; 78:781–787.

66. Kelley LL, Green WF, Hicks GG, Bondurant MC, Koury MJ, Ruley HE. Apoptosis in erythroid progenitors deprived of erythropoietin occurs during the G1 and S phases of the cell cycle without growth arrest or stabilization of wild-type p53. Mol Cell Biol 1994; 14:4183–4192.

67. Kelley LL, Koury MJ, Bondurant MC, Koury ST, Sawyer ST, Wickrema A. Survival or death of individual proerythroblasts results from differing erythropoietin sensitivities: a mechanism for controlled rates of erythrocyte production. Blood 1993; 82:2340–2352.

68. Sui X, Krantz SB, Zhao ZJ. Stem cell factor and erythropoietin inhibit apoptosis of human erythroid progenitor cells through different signalling pathways. Br J Haematol 2000; 110:63–70.

69. Millot GA, Svinarchuk F, Lacout C, Vainchenker W, Dumenil D. The granulocyte colony-stimulating factor receptor supports erythroid differentiation in the absence of the erythropoietin receptor or Stat5. Br J Haematol 2001; 112:449–458.

70. Cazzola M, Ponchio L, Pedrotti C, Farina G, Cerani P, Lucotti C, Novella A, Rovati A. Prediction of response to recombinant human erythropoietin (rHuEpo) in anemia of malignancy. Haematologica 1996; 81:434–441.

71. Musto P, Modoni S, Alicino G, Savino A, Longo A, Bodenizza C, Falcone A, D'Arena G, Scalzulli P, Perla G, et al. Modifications of erythropoiesis in myelodysplastic syndromes treated with recombinant erythropoietin as evaluated by soluble transferrin receptor, high fluorescence reticulocytes and hypochromic erythrocytes. Haematologica 1994; 79:493–499.

72. Economopoulos T, Mellou S, Papageorgiou E, Pappa V, Kokkinou V, Stathopoulou E, Pappa M, Raptis S. Treatment of anemia in low risk myelodysplastic syndromes with granulocyte-macrophage colony-stimulating factor plus recombinant human erythropoietin. Leukemia 1999; 13:1009–1012.

73. Stasi R, Pagano A, Terzoli E, Amadori S. Recombinant human granulocyte-macrophage colony-stimulating factor plus erythropoietin for the treatment of cytopenias in patients with myelodysplastic syndromes. Br J Haematol 1999; 105:141–148.

74. Hansen PB, Johnsen HE, Hippe E, Hellstrom-Lindberg E, Ralfkiaer E. Recombinant human granulocyte-macrophage colony-stimulating factor plus recombinant human erythropoietin may improve anemia in selected patients with myelodysplastic syndromes. Am J Hematol 1993; 44:229–236.

75. Thompson JA, Gilliland DG, Prchal JT, et al. Effect of recombinant human erythropoietin combined with granulocyte/macrophage colony-stimulating factor in the treatment of patients with myelodysplastic syndrome. GM/EPA Study Group. Blood 2000; 95:1175–1179.

76. Takeda Y, Sawada H, Sawai H, Toi-Matsuda T, Tashima M, Okuma M, Watanabe S, Ohmori S, Kondo M. Acquired hypochromic and microcytic sideroblastic anaemia responsive to pyridoxine with low value of free erythrocyte protoporphyrin: a possible subgroup of idiopathic acquired sideroblastic anaemia (IASA). Br J Haematol 1995; 90:207–209.

77. Anzai N, Kawabata H, Hirama T, Masutani H, Ohmori M, Yoshida Y, Okuma M. Marked apoptosis of human myelomonocytic leukemia cell line P39: significance of cellular differentiation. Leukemia 1994; 8:446–453.

78. Clark RE, Jacobs A, Lush CJ, Smith SA. Effect of 13-cis-retinoic acid on survival of patients with myelodysplastic syndrome. Lancet 1987; 1:763–765.

79. Koeffler HP, Heitjan D, Mertelsmann R, Kolitz JE, Schulman P, Itri L, Gunter P, Besa E. Randomized study of 13-cis retinoic acid v placebo in the myelodysplastic disorders. Blood 1988; 71:703–708.

80. Ohno R, Naoe T, Hirano M, Kobayashi M, Hirai H, Tubaki K, Oh H. Treatment of myelodysplastic syndromes with all-trans retinoic acid. Leukemia Study Group of the Ministry of Health and Welfare. Blood 1993; 81:1152–1154.

81. Motomura S, Kanamori H, Maruta A, Kodama F, Ohkubo T. The effect of 1-hydroxyvitamin D3 for prolongation of leukemic transformation-free survival in myelodysplastic syndromes. Am J Hematol 1991; 38:67–68.

82. Petti MC, Latagliata R, Avvisati G, Spiriti MA, Montefusco E, Spadea A, Mandelli F. Treatment of high-risk myelodysplastic syndromes with lymphoblastoid alpha interferon. Br J Haematol 1996; 95:364–367.

83. Gisslinger H, Chott A, Linkesch W, Fritz E, Ludwig H. Long-term alpha-interferon therapy in myelodysplastic syndromes. Leukemia 1990; 4:91–94.

84. Hellstrom E, Robert KH, Gahrton G, Mellstedt H, Lindemalm C, Einhorn S, Bjorkholm M, Grimfors G, Uden AM, Samuelsson J, et al. Therapeutic effects of low-dose cytosine arabinoside, alpha-interferon, 1 alpha-hydroxyvitamin D3 and retinoic acid in acute leukemia and myelodysplastic syndromes. Eur J Haematol 1988; 40:449–459.

85. Catalano L, Majolino I, Musto P, Fragrasso A, Molica S, Cirincione S, Selleri C, Luciano L, DeRenzo A, Vecchione R, et al. Alpha interferon in the treatment of chronic myelomonocytic leukemia. Haematologica 1989; 74:577–581.

86. Maiolo AT, Cortelezzi A, Calori R, Polli EE. Recombinant gamma-interferon as first line therapy for high-risk myelodysplastic syndromes. Italian MDS Study Group. Leukemia 1990; 4:480–485.

87. Andreeff M, Stone R, Michaeli J, Young CW, Tong WP, Sogoloff H, Ervin T, Kufe D, Rifkind RA, Marks PA. Hexamethylene bisacetamide in myelodysplastic syndrome and acute myelogenous leukemia: a phase II clinical trial with a differentiation-inducing agent. Blood 1992; 80:2604–2609.
88. Rowinsky EK, Conley BA, Jones RJ, Spivak JL, Auerbach M, Donehower RC. Hexamethylene bisacetamide in myelodysplastic syndrome: effect of five-day exposure to maximal therapeutic concentrations. Leukemia 1992; 6:526–534.
89. Richon VM, Emiliani S, Verdin E, Webb Y, Breslow R, Rifkind RA, Marks PA. A class of hybrid polar inducers of transformed cell differentiation inhibits histone deacetylases. Proc Natl Acad Sci USA 1998; 95:3003–3007.
90. Gore SD, Samid D, Weng LJ. Impact of the putative differentiating agents sodium phenylbutyrate and sodium phenylacetate on proliferation, differentiation, and apoptosis of primary neoplastic myeloid cells. Clin Cancer Res 1997; 3:1755–1762.
91. Timonen TT, Kauma H. Therapeutic effect of heme arginate in myelodysplastic syndromes. Eur J Haematol 1992; 49:234–238.
92. Bagby GC Jr. Mechanisms of glucocorticosteroid activity in patients with the preleukaemic syndrome (hematopoietic dysplasia). Leuk Res 1980; 4:571–580.
93. Watts EJ, Majer RV, Green PJ, Mavor WO. Hyperfibrotic myelodysplasia: a report of three cases showing haematological remission following treatment with prednisolone. Br J Haematol 1991; 78:120–122.
94. Molldrem JJ, Caples M, Mavroudis D, Plante M, Young NS, Barrett AJ. Antithymocyte globulin for patients with myelodysplastic syndrome. Br J Haematol 1997; 99:699–705.
95. Killick SB, Marsh JC, Cavenagh JD, Mijovic A, Mufti G, Gordon-Smith EC, Bowen D. Antithymocyte globulin for the treatment of patients with "low risk" myelodysplastic syndromes. Blood 1999; 94(suppl 1):306a.
96. Dunn DE, Tanawattanacharoen P, Boccuni P, Nagakura S, Green SW, Kirby MR, Kumar MS, Rosenfeld S, Young NS. Paroxysmal nocturnal hemoglobinuria cells in patients with bone marrow failure syndromes. Ann Intern Med 1999; 131:401–408.
97. Saunthararajah Y, Nakamura R, Robyn J, Loberiza F, Brown KE, Young NS, Barrett AJ. HLA DR15 (DR2) is over-represented in myelodysplastic syndrome (MDS) and is associated with a response to immunosuppression. Blood 2000; 96(suppl 1): 546a.
98. Jonásova A, Neuwirtová R, Cermák J, Vozobulová V, Mociková K, Sisková M, Hochova I. Cyclosporin A therapy in hypoplastic MDS patients and certain refractory anaemias without hypoplastic bone marrow. Br J Haematol 1998; 100:304–309.
99. Catalano L, Selleri C, Califano C, Luciano L, Volpicelli M, Rocco S, Varriale G, Ricci P, Rotoli B. Prolonged response to cyclosporin-A in hypoplastic refractory anemia and correlation with in vitro studies. Haematologica 2000; 85:133–138.
100. Hassan Z, Fadeel B, Zhivotovsky B, Hellstrom-Lindberg E. Two pathways of apoptosis induced with all-trans retinoic acid and etoposide in the myeloid cell line P39. Exp Hematol 1999; 27:1322–1329.
101. List AF, Heaton R, Glinsmann-Gibson B, Capizzi RL. Amifostine stimulates for-

mation of multipotent and erythroid bone marrow progenitors. Leukemia 1998; 12: 1596–1602.

102. List AF, Holmes H, Greenberg PL, Bennett JM, Oster W. Phase II study of amifostine in patients with myelodysplastic syndromes. Blood 1999; 94(suppl 1):305a.

103. Bowen DT, Denzlinger C, Brugger W, Culligan D, Gelly K, Adlakha S, Groves M, Hepburn M, Kanz L. Poor response rate to a continuous schedule of Amifostine therapy for 'low/intermediate risk' myelodysplastic patients. Br J Haematol 1998; 103:785–787.

104. Cortelezzi A, Cattaneo C, Cristiani S, Duca L, Sarina B, Deliliers GL, Fiorelli G, Cappellini MD. Non-transferrin-bound iron in myelodysplastic syndromes: a marker of ineffective erythropoiesis? Hematol J 2000; 1:153–158.

105. Nemunaitis J, Rosenfeld C, Getty L, Boegel F, Meyer W, Jennings LW, Zegler A, Snadduck R. Pentoxifylline and ciprofloxacin in patients with myelodysplastic syndrome. A phase-II trial. Am J Clin Oncol 1995; 18:189–193.

106. Novitzky N, Mohamed R, Finlayson J, du Toit C. Increased apoptosis of bone marrow cells and preserved proliferative capacity of selected progenitors predict for clinical response to anti-inflammatory therapy in myelodysplastic syndromes. Exp Hematol 2000; 28:941–949.

107. Raza A, Qawi H, Lisak L, Andric T, Dar S, Andrews C, Venugopal P, Gezer S, Gregory S, Loew J, Robin E, Rifkin S, Hsu WT, Huang RW. Patients with myelodysplastic syndromes benefit from palliative therapy with amifostine, pentoxifylline, and ciprofloxacin with or without dexamethasone. Blood 2000; 95:1580–1587.

108. Miller KB, Kim K, Morrison FS, Winter JN, Bennett JM, Neiman RS, Head DR, Cassileth PA, O'Connell MJ, Kyungmann K. The evaluation of low-dose cytarabine in the treatment of myelodysplastic syndromes: a phase-III intergroup study [published erratum appears in Ann Hematol 1993; 66:164]. Ann Hematol 1992; 65:162–168.

109. Hellstrom-Lindberg E, Robert KH, Gahrton G, Lindberg G, Forsblom AM, Kock Y, Ost A. A predictive model for the clinical response to low dose ara-C: a study of 102 patients with myelodysplastic syndromes or acute leukemia. Br J Haematol 1992; 81:503–511.

110. Juneja HS, Jodhani M, Gardner FH, Trevarthen D, Schottstedt M. Low-dose ARA-C consistently induces hematologic responses in the clinical 5q-syndrome. Am J Hematol 1994; 46:338–342

111. Denzlinger C, Bowen D, Benz D, Gelly K, Brugger W, Kanz L. Low-dose melphalan induces favourable responses in elderly patients with high-risk myelodysplastic syndromes or secondary acute myeloid leukaemia. Br J Haematol 2000; 108:93–95.

112. Omoto E, Deguchi S, Takaba S, Kojima K, Yano T, Katayama Y, Sunami K, Takeuchi M, Kimura F, Harada M, Kimura I. Low-dose melphalan for treatment of high-risk myelodysplastic syndromes. Leukemia 1996; 10:609–614.

113. Kerr R, Cunningham J, Bowen DT. Low-dose melphalan in elderly acute myeloid leukaemia: complete remissions but resistant relapse with therapy-related karyotypes. Leukemia 2000; 14:953.

114. Silverman LR, Holland JF, Weinberg RS, Alter BP, Davis RB, Ellison RR, Demakos EP, Cornell CJ Jr, Carey RW, Schiffer C, et al. Effects of treatment with

5-azacytidine on the in vivo and in vitro hematopoiesis in patients with myelodysplastic syndromes. Leukemia 1993; 7(suppl 1):21–29.

115. Wijermans P, Lubbert M, Verhoef G, Bosly A, Ravoet C, Andre M, Ferrant A. Low-dose 5-aza-2'-deoxycytidine, a DNA hypomethylating agent, for the treatment of high-risk myelodysplastic syndrome: a multicenter phase II study in elderly patients. J Clin Oncol 2000; 18:956–962.

116. Rose EH, Abels RI, Nelson RA, McCullough DM, Lessin L. The use of rHuEpo in the treatment of anemia related to myelodysplasia (MDS). Br J Haematol 1995; 89:831–837.

# 14

# Immune Mediation of Pancytopenia in Myelodysplastic Syndromes: Pathophysiology and Treatment

**Neal S. Young and A. John Barrett**
*National Heart, Lung, and Blood Institute, Bethesda, Maryland*

## I. INTRODUCTION

Recent clinical observations and laboratory studies suggest that the myelodys-plastic syndromes (MDS) belong to a group of related diseases (Fig. 1) in which the pathophysiology of bone marrow failure is mediated, at least in part, by the immune system. In this chapter, we will review the relationship between MDS and aplastic anemia, the data supporting a role for lymphocytes and cytokines in suppression of hematopoiesis, and the results of therapeutic trials employing immunosuppression to treat pancytopenia in MDS (for helpful reviews and other approaches to this subject, see Refs. 1–4).

Aplastic anemia is a far more uniform clinical entity than is the MDS group-ing. With aplastic anemia, blood count findings are usually striking, the bone marrow morphology is unambiguous, typical clinical patterns are easily de-scribed, and the response to therapy is relatively predictable (5). Although impor-tant questions as to inciting events and long-term progression are unanswered, the essential pathophysiology of acquired aplastic anemia also has been delineated, at least in outline (6,7). In most patients, the empty bone marrow is the result of efficient and specific immune system attack on hematopoietic targets, including both stem and progenitor cells: T cells of $T_H1$ cytokine profile, producing inter-feron and tumor necrosis factor, induce apoptosis in their marrow targets through activation of the Fas receptor, leading to destruction of the hematopoietic cell compartment. At the time of presentation with severe pancytopenia this process

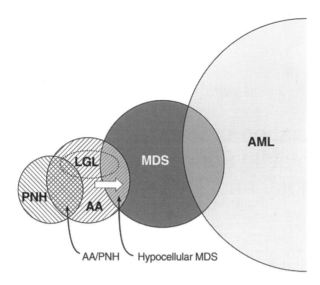

**Fig. 1** Overlapping diagnostic and etiological relationships among bone marrow failure syndromes and acute leukemia. AA, aplastic anemia; AML, acute myeloid leukemia; LGL, large granular lymphocytic leukemia; MDS, myelodysplastic syndromes; PNH, paroxysmal nocturnal hemoglobinuria.

is advanced; measurements in surrogate stem cell assays suggest that the stem cell pool is reduced to a few percentage or less of normal. Most patients do respond with hematological improvement to immunosuppressive therapies, now usually a combination of an antilymphocyte globulin and cyclosporine, but both relapse of pancytopenia and a requirement for continued cyclosporine administration to maintain adequate blood counts are common.

## II. MDS AND APLASTIC ANEMIA

MDS and aplastic anemia are closely related and clinically often difficult to distinguish. Aplastic anemia has been defined historically by extremely low bone marrow cellularity on biopsy. Although not separately considered in the initial French-American-British definition and categorization of MDS, a significant proportion of MDS also shows marrow hypocellularity, with large series averaging about 20% of cases; hypocellular MDS have not been reported to be markedly different in clinical characteristics such as age, FAB subtypes, or prognosis from the more common cellular disease (8). However, the differential diagnosis between aplasia and MDS often relies on "soft" histological criteria, such as myeloid cells lacking granules (an appearance that can also arise from technical staining artifact), dyserythropoiesis (with megaloblastoid changes frequently seen in aplasia), or dysmorphic megakaryocytes (usually infrequent in hypocellular aspirate smears). Histological dysplasia can be found not only in aplastic anemia but also in hemophagocytic lymphohistocytosis (9). In practice, with severely hypocellular marrows, aplasia usually becomes the diagnosis of default for lack of sufficient cells on which to base a morphological diagnosis of MDS. Cytogenetic abnormalities of bone marrow cells are more objective evidence of myelodysplasia, but some authorities regard findings such as trisomy 6 or 8 as simply delineating a subset of otherwise typical aplastic anemias (10).

The border between MDS and aplastic anemia becomes further blurred because of the late evolution of some aplastic anemia to MDS. A significant proportion of aplastic anemia patients who undergo immunosuppressive therapy later manifest features of MDS, with recurrent pancytopenia associated with bone marrow dysplasia or chromosomal aberrations or evidence of a new cytogenetic abnormality. In our series of 122 patients having severe aplastic anemia and treated with antithymocyte globulin and cyclosporine, 22% were diagnosed as having MDS at 5 years. The risk of evolution was much higher in adults than in children (20 years or younger). In the large European Group for Bone Marrow Transplantation experience, the risk for evolution to MDS was estimated at about 12% at 12 years posttreatment (11) (clinical diagnostic criteria and protocols for serial monitoring differ between the American single-center study and the multicenter European registry).

The clinical characteristics of MDS evolved from aplastic anemia have been less fully described. In our experience, cytogenetic abnormalities can appear as soon as the 3-month follow-up visit, suggesting that they likely were present at diagnosis but missed owing to sampling error. For chromosomal changes, there are two stereotypical patterns (12,129). Monosomy 7, associated with refractory pancytopenia, more frequently emerges in patients who have not responded to immunosuppressive treatment; its appearance is a poor prognostic sign and may herald leukemic conversion. In contrast, trisomy 8 typically is observed in patients who have adequate blood counts, the maintenance of which is dependent on continued cyclosporine therapy.

## III. THE ORIGIN OF HEMATOPOIETIC FAILURE IN MDS

The concept of MDS originated in the merger of two ill-defined but clearly different hematological processes, "preleukemia" and "refractory anemia." As is discussed in other chapters in this volume, the pathophysiology of preleukemic MDS presumably reflects a process of accumulation of genetic alterations within a hematopoietic stem cell clone, leading to a combination of proliferative advantage, defect in apoptosis, and stunted differentiation, as occurs in acute myelogenous leukemia; indeed, the recent World Health Organization classification has abolished the MDS subgroup refractory anemia with excess blasts, which is now viewed as equivalent to acute myelogenous leukemia in the elderly. However, pancytopenia and not leukemia is the proximate cause of death in most whose MDS is terminal. Why hematopoiesis fails, and especially the development of bone marrow hypocellularity that accompanies this failure, is not clearly understood. Contributing to this lack of understanding is that the interpretation of the laboratory studies (reviewed below) is confounded by the heterogeneity of the clinical entities within MDS, the coexistence of normal and abnormal hematopoietic stem cells and their progeny in many MDS patients, and the limited correlation between in vitro data and in vivo clinical behavior.

## A. MDS Hematopoiesis in Tissue Culture

The highly varied pattern of hematopoiesis in tissue culture in MDS should be contrasted with a monotonous picture in aplastic anemia, in which both mature and primitive progenitors are uniformly and severely decreased, often to undetectable levels. In MDS, measurements of hematopoietic cell proliferation and progenitor cell number and function show more paradoxical features. Cell proliferation rates are often elevated, as measured by in vitro nucleotide incorporation (13), autonomous colony formation (14), or expression of specific cell markers like MIB-1 (15), reflective of the cellular character of most MDS bone marrows. Hematopoietic progenitor-derived colony formation, in contrast, is usually deficient. For example, erythropoiesis, as measured by BFU-E (burst-forming units–erythrocytes) and CFU-E (colony-forming units–erythrocytes) in semisolid medium, is diminished in most patients with MDS, consistent with the high frequency of anemia; megakaryocytic colony formation has generally paralleled erythroid results (16–23) while myeloid colony growth from CFU-GM (granulocyte, monocyte) may be near normal in the majority of the same cases (16,17). Additionally, CFU-GEMM (granulocyte, erythrocyte, monocyte, megakaryocyte), progenitor cells capable of giving rise to mixed colonies, have been generally reduced in MDS marrow (24,25). In our study of marrow long-term culture-initiating cells (LTC-IC), numbers of secondary colonies formed in vitro were on average low, but a quarter of patients nevertheless retained normal numbers (by comparison, numbers of marrow LTC-IC are uniformly severely decreased in aplastic anemia) (26). Cells capable of forming blast colonies were normal in another study, but they gave rise to deficient numbers of secondary erythroid cells (27). Phenotypic analyses of CD34 cells have shown deficiencies mainly in erythroid antigen expression (28) or reduced CD34 expression in the case of patients with hypocellular marrow morphology (29). Most studies have suggested that entirely normal colony formation, as occurs in a significant proportion of patients, is found in good prognostic subtypes, like 5q- and ringed sideroblastic anemia. Conversely, patients with low CFU-GM numbers, aberrant myeloid maturation in vitro, predominant cluster over colony formation, and abnormal immunophenotypes of progenitors, all findings seen in acute myelogenous leukemia, have an expectedly poor prognosis (16,22,30,31).

The response of progenitors to hematopoietins in vitro is generally subnormal, with poor colony formation despite high concentrations of purified or recombinant factors, alone or in combination. Tissue culture studies have not consistently been predictive of therapeutic outcomes in clinical interventional trials: for example, high concentrations of erythropoietin marginally improved erythropoiesis in vitro in several studies (32,33), but colony numbers have not consistently increased in patients whose anemia responded to erythropoietin treatment (34). In some experiments, very high concentrations of erythropoietin were required to improve erythroid colony formation (35), consistent with the pharmacological efficacy in clinical trials. Both G-CSF (granulocyte colony-stimulating factor) and GM-CSF (granulocyte-monocyte colony-stimulating factor) increase myeloid colony growth, at least in a subset of patients (33,36). In systematic studies of Nagler and colleagues (34,37), GM-CSF was a more potent proliferation stimulator and G-CSF was more efficient at driving granulocytic differentiation although the effects of the two growth factors overlapped. Purified CD34 cells from MDS patients have generally provided normal response profiles to early acting growth factors like stem cell factor and the interleukins IL-3 and IL-6 (38,39), but primitive colony formation when low has been unaffected by addition of exogenous factors (36).

There are few studies of bone marrow stroma in MDS, but adherent cell layers from some, but not all, patients with MDS have been defective in their ability to sustain normal hematopoietic progenitors in long-term culture (40–42).

## B. Cell Death in the Dysplastic Marrow

The occurrence in MDS of pancytopenia, despite normal to increased numbers of marrow precursor cells, has led to the obvious inference that cell death in the hematopoietic cell compartment is dominant over cell proliferation. That the histological abnormalities of MDS might reflect not only a process of intramedullary cellular destruction but specifically apoptosis or programmed cell death was first proposed by Clark and Lampert (43), and more recent, quantitative studies have supported this conclusion: for example, an elevated apoptotic index of 3% in MDS contrasted with normal marrow values of 1%, as based on morphological and ultrastructural changes on thin section biopsies (44). The Pelger-Huet abnormality may represent apoptotic polymorphonuclear granulocytes (45). In short-term tissue culture, the poor growth of colonies and the dominance of clusters also has been argued to reflect a high initial rate of growth followed by failure of both proliferation and differentiation (46), and a leukemic cell line from a patient with myelomonocytic leukemia showed high susceptibility to the induction of cell suicide (47). However, cultured MDS cells may also manifest much more striking degrees of apoptosis than fresh cells, so artifactual results due to in vitro cell manipulations may influence both quantitative and qualitative conclusions (48). In biopsy specimens, single cells can be examined for evidence of apoptosis but their exact lineage usually cannot be confidently determined, and not only hematopoietic precursors but also stromal cells, endothelium, and fat may score positive (49).

Other more specific measurements of apoptosis have been abnormally elevated in MDS: in situ end labeling (ISEL) detection of DNA strand breaks; terminal deoxynucleotide transferase incorporation of nucleotides on 3′ ends of DNA (TUNEL); detection of subgenomic DNA in histograms of cell populations subjected to fluorescence-activated flowcytometry; binding of annexin-V to exposed phosphotidylserine of cell membranes, also assessed by flow cytometry; and the detection of apoptosis-related proteins like Bcl-2 in individual permeabilized cells (1,4). These techniques all measure relatively early events in programmed cell death; most investigators have been unable to demonstrate the typical laddering pattern seen late as a result of DNA fragmentation. In general, despite the diversity of the methods employed, there is agreement that apoptosis is increased in MDS as compared with both normal specimens and bone marrows from patients with acute leukemia. Mechanistically, low Bcl-2 expression has correlated with high apoptotic rates in total bone marrow (14,50) or fractionated cell populations (51,52), and enhanced Bcl-2 expression has been linked to leukemic transformation; sequential caspase activation consistent with appropriate death signal transduction also has been reported for MDS marrow specimens (53). Additionally, a few serial studies have lent credibility to the biological significance of apoptosis measurements as improvements in blood counts with growth factor therapy (54) and anti-inflammatory agents such as pentoxifylline and corticosteroids (42) have correlated with lowered rates of apoptosis. However, the MDS patient populations examined have been very heterogeneous, and the range of results broad; for example, in one large study of 175 patients, 71 showed high and 43 low levels of apoptosis by ISEL, and 61 were normal (55).

More detailed conclusions have remained controversial, with opposite results presented in the literature. First, one appealing hypothesis proposed that programmed cell death dominated early in the pancytopenic phase of MDS, and that leukemic transformation represented escape from the apoptotic (intracellular) process or (extracellular) environment. Higher rates of apoptosis have been observed in refractory anemia and refractory anemia with excess blasts compared with transforming MDS or acute leukemia, including measurements by TUNEL (56) and flow cytometry for annexin-V binding, subgenomic DNA, and staining for apoptosis-related proteins (57–59). Using ISEL, some investigators have found a similar correlation with stage of disease (50) while others using the same technique have found increased rates in late stages of disease (60,61). Second, a question remains as to the extent of apoptosis in MDS, with quantitative inferences ranging from minimally or modestly increased (48) to massive destruction (45). These arguments are confounded by: significant levels of apoptosis in normal bone marrow specimens, and often relatively small differences between MDS and normal specimens; the likelihood that apoptosis occurs normally in hematopoietic differentiation and that measurements might be influenced by the relative myeloid and erythroid distribution of a marrow specimen and its overall state of differentiation; the possibility that apoptotic cells are rapidly removed from the marrow; and the lack of information as to the biological kinetic significance of even low levels of apoptosis in a highly dynamic marrow composed of cell population of different lineages, stages of differentiation, and containing normal as well as abnormal progenitors. Third, apoptosis may be restricted to certain hematopoietic cells in MDS. Evidence from flow cytometric analysis of individual cells supports apoptosis in the CD34 cell compartment (57–59,62) while others have suggested that cell death is far more frequent among mature cells (of high compared with low density) (45) and rare by TUNEL measurements in CD34 cells within biopsies (63).

## C. Immune Triggering of Apoptosis in MDS

In aplastic anemia, hematopoietic destruction by the immune system appears to occur at least in part by lymphokine-mediated triggering of Fas expression on CD34 cell markers with induction of apoptosis (6,7). Similar mechanisms hypothesized to operate in MDS have support from laboratory study (for reviews, see Refs. 3,64,65). Early observations included measurements of overexpression by cultured MDS patients' blood (66) and marrow cells (67) of cytokines such as tumor necrosis factor (TNF) and interferon. TNF levels have been elevated in MDS marrow biopsies (53,68). Using multiplex polymerase chain reactions, elevated levels of marrow mRNA for TNF among other cytokines have been reported for a subset of MDS patients (70). Increased levels of TNF (71–74) and also of the soluble form of the TNF receptor (72,75) have been measured in MDS sera (and appear to decline in patients treated with anticytokine therapies [amifostine (74) and pentoxifylline plus ciprofloxacin (73)]). The presence of TNF, as determined by histochemistry of the bone marrow of MDS patients, also showed caspase activity, as expected if TNF were triggering apoptosis (53). Other downstream consequences of TNF activation, the induction of nitric oxide synthase (76), and intracellular redox changes leading to DNA damage (77) have also been reported for MDS marrows. As with levels of apoptosis, different groups have reported variable correlations between TNF expression and MDS diagnostic categories, for example, elevated with refractory anemia (72), with disease transforming to leukemia (78), or unrelated to subtypes (79).

The source of TNF in MDS marrow has been assumed to be the macrophage (78), but macrophages that inhibited hematopoiesis have not always been shown to produce this or related cytokines (80). Despite generally diminished functioning of natural killer cells, one early investigator reported autologous restricted killing of CFU-GM by patients' cells (81). Toxicity of stroma cells, dependent on cell-cell contact, has been described for adherent cells and a stromal cell line from an MDS patient (82). In our own laboratory work, we identified T cells functionally inhibitory of the growth of autologous marrow progenitor cells, with appropriate class I histocompatibility restriction and with diminished activity after successful immunosuppressive therapy (see below) (83). Additionally, MDS patients may have a skewed T-cell repertoire, as assessed by T-cell receptor (TCR) V-β analysis as has been observed in immunologically mediated diseases (83).

To link an immune cytokine to increased apoptosis in MDS, TNF expression has been studied in relationship to induction on hematopoietic target cells of Fas, a cell surface protein and member of the tumor necrosis factor receptor family, the triggering of which initiates the signal transduction pathway for programmed cell death. Deeg and colleagues, using flowcytometry, measured increased Fas and Fas-ligand surface expression on MDS CD34 cells and, in functional assays, monoclonal antibody-mediated blockade of Fas, Fas ligand, or TNF-enhanced hematopoiesis in long-term bone marrow colony culture and in hematopoietic progenitor assays (72). Addition of anti-Fas ligand antibody in other experiments also decreased apoptosis in marrow samples from MDS patients (84). Flowcytometric results for Fas and Fas-ligand expression have been confirmed by amplification of cDNA from mRNA (69,85) and immunohistochemistry of fixed specimens (56,85). In some studies, increased Fas expression has been correlated to the degree of apoptosis in clinical specimens (65) while others have found no such relationship (86,87). Fas expression has been more striking in refractory anemia than in other MDS subtypes (69) and may decrease in the marrow during transformation to leukemia (56); conversely, Fas-ligand expression has been high in leukemic blast cells (88).

In summary, a current popular model to explain ineffective hematopoiesis in MDS postulates that, despite evident proliferation in the hypercellular bone marrows of most patients, higher rates of apoptosis predominate. Owing to excessive production of TNF and related inhibitory cytokines, Fas is up-regulated on hematopoietic target cells. Apoptosis then is induced by triggering of the Fas pathway, presumably by local Fas ligand, present constitutively or produced by lymphocytes, stromal cells, or even CD34 cells themselves. However, as indicated above, considerable disagreement exists among the results from various laboratories, correlations are inconsistent, and the clinical heterogeneity of MDS is reflected in abnormalities occurring only in a subset of patients. Further complicating biological factors include the complex bifunctionality of TNF for hematopoiesis, where this factor can act to both stimulate and inhibit cell growth, and the uncertain physiological role of TNF, which is produced in normal bone marrow and regulated in response to infection or hematopoietic stress. Technically, accurate quantitation and correlation of apoptosis, cytokine production and expression, and Fas-Fas ligand expression can be confounded by the mixture of cell types and stages of differentiation in normal and MDS marrow, intrinsic limitations of some of the methodologies employed, and nonspecificity of reagents. Finally, most experiments have required examination of a few molecules and cell types, and whether the results obtained are primary to the pathophysiology or epiphenomenal remains an open question: is apoptosis induced by lymphokines produced in response to aberrant proteins expressed in a genetically abnormal stem cell and its progeny, or are the immune abnormalities secondary to excessive apoptosis of an intrinsically abnormal bone marrow? In this respect, correlation with clinical aspects of MDS, especially relating to evidence for systemic evidence of immune system dysfunction and to the results of therapeutic interventions, may be helpful.

## D.  Clinical Immune Dysfunction in MDS

Global abnormalities of immune system function have been reported, but because most studies were published in the 1980s as "preleukemia," modern clinical descriptions are lacking. For the cellular immune system, decreased natural killer cell activity was consistently observed (89–93) while abnormalities of antibody-dependent cell killing (92,94), mitogenic response (95,96), and diminished CD4-helper cell numbers (97,98) were more variable. For B-cell function, abnormalities in series of MDS patients have included polyclonally increased and decreased levels of immunoglobulins as well as monoclonal gammopathies; additionally, patients with MDS may have a higher frequency of autoantibodies to erythrocytes, gastric intrinsic factor, and thyroglobulin (99–101). In a large group of 153 Japanese patients at a single institution, 63% had some abnormal immunological test: hypergammaglobulinemia was most frequent (in 39%) followed by hypoglobulinemia and the presence of antinuclear antibodies, rheumatoid factor, anti-DNA antibodies, and positive Coombs test (98). Such findings may reflect immune dysfunction and especially a propensity to autoimmune disease; unfortunately, many of these abnormalities are more frequent in older individuals and few MDS series have been controlled for age.

Case reports and small series suggest that autoimmune diseases are increased in patients with MDS (for review, see Ref. 102). Again, some, such as rheumatoid arthritis, may be coincidentally associated owing to the advanced age of patients. Nevertheless, other syndromes are observed with apparently increased frequency, including autoimmune hemolytic anemia, pernicious anemia, hypothyroidism, pure red cell aplasia, immune thrombocytopenia, pyoderma gangrenosum, eosinophilic fasciitis (prominent also as an association with aplastic anemia), erythema nodosum, Behçet's syndrome, and immune vasculitis (102). In the large series of Japanese patients described above, 12% of 153 patients developed some autoimmune disorder (98). Of 30 patients from the University of Minnesota, 18 showed systemic acute autoimmune phenomena (various combinations of skin vasculitis, arthritis, pleuritis, pericarditis, and myositis), neurological symptoms such as seizures and peripheral neuropathy, and more classic collagen vascular disorders (103). Many cases of coincident lymphoid and plasma cell neoplasms with MDS have been collected (102,104,105). Although not well documented in the literature, expanded populations of histologically recognizable large granular lymphocytes (LGL) in the marrow also coexist with MDS (102,106). Interestingly, MDS and LGL leukemia are associated; in a survey of 83 recent referrals, we found nine patients with MDS who also had a clonal expansion of circulating CD8+, CD57+, CD56+ cells, consistent with the diagnosis of LGL leukemia (107).

## IV. TRIALS OF IMMUNOSUPPRESSION IN MDS

Figure 2 illustrates the rationale behind several experimental treatment approaches in MDS aimed at preventing lymphocyte-mediated marrow suppression either by targeting lymphocytes or the cytokines they produce either directly or by stimulation of accessory cells such as macrophages.

### A. Prednisone

An early study showed that prednisone alone improved low blood counts in a minority of patients with MDS and that the response could be predicted in vitro by enhancement of CFU-GM growth (108). Subsequent to this report, it became customary to use corticosteroids to treat MDS. However, low response rates and increased risk of infection make them unattractive agents in MDS and their mode of action remains unclear.

### B. Antithymocyte Globulin

Because of the similarity of hypoplastic MDS to severe aplastic anemia, antithymocyte globulin (ATG) was used occasionally to treat hypoplastic MDS with severe cytopenia. A summary of case reports and small series reveals hematological responses in eight of 13 hypoplastic MDS patients (109,110). Based on these

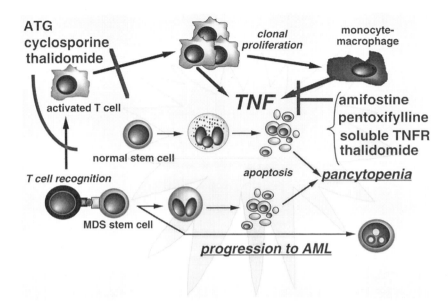

**Fig. 2**   Immune-mediated myelosuppression in MDS and the therapeutic role of immuno-suppressive agents. T cells recognizing antigens on MDS stem cells initiate a cytotoxic immune response, which involves direct cell-mediated toxicity and TNF, in addition to clonal T-cell expansions. Autoaggressive T cells increase apoptosis in MDS cells and in residual normal marrow function, leading to pancytopenia. Progression to acute leukemia is an intrinsic process in the MDS stem cell probably unaffected by the autologous T-cell response. The presumed site of action of several immunosuppressive agents is illustrated. MDS, myelodysplastic syndromes; ATG, anti-thymocyte globulin; TNF, tumor necrosis factor; TNFR, TNF receptor; AML, acute myeloid leukemia.

reports, unpublished observations, and the hypothesis that a T-cell-mediated process may cause pancytopenia, we evaluated ATG as immunosuppressive treatment to improve marrow function in MDS (111). This study, now completed, involved 61 patients. Study entry criteria were red-cell or platelet-transfusion dependence and no concurrent treatment with immunosuppressives, chemotherapy, or growth factors. Thirty-seven patients had refractory anemia (RA), 14 had RA with excess of blasts (RAEB), and 10 had RA with ringed sideroblasts (RARS). Marrow cellularity varied from hypo- to hypercellular. Most patients (75%) had failed previous treatment with single or multiple agents, including cyclosporine, amifostine, and growth factors. The interval between diagnosis and entry to the study was 3–300 months, with a median of 24 months. Twenty-three patients had hypoplastic MDS, seven had a paroxysmal nocturnal hemoglobinuria

(PNH) abnormality as determined by flow cytometry, and 23 had karyotypic abnormalities characteristic of MDS. Patients received ATG at 40 mg/kg/day for 4 days and were periodically evaluated for 38 (range 20–58) months. The main criterion for response was independence from the requirement for red-cell transfusions. Twenty-one patients (33%) became red-cell-transfusion-independent within 8 months of treatment (median 75 days). Transfusion-independence was maintained in 76% of responding patients for a median of 32 months (range 20–58). Twenty-three of 41 severely thrombocytopenic patients (56%) had sustained platelet count increases between 25,000 and 290,000/µl and 18 of 41 severely neutropenic patients (44%) achieved sustained neutrophil counts $> 1000/$ µl. At last follow-up, 39 patients were alive with an actuarial survival of 64% at a median of 34 (range 18–72) months. Of the 21 responders, 20 survive and one died following progression to AML. In the 20 survivors, no significant alteration in the bone marrow appearance or cellularity was observed and cytogenetic abnormalities, present in four, persisted after treatment. Three relapsed with transfusion-dependence but one regained red-cell-transfusion-independence after a second course of ATG. Of the 40 nonresponders, 21 died, 15 from cytopenia and six from progression to AML.

In a multivariate analysis of 82 RA or RAEB patients treated with either ATG alone or cyclosporine alone, younger age, shorter duration of red-cell-transfusion-dependence, and the presence of HLA-DR15 correlated with a response to immunosuppression. In other words, to maximize the probability of response to immunosuppression, patients should be treated sooner rather than later. Furthermore, this strategy appears to be particularly appropriate and effective in RA or RAEB patients who are young and/or have HLA-DR15. Factors predicting a response to immunosuppression are summarized in Table 1. Responses were associated with a significant survival benefit at 4 years (95% vs. 38% for nonresponders, $p = 0.006$). In the subset of 41 responders out of 61 patients categorized as "Intermediate-1" according to the International Prognostic Scoring System (112) and who were given ATG, 100% of the responders survived at 3 years with no disease progression versus 45% of the nonresponders survived ($p < 0.0004$) and 51% of the nonresponders suffered disease progression ($p = 0.02$). Since we previously found correlation between response to ATG treatment and normalization of TCR (113), we studied 15 patients with MDS receiving immunosuppression for biological markers of response. Abnormalities in TCR $V_\beta$ were common and occurred in both responders and nonresponders, rendering $V_\beta$ analysis of no prognostic value.

## C. Cyclosporine

Jonasova and co-workers reported a high proportion of hematological responses following cyclosporine treatment in MDS (114). Sixteen patients with RA and

**Table 1**  Factors Predictive of Myelodysplastic
Syndrome Response to Immunosuppression

| Predictive factor[a] | Measure or type for greatest response |
|---|---|
| Age | Less than 60 years |
| Disease type | Refractory anemia |
| Cytopenia | Pancytopenia |
| Duration of transfusion dependence | Less than 2 years |
| HLA type | HLA-DR15 |
| PNH defect | CD55 loss[b] |

[a] Factors not predictive of response include karyotype, IPSS
score, and marrow cellularity.
[b] Detectable in granulocytes by flow cytometry.
HLA, human leukocyte antigen; PNH, paroxysmal nocturnal
hemogloburinia; CD55, decay accelerating factor; IPSS, International Prognostic Scoring System.

one with RAEB were given standard doses of cyclosporine for 5–31 months.
Substantial hematological responses were observed in 33 months, mostly occurring around 3 months. Transfusion-independence was achieved in all 12 patients who had required red cells before cyclosporine administration, and significant increases in leukocyte and platelet counts also occurred. Responses occurred
in the RAEB patient as well as in the RA patients and in those with hyper- or
normally cellular MDS (six of eight responders) as well as in those with hypocellular MDS (seven of nine responders). Of six patients with abnormal karyotype,
three responded (all were 5q-). These clinical studies provide strong evidence to
support an immune mechanism of marrow suppression in patients with MDS.

Based on these preliminary findings for cyclosporine as well as the finding
for ATG, several trials evaluating immunosuppressive treatment for MDS are
underway in the United States and in Europe. Collectively these studies should
better define the potential benefit for immunosuppression by comparing ATG
treatment with a control arm of conventionally supported patients. Prospective
randomized trials will evaluate the relative effects of different ATG types and
different immunosuppressive combinations in improving marrow function and
prolonging survival.

## D.  Amifostine

Amifostine is a phosphorylated organic thiol that is metabolized to intermediates
with antioxidant activity. The drug has two actions: (1) it protects cells from

oxidative stress after exposure to cytokines including TNF-α; and (2) it suppresses inflammatory cytokine release. Since amifostine reduces apoptotic marrow cell death following chemotherapy, it may also reduce apoptosis in MDS (115). Indeed, incubation of MDS marrow cells with amifostine was found to improve colony growth (116). In a study reported by List et al. (117), five of 18 patients with MDS who were given amifostine had single or multilineage hematological responses. These results were recently updated for 75 patients; 40% experienced platelet responses, 24% absolute-neutrophil count responses, and 20% had greater than 50% reduction in transfusion requirements (118). Ongoing studies on the use of amifostine in combination with growth factors and chemotherapeutic agents should add more information on its efficacy.

### E. Pentoxifylline

The observation that three proinflammatory cytokines, TNF-α, TGF-β (transforming growth factor β), and IL-1α, are implicated in the increased apoptosis of MDS (60,61), led Raza et al. to treat MDS patients with pentoxifylline (PTX), a xanthine derivative known to interfere with the lipid signaling pathway used by these cytokines (119). Ciprofloxacin was added because it reduced hepatic degradation of PTX, and dexamethasone was used to further down-regulate TNF production by reducing translation of TNF mRNA. Eighteen of 43 patients had hematopoietic responses, which correlated with a reduction in blood levels of TNF. In a subsequent study, a four-drug combination of amifostine, PTX, ciprofloxacin, and dexamethasone was used to optimize the anticytokine effect (120). Of 29 patients given this combination, evaluable because they survived 12 or more weeks, 22 (76%) showed partial responses, 19 with improvement in neutrophils, 11 with a reduction in transfusion requirement or a rise in hemoglobin, and 7 with improvements in platelet counts. However, these improvements were not sustained or statistically significant at 24 weeks and are similar to those reported for amifostine alone. There were no complete responses or conversions to transfusion-independence. In contrast, in a study of 14 patients given PTX and ciprofloxacin, Nemunaitis et al. found a trend to lower TNF levels with treatment but no hematological response in any patient (121).

### F. TNF Receptor (Etanercept)

Excessive amounts of soluble receptor can effectively block the function of TNF by competitive binding. In a recent report, the soluble receptor etanercept was reported to be well tolerated and to reduce plasma TNF concentrations. However, clinical responses were modest (122).

## G.  Thalidomide

Thalidomide is an immunosuppressive drug that switches helper T cells from a $T_H1$ to a $T_H2$ cytokine profile, thereby inhibiting production of TNF-$\alpha$ (123) by monocytes (124). The drug has also been found to strongly inhibit angiogenesis in animal experiments and in in vitro cultures of human cells (125,126). Thalidomide has produced surprisingly substantial responses in patients with myeloma, possibly because of its effects on marrow angiogenesis. Both the immunosuppression and the angiogenesis inhibition of thalidomide might be beneficial in MDS.

Raza has recently completed a study of thalidomide in 83 patients with MDS (127). The drug was started at a dose of 100 mg daily and increased to a maximum, when tolerated, of 400 mg daily. Despite this approach, 26 patients stopped treatment within 12 weeks because of toxicity. Twenty-one of the 57 patients who continued treatment responded, 15 showing an erythroid, 13 a platelet, and seven a neutrophil response, with a median time to response of 10 weeks. By intention-to-treat analysis, 37% of patients became responders. Of note, eight of the 15 erythroid responses were patients who became transfusion-independent. There was no evidence that thalidomide favorably or unfavorably affected disease progression, but follow-up was short. Patients most likely to respond to thalidomide had fewer blast cells in the marrow. These findings suggest that thalidomide can improve marrow function in some patients with MDS.

## V.  FUTURE DIRECTIONS

We still know very little about the interaction of the immune system, the marrow microenvironment and the MDS stem cell. The antigens evoking the T-cell response are unknown and the mechanism of T-cell-mediated myelosuppression is not defined. Furthermore, the etiology of MDS remains unclear. Similarities between MDS and aplastic anemia, including the response to immunosuppressive treatment, raise questions about the relationship between these two diseases (128). Are they different entities sharing a common autoimmune pathology or are they two ends of a spectrum of a marrow failure syndrome differing only in their tendency to evolve to acute leukemia? Possibly the abnormal immune response environment in aplastic anemia is the initiator of genetic instability in the stem cell target leading to clonal evolution and leukemia (7). Also, this abnormal milieu may act as selective pressure in favor of the abnormal MDS clone. In these scenarios, immune modulation at an early stage of clonal evolution might be expected to maintain disease stability. Finally, the relationship between the MDS stem cell and the marrow microenvironment deserves further study. In this regard, it will be important to determine whether thalidomide exerts its beneficial effect through inhibition of angiogenesis as well as through immunosuppression.

## REFERENCES

1. Yoshida Y, Mufti GJ. Apoptosis and its significance in MDS: controversies revisited. Leuk Res 1999; 23:777–785.
2. Parker JE, Mufti GJ. Ineffective haemopoiesis and apoptosis in myelodysplastic syndromes. Br J Haematol 1998; 101:220–230.
3. Rosenfeld C, List A. A hypothesis for the pathogenesis of myelodysplastic syndromes: implications for new therapies. Leukemia 2000; 14:2–8.
4. Greenberg PL. Apoptosis and its role in the myelodysplastic syndromes: implications for disease natural history and treatment. Leuk Res 1998; 22:1123–1136.
5. Young NS. Aplastic anaemia. Lancet 1995; 346:228–232.
6. Young NS, Maciejewski J. The pathophysiology of acquired aplastic anemia. N Engl J Med 1997; 336:1365–1372.
7. Young NS. Hematopoietic cell destruction by immune mechanisms in acquired aplastic anemia. Semin Hematol 2000; 37:3–14.
8. Tuzuner N, Cox C, Rowe JM, Watrous D, Bennett JM. Hypocellular myelodysplastic syndromes (MDS): new proposals. Br J Haematol 1995; 91:612–617.
9. Imashuku S, Kitazawa K, Ishii M, Kataoka S, Asami K, Ishii E, Fukushima K, Sako M, Matsubayashi T, Teramura GT, Hibi S. Bone marrow changes mimicking myelodysplasia in patients with hemophagocytic lymphohistiocytosis. Int J Hematol 2000; 72:353–357.
10. Geary CG, Marsh JC, Gordon-Smith EC. Hypoplastic myelodysplasia (MDS). Br J Haematol 1996; 94:582–583.
11. Socié G, Henry-Amar M, Bacigalupo A, Hows J, Tichelli A, Ljungman P, McCann SR, Frickhofen N, Van't Veer-Korthof E, Gluckman E. Malignant tumors occurring after treatment of aplastic anemia. European Bone Marrow Transplantation-Severe Aplastic Anaemia Working Party. N Engl J Med 1993; 329:1152–1157.
12. Mikhailova N, Sessarego M, Fugazza G, Caimo A, De Filippi S, van Lint MT, Bregante S, Valeriani A, Mordini N, Lamparelli T, Gualandi F, Occhini D, Bacigalupo A. Cytogenetic abnormalities in patients with severe aplastic anemia. Haematologica 1996; 81:418–422.
13. Raza A, Alvi S, Borok RZ, Span L, Parcharidou A, Alston D, Rifkin S, Robin E, Shah R, Gregory SA. Excessive proliferation matched by excessive apoptosis in myelodysplastic syndromes: the cause-effect relationship. Leuk Lymphoma 1997; 27:111–118.
14. Bincoletto C, Saad ST, Soares da Silva E, Queiroz ML. Autonomous proliferation and bcl-2 expression involving haematopoietic cells in patients with myelodysplastic syndrome. Br J Cancer 1998; 78:621–624.
15. Shimazaki K, Ohshima K, Suzumiya J, Kawasaki C, Kikuchi M. Evaluation of apoptosis as a prognostic factor in myelodysplastic syndromes. Br J Haematol 2000; 110:584–590.

16. Ruutu T, Partanen S, Lintula R, Teerenhovi L, Knuutila S. Erythroid and granulo-cyte-macrophage colony formation in myelodysplastic syndromes. Scand J Haematol 1984; 32:395–402.

17. Maciejewski JP, Kim S, Sloand E, Selleri C, Young NS. Sustained long-term hematologic recovery despite a marked quantitative defect in the stem cell compartment of patients with aplastic anemia after immunosuppressive therapy. Am J Hematol 2000; 65:123–131.

18. Dan K, An E, Futaki M, Inokuchi K, Gomi S, Yamada T, Ogata K, Tanabe Y, Ohki I, Shinohara T, et al. Megakaryocyte, erythroid and granulocyte-macrophage colony formation in myelodysplastic syndromes. Acta Haematol 1993; 89:113–118.

19. Fukushima Y, Kanno Y, Miura AB. Three-lineage hemopoietic precursor cells and effectiveness of recombinant human erythropoietin in patients with myelodysplastic syndromes. Tohoku J Exp Med 1992; 166:375–385.

20. Juvonen E, Partanen S, Knuutila S, Ruutu T. Megakaryocyte colony formation by bone marrow progenitors in myelodysplastic syndromes. Br J Haematol 1986; 63: 331–334.

21. Juvonen E, Partanen S, Knuutila S, Ruutu T. Colony formation by megakaryocyte progenitors in myelodysplastic syndromes. Eur J Haematol 1989; 42:389–395.

22. Juvonen E, Aimolahati A, Volin L, Ruutu T. The prognostic value of in vitro cultures of erythroid and megakaryocytic progenitors in myelodysplastic syndromes. Leuk Res 1999; 23:889–894.

23. Geissler D, Zwierzina H, Pechlaner C, Gaggl S, Schmalzl F, Konwalinka G, Braun-steiner H. Abnormal megakaryopoiesis in patients with myelodysplastic syndromes: analysis of cellular and humoral defects. Br J Haematol 1989; 73:29–35.

24. Broxmeyer HE, Cooper S, Williams DE, Hangoc G, Gutterman JU, Vadhan-Raj S. Growth characteristics of marrow hematopoietic progenitor/precursor cells from patients on a phase I clinical trial with purified recombinant human granulocyte-macrophage colony-stimulating factor. Exp Hematol 1988 Aug; 16(7):594–602.

25. Carlo-Stella C, Cazzola M, Bernasconi P, Bergamaschi G, Dezza L, Pedrazzoli P, Rosti V, Tomaselli S, Zappone E. In vitro growth of bone marrow-derived multipotent and lineage-restricted hematopoietic progenitor cells in myelodysplastic syndromes. Haematologica 1989; 74:181–186.

26. Maciejewski JP, Selleri C, Sato T, Anderson S, Young NS. A severe and consistent deficit in marrow and circulating primitive hematopoietic cells (long-term culture-initiating cells) in acquired aplastic anemia. Blood 1996; 88:1983–1991.

27. Backx B, Broeders L, Touw I, Lowenberg B. Blast colony-forming cells in myelo-dysplastic syndrome: decreased potential to generate erythroid precursors. Leukemia 1993; 7:75–79.

28. Sawada K, Sato N, Notoya A, Tarumi T, Hirayama S, Takano H, Koizumi K, Yasukouchi T, Yamaguchi M, Koike T. Proliferation and differentiation of myelo-dysplastic CD34+ cells: phenotypic subpopulation of marrow CD34+ cells. Blood 1995; 85:194–202.

29. Maciejewski JP, Anderson S, Katevas P, Young NS. Phenotypic and functional analysis of bone marrow progenitor cell compartment in bone marrow failure. Br J Haematol 1994; 87:227–234.

30. Schouten HC, Delwel R, Bot FJ, Hagemeijer A, Touw IP, Lowenberg B. Characterization of clonogenic cells in refractory anemia with excess of blasts (RAEB-CFU): response to recombinant hematopoietic growth factors and maturation phenotypes. Leuk Res 1989; 13:245–251.

31. Shihab-el-Deen A, Guevara C, Prchal JF. Bone marrow cultures in dysmyelopoietic syndrome: diagnostic and prognistic evaluation. Acta Haematol 1987; 78:17–22.

32. Mayani H, Baines P, Bowen DT, Jacobs A. In vitro growth of myeloid and erythroid progenitor cells from myelodysplastic patients in response to recombinant human granulocyte-macrophage colony-stimulating factor. Leukemia 1989; 3:29–32.

33. Baines P, Bowen D, Jacobs A. Clonal growth of haematopoietic progenitor cells from myelodysplastic marrow in response to recombinant haemopoietins. Leuk Res 1990; 14:247–253.

34. Nagler A, MacKichan ML, Negrin RS, Donlon T, Greenberg PL. Effects of granulocyte colony-stimulating factor therapy on in vitro hemopoiesis in myelodysplastic syndromes. Leukemia 1995; 9:30–39.

35. Merchav S, Nielson OJ, Rosenbaum H, Sharon R, Brenner B, Tatarsky I, Scigalla P, Wieczorek L. In vitro studies of erythropoietin-dependent regulation of erythropoiesis in myelodysplastic syndromes. Leukemia 1990; 4:771–774.

36. Carlo-Stella C, Cazzola M, Bergamaschi G, Bernasconi P, Dezza L, Invernizzi R, Pedrazzoli P. Growth of human hematopoietic colonies from patients with myelodysplastic syndromes in response to recombinant human granulocyte-macrophage colony-stimulating factor. Leukemia 1989; 3:363–366.

37. Nagler A, Binet C, MacKichan ML, Negrin R, Bangs C, Donlon T, Greenberg P. Impact of marrow cytogenetics and morphology on in vitro hematopoiesis in the myelodysplastic syndromes: comparison between recombinant human granulocyte colony-stimulating factor (CSF) and granulocyte-monocyte CSF. Blood 1990; 76: 1299–1307.

38. Soligo D, Servida F, Cortelezzi A, Pedretti D, Uziel L, Morgutti M, Pogliani E, Lambertenghi Deliliers G. Effects of recombinant human stem cell factor (rh-SCF) on colony formation and long-term bone marrow cultures (LTBMC) in patients with myelodysplastic syndromes. Eur J Haematol 1994; 52:53–60.

39. Asano H, Hotta T, Ichihara M, Murate T, Kobayashi M, Saito H. Growth analysis of marrow CD34-positive hematopoietic progenitor cells in patients with myelodysplastic syndromes. Leukemia 1994; 8:833–838.

40. Coutinho LH, Geary CG, Chang J, Harrison C, Testa NG. Functional studies of bone marrow haematopoietic and stromal cells in the myelodysplastic syndrome (MDS). Br J Haematol 1990; 75:16–25.

41. Aizawa S, Nakano M, Iwase O, Yaguchi M, Hiramoto M, Hoshi H, Nabeshima R, Shima D, Handa H, Toyama K. Bone marrow stroma from refractory anemia of myelodysplastic syndrome is defective in its ability to support normal CD34-positive cell proliferation and differentiation in vitro. Leuk Res 1999; 23:239–246.

42. Novitzky N, Mohamed R, Finlayson J, du Toit C. Increased apoptosis of bone marrow cells and preserved proliferative capacity of selected progenitors predict for clinical response to anti-inflammatory therapy in myelodysplastic syndromes. Exp Hematol 2000; 28:941–949.

43. Clark DM, Lampert IA. Apoptosis is a common histopathological finding in myelo-

dysplasia, the correlate of ineffective hematopoiesis. Leuk Lymphoma 1990; 2: 415–418.

44. Bogdanovic AD, Trpinac DP, Jankovic GM, Bumbasirevic VZ, Obradovic M, Colovic MD. Incidence and role of apoptosis in myelodysplastic syndrome: morphological and ultrastructural assessment. Leukemia 1997; 11:656–659.

45. Shetty V, Hussaini S, Broady-Robinson L, Allampallam K, Mundle S, Borok R, Broderick E, Mazzoran L, Zorat F, Raza A. Intramedullary apoptosis of hematopoietic cells in myelodysplastic syndrome patients can be massive: apoptotic cells recovered from high-density fraction of bone marrow aspirates. Blood 2000; 96: 1388–1392.

46. Ohmori M, Ohmori S, Ueda Y, Yoshida Y, Okuda M. Ineffective hematopoiesis in the myelodysplastic syndromes (MDS) as studied by daily in situ observation of colony-cluster formation. Int J Cell Cloning 1990; 9:521–530.

47. Anzai N, Kawabata H, Hirama T, Masutani H, Ohmori M, Yoshida Y, Okuma M. Marked apoptosis of human myelomonocytic leukemia cell line P39: significance of cellular differentiation. Leukemia 1994; 8:446–453.

48. Lepelley P, Campergue L, Grardel N, Preudhomme C, Cosson A, Fenaux P. Is apoptosis a massive process in myelodysplastic syndromes? Br J Haematol 1996; 95:368–371.

49. Parcharidou A, Raza A, Economopoulos T, Papageorgiou ES, Anagnostou D, Papadaki T, Raptis S. Extensive apoptosis of bone marrow cells as evaluated by the in situ end-labelling (ISEL) technique may be the basis for ineffective haematopoiesis in patients with myelodysplastic syndromes. Eur J Haematol 1999; 62:19–26.

50. Kurotaki H, Tsushima Y, Nagai K, Yagihashi S. Apoptosis, bcl-2 expression and p53 accumulation in myelodysplastic syndrome, myelodysplastic-syndrome-derived acute myelogenous leukemia and de novo acute myelogenous leukemia. Acta Haematol 2000; 102:115–123.

51. Cortelezzi A, Di Stefano M, Sarina B, Giannini S, Pomas M, Silvestris L, et al. Apoptosis in myelodysplastic syndromes (MDS): putative role of the bcl2 proto-oncogene. Blood 1996; 88:95a.

52. Davis RE, Greenberg PL. Bcl-2 expression by myeloid precursors in myelodysplastic syndromes: relation to disease progression. Leuk Res 1998; 22:767–777.

53. Mundle SD, Reza S, Ali A, Mativi BY, Shetty V, Venugopal P, Gregory SA, Raza A. Correlation of tumor necrosis factor alpha (TNF alpha) with high caspase 3–like activity in myelodysplastic syndromes. Cancer Lett 1999; 140:201–207.

54. Hellström-Lindberg E, Kanter-Lewensohn L, Öst Å. Morphological changes and apoptosis in bone marrow from patients with myelodysplastic syndromes treated with granulocyte-CSF and erythropoietin. Leuk Res 1997; 21:415–425.

55. Dar S, Mundle S, Andric T, Qawi H, Shetty V, Reza S, Mativi BY, Allampallam K, Ali A, Venugopal P, Gezer S, Broady-Robinson L, Cartlidge J, Showel M, Hussaini S, Ragasa D, Ali I, Chaudhry A, Waggoner S, Lisak L, Huang RW, Raza A. Biological characteristics of myelodysplastic syndrome patients who demonstrated high versus no intramedullary apoptosis. Eur J Haematol 1999; 62:90–94.

56. Bouscary D, De Vos J, Guesnu M, Jondeau K, Viguier F, Melle J, Picard F, Dreyfus F, Fontenay-Roupie M. Fas/Apo-1 (CD95) expression and apoptosis in patients with myelodysplastic syndromes. Leukemia 1997; 11:839–845.

57. Rajapaksa R, Ginzton N, Rott LS, Greenberg PL. Altered oncoprotein expression and apoptosis in myelodysplastic syndrome marrow cells. Blood 1996; 88:4275–4287.

58. Parker JE, Mufti GJ, Rasool F, Mijovic A, Devereux S, Pagliuca A. The role of apoptosis, proliferation, and the Bcl-2-related proteins in the myelodysplastic syndromes and acute myeloid leukemia secondary to MDS. Blood 2000; 96:3932–3938.

59. Ricciardi MR, Petrucci MT, Ariola C, Gregorj F, Mazzola F. High levels of apoptosis characterize RAEB and are lost during leukemic transformation. Blood 1998; 90:520a.

60. Raza A, Mundle S, Shetty V, Alvi S, Chopra H, Span L, Parcharidou A, Dar S, Venugopal P, Borok R, Gezer S, Showel J, Loew J, Robin E, Rifkin S, Alston D, Hernandez B, Shah R, Kaizer H, Gregory S. Novel insights into the biology of myelodysplastic syndromes: excessive apoptosis and the role of cytokines. Int J Hematol 1996; 63:265–278.

61. Raza A, Gezer S, Mundle S, Gao XZ, Alvi S, Borok R, Rifkin S, Iftikhar A, Shetty V, Parcharidou A, et al. Apoptosis in bone marrow biopsy samples involving stromal and hematopoietic cells in 50 patients with myelodysplastic syndromes. Blood 1995; 86:268–276.

62. Tsoplou P, Kouraklis-Symeonidis A, Thanopoulou E, Zikos P, Orphanos V, Zoumbos NC. Apoptosis in patients with myelodysplastic syndromes: differential involvement of marrow cells in ''good'' versus ''poor'' prognosis patients and correlation with apoptosis-related genes. Leukemia 1999; 13:1554–1563.

63. Mundle S, Venugopal P, Shetty V, Ali A, Chopra H, Handa H, Rose S, Mativi BY, Gregory SA, Preisler HD, Raza A. The relative extent and propensity of CD34+ vs. CD34− cells to undergo apoptosis in myelodysplastic marrows. Int J Hematol 1999; 69:152–159.

64. Laveder F, Marcolongo R. Uncontrolled triggering of programmed cell death (apoptosis) in haematopoietic stem cells: a new hypothesis for the pathogenesis of aplastic anaemia. Immunol Cell Biol 1996; 74:159–162.

65. Raza A, Mundle S, Shetty V, Alvi S, Chopra H, Span L, Parcharidou A, Dar S, Venugopal P, Borok R, Gezer S, Showel J, Loew J, Robin E, Rifkin S, Alston D, Hernandez B, Shah R, Kaizer H, Gregory S, Preisler H. A paradigm shift in myelodysplastic syndromes. Leukemia 1996; 10:1648–1652.

66. Koike M, Ishiyama T, Tomoyasu S, Tsuruoka N. Spontaneous cytokine overproduction by peripheral blood mononuclear cells from patients with myelodysplastic syndromes and aplastic anemia. Leuk Res 1995; 19:639–644.

67. Kitagawa M, Saito I, Kuwata T, Yoshida S, Yamaguchi S, Takahashi M, Tanizawa T, Kamiyama R, Hirokawa K. Overexpression of tumor necrosis factor (TNF)-alpha and interferon (INF)-gamma by bone marrow cells from patients with myelodysplastic syndromes. Leukemia 1997; 11:2049–2054.

68. Molnar L, Berki T, Hussain A, Nemeth P, Losonczy H. Detection of TNF alpha expression in the bone marrow and determination of TNF alpha production of peripheral blood mononuclear cells in myelodysplastic syndrome. Pathol Oncol Res 2000; 6:18–23.

69. [Deleted in proof.]

70. Allampallam K, Shetty V, Hussaini S, Mazzoran L, Zorat F, Huang R, Raza A. Measurement of mRNA expression for a variety of cytokines and its receptors in bone marrows of patients with myelodysplastic syndromes. Anticancer Res 1999; 19:5323–5328.

71. Verhoef GE, De Schouwer P, Ceuppens JL, Van Damme J, Goossens W, Boogaerts MA. Measurement of serum cytokine levels in patients with myelodysplastic syndromes. Leukemia 1992; 6:1268–1272.

72. Gersuk GM, Beckham C, Loken MR, Kiener P, Anderson JE, Farrand A, Troutt AB, Ledbetter JA, Deeg HJ. A role for tumour necrosis factor-alpha, Fas and Fas-Ligand in marrow failure associated with myelodysplastic syndrome. Br J Haematol 1998; 103:176–188.

73. Reza S, Shetty V, Dar S, Qawi H, Raza A. Tumor necrosis factor-alpha levels decrease with anticytokine therapy in patients with myelodysplastic syndromes. J Interferon Cytokine Res 1998; 18:871–877.

74. Hofmann WK, Seipelt G, Ottmann OG, Kalina U, Koschmieder S, Brucher J, Frickhofen N, Klausmann M, Mitrou PS, Hoelzer D. Effect of treatment with amifostine used as a single agent in patients with refractory anemia on clinical outcome and serum tumor necrosis factor alpha levels. Ann Hematol 2000; 79: 255–258.

75. Shinohara K, Muraki K, Ota I, Nawata R, Oeda E, Takahashi T. Increased levels of soluble tumor necrosis factor receptors in patients with aplastic anemia and myelodysplastic syndrome. Am J Hematol 2000; 65:326–327.

76. Kitagawa M, Takahashi M, Yamaguchi S, Inoue M, Ogawa S, Hirokawa K, Kamiyama R. Expression of inducible nitric oxide synthase (NOS) in bone marrow cells of myelodysplastic syndromes. Leukemia 1999; 13:699–703.

77. Peddie CM, Wolf CR, McLellan LI, Collins AR, Bowen DT. Oxidative DNA damage in CD34+ myelodysplastic cells is associated with intracellular redox changes and elevated plasma tumour necrosis factor-alpha concentration. Br J Haematol 1997; 99:625–631.

78. Reza S, Dar S, Andric T, Qawi H, Mundle S, Shetty V, Venugopal P, Ali I, Lisak L, Raza A. Biologic characteristics of 164 patients with myelodysplastic syndromes. Leuk Lymphoma 1999; 33:281–287.

79. Deeg HJ, Beckham C, Loken MR, Bryant E, Lesnikova M, Shulman HM, Gooley T. Negative regulators of hemopoiesis and stroma function in patients with myelodysplastic syndrome. Leuk Lymphoma 2000; 37:405–414.

80. Ohmori M, Ohmori S, Ueda Y, Tohyama K, Yoshida Y, Uchino H. Myelodysplastic syndrome (MDS)-associated inhibitory activity on haemopoietic progenitor cells. Br J Haematol 1990; 74:179–184.

81. Kerndrup G, Hokland P. Natural killer cell-mediated inhibition of bone marrow colony formation (CFU-GM) in refractory anaemia (preleukaemia): evidence for patient-specific cell populations. Br J Haematol 1988; 69:457–462.

82. Aizawa S, Hiramoto M, Hoshi H, Toyama K, Shima D, Handa H. Establishment of stromal cell line from an MDS RA patient which induced an apoptotic change in hematopoietic and leukemic cells in vitro. Exp Hematol 2000; 28:148–155.

83. Molldrem JJ, Jiang YZ, Stetler-Stevenson M, Mavroudis D, Hensel N, Barrett AJ. Haematological response of patients with myelodysplastic syndrome to antithymocyte globulin is associated with a loss of lymphocyte-mediated inhibition of CFU-GM and alterations in T-cell receptor Vbeta profiles. Br J Haematol 1998; 102: 1314–1322.

84. Mundle SD, Mativi BY, Bagai K, Feldman G, Cheema P, Gautam U, Reza S, Cartlidge JD, Venugopal P, Shetty V, Gregory SA, Robin E, Rifkin S, Shah R, Raza A. Spontaneous down-regulation of Fas-associated phosphatase-1 may contribute to excessive apoptosis in myelodysplastic marrows. Int J Hematol 1999; 70: 83–90.

85. Kitagawa M, Yamaguchi S, Takahashi M, Tanizawa T, Hirokawa K, Kamiyama R. Localization of Fas and Fas ligand in bone marrow cells demonstrating myelodysplasia. Leukemia 1998; 12:486–492.

86. Lepelley P, Grardel N, Emy O, Iaru T, Obein V, Cosson A, Fenaux P. Fas/APO-1 (CD95) expression in myelodysplastic syndromes. Leuk Lymphoma 1998; 30: 307–312.

87. Won JH, Yu BW, Hong DS, Suh WS, Jeon JW, Baick SH, et al. The expression of the Fas antigen and apoptosis in patients with myelodysplastic syndromes and its clinical relevance. Blood 1996; 88:95a.

88. Gupta P, Niehans GA, LeRoy SC, Gupta K, Morrison VA, Schultz C, Knapp DJ, Kratzke RA. Fas ligand expression in the bone marrow in myelodysplastic syndromes correlates with FAB subtype and anemia, and predicts survival. Leukemia 1999; 13:44–53.

89. Porzsolt F, Heimpel H. Impaired T-cell and NK-cell function in patients with preleukemia. Blut 1982; 45:243–248.

90. Anderson RW, Volsky DJ, Greenberg B, Knox SJ, Bechtold T, Kuszynski C, Harada S, Purtilo DT. Lymphocyte abnormalities in preleukemia. 1. Decreased NK activity, anomalous immunoregulatory cell subsets and deficient EBV receptors. Leuk Res 1983; 7:389–395.

91. Takagi S, Kitagawa S, Takeda A, Minato N, Takaku F, Miura Y. Natural killer-interferon system in patients with preleukaemic states. Br J Haematol 1984; 58: 71–81.

92. Kerndrup G, Meyer K, Ellegaard J, Hokland P. Natural killer (NK)-cell activity and antibody-dependent cellular cytotoxicity (ADCC) in primary preleukemic syndrome. Leuk Res 1984; 8:239–247.

93. Okabe M, Minagawa T, Nakane A, Sakurada K, Miyasaki T. Impaired alpha-interferon production and natural killer activity in blood mononuclear cells in myelodysplastic syndromes. Scand J Haematol 1986; 37:111–117.

94. Janowska-Wieczorek A, Jakobisiak M, Dobaczewska H. Decreased antibody-dependent cellular cytotoxicity in preleukemic syndromes. Acta Haematol 1983; 69:132–135.

95. Baumann MA, Milson TJ, Patrick CW, Libnoch JA, Keller RH. Immunoregulatory abnormalities in myelodysplastic disorders. Am J Hematol 1986; 22:17–26.

96. Colombat PH, Renoux M, Lamagnere JP, Renoux G. Immunologic indices in myelodysplastic syndromes. Cancer 1988; 61:1075–1081.

97. Bynoe AG, Scott CS, Ford P, Roberts BE. Decreased T helper cells in the myelo-dysplastic syndromes. Br J Haematol 1983; 54:97–102.

98. Okamoto T, Okada M, Mori A, Saheki K, Takatsuka H, Wada H, Tamura A, Fuji-mori Y, Takemoto Y, Kanamaru A, Kakishita E. Correlation between immunologi-cal abnormalities and prognosis in myelodysplastic syndrome patients. Int J Hema-tol 1997; 66:345–351.

99. Economopoulos T, Economidou J, Giannopoulos G, Terzoglou C, Papageorgiou E, Dervenoulas J, Arseni P, Hadjioannou J, Raptis S. Immune abnormalities in myelodysplastic syndromes. J Clin Pathol 1985; 38:908–911.

100. Mufti GJ, Figes A, Hamblin TJ, Oscier DG, Copplestone JA. Immunological abnor-malities in myelodysplastic syndromes. I. Serum immunoglobulins and autoanti-bodies. Br J Haematol 1986; 63:143–147.

101. Sokol RJ, Hewitt S, Booker DJ. Erythrocyte autoantibodies, autoimmune haemoly-sis, and myelodysplastic syndromes. J Clin Pathol 1989; 42:1088–1091.

102. Hamblin T. Immunologic abnormalities in myelodysplastic syndromes. Hematol Oncol Clin North Am 1992; 6:571–586.

103. Enright H, Jacob HS, Vercellotti G, Howe R, Belzer M, Miller W. Paraneoplastic autoimmune phenomena in patients with myelodysplastic syndromes: response to immunosuppressive therapy. Br J Haematol 1995; 91:403–408.

104. Copplestone JA, Mufti GJ, Hamblin TJ, Oscier DG. Immunological abnormalities in myelodysplastic syndromes. II. Coexistent lymphoid or plasma cell neoplasms: a report of 20 cases unrelated to chemotherapy. Br J Haematol 1986; 63:149–159.

105. Katsuki K, Shinohara K, Kameda N, Yamada T, Takeda K, Kamei T. Two cases of myelodysplastic syndrome with extramedullary polyclonal plasma cell prolifera-tion and autoantibody production: possible role of soluble Fas antigen for produc-tion of excessive self-reactive B cells. Intern Med 1998; 37:973–977.

106. Shiozawa S, Ogawa R, Morimoto I, Tanaka Y, Kanda N, Tatsumi E, Yamaguchi N, Fujita T. Polyarthritis, mononeuritis multiplex and eczematous ulcerative skin rash in a patient with myelodysplastic syndrome and peripheral large granular lym-phocytosis. Clin Exp Rheumatol 1991; 9:629–633.

107. Saunthararajah Y, Molldrem JL, Rivera M, Williams A, Stetler-Stevenson M, Sorb-ara L, Young NS, Barrett AJ. Coincident myelodysplastic syndrome and T-cell large granular lymphocytic disease: clinical and pathophysiological features. Br J Haematol 2001; 112:195–200.

108. Bagby GC Jr, Gabourel JD, Linman JW. Gluticocorticoid therapy in the preleuke-mic syndrome (hemopoietic dysplasia): identification of responsive patients using in-vitro techniques. Ann Intern Med 1980; 92:55–58.

109. Tichelli A, Gratwohl A, Wuersch A, Nissen C, Speck B. Antilymphocyte globulin for myelodysplastic syndrome. Br J Haematol 1988; 68:139–140.

110. Biesma DH, van den Tweel JG, Verdonck LF. Immunosuppressive therapy for hypoplastic myelodysplastic syndrome. Cancer 1997; 79:1548–1551.

111. Molldrem JJ, Caples M, Mavroudis D, Plante M, Young NS, Barrett AJ. Antithy-mocyte globulin for patients with myelodysplastic syndrome. Br J Haematol 1997; 99:699–705.

112. Greenberg P, Cox C, LeBeau MM, Fenaux P, Morel P, Sanz G, Sanz M, Vallespi T, Hamblin T, Oscier D, Ohyashiki K, Toyama K, Aul C, Mufti G, Bennett J. International scoring system for evaluating prognosis in myelodysplastic syndromes. Blood 1997; 89:2079–2088.

113. Molldrem JJ, Jiang YZ, Stetler-Stevenson M, Mavroudis D, Hensel N, Barrett AJ. Haematological response of patients with myelodysplastic syndrome to antithymocyte globulin is associated with a loss of lymphocyte-mediated inhibition of CFU-GM and alterations in T-cell receptor Vbeta profiles. Br J Haematol 1998; 102: 1314–1322.

114. Jonasova A, Neuwirtova R, Cermak J, Vozobulova V, Mocikova K, Siskova M, Hochova I. Cyclosporin A therapy in hypoplastic MDS patients and certain refractory anaemias without hypoplastic bone marrow. Br J Haematol 1998; 200:304–309.

115. Kemp G, Rose P, Lurain J, Berman M, Manetta A, Roullet B, Homesley H, Belpomme D, Glick J. Amifostine pretreatment for protection against cyclophosphamide-induced and cisplatin-induced toxicities: results of a randomized control trial in patients with advanced ovarian cancer. J Clin Oncol 1996; 14:2101–2112.

116. List AF, Heaton R, Glinsmann-Gibson B, Capizzi RL. Amifostine protects primitive hematopoietic progenitors against chemotherapy cytotoxicity. Semin Oncol 1996; 23(4 suppl):58–63.

117. List AF, Brasfield F, Heaton R, Glinsmann-Gibson B, Crook L, Taetle R, Capizzi R. Stimulation of hematopoiesis by amifostine in patients with myelodysplastic syndrome. Blood 1997; 90:3364–3369.

118. List AF, Holmes H, Greenberg PL, Bennett JM, Oster W. Phase II study of amifostine in patients with myelodysplastic syndromes. Blood 1999; 94(suppl 1):305a.

119. Raza A, Qawi H, Andric T, Dar S, Lisak L, Huang RW, Venugopal P, Gezer S, Gregory SA, Hsu WT, Loew J, Robin E, Rifkin S, Shah R, Divgi A, Taylor R, Grosset A. Pentoxifylline, ciprofloxacin and dexamethasone improve the ineffective hematopoiesis in myelodysplastic syndrome patients' malignancy. Hematology 2000; 5:275–284.

120. Raza A, Qawi H, Lisak L, Andric T, Dar S, Andrews C, Venugopal P, Gezer S, Gregory S, Loew J, Robin E, Rifkin S, Hsu WT, Huang RW. Patients with myelodysplastic syndromes benefit from palliative therapy with amifostine, pentoxifylline, and ciprofloxacin with or without dexamethasone. Blood 2000; 95:1580–1587.

121. Nemunaitis J, Rosenfeld C, Getty L, Boegel F, Meyer W, Jennings LW, Zeigler Z, Shadduck R. Pentoxifylline and ciprofloxacin in patients with myelodysplastic syndrome. A phase II trial. Am J Clin Oncol 1995; 18:189–193.

122. Raza A, Allampallam K, Shetty V, Mundle S, Borok R, Lisak L et al. Biologic and clinical response to recombinant human soluble tumor necrosis factor receptor (Enbrel) in patients with myelodysplastic syndromes. Blood 1999; 94(suppl 1): 171a.

123. McHugh SM, Rifkin IR, Deighton J, Wilson AB, Lachmann PJ, Lockwood CM, Ewan PW. The immunosuppressive drug thalidomide induces T helper cell type 2 (Th2) and concomitantly inhibits Th1 cytokine production in mitogen- and antigen-stimulated human peripheral blood mononuclear cell cultures. Clin Exp Immunol 1995; 99:160–167.

124. Sampaio EP, Sarno EN, Galilly R, Cohn ZA, Kaplan G. Thalidomide selectively inhibits tumor necrosis factor alpha production by stimulated human monocyte. J Exp Med 1991; 173:699–703.
125. Klausner JD, Freedman VH, Kaplan G. Thalidomide as an anti-TNF-alpha inhibitor: implications for clinical use. Clin Immunol Immunopathol 1996; 81:219–223.
126. Amato RJ, Loughnan MSFE, Folkman J. Thalidomide is an inhibitor of angiogenesis. Proc Natl Acad Sci USA 1994; 91:4082–4085.
127. Raza A. Anti-TNF therapies in rheumatoid arthritis, Crohn's disease, sepsis, and myelodysplastic syndromes. Microsc Res Tech 2000; 50:229–235.
128. Barrett AJ, Saunthararajah Y. Myelodysplastic syndrome and aplastic anemia: distinct entities or diseases linked by a common pathophysiology? Semin Hematol 2000; 37:15–29.
129. Maciejewski JP, Risitano AM, Nunez O, Young NS. Distinct clinical outcomes for cytogenetic abnormalities evolving from aplastic anemia. Blood. 2002; in press.

# 15

# New Investigational Strategies in Patients with Myelodysplastic Syndromes

**Guillermo Garcia-Manero and Hagop M. Kantarjian**
*University of Texas M.D. Anderson Cancer Center,*
*Houston, Texas*

## I.  INTRODUCTION

Therapeutic decisions in myelodysplastic syndromes (MDS) are complex owing to the gradual realization that not all patients with MDS have an indolent course. MDS is recognized as a heterogeneous group of disorders with different natural histories and is generally classified using the French-American-British (FAB) classification scheme (1) or the more recent International Prognostic Scoring System (IPSS) (2). Low-risk patients, as classified according to the FAB system, are those with refractory anemia (RA) or RA with ringed sideroblasts (RARS) or those classified according to the IPSS as being in the low or intermediate-1 risk groups. High-risk patients are those having RA with excess blasts in transformation (RAEB-t by FAB classification) or those in the high-risk group (IPSS). Categorization of patients having RA with excess blasts (RAEB by FAB classification) or those in the intermediate-2 risk group (IPSS) may depend on whether the categorization is at diagnosis (low risk) or is following referral to a tertiary-care center, with initial therapy having failed (high risk) (3) (Table 1). For the practical purposes of this review regarding investigational options, low-risk MDS patients are generally those with less than 10% blasts while high-risk MDS patients are those with more than 10% blasts. As the percentage of marrow blasts

**Table 1**  Differences in Median Survival When MDS Patients Are Classified at
Diagnosis Versus at a Tertiary Care Center

| | MDS patients classified at diagnosis[a] (n = 816) | | MDS patients classified at a tertiary care center[b] (n = 219) | |
|---|---|---|---|---|
| IPSS risk group | % of total | Median survival (years) | % of total | Median survival (years) |
| Low | 33 | 5.7 | 13 | 2.1 |
| Intermediate-1 | 38 | 3.5 | 41 | 1.2 |
| Intermediate-2 | 22 | 1.2 | 30 | 0.7 |
| High | 7 | 0.4 | 16 | 0.4 |

[a] Data of untreated patients from which the IPSS was developed (2).
[b] Patient data from the M.D. Anderson Cancer Center (3).
MDS, myelodysplastic syndromes; N, number; IPSS, International Prognostic Scoring System.

is the most weighted prognostic factor in both the FAB and IPSS classification
systems, this simplified categorization is reasonable.

Current therapeutic strategies for patients with MDS vary depending on
the risk category (Table 2). Patients with low-risk MDS are generally observed
or are given supportive care measures appropriate to their cytopenias, such as

**Table 2**  Possible Therapeutic Approaches for Myelodysplastic Syndromes

| Presentation | Therapy |
|---|---|
| Low-risk MDS | |
|   Mild cytopenia | Observation |
|   Anemia | Erythropoietin ± G-CSF |
|   Granulocytopenia ± infections | Antibiotics ± G-CSF |
|   Thrombocytopenia | Low-dose interleukin 11, thrombopoietin |
|   Multiple cytopenias | Combinations of growth factors |
|   Cytopenias ± hypocellularity | Immunomodulation (steroids, cyclosporine A, anti-thymocyte globulin) |
|   Refractoriness to above | Topotecan + cytosine arabinoside, AML-type therapy, investigational therapies (see text) |
| High-risk MDS | |
|   Any presentation | AML-type regimens, topotecan + cytosine arabinoside, allogeneic stem cell transplantation, investigational therapies (see text) |

G-CSF, granulocyte colony-stimulating factor, AML, acute myeloid leukemia.

blood or platelet transfusions, antibiotics, or growth factors [erythropoietin, granulocyte colony-stimulating factor (G-CSF), granulocyte-macrophage colony-stimulating factor (GM-CSF), and interleukin-11]. Those with high-risk MDS are offered intensive chemotherapy programs, similar to those used for the treatment of acute myeloid leukemia (AML), or marrow ablative therapies and stem cell transplant. In this chapter, we review the results of several new therapeutic agents for patients with MDS. Since the mechanisms of action are novel, these agents may provide for the development of new combination programs for the treatment of these syndromes.

## II. HYPOMETHYLATING AGENTS

Global and gene-specific DNA methylation abnormalities are frequent in leukemias (4) and MDS (5). DNA methylation, or CpG-island methylation, is the addition of a methyl group to the fifth-position of the cytosine ring in a cytosine-guanine dinucleotide (CpG). The methylation of promoter-associated CpG-islands has been associated with DNA transcription inactivation and gene silencing (6). The mechanisms and regulation of DNA methylation-mediated gene silencing are poorly understood but probably involve a complex interplay of multiple proteins, including DNA-methyltransferases (DNMT) and histone acetyl transferases and deacetylases, as well as the replication machinery. Aberrant DNA methylation, through the silencing of the expression of genes crucial for cell function such as tumor suppressor genes, has been implicated in oncogenesis (7); this mechanism is a molecular alternative to gene mutation and/or deletion and is frequently observed in acute leukemias and myelodysplasia (4,5).

Several genes are known to be abnormally methylated in human leukemias (4,8–10). In MDS, the calcitonin gene (11,12) and the cell cycle inhibitor P15$^{INK4b}$ (13–15) have been found to be frequently hypermethylated, especially in high-risk MDS. Recently, a hypermethylator phenotype has been identified in several malignancies (16–18), including AML (9) and acute lymphocytic leukemia (ALL) (10). This hypermethylator phenotype is characterized by the aberrant methylation of multiple promoter-associated CpG islands in a subset of patients. It is possible that a subgroup of patients with MDS may be characterized by a similar phenotype and that these patients could potentially benefit from hypomethylating treatments.

The association between aberrant DNA methylation and leukemia has generated interest in the use of hypomethylating agents, for example, 5-azacytidine and 5-aza-2′-deoxycytidine (decitabine) (19). Intravenous and subcutaneous schedules of 5-azacytidine, a pyrimidine-nucleoside cytosine analog, were investigated by Silverman et al. in pilot studies. In the first study, 5-azacytidine was given by continuous infusion at 75 mg/m$^2$ per day for 7 days every 4 weeks.

Among 43 patients with RAEB or RAEB-t, responses were noted in 21 (49%): five (12%) complete remissions (CR), 11 (25%) partial remissions (PR), and five (12%) hematological improvements (HI). Trilineage responses were observed in 33% of all treated patients. The most frequent toxicity was mild to moderate nausea and vomiting (63%), and dose reductions due to myelosuppression were required in 33% of the patients. The median survival was 13 months and the median duration of remission was 14 months (20). In another study of 36 patients (21), the same schedule was administered subcutaneously (s.q.) and responses were observed in 12 of those patients (33%): four CR and eight PR. Again, 33% of the patients had trilineage responses, but no marrow hypoplasia was induced. Based on these results, the Cancer and Leukemia Group B (CALGB) developed a multiinstitutional, randomized trial that compared observation ($n = 92$) versus 5-azacytidine at 75 mg/m$^2$ s.q. daily for 7 days ($n = 99$) every 4 weeks. Responses were observed in 63% of evaluable patients receiving 5-azacytidine (6% CR, 10% PR, and 47% HI) versus only 7% in the observation arm. Patients receiving 5-azacytidine had longer time to leukemia transformation (22 months vs. 12 months; $p < 0.01$) and longer median survival (18 vs. 14 months), which was not statistically significant, perhaps owing to the crossover design (22) (Table 3). Patients treated with 5-azacytidine also had a better quality of life (23).

Decitabine has a similar structure to 5-azacytidine (Fig. 1) but has more potent hypomethylating activity. This hypomethylating activity is mediated by inhibition of DNMT (24) and is dose-dependent. At low doses, decitabine is incorporated into DNA where it forms covalent bonds with DNMT, thereby inducing hypomethylation, gene activation, and cell differentiation (25,26). At high doses, decitabine is cytotoxic (27), probably owing to the formation of bulky

**Table 3**  Results of the Randomized Study of 5-Azacytidine Versus Observation in Myelodysplastic Syndromes

| Parameter | 5-Azacytidine | Observation | $p$ value |
|---|---|---|---|
| Number of treated patients | 99 | 92 | |
| Responses | | | |
|   Overall (%) | 63 | 7 | 0.0001 |
|   Complete remission (%) | 6 | 0 | |
|   Partial remission (%) (with % hematological improvement) | 10 (47) | 0 (7) | |
|   Median time to leukemia transformation (months) | 22 | 12 | 0.003 |
| Median survival (months) | 18 | 14 | 0.1 |
| Quality of life | Better | Worse | 0.001 |

*Source*: Data from Ref. 22.

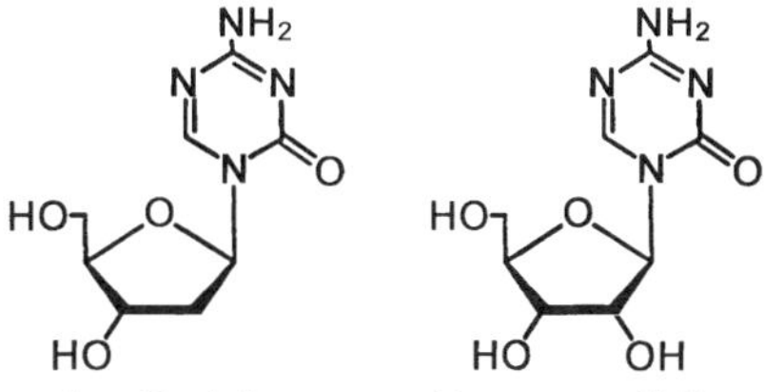

decitabine    5-azacytidine

**Fig. 1** Molecular structures of decitabine and 5-azacytidine are similar.

DNA adducts. However, some studies have indicated that decitabine cell toxicity was mediated by the covalent trapping of DNMT since cells devoid of DNMT were resistant to decitabine (28).

Studies have been conducted to determine effective and tolerable doses of decitabine. Initial studies on leukemia patients (29) established the tolerable antileukemic dose to be in the range of 36–80 mg/kg given as a continuous infusion. Subsequently, a schedule of 1 mg/kg/hr for 36–50 hr was shown, however, to have short-lived activity in patients with advance acute leukemias (30). The European Organization for Research in the Treatment of Cancer (EORTC) later reported their experience with decitabine at different doses and schedules in patients with refractory leukemia; prolonged pancytopenia and cardiopulmonary toxicities were associated with the treatments (31). In a different study, Richel et al. combined decitabine, at 125–500 mg/m$^2$ infused over 6 hr, with amsacrine. This treatment resulted in durable CR for relapsed leukemia in eight of 11 patients. The associated toxicities included pancytopenia, which lasted for 3–4 weeks, nonbacterial peritonitis, and neurotoxicity, with the latter only at higher doses (32). More recent studies have shown response rates of 5–40% when decitabine was used as a single agent for AML salvage and response rates of 30–60% when it was used in combination with amsacrine or anthracyclines (33–35).

The concept that decitabine may be a more effective anticancer agent if used at low doses that induce hypomethylation has triggered interest in developing prolonged-exposure, low-dose schedules. This concept was supported by (1) the excessive myelosuppressive toxicity that occurs at higher doses of decitabine, (2) the short half-life of decitabine, and (3) the need for cell division to achieve hypomethylation. The effectiveness of low-dose, prolonged exposure has been shown in several studies conducted on MDS. A pilot study of decitabine administered at 15–30 mg/m$^2$ over 4 hr 3 times a day for 3 consecutive days showed significant activity (one CR and three PR in nine MDS patients treated). Additionally, immunophenotypic changes suggestive of cell differentiation were observed (36,37), including the down-regulation of cell markers CD34 and CD33 on bone marrow leukemic cells (38). Wijermans et al. subsequently conducted several studies of decitabine in elderly patients with high-risk MDS. In the initial study, decitabine was given at 40–50 mg/m$^2$ as a continuous infusion over 24 hr for 3 days. Responses were observed in 54% of the 29 patients, including eight CR and five PR, and the median survival was 46 weeks. At this dose schedule, the major toxicity was myelosuppression, which induced toxic deaths in five patients. Prophylactic antibiotics and lower-dose schedules made therapy safer in subsequent studies.

The same investigators recently reported the results of a multicenter phase II study of lower-dose decitabine (15 mg/m$^2$ over 4 hr 3 times a day for 3 consecutive days) in 66 elderly patients (median age of 68 years with a range of 38–84 years) having MDS [eight RA/RARS, 29 RAEB, 20 RAEB-t, nine chronic myelomonocytic leukemia (CMML)] of which 25 patients (37%) had high-risk IPSS scores (39). Thirteen patients (20%) achieved CR, three (4%) had PR, and 16 (24%) had HI. Response rates were higher in RAEB-t than with RA (70% vs. 25%) and with higher IPSS risk score (64% vs. 25%), and responses were usually observed during the first three courses. Of interest, 36% of patients had an increase (over $100 \times 10^9$/L) in platelet counts. The median response duration was 7 months and the median survival 15 months, although patients who achieved CR had a median survival of 19 months. Toxicities included fever (27%), infections (20%), and sepsis (11%), and five patients (8%) suffered toxic deaths, three from drug-induced myelosuppression. Although the frequent occurrence of myelosuppression suggested a cytotoxic mode of action, the authors observed slow responses and demethylation of p15 (40), indicating that the activity of decitabine may indeed be mediated through hypomethylation. In a recent summary of the three studies conducted by Wijermans et al., the overall response rate was 49%, the actuarial response duration 38 weeks, and the median survival 15 months (Table 4).

With this knowledge, a phase I study of low-dose decitabine was initiated at the University of Texas M.D. Anderson Cancer Center (UTMDACC) in patients with relapsed leukemia or myelodysplasia. The starting dose was 5 mg/m$^2$ infused over 1 hr daily for 10 days (50 mg/m$^2$/course), with dose escalation to 10, 15, and 20 mg/m$^2$ daily. The study aims were to provide a safe low-dose schedule that targets hypomethylation and correlate this with response. Preliminary results indicate that a dose of 15 mg/m$^2$ daily for 10 days (150 mg/m$^2$/course) was active, especially in patients with relapsed AML [four CR (16%) among 20 patients treated] and was well tolerated in an outpatient setting. In addition to the clinical results, the methylation status of multiple genes was measured prior to therapy and at different time intervals during treatment; these data should provide insights into the mechanism of action of decitabine and as to which patients may benefit from this treatment. Future strategies with decitabine,

**Table 4**   Experience with 5-Aza-2′-deoxycytidine
(Decitabine) in Myelodysplastic Syndromes

| Parameter | Measure |
|---|---|
| Patients (number) | 125 |
| Median age and range (years) | 70 (39–89) |
| IPSS risk group (number of patients) | |
|    Intermediate-1 | 35 |
|    Intermediate-2 | 38 |
|    High | 52 |
| Overall response rate (%) | 49 |
|    Complete remission | 20 |
|    Partial remission (with % hemato-<br>     logical improvement) | 10 (19) |
| Response (%) by IPSS risk group | |
|    Intermediate-1 | 39 |
|    Intermediate-2 | 45 |
|    High | 58 |
| Median response duration (months) | 10 |
| Median survival (months) | 15 |
|    Intermediate-1 | 19 |
|    Intermediate-2 | 13 |
|    High | 14 |

*Source*: Data from Ref. 106.

besides its use on patients selected according to their methylation characteristics, include combinations with other agents such as topoisomerase I inhibitors, retinoic acid, and histone deacetylase inhibitors.

## III.   DNA TOPOISOMERASE I INHIBITORS

The regulation of chromatin structure and DNA topology, or tridimensional conformation, is fundamental for cell function and is therefore tightly regulated (41). DNA topoisomerases are enzymes with the capacity of forming covalent DNA bonds while inducing double-strand DNA breaks (DNA topoisomerase II) or single-strand breaks [DNA topoisomerase I (topo I)] (42). Several inhibitors of topo I have been developed and have shown activity in a variety of solid tumors (43) and leukemias (44).

Topotecan is an alkaloid camptothecin that acts as a specific topo I inhibitor. It was first studied in 60 MDS patients (30 RAEB/RAEB-t, 30 CMML) as a single agent at a dose of 2 mg/m$^2$ by continuous infusion daily for 5 days (45,46). CR was achieved in 19 patients (31%). Further, remissions were associated with disappearance of chromosomal abnormalities and patients classified as having RAEB/RAEB-t had a higher response rate than those having CMML (37% vs. 27%). Median CR duration was 7.5 months and median survival 10.5 months. Frequent toxicities included severe mucositis (23%) and severe diarrhea (17%).

Subsequently, topotecan has been combined with cytosine arabinoside (ara-C) in several treatment programs. Initially, topotecan was infused at 1.25 mg/m$^2$ daily for 5 days along with ara-C at 1 g/m$^2$ over 2 hr daily (47). Induction chemotherapy was given with intensive supportive care and prophylactic antibiotics and patients older than 50 years of age were treated while in laminar flow rooms. A total of 86 patients had been treated, 59 with MDS and 27 with CMML. The median age of the patients was 64 years, 35% of the patients had received prior therapy, and 50% had poor-prognosis chromosomal abnormalities. CR was observed in 56% of the patients, median duration of CR was 8 months, and median survival was 14 months. As with single-agent topotecan, responses were more frequent in MDS than in CMML (61% vs. 44%). Induction mortality occurred in 7% of the patients and mucositis and diarrhea were observed in only 3% of patients. Thus, the high response rate suggested that topo I inhibitors could be alternatives to anthracyclines in elderly patients, particularly those with high multidrug-resistance (MDR) expression. As a result, several induction programs devoid of anthracyclines, such as the CAT program (cyclophosphamide, ara-C, topotecan), were developed for AML and high-risk MDS (48). A program combining topotecan, fludarabine, ara-C, and G-CSF has since shown encouraging activity and toxicity in a cohort of elderly high-risk patients as reported by Besa et al. (49).

Another topo I inhibitor, 9-nitro-20-(S)-camptothecin (9-NC), is an alkaloid camptothecin that can be administered orally. An oral route has the advantage of facilitating prolonged exposure schedules, which, in turn, may result in higher levels of DNA–topo I complex formation. The dose-limiting toxicity of 9-NC was myelosuppression and gastrointestinal complications. The maximally tolerated dose (MTD) was initially suggested to be 2.0 mg/m$^2$ orally daily for 5 days every week, but was later reduced to 1.5 mg/m$^2$ owing to severe diarrhea (50). Eight patients with MDS were treated (seven CMML, one RAEB) and seven responded (one CR, two PR, four HI) (51).

DX-8951f is a water-soluble, nonprodrug analog of camptothecin with in vitro cytotoxicity against various human cancer cell lines (52). DX-8951f has also shown significant activity against human AML cells transplanted into severe combined immunodeficient (SCID) mice (53). A phase I study performed at UT-MDACC in patients with relapsed or refractory AML or advanced MDS showed that DX-8951f induced marrow hypoplasia in 60% of patients. The dose-limiting toxicity was stomatitis and the calculated MTD was 0.9 mg/m²/day for 5 days (54). Future studies may investigate combinations of DX-8951f with other agents for treatment of advanced MDS and AML, or liposomal formulations of topo I inhibitors.

## IV. HOMOHARRINGTONINE

Homoharringtonine (HHT) is a cephalotaxime plant alkaloid with activity in AML and chronic myelogenous leukemia (CML) (55,56). Initial studies in MDS used HHT at a dose of 5 mg/m² continuous infusion daily for 9 days (57). Among 28 patients evaluated (16 with MDS and 12 with AML), responses were observed in four patients with MDS. Therapy was associated with severe pancytopenia, resulting in 13 deaths among the 28 patients treated. Current studies in CML have used HHT at a dose of 2.5 mg/m² for 7 days and successfully combined HHT with ara-C (58). Thus, lower dose schedules of HHT, alone or with low-dose ara-C, may produce effective anti-MDS activity without the previously observed myelosuppression. In addition, several new synthetic HHT derivatives have shown promising in vitro activity (59) and may expand the potential applications of HHT in MDS.

## V. TARGETED THERAPY WITH MYLOTARG

Mylotarg (formerly CMA 676), a conjugate of an anti-CD33 monoclonal antibody and calicheamicin (60), has been approved for the treatment of elderly patients with relapsed AML whose first CR duration was longer than 3 months. The approval was based on a multicenter phase II study of 142 patients in which the overall response rate to Mylotarg was 29% (16% CR, 13% marrow CR with low platelets). CD33 is present on blasts in the vast majority of patients with MDS and is exclusively present in hematopoietic cells; this feature presumably underlies the relatively low incidence of extramedullary toxicity observed with single-agent Mylotarg in relapsed AML. However, a few adverse events have been observed, including liver dysfunction in 10% of the cases and veno-occlusive disease in rare instances.

Mylotarg has been investigated in pilot trials in relapsed and high-risk frontline MDS at our institution (E. Estey, unpublished data). Mylotarg was given as a single agent at a dose of 9 mg/m² IV on days 1 and 15 to newly diagnosed patients having high risk of mortality from combination chemotherapy (e.g., age ≥ 65 years; poor performance status). Among those patients with diploid karyotype, a CR rate of 50% was observed. However, in patients with unfavorable karyotype [any abnormality excluding t(8;21), inv(16), and −Y], the CR rate was

**Table 5**  Results of Single-Agent Mylotarg in Frontline High-Risk MDS and AML: The University of Texas M.D. Anderson Cancer Center Experience

| Diagnosis | Karyotype[a] | Number of treated[b] patients | Number of CR (%) | Number of deaths (%) |
|---|---|---|---|---|
| MDS | Diploid | 4 | 1 (25) | 1 (25) |
|  | Poor karyotype | 9 | 0 (0) | 2 (22) |
| AML | Diploid | 15 | 8 (53) | 1 (6) |
|  | Poor karyotype | 21 | 1 (4) | 13 (61) |

[a] Poor karyotype refers to any abnormality excluding t(8;21), inv(16), and −Y.
[b] As part of their treatment, all patient were randomized to receive interleukin-11.
MDS, myelodysplastic syndromes; AML, acute myeloid leukemia; CR, complete remission.

very low and induction mortality remained high owing to ineffective antileukemic activity and high incidences of myelosuppression and resistance (Table 5). Currently, several trials at our institution are investigating the safety and efficacy of Mylotarg in combination with anthracyclines plus ara-C, fludarabine plus ara-C plus cyclosporine, and topotecan plus ara-C for patients with relapsed or frontline AML or high-risk MDS.

## VI.  THALIDOMIDE

Thalidomide was developed as a sedative-hypnotic with antiemetic activity, but unfortunately was associated with fetal malformations in the offspring of mothers who used the drug during pregnancy (61), which led to its abandonment in the mid-1960s. Thalidomide was also shown to have activity against lepromatous leprosy (62) and against several cutaneous and rheumatological disorders (63), particularly recurrent aphthous ulcers in patients with acquired immunodeficiency syndrome (AIDS) (64). Thalidomide was additionally used in the treatment of refractory graft-versus-host disease in patients receiving allogeneic bone marrow transplantation (65). The effects of thalidomide on lymphocytes included stimulation of CD8+ T cells, a shift to $T_H2$ responses, and inhibition of T-cell proliferation (66–68). Thalidomide also inhibits the production of tumor necrosis factor (TNF)-$\alpha$ (69) and other cytokines.

The limb malformations observed in offsprings of pregnant women who received thalidomide suggested it could promote inhibition of normal neovascularization of the fetal limb bud. Thalidomide was subsequently shown to inhibit angiogenesis (70), a fundamental process in of tumor development (71) and a process that may also be pathophysiological in leukemia and MDS (72). Thalidomide has already been shown to be active in several solid tumors and in multiple myeloma (73,74).

Studies of the use of thalidomide for refractory hematological malignancies have been conducted (Table 6). In a trial involving 28 patients, nine patients had MDS [six RAEB, two RAEB-t, one CMML in transformation (CMML-t)]. The initial dose of thalidomide was 200 mg at bedtime, and increased to 800 mg daily or the maximally tolerated dose. One patient with RAEB achieved CR. Toxicities included fatigue, which was dose-limiting, constipation, and skin rashes (75). In another trial, Raza et al. reported more encouraging results with thalidomide for treatment of patients with low-risk MDS (76). In this trial, 61 patients (22 RA, 13 RARS, 19 RAEB, four RAEB-t, three CMML) were treated with thalidomide at doses of 100–400 mg daily. Seventeen of 25 evaluable patients (68%) responded, but response criteria included "softer" end points. Transfusion independence was reported in patients with RA, and the authors emphasized the importance of delayed responses (3 months) and the need to continue the therapy. Dourado et al. reported their preliminary results of a study in which responses were observed in six of nine MDS patients treated with thalidomide; three patients became red cell transfusion-independent. Only patients with early MDS responded in this study (77). An ongoing multi-institutional phase II trial of thalido-

**Table 6** Thalidomide Therapy in Myelodysplastic Syndromes

| Investigators (publication) | Number of treated patients | MDS category (number of treated patients) | Number of responses[a] (% of treated patients) |
|---|---|---|---|
| Thomas et al. (75) | 9 | RAEB (6) RAEB-t (2) CMML-t (1) | 1 CR (11) |
| Raza et al. (76) | 25[b] | RA (22) RARS (13) RAEB (19) RAEB-t (4) CMML (3) | 17 (68) |
| Dourado et al. (77) | 9 | RARS (2) CMML (1) RAEB-t/AML (6) | 6 (66) |

[a] Response definitions variable between studies.
[b] Twenty-five evaluable patients out of 61 patients treated.
RA, refractory anemia; RAEB, refractory anemia with excess blasts; RAEB-t, refractory anemia with excess blasts in transformation; RARS, refractory anemia with ringed sideroblasts; CMML, chronic myelomonocytic leukemia; CMML-t, chronic myelomonocytic leukemia in transformation; AML, acute myeloid leukemia; CR, complete remission.

mide therapy for treating MDS may potentially lead to FDA approval. In addition, the benefit of combining thalidomide with other agents, including topotecan, is also under study (78). Of note, severe dermatological toxicity has been occasionally reported with thalidomide in combination with steroids (79) but more frequent and as yet not-well-publicized toxicities associated with thalidomide include hypothyroidism and thromboembolic complications.

## VII. AMIFOSTINE

Amifostine (WR-2721) is a phosphorylated aminothiol originally developed as a radioprotectant. Animal studies showed differential protection of normal tissues by amifostine with no increase in the radioresistance of tumors, as well as protection against the development of secondary neoplasms in irradiated animals (80,81). Amifostine has also been shown to protect normal tissues from the cytotoxic effects of alkylating agents and platinum-based drugs (82,83). The action of amifostine depends on the dephosphorylation of the parent compound by membrane-bound alkaline phosphatase in normal tissues and the transport to the intracellular space of the active metabolite (84). The relative lower level of membrane-bound alkaline phosphatase in tumors as compared with that of normal tissues may explain the selective cytoprotection of amifostine.

Several clinical trials have confirmed the cytoprotective effects of amifostine. For example, a phase I study of dose escalation of 3 days of idarubicin with 7 days of ara-C combined with amifostine for induction treatment of elderly patients with AML showed that the dose of idarubicin could be increased up to 19 $mg/m^2$ daily for three doses, resulting in minimal toxicities (marked reduction of mucositis and delayed alopecia) (85). Amifostine has also been shown to improve the therapeutic index of mafosfamide (86). Common toxicities of amifostine include hypotension (especially at higher doses, such as 910 $mg/m^2$ infused over 15 min), nausea, vomiting, flushed feeling, sneezing, hypocalcemia, and allergic reactions (87).

Amifostine is also being investigated for treatment of MDS. Clonogenic assays in which amifostine is preincubated with bone marrow cells from patients with MDS showed increased colony formation (88). An initial phase I study of amifostine in 18 patients with MDS (12 RA/RARS, four RAEB, two RAEB-t) showed single or multilineage improvements in 83% of the patients and concomitant increases in CFU-GEMM (colony-forming units–granulocyte, erythrocyte, monocyte, megakaryocyte) and BFU-E (burst-forming units–erythrocyte) colonies in a subset of patients. A dose of 200 $mg/m^2$ administered three times a week was well tolerated (89). Subsequently, in a multicenter study of 75 evaluable patients (27 RA/RARS, 37 RAEB, four RAEB-t, four CMML, three under review), hematological responses were observed in 36% of the patients and 10 patients had 50% reduction of bone marrow blasts (90).

In a smaller study, investigators analyzed the impact of amifostine, 300 mg/m$^2$, in 12 patients. CR was achieved in two patients and PR in two other patients. No differences were observed between patients treated with this dose or those receiving 400 mg/m$^2$ (91). More modest responses to amifostine in MDS have been reported by other investigators (92,93). Again, as with thalidomide and other investigational agent studies, differences in response rates reported may have been due to differences in dose schedules and duration, study group characteristics, or response definitions. The latter issue (i.e., objectivity and clinical significance of responses) has been recently addressed (94) and is critical for the comparative evaluation of new strategies in MDS. The role of amifostine in MDS has not yet been defined.

## VIII.  OTHER STRATEGIES

### A.  Anti-TNF/Antiapoptosis Approaches

Based on known molecular abnormalities, several new treatments are being developed in MDS. TNF has been shown to be up-regulated in MDS (95) while apoptosis is prominent in early MDS. Raza et al. reported initial encouraging results using pentoxifylline, ciprofloxacin, amifostine, and steroids; among 29 evaluable patients, 76% showed some form of response (96). However, Nemunaitis et al. reported poor results with pentoxifylline combinations (97). Potential combination programs include the incorporation of amifostine and pentoxifylline or utilization of soluble TNF receptors alone or in combination with amifostine, pentoxifylline, and anti-Fas ligand. A program using a soluble TNF-receptor (Enbrel) is being investigated at several institutions with preliminary results showing responses in six of 10 evaluable patients (98).

### B.  p53-Mediated Approaches

Mutations of p53 are common in MDS (99). An approach using antisense oligonucleotides to inactivate p53 RNA has been generated. So far, however, results have been disappointing; only one of 10 high-risk MDS patients treated with antisense oligonucleotides had a transient response (100).

### C.  Anti-ras or Farnesyl Transferase Inhibitors

Activation of ras oncogenes has been described in 20–30% of patients with AML (101). Inhibitors of the Ras-MAPK (mitogen-activated protein kinase) pathway act by inhibiting farnesyl transferases, enzymes necessary for Ras localization to the cell membrane. These inhibitors are undergoing clinical trials for MDS, the results of which will be used to direct phase II trials in the near future.

## D.  Differentiating Agents

Agents with interesting differentiation properties include hexamethylene bisacetamid (HMBA) and sodium phenylbutyrate. In two studies, HMBA was given by continuous infusion to 57 MDS patients, which induced CR in three patients and PR in six patients (objective response rate 17%) (102,103). Sodium phenylbutyrate, a histone deacetylase inhibitor, was given to 27 patients at doses up to 440 mg/kg daily for 7 days every 4 weeks; 17 patients had improvements in granulocyte counts and three had improvements in platelet counts (104). Both HMBA and sodium phenylbutyrate work by inhibiting deacetylation of histones, a mechanism involved in gene silencing. Study of the interactions between histone acetylation metabolism, DNA methylation, and DNA topoisomerases may lead to the development of combination programs using inhibitors of these different molecular mechanisms.

## E.  Arsenicals

The role of arsenicals, particularly arsenic trioxide, is being evaluated in leukemias. Data for acute promyelocytic leukemia (APL) suggest that arsenic trioxide has significant anti-APL activity in the frontline and salvage settings. In addition, arsenicals were modestly active against CML. Anecdotal experience suggests that arsenic trioxide (105) may be active in MDS. As with retinoic acid, combinations with hypomethylating agents are of potential interest.

## IX.  SUMMARY

MDS are a complex group of hematopoietic disorders. Several molecular abnormalities have been identified in subsets of patients. These include aberrant methylation, increased apoptosis (early MDS), immune dysregulation, abnormal angiogenesis, increased expression of cytokines, and mutations of different oncogenes, among others. Several therapeutic agents have shown promising activity in subsets of patients with MDS. Better understanding of the mechanisms of action of these drugs may allow the development of targeted therapies for specific subgroups of patients with defined molecular abnormalities and the generation of combination programs using therapies that act via different and synergistic mechanisms.

## REFERENCES

1. Bennett JM, Catovsky D, Daniel MT, Flandrin G, Galton DA, Gralnick HR, Sultan C. Proposals for the classification of the myelodysplastic syndromes. Br J Haematol 1982; 51:189–199.
2. Greenberg P, Cox C, LeBeau MM, Fenaux P, Morel P, Sanz G, Sanz M, Vallespi T, Hamblin T, Oscier D, Ohyashiki K, Toyama K, Aul C, Mufti G, Bennett J. International scoring system for evaluating prognosis in myelodysplastic syndromes. Blood 1997; 89:2079–2088.
3. Estey E, Keating M, Pierce S, Beran M. Application of the International Scoring System for myelodysplasia to M.D. Anderson patients. Blood 1997; 90:2843–2846.
4. Issa JP, Baylin SB, Herman JG. DNA methylation changes in hematologic malignancies: biologic and clinical implications. Leukemia 1997; 11(suppl 1):S7–11.
5. Baylin SB, Herman JG, Graff JR, Vertino PM, Issa JP. Alterations in DNA methylation: a fundamental aspect of neoplasia. Adv Cancer Res 1998; 72:141–196.
6. Wolffe AP, Matzke MA. Epigenetics: regulation through repression. Science 1999; 286:481–486.
7. Jones PA, Laird PW. Cancer epigenetics comes of age. Nat Genet 1999; 21:163–167.
8. Melki JR, Vincent PC, Clark SJ. Concurrent DNA hypermethylation of multiple genes in acute myeloid leukemia. Cancer Res 1999; 59:3730–3740.
9. Toyota M, Kopecky KJ, Toyota MO, Jair KW, Willman CL, Issa JP. Methylation profiling in acute myelogenous leukemia. Blood 2001; 97:2823–2829.
10. Garcia-Manero G, Daniels J, Pierce S, et al. Aberrant methylation of multiple genes in ALL. Blood 2000; 96:102a.
11. Ihalainen J, Pakkala S, Savolainen ER, Jansson SE, Palotie A. Hypermethylation of the calcitonin gene in the myelodysplastic syndromes. Leukemia 1993; 7:263–267.
12. Dhodapkar M, Grill J, Lust JA. Abnormal regional hypermethylation of the calcitonin gene in myelodysplastic syndromes. Leuk Res 1995; 19:719–726.
13. Uchida T, Kinoshita T, Nagai H, Nakahara Y, Saito H, Hotta T, Murate T. Hypermethylation of the p15INK4B gene in myelodysplastic syndromes. Blood 1997; 90:1403–1409.
14. Aoki E, Uchida T, Ohashi H, Nagai H, Murase T, Ichikawa A, Yamao K, Hotta T, Kinoshita T, Saito H, Murate T. Methylation status of the p15INK4B gene in hematopoietic progenitors and peripheral blood cells in myelodysplastic syndromes. Leukemia 2000; 14:586–593.
15. Quesnel B, Guillerm G, Vereecque R, Wattel E, Preudhomme C, Bauters F, Vanrumbeke M, Fenaux P. Methylation of the p15(INK4b) gene in myelodysplastic syndromes is frequent and acquired during disease progression. Blood 1998; 91:2985–2990.
16. Toyota M, Ahuja N, Ohe-Toyota M, Herman JG, Baylin SB, Issa JP. CpG island methylator phenotype in colorectal cancer. Proc Natl Acad Sci USA 1999; 96:8681 8686.

17. Toyota M, Ahuja N, Suzuki H, Itoh F, Ohe-Toyota M, Imai K, Baylin SB, Issa JP. Aberrant methylation in gastric cancer associated with the CpG island methylator phenotype. Cancer Res 1999; 59:5438–5442.

18. Ueki T, Toyota M, Sohn T, Yeo CJ, Issa JP, Hruban RH, Goggins M. Hypermethylation of multiple genes in pancreatic adenocarcinoma. Cancer Res 2000; 60:1835–1839.

19. Lubbert M. DNA methylation inhibitors in the treatment of leukemias, myelodysplastic syndromes and hemoglobinopathies: clinical results and possible mechanisms of action. Curr Top Microbiol Immunol 2000; 249:135–164.

20. Silverman LR, Holland JF, Weinberg RS, Alter BP, Davis RB, Ellison RR, Demakos EP, Cornell CJ Jr, Carey RW, Schiffer C, et al. Effects of treatment with 5-azacytidine on the in vivo and in vitro hematopoiesis in patients with myelodysplastic syndromes. Leukemia 1993; 7(suppl 1):21–29.

21. Silverman LR, Holland JF, Demakos EP, Gattani A, Cuttner J. 5-azacytidine in myelodysplastic syndromes (MDS): the experience at Mount Sinai Hospital, New York. Leukemia Res 1993; 18:21.

22. Silverman LR, Demakos EP, Peterson B, et al. A randomized controlled trial of subcutaneous azacytidine (aza c) in patients with myelodysplastic syndrome (MDS): a study of the cancer and leukemia group B (CALGB). Proc Am Soc Clin Oncol 1998; 34:12a.

23. Kornblith A, Silverman LR. The impact of 5-azacytidine on the quality of life of patients with myelodysplastic syndromes (MDS) treated in a randomized phase III trial of the Cancer and Leukemia Group B. Proc Am Soc Clin Oncol 1998; 34: 189.

24. Jones PA, Taylor SM. Cellular differentiation, cytidine analogs and DNA methylation. Cell 1980; 20:85–93.

25. Pinto A, Attadia V, Fusco A, Ferrara F, Spada OA, Di Fiore PP. 5-Aza-2′-deoxycytidine induces terminal differentiation of leukemic blasts from patients with acute myeloid leukemias. Blood 1984; 64:922–929.

26. Koshy M, Dorn L, Bressler L, Molokie R, Lavelle D, Talischy N, Hoffman R, van Overveld W, DeSimone J. 2-Deoxy 5-azacytidine and fetal hemoglobin induction in sickle cell anemia. Blood 2000; 96:2379–2384.

27. Willemze R, Suciu S, Archimbaud E, Muus P, Stryckmans P, Louwagie EA, Berneman Z, Tjean M, Wijermans P, Dohner H, Jehn U, Labar B, Jaksic B, Dardenne M, Zittoun R. A randomized phase II study on the effects of 5-Aza-2′-deoxycytidine combined with either amsacrine or idarubicin in patients with relapsed acute leukemia: an EORTC Leukemia Cooperative Group phase II study (06893). Leukemia 1997; 11(suppl 1):S24–27.

28. Juttermann R, Li E, Jaenisch R. Toxicity of 5-aza-2′-deoxycytidine to mammalian cells is mediated primarily by covalent trapping of DNA methyltransferase rather than DNA demethylation. Proc Natl Acad Sci USA 1994; 91:11797–11801.

29. Rivard GE, Momparler RL, Demers J, Benoit P, Raymond R, Lin K, Momparler LF. Phase I study on 5-aza-2′-deoxycytidine in children with acute leukemia. Leuk Res 1981; 5:453–462.

30. Momparler RL, Rivard GE, Gyger M. Clinical trial on 5-aza-2′-deoxycytidine in patients with acute leukemia. Pharmacol Ther 1985; 30:277–286.

31. Debusscher L, Marie JP, Dodion P, et al. Phase I, II trial of 5-aza-deoxycytidine (NSC127, 716) in adult patients with acute leukemias. In: Momparler RL, de Vos D, eds. Decitabine, Preclinical and Clinical Studies. Haarlem, The Netherlands: PCH Publications, 1990:131–143.

32. Richel DJ, Colly LP, JC Kluin-Nelemans, Willemze R. The antileukaemic activity of 5-Aza-2 deoxycytidine (Aza-dC) in patients with relapsed and resistant leukaemia. Br J Cancer 1991; 64:144–148.

33. Petti MC, Mandelli F, Zagonel V, De Gregoris C, Merola MC, Latagliata R, Gattei V, Fazi P, Monfardini S, Pinto A. Pilot study of 5-aza-2'-deoxycytidine (Decitabine) in the treatment of poor prognosis acute myelogenous leukemia patients: preliminary results. Leukemia 1993; 7(suppl 1):36–41.

34. Willemze R, Archimbaud E, Muus P. Preliminary results with 5-aza-2'-deoxycytidine (DAC)-containing chemotherapy in patients with relapsed or refractory acute leukemia. The EORTC Leukemia Cooperative Group. Leukemia 1993; 7(suppl 1): 49–50.

35. Zagonel V, Bullian PL, Sardeo G, et al. 5-aza-2'-deoxycytidine (decitabine): an effective agent in the treatment of myelodysplastic syndrome (MDS). Hematologica 1991; Abstract 160. 76(suppl 4): p. 76.

36. Zagonel V, Lo Re G, Marotta G, Barbare R, Sardeo G, Gattei V, De Angelis V, Monfardini S, Pinto A. 5-Aza-2'-deoxycytidine (Decitabine) induces trilineage response in unfavourable myelodysplastic syndromes. Leukemia 1993; 7(suppl 1): 30–35.

37. Pinto A, Zagonel V, Attadia V, Bullian PL, Gattei V, Carbone A, Monfardini S, Colombatti A. 5-Aza-2'-deoxycytidine as a differentiation inducer in acute myeloid leukaemias and myelodysplastic syndromes of the elderly. Bone Marrow Transplant 1989; 4(suppl 3):28–32.

38. Richel DJ, Colly LP, Willemze R. Decitabine in patients with relapsed acute leukemia. Proc Am Soc Clin Oncol 1989; 9:214.

39. Wijermans P, Lubbert M, Verhoef G, Bosly A, Rauoet C, Andre M, Ferront A. Low-dose 5-aza-2'-deoxycytidine, a DNA hypomethylating agent, for the treatment of high-risk myelodysplastic syndrome: a multicenter phase II study in elderly patients. J Clin Oncol 2000; 18:956–962.

40. Daskalakis M, Nguyen TT, Wijermans PW, et al. Reduction of p15 hypermethylation in bone marrow cells from patients with MDS following treatment with a methyltransferase inhibitor, decitabine. Blood 1998; 94:306a.

41. Wang JC, Caron PR, Kim RA. The role of DNA topoisomerases in recombination and genome stability: a double-edged sword? Cell 1990; 62:403–406.

42. Wang JC. DNA topoisomerases (review). Annu Rev Biochem 1996; 65:635–692.

43. Saltz LB, Cox JV, Blanke C, Rosen LS, Fehrenbacher L, Moore MJ, Moroun JA, Ackland SP, Locker PK, Pirotta N, Elfring GL, Miller LL. Irinotecan plus fluorouracil and leucovorin for metastatic colorectal cancer. Irinotecan Study Group. N Engl J Med 2000; 343:905–914.

44. Beran M, Kantarjian H. Topotecan in the treatment of hematologic malignancies. Semin Hematol 1998; 35(suppl 4):26–31.

45. Beran M, Kantarjian H, O'Brien S, Koller C, al-Bitar M, Arbuck S, Pierce S, Moore M, Abbruzzese JL, Andreeff M, Keating M, Estey E. Topotecan, a topoisomerase

I inhibitor, is active in the treatment of myelodysplastic syndrome and chronic mye-lomonocytic leukemia. Blood 1996; 88:2473–2479.

46. Beran M, Estey E, O'Brien SM, Giles FJ, Koller CA, Komblau S, Keating M, Kantarjian HM. Results of topotecan single-agent therapy in patients with myelo-dysplastic syndromes and chronic myelomonocytic leukemia. Leuk Lymphoma 1998; 31:521–531.

47. Beran M, Kantarjian H. Results of topotecan-based combination therapy in patients with myelodysplastic syndromes and chronic myelomonocytic leukemia. Semin Hematol 1999; 36(suppl 8):3–10.

48. Cortes J, Estey E, Beran M, O'Brien S, Giles F, Koller C, Keating M, Kantarjian H. Cyclophosphamide, ara-C and topotecan (CAT) for patients with refractory or relapsed acute leukemia. Leuk Lymphoma 2000; 36:479–484.

49. Besa EC, Roda P, Woodland C, Dourado C. Topotecan, fludarabine, ara-C and G-CSF (T-FLAG) for aggressive myelodysplastic syndromes and acute myelogenous leukemia in the elderly: a dose finding for topotecan study. Blood 2000; 96:259b.

50. Vey N, Kantarjian H, Tran H, Beran M, O'Brien S, Cortes J, Koller C, Estey E. Phase I and pharmacologic study of 9-aminocamptothecin colloidal dispersion for-mulation in patients with refractory or relapsed acute leukemia. Ann Oncol 1999; 10:577–583.

51. Cortes JE, O'Brien S, Giles F, et al. 9-Nitro-20-(s)-camptothecin (9-NC, RFS2000) in chronic myeloid leukemia (CML), chronic myelomonocytic leukemia (CMML) and myelodysplastic syndromes (MDS). Proc Am Soc Clin Oncol 2000; 19:7a.

52. Nomoto T, Nishio K, Ishida T, Mori M, Saijo N. Characterization of a human small-cell lung cancer cell line resistant to a new water-soluble camptothecin deriv-ative, DX-8951f. Jpn J Cancer Res 1998; 89:1179–1186.

53. Vey N, Giles FJ, Kantarjian H, Smith TL, Beran M, Jeha S. The topoisomerase I inhibitor DX-8951f is active in a severe combined immunodeficient mouse model of human acute myelogenous leukemia. Clin Cancer Res 2000; 6:731–736.

54. Giles FJ, Cortes JE, Thomas DA, et al. Phase I study of exatecan mesylate (DX-8951f), a novel topoisomerase I (TOPO 1) inhibitor. Blood 2000; 96:121a.

55. Kantarjian HM, Keating MJ, Walters RS, Koller CA, McCredie KB, Freireich EJ. Phase II study of low-dose continuous infusion homoharringtonine in refractory acute myelogenous leukemia. Cancer 1989; 63:813–817.

56. O'Brien S, Kantarjian H, Keating M, Beran M, Koller C, Robertson LE, Hester J, Rios MB, Andreeff M, Talpaz M. Homoharringtonine therapy induces responses in patients with chronic myelogenous leukemia in late chronic phase. Blood 1995; 86:3322–3326.

57. Feldman FJ, Seiter KP, Ahmed T, Baskind P, Arlin ZA. Homoharringtonine in patients with myelodysplastic syndrome (MDS) and MDS evolving to acute my-eloid leukemia. Leukemia 1996; 10:40–42.

58. Bian S, Xue Y, Zhao Y, et al. Comparison of four regimens composed of three drugs in treatment of untreated acute myeloid leukemia. Blood 2000; 96:326a.

59. Robin JP, Radosevic N, Pasco S, et al. A new series of synthetic homoharringtonine (HHT) analogs exhibiting potent antileukemic activity in vitro. Blood 2000; 96: 1372.

60. Sievers EL, Appelbaum FR, Spielberger RT, Forman SJ, Flowers D, Smith FO, Shannon-Dorcy K, Berger MS, Bernstein ED. Selective ablation of acute myeloid leukemia using antibody-targeted chemotherapy: a phase I study of an anti-CD33 calicheamicin immunoconjugate. Blood 1999; 93:3678–3684.

61. Mellin GW, Katzenstein M. The saga of thalidomide (concluded): neuropathy to embryopathy, with case reports of congenital anomalies. N Engl J Med 1962; 267: 1238–1244.

62. Sheskin J. Further observation with thalidomide in lepra reactions. Lepr Rev 1965; 36:183–187.

63. Calderon P, Anzilotti M, Phelps R. Thalidomide in dermatology. New indications for an old drug (review). Int J Dermatol 1997; 36:881–887.

64. Jacobson JM, Greenspan JS, Spritzler J, Ketter N, Fahey JL, Jackson JB, Fox L, Chernoff M, Wu AW, MacPhail LA, Vasquez GJ, Wohl DA. Thalidomide for the treatment of oral aphthous ulcers in patients with human immunodeficiency virus infection. National Institute of Allergy and Infectious Diseases AIDS Clinical Trials Group. N Engl J Med 1997; 336:1487–1493.

65. Parker PM, Chao N, Nademanee A, O'Donnell MR, Schmidt GM, Snyder DS, Stein AS, Smith EP, Molina A, Stepon DE, et al. Thalidomide as salvage therapy for chronic graft-versus-host disease. Blood 1995; 86:3604–3609.

66. Haslett PA, Corral LG, Albert M, Kaplan G. Thalidomide costimulates primary human T lymphocytes, preferentially inducing proliferation, cytokine production, and cytotoxic responses in the CD8+ subset. J Exp Med 1998; 187:1885–1892.

67. McHugh SM, Rifkin IR, Deighton J, Wilson AB, Lachmann PJ, Lockwood CM, Ewan PW. The immunosuppressive drug thalidomide induces T helper cell type 2 (Th2) and concomitantly inhibits Th1 cytokine production in mitogen- and antigen-stimulated human peripheral blood mononuclear cell cultures. Clin Exp Immunol 1995; 99:160–167.

68. Keenan RJ, Eiras G, Burckart GJ, Stuart RS, Hardesty RL, Vogelsang G, Griffith BP, Zeevi A. Immunosuppressive properties of thalidomide. Inhibition of in vitro lymphocyte proliferation alone and in combination with cyclosporine or FK506. Transplantation 1991; 52:908–910.

69. Turk BE, Jiang H, Liu JO. Binding of thalidomide to alpha 1-acid glycoprotein may be involved in its inhibition of tumor necrosis factor alpha production. Proc Natl Acad Sci USA 1996; 93:7552–7556.

70. D'Amato RJ, Loughnan MS, Flynn E, Folkman J. Thalidomide is an inhibitor of angiogenesis. Proc Natl Acad Sci USA 1994; 91:4082–4085.

71. Folkman J. Angiogenesis in cancer, vascular, rheumatoid and other disease. Nat Med 1995; 1:27–31.

72. Aguayo A, Kantarjian H, Manshouri T, Gidel C, Estey E, Thomas D, Koller C, Estrov Z, O'Brien S, Keating M, Freireich E, Albitar M. Angiogenesis in acute and chronic leukemias and myelodysplastic syndromes. Blood 2000; 96:2240–2245.

73. Thomas DA, Kantarjian HM. Current role of thalidomide in cancer treatment. Curr Opin Oncol 2000; 12:564–573.

74. Singhal S, Mehta J, Desikan R, Ayers D, Roberson P, Eddlemon P, Munshi N, Anaissie E, Wilson C, Dhodapkar M, Zeddis J, Barlogie B. Antitumor activity

      of thalidomide in refractory multiple myeloma. N Engl J Med 1999; 341:1565–
      1571.
75.   Thomas DA, Aguayo A, Estey E, et al. Thalidomide as anti-angiogenesis therapy
      (RX) in refractory and relapsed leukemias. Blood 1999; 94:2269a.
76.   Raza A, Lisak L, Andrews C, et al. Encouraging improvement in cytopenias of
      patients with myelodysplastic syndromes (MDS) with thalidomide. Proc Am Soc
      Clin Oncol 2000; 19:30a.
77.   Dourado CMC, Seixas-Silva J, Besa EC. Response to thalidomide in 9 patients
      with myelodysplastic syndromes: a promising treatment for early and postchemo-
      therapy in late forms of MDS. Blood 2000; 96:260b.
78.   Raza A, Lisak L, Little L, et al. Thalidomide as a single agent or in combination
      with topotecan, pentoxifylline and/or enbrel in myelodysplastic syndromes. Blood
      2000; 96:146a.
79.   Rajkumar SV, Gertz MA, Witzig TE. Life-threatening toxic epidermal necrolysis
      with thalidomide therapy for myeloma. N Engl J Med 2000; 343:972–973.
80.   Harris JW, Phillips TL. Radiobiological and biochemical studies of thiophosphate
      radioprotective compounds related to cysteamine. Radiat Res 1971; 46:362–379.
81.   Stewart FA, Rojas A, Denekamp J. Radioprotection of two mouse tumors by WR-
      2721 in single and fractionated treatments. Int J Radiat Oncol Biol Phys 1983; 9:
      507–513.
82.   Wasserman TH, Phillips TL, Ross G, Kane LJ. Differential protection against cyto-
      toxic chemotherapeutic effects on bone marrow CFUs by Wr-2721. Cancer Clin
      Trials 1981; 4:3–6.
83.   Yuhas JM, Culo F. Selective inhibition of the nephrotoxicity of cisdichlorodiammi-
      neplatinum(II) by WR-2721 without altering its antitumor properties. Cancer Treat
      Rep 1980; 64:57–64.
84.   Capizzi R. Amifostine: the preclinical basis for broad-spectrum selective cytopro-
      tection of normal tissues from cytotoxic therapies. Semin Oncol 1996; 23(4 suppl
      8):2–17.
85.   Garcia-Manero G, Grosso D, Beardell F, Grabchet F, Martinez J, Schuster SJ, Fil-
      icko J, Brunner J, Flomenberg N, Capizzi R. High complete remission rate and
      normal organ cytoprotection using dose escalation of idarubicin with amifostine in
      high risk patients with acute myelogenous leukemia. Blood 1999; 92:216b.
86.   Douay L, Hu C, Giarratana MC, Bouchet S, Conlon J, Capizzi RL, Gorin NC.
      Amifostine improves the antileukemic therapeutic index of mafosfamide: implica-
      tions for bone marrow purging. Blood 1995; 86:2849–2855.
87.   Schuchter LM. Guidelines for the administration of amifostine. Semin Oncol 1996;
      23(4 suppl 8):40–43.
88.   List AF, Heaton R, Glinsmann-Gibson B, Capizzi R. Amifostine stimulates forma-
      tion of multipotent progenitors and generates macroscopic colonies in normal and
      myelodysplastic bone marrow. Proc Am Soc Clin Oncol 1996; 15:449.
89.   List AF, Brasfield F, Heaton R, Glinsmann-Gibson B, Crook L, Taitle R, Capizzi
      R. Stimulation of hematopoiesis by amifostine in patients with myelodysplastic
      syndrome. Blood 1997; 90:3364–3369.
90.   List A, Holmes H, Greenberg P, Bennet J, Oster W. Phase II study of amifostine
      in patients with myelodysplastic syndromes. Blood 1999; 94:305a.

91.  Anagnostopoulos NI, Viniou N-A, Galanopoulo A, et al. Treatment of anemia in myelodysplastic syndromes with amifostine. In vitro testing response. Blood 2000; 96:259b.

92.  Bowen DT, Denzlinger C, Brugger W, Culligan D, Gelly K, Adlakha S, Groves M, Hepburn M, Kanz L. Poor response rate to a continuous schedule of Amifostine therapy for 'low/intermediate risk' myelodysplastic patients. Br J Haematol 1998; 103:785–787.

93.  Schuster SJ, Crook L, Matthwes A, et al. Crossover trial of subcutaneous versus intravenous amifostine in patients with de novo myelodysplastic syndromes: preliminary results. Blood 1998; 92:362a.

94.  Cheson BD, Bennett JM, Kantarjian H, Pinto A, Schiffer CA, Nimer SD, Lowenberg B, Beran M, de Witte TM, Stone RM, Mittelman M, Sanz GF, Wijermans PW, Gore S, Greenberg PL. Report of an international working group to standardize response criteria for myelodysplastic syndromes. Blood 2000; 96:3671–3674.

95.  Kitagawa M, Saito I, Kuwata T, Yoshida S, Yamaguchi S, Takahashi M, Tanizawa T, Kamiyama R, Hirokawa K. Overexpression of tumor necrosis factor (TNF)-alpha and interferon (IFN)-gamma by bone marrow cells from patients with myelodysplastic syndromes. Leukemia 1997; 11:2049–2054.

96.  Raza A, Qawi H, Lisak L, Andric T, Dar S, Andrews C, Venugopal P, Gezer S, Gregory S, Loew J, Robin E, Rifkin S, Hsu WT, Huang RW. Patients with myelodysplastic syndromes benefit from palliative therapy with amifostine, pentoxifylline, and ciprofloxacin with or without dexamethasone. Blood 2000; 95:1580–1587.

97.  Nemunaitis J, Rosenfeld C, Getty L, Boegel F, Meyer W, Jennings LW, Zeigler Z, Shadduck R. Pentoxifylline and ciprofloxacin in patients with myelodysplastic syndrome. A phase II trial. Am J Clin Oncol 1995; 18:189–193.

98.  Deeg HJ, Gotlib J, Beckham C, Dugan K, Appelbaum F. Soluble TNF receptor fusion protein (TNFR:Fc; Enbrel) in the treatment of patients with myelodysplastic syndromes (MDS). Blood 2000; 96:146a.

99.  Sugimoto K, Hirano N, Toyoshima H, Chiba S, Mano H, Takaku F, Yazaki Y, Hirai H. Mutations of the p53 gene in myelodysplastic syndrome (MDS) and MDS-derived leukemia. Blood 1993; 81:3022–3026.

100.  Bishop MR, Iversen PL, Bayever E, Sharp JG, Greiner TC, Copple BL, Ruddon R, Zon G, Spinolo J, Arneson M, Armitage JO, Kessinger A. Phase I trial of an antisense oligonucleotide OL(1)p53 in hematologic malignancies. J Clin Oncol 1996; 14:1320 1326.

101.  Reuter CW, Morgan MA, Bergmann L. Targeting the Ras signaling pathway: a rational, mechanism-based treatment for hematologic malignancies? (review). Blood 2000; 96:1655–1669.

102.  Andreeff M, Stone R, Michaeli J, Young CW, Tong WP, Sogoloff H, Ervin T, Kufe D, Rifkind RA, Marks PA. Hexamethylene bisacetamide in myelodysplastic syndrome and acute myelogenous leukemia: a phase II clinical trial with a differentiation-inducing agent. Blood 1992; 80:2604–2609.

103.  Rowinsky EK, Conley BA, Jones RJ, Spivak JL, Auerbach M, Donehower RC. Hexamethylene bisacetamide in myelodysplastic syndrome: effect of five-day exposure to maximal therapeutic concentrations. Leukemia 1992; 6:526–534.

104.  Gore SD, Miller CB, Weng LJ, et al. Clinical development of sodium phenylbuty-

rate as a putative differentiating agent in myeloid malignancies. Anticancer Res 1997; 17:3938a.

105. Dutcher JP, Wiernik PH, Novik Y, Garl S, Hughes J, Arezz J. Major hematologic response in a patient with myelodysplasia (MDS) to arsenic trioxide (ATO). Blood 2000; 96:260b.

106. Wijermans P, Luebbert M, Verhoef G, et al. DNA demethylating therapy in MDS: the experience with 5-aza-2′-deoxycytidine (decitabine). Blood 1999; 94:306a.

# 16

# Intensive Chemotherapy, Including Autologous Stem Cell Transplantation, in the Myelodysplastic Syndromes

**Theo M. de Witte and Margriet Oosterveld**
*University Medical Center, Nijmegen, The Netherlands*

## I. INTRODUCTION

The myelodysplastic syndromes (MDS) are a heterogeneous group of disorders with a variable prognosis. Refractory anemia (RA) and RA with ringed sideroblasts (RARS) are characterized by a low risk of transformation to acute myeloid leukemia (AML) and a median survival usually in excess of 30 months (1). In contrast, the median survival of patients with refractory anemia with excess blasts (RAEB) or RAEB in transformation (RAEB-t) is less than 12 months (2,3). The prognosis for patients with therapy-related MDS, or secondary acute myeloblastic leukemia (secondary leukemia), is also poor, with median survivals of less than 12 months (3,4). In addition to the MDS subtype, the patient's karyotype is a valuable prognosticator of survival (5,6); see Chapter 5 for a detailed discussion.

Various criteria have been developed to predict the prognosis of patients with MDS. The most widely accepted evaluation or scoring method is the International Prognostic Scoring System (IPSS), which is based on the number of blasts in the bone marrow, karyotype, and the number of peripheral blood cytopenias (7). The IPSS outlines four distinct risk categories (low, intermediate-1, intermediate-2, and high risk), from which survival probabilities can be estimated. It is important to note that the IPSS was developed using MDS patients treated with transfusions, biological response modifiers, and/or low-dose oral chemotherapy.

...iotherapy, including stem cell transplantation, ...ialysis. Thus, it is still unknown whether the IPSS ...ated with intensive treatment strategies as well (8).

...ity of individuals with MDS are of advanced age, most ...have ...receive supportive therapy, which mainly consists of antibi- ...is a...nsfusions (9). If patients with these disorders are treated with ...motherapy, about 50–60% may achieve complete remission (CR), ...edian remission duration is less than 8 months despite maintenance ...herapy (4,10).

Young patients (≤60–65 years of age) can be treated successfully by allogeneic bone marrow transplantation if a histocompatible sibling donor is available (11–14). The role of remission-induction chemotherapy, prior to allogeneic stem cell transplantation, for patients with advanced stages of MDS is discussed in Chapter 17. Intensive chemotherapy followed by autologous bone marrow transplantation may provide an alternative therapy for patients lacking a suitable donor, as discussed below. To date, autologous bone marrow transplantation has been reported for only a relatively small number of patients (15–18).

## II. CHEMOTHERAPY

MDS patients with poor risk features may be candidates for treatment with combination chemotherapy. Conventional chemotherapy, such as that administered to induce CR in de novo AML, was demonstrated to be effective in MDS in the early 1980s (19,20); CR rates for AML and MDS are 15% and 51%, respectively. Later results obtained with intensive chemotherapy regimens, such as high-dose single-agent therapy or combinations of cytosine arabinoside (Ara-C), daunorubicin, thioguanine, and/or vincristine, yielded CR rates in diverse MDS patient populations varying from 15% to 64% (3,4,10,21,22). Preisler et al. attempted to treat 15 MDS patients with high-dose Ara-C, but only two patients responded completely and more than 40% died from the toxicity of this intensive regimen (23).

CR rates of patients with MDS or MDS/AML are generally lower than those of patients with de novo AML treated with similar chemotherapy regimens. The higher failure rate associated with MDS or MDS/AML can be explained in part by the longer duration of hypoplasia after chemotherapy in these patients. A longer duration of hypoplasia after remission-induction therapy has been reported by several groups that showed a toxic death rate ranging from 14% to 21% (10,23,24); however, this toxicity appeared to be a function of age (10). Moreover, the prolonged period of hypoplasia has not been demonstrated consistently in all studies (25,26).

# 16

# Intensive Chemotherapy, Including Autologous Stem Cell Transplantation, in the Myelodysplastic Syndromes

**Theo M. de Witte and Margriet Oosterveld**
*University Medical Center, Nijmegen, The Netherlands*

## I. INTRODUCTION

The myelodysplastic syndromes (MDS) are a heterogeneous group of disorders with a variable prognosis. Refractory anemia (RA) and RA with ringed sideroblasts (RARS) are characterized by a low risk of transformation to acute myeloid leukemia (AML) and a median survival usually in excess of 30 months (1). In contrast, the median survival of patients with refractory anemia with excess blasts (RAEB) or RAEB in transformation (RAEB-t) is less than 12 months (2,3). The prognosis for patients with therapy-related MDS, or secondary acute myeloblastic leukemia (secondary leukemia), is also poor, with median survivals of less than 12 months (3,4). In addition to the MDS subtype, the patient's karyotype is a valuable prognosticator of survival (5,6); see Chapter 5 for a detailed discussion.

Various criteria have been developed to predict the prognosis of patients with MDS. The most widely accepted evaluation or scoring method is the International Prognostic Scoring System (IPSS), which is based on the number of blasts in the bone marrow, karyotype, and the number of peripheral blood cytopenias (7). The IPSS outlines four distinct risk categories (low, intermediate-1, intermediate-2, and high risk), from which survival probabilities can be estimated. It is important to note that the IPSS was developed using MDS patients treated with transfusions, biological response modifiers, and/or low-dose oral chemotherapy.

Patients treated with intensive chemotherapy, including stem cell transplantation, have been excluded from this analysis. Thus, it is still unknown whether the IPSS is applicable to patients treated with intensive treatment strategies as well (8).

Because the majority of individuals with MDS are of advanced age, most MDS patients usually receive supportive therapy, which mainly consists of antibiotics or blood transfusions (9). If patients with these disorders are treated with intensive chemotherapy, about 50–60% may achieve complete remission (CR), but the median remission duration is less than 8 months despite maintenance chemotherapy (4,10).

Young patients (≤60–65 years of age) can be treated successfully by allogeneic bone marrow transplantation if a histocompatible sibling donor is available (11–14). The role of remission-induction chemotherapy, prior to allogeneic stem cell transplantation, for patients with advanced stages of MDS is discussed in Chapter 17. Intensive chemotherapy followed by autologous bone marrow transplantation may provide an alternative therapy for patients lacking a suitable donor, as discussed below. To date, autologous bone marrow transplantation has been reported for only a relatively small number of patients (15–18).

## II. CHEMOTHERAPY

MDS patients with poor risk features may be candidates for treatment with combination chemotherapy. Conventional chemotherapy, such as that administered to induce CR in de novo AML, was demonstrated to be effective in MDS in the early 1980s (19,20); CR rates for AML and MDS are 15% and 51%, respectively. Later results obtained with intensive chemotherapy regimens, such as high-dose single-agent therapy or combinations of cytosine arabinoside (Ara-C), daunorubicin, thioguanine, and/or vincristine, yielded CR rates in diverse MDS patient populations varying from 15% to 64% (3,4,10,21,22). Preisler et al. attempted to treat 15 MDS patients with high-dose Ara-C, but only two patients responded completely and more than 40% died from the toxicity of this intensive regimen (23).

CR rates of patients with MDS or MDS/AML are generally lower than those of patients with de novo AML treated with similar chemotherapy regimens. The higher failure rate associated with MDS or MDS/AML can be explained in part by the longer duration of hypoplasia after chemotherapy in these patients. A longer duration of hypoplasia after remission-induction therapy has been reported by several groups that showed a toxic death rate ranging from 14% to 21% (10,23,24); however, this toxicity appeared to be a function of age (10). Moreover, the prolonged period of hypoplasia has not been demonstrated consistently in all studies (25,26).

Another contribution to treatment failure with chemotherapy is the higher intrinsic biological drug resistance of the malignant clone (27). The addition of drugs that are less dependent on P-glycoprotein for uptake, such as idarubicin, or the use of granulocyte colony-stimulating factor (G-CSF) for induction into proliferation of leukemic stem cells may overcome this drug resistance (28,29).

Maintaining remission after remission-induction chemotherapy is a difficult issue. Patients who are not eligible for allogeneic bone marrow transplantation could be treated with postremission chemotherapy. Some patients may achieve prolonged, disease-free survival with this approach (19,30), but in several studies, the overall median remission duration was usually less than 12 months (10,30,31). Patients without cytogenetic abnormalities appeared to have a better outcome after antileukemic chemotherapy compared with patients with cytogenetic abnormalities (4).

## III. PROGNOSTIC FACTORS AFFECTING OUTCOME AFTER CHEMOTHERAPY

### A. Morphological Subtypes and Clinical Features

Too few patients with RA or RARS have been treated with combination remission-induction chemotherapy for conclusions to be drawn and recommendations made. Patients with the morphological picture of RAEB (19) and RAEB-t (33) appeared to respond favorably to intensive chemotherapy, with remission rates approaching those associated with de novo AML. Patients with chronic myelomonocytic leukemia (CMML) have not been treated with intensive chemotherapy in large numbers. Findings from one small clinical trial conducted by the Memorial Sloan Kettering group revealed CR in nine of 14 CMML patients treated with remission-induction chemotherapy (20). Patients with RAEB, RAEB-t, and de novo AML showed no difference in treatment outcome when matched for such prognostic factors as a history of cytopenias and cytogenetic characteristics (32,33). However, this lack of a difference may reflect inconsistencies in the definitions of and the distinction between MDS and de novo AML. A patient with the morphological picture of RAEB-t, but without cytogenetic abnormalities and a short history of cytopenias, may respond to intensive antileukemic therapy as would the average patient with de novo AML. Similarly, a patient with de novo AML, trilineage dysplasia, and monosomy 7 may respond as would the average patient with MDS (34). Auer rod–positive patients, regardless of karyotype, have a better prognosis than Auer rod–negative patients (35).

Some analyses evaluating response to therapy reported data on patients initially diagnosed with de novo AML but retrospectively diagnosed with MDS (20,33,36). These patients may represent a subcategory of MDS: individuals with a short history of cytopenia and clinical and/or cytogenetic features resembling de novo AML. The efficacy of combination chemotherapy in this category of patients may be better than in the overall population of MDS patients. Bernstein et al. (33) observed no relevant differences in response rates and survival time among patients retrospectively rediagnosed as having RAEB, RAEB-t, or AML when treated with frontline AML protocols.

The timing of initiation of chemotherapy after diagnosis and the duration of cytopenia appear to influence treatment outcome. Compared with patients who initiated intensive chemotherapy more than 3 months after their diagnosis, MDS patients treated within 3 months of diagnosis showed a better response to intensive chemotherapy (28). A long preceding phase of cytopenias appears to have a negative impact on the outcome after combination chemotherapy (28).

Patients with secondary AML (sAML) that evolved from MDS respond less well to chemotherapy than do those with de novo leukemias, and long-term remissions are rare (10,25,37). Certain subcategories of patients with sAML may have response rates similar to de novo AML (10,25,37).

The clinical outcome after intensive chemotherapy for therapy-related MDS and AML (tMDS and tAML, respectively) is usually poor, with only the exceptional patient surviving beyond 1 year (19,38). These exceptional patients are characterized by specific chromosomal rearrangements typical of de novo AML or no cytogenetic abnormalities and their disease presents as AML not preceded by MDS (37).

## B.  Age

Patients younger than 45–50 years of age respond better to combination chemotherapy than older patients. CR rates in patients <45–50 years old ranged from 71% to 86% in several studies, whereas the remission rates in older patients (>50 years of age) ranged from 25% to 45% (10,25,30).

The principal cause of treatment failure in MDS is similar to that identified in elderly AML patients (39). Estey (39) characterized elderly AML patients as those of older age (>55 years) with an abnormal karyotype characteristic of MDS, high rate of multiple drug resistance (MDR) expression, or a long preceding phase of cytopenias. As with elderly AML patients, MDS patients who are fit enough to be treated by combination chemotherapy should receive treatment that focuses on overcoming primary drug resistance. New approaches in this field are angiogenesis inhibitors, such as thalidomide and the tyrosine kinase inhibitors. Vascularity and angiogenic factors are increased in MDS and may be targets for novel therapeutic approaches in MDS (40). The new formulations of the anthracyclines—liposomal daunorubicin or calicheamycin coupled to an anti-CD33 monoclonal antibody (Mylotarg)—may overcome the intrinsic drug resistance and allow for lower chemotherapeutic drug doses thus reducing systemic toxicities (41).

## C. Cytogenetic Features

The presence of cytogenetic abnormalities characteristic of MDS, such as abnormalities of chromosomes 5 or 7, has a major negative impact on the prognosis after combination chemotherapy. Fenaux et al. observed a CR rate of 57% in patients with a normal karyotype, which contrasts with the 31% CR rate for patients with abnormalities of chromosomes 5 or 7 (28). None of the five patients with multiple chromosomal abnormalities achieved CR in a Leukemia Cooperative Group study of the European Organisation for Research and Treatment in Cancer (EORTC-LCG) (4).

## IV. RESIDUAL NORMAL STEM CELLS AFTER CHEMOTHERAPY

Myelodysplastic syndromes are clonal stem cell disorders, which raises the concern about the presence of sufficient numbers of residual normal stem cells to perform autologous stem cell transplantation. However, chemotherapy is capable of inducing a cytogenetically normal CR in patients with a detectable cytogenetic marker of the malignant clone. In a pilot study of intensive chemotherapy for poor-prognosis MDS/sAML patients, seven of eight patients with cytogenetic abnormalities in CR after chemotherapy appeared to have a cytogenetically normal bone marrow (4). Indeed, some patients may achieve long-term, polyclonal remissions after intensive combination chemotherapy (42). In addition, polymerase chain reaction (PCR) techniques, based on X-chromosome inactivation patterns, have demonstrated polyclonality in the peripheral stem cell harvests of three MDS patients with a poor prognosis (43).

In the analysis from the European Group for Blood and Marrow Transplantation (EBMT) registries (44), only seven of the 79 patients who underwent autologous stem cell transplantation during their first CR died owing to complications of the transplant. However, the transplant-related mortality was not higher than that of a matched control group of patients transplanted for de novo AML in first CR. Together, these findings suggest that the engraftment capabilities of stem cells derived from patients with MDS are usually sufficient to restore hematopoiesis to levels that prevent fatal infectious and hemorrhagic complications.

The administration of a higher number of stem cells, obtained by mobilization of the stem cells into the peripheral blood, may improve the speed of engraftment. Pilot studies have shown the feasibility to collect peripheral stem cells in MDS or sAML patients in CR (45,46). Although the engraftment appeared to be much faster, this approach is not likely to substantially improve the treatment-related mortality of autologous transplantation in MDS since the mortality is already less than 10% after the use of autologous bone marrow stem cells.

## V. AUTOLOGOUS STEM CELL TRANSPLANTATION

Until recently, the experience with autologous stem cell transplantation in MDS or leukemia secondary to MDS has been limited (15,16). From a large series of 82 adult patients with AML, six patients with a known preceding myelodysplastic state received autologous bone marrow transplantation during their first remission. After the transplant, three patients relapsed and the overall leukemia-free survival was worse than that of a control group without an antecedent hematological disorder (18). A preliminary analysis from the EBMT in 1989 reported the results of autologous bone marrow transplantation in 17 patients with MDS (17). Engraftment occurred in 15 of 16 evaluable patients, and the median relapse-free survival was 11 months. Transplant-related mortality and death due to regeneration failure did not appear to occur more often than that observed after autologous bone marrow transplantation for de novo AML. Hematopoietic engraftment was slow despite the sufficient number of colony-forming units–granulocyte macrophage (CFU-GM) being collected per kilogram body weight ($5 \times 10^4$/kg) (17).

Laporte et al. reported the results of autologous bone marrow transplantation with mafosfamide-treated marrow in patients with AML following MDS. The hematopoietic engraftment was also slow in these seven patients, but all patients engrafted except for one patient who died of treatment-related causes before engraftment (18).

The EBMT recently reported the results for 79 patients with MDS/sAML transplanted with autologous marrow in first CR (44). The 2-year survival, disease-free survival, and relapse rates for the 79 patients transplanted in first CR were 39%, 34%, and 64%, respectively. The main reason for treatment failure was a high relapse risk after the autologous stem cell procedure, which was higher than 55% for all stages and all disease categories. Late relapses beyond 2 years were rare events; only 15 patients were at risk beyond this time. Age appeared to influence relapse risk, as age less than 40 years at the time of transplantation was associated with a significantly better prognosis, with a disease-free survival of 39%. The lower relapse risk in the younger age group may be due to several factors, such as duration of disease prior to treatment and the absence of cytogenetic abnormalities. However, the limited number of patients in this study and the lack of cytogenetic data precluded an analysis on cytogenetic prognostic criteria.

Within the EBMT analysis (44), a cohort of 55 patients for whom the duration of first CR was known was compared with a matched control group of 110 patients with de novo AML. The disease-free survival at 2 years was 28% for the cohort of 55 patients transplanted for MDS/sAML and 51% for those transplanted for de novo AML ($p = 0.025$). The relapse rates were 69% for patients with MDS/sAML and 40% for those with de novo AML ($p = 0.007$). The difference in disease-free survival between autologous bone marrow transplantation in MDS/sAML and autologous bone marrow transplantation for de novo AML was mainly due to a higher relapse rate in the MDS/sAML group since the mortality rate was low in both patient groups. The higher relapse rate in patients treated for MDS or secondary leukemia suggests a higher burden of residual disease in these patients. For that reason, it is important to carefully monitor residual disease in future studies by both cytogenetic and molecular techniques.

The EBMT recently updated the results of autologous stem cell transplantation in a larger cohort of patients (unpublished data). The 3-year disease-free survival of the 173 patients transplanted with autologous stem cells was 30% (Table 1). The majority of autologous transplants were performed in first CR, with a 33% disease-free survival for the 126 patients transplanted in first CR. Treatment failure was mainly due to a high relapse risk (55%); nonrelapse mortality was 25%. The disease-free survival of patients transplanted beyond first CR was 18%. Age had only a borderline significant effect on treatment outcome. The disease-free survival was 46% in patients younger than 20 years at time of

**Table 1**   The Influence of Age on Treatment Outcome: For Patients with Myelodysplastic Syndromes or Secondary Acute Myeloid Leukemia Treated with Autologous Stem Cell Transplantation, the 3-Year Actuarial Probability of Disease-Free Survival, Survival, Treatment-Related Mortality, and Relapse

| Patient category | Number of patients | Disease-free survival (%) | Overall survival (%) | Treatment-related mortality (%) | Relapse (%) |
|---|---|---|---|---|---|
| Autologous transplants | 173 | 30 | 32 | 29 | 58 |
| CR-1 | 126 | 33 | 38 | 25 | 55 |
| No CR-1 | 47 | 18 | 14 | 51 | 64 |
| $p$ value | | 0.06 | 0.01 | 0.07 | 0.32 |
| Age | | | | | |
| <20 years[a] | 12 | 46 | 58 | 17 | 44 |
| 20–40 years[a] | 48 | 36 | 41 | 15 | 58 |
| >40 years[a] | 66 | 29 | 29 | 39 | 51 |
| $p$ value | | 0.08 | 0.05 | 0.22 | 0.27 |

[a] Only patients in first complete remission.
CR, complete remission; P, probability.
*Source*: Unpublished data: European Group for Blood and Marrow Transplantation.

transplant, and 29% in patients older than 40 years. This difference can be explained by a higher treatment-related mortality in the older age group. The relapse incidence was similar for all age groups.

A French prospective study assessed the value of autologous stem cell transplantation in MDS (47). CR was attained in 51% of patients (42 of 83). Three patients were allografted. In 39 of these patients, 24 had either transplantation with autologous bone marrow cells (16 patients) or autologous peripheral stem cells (eight patients). Importantly, hematological reconstitution occurred in all autografted patients. However, this study did not establish a faster hemopoietic recovery for peripheral blood stem cells compared with bone marrow cells. The median disease-free survival of the autografted patients was 29 months from transplantation.

A recently completed joint study of the EORTC-LCG and EBMT prospectively evaluated the role of autologous stem cell transplantation in 196 patients with MDS and secondary leukemia (48). The CR rate after remission-induction chemotherapy was 54%. (Both allogeneic and autologous stem cell transplantation were utilized as postconsolidation treatment.) The overall and disease-free survival at 4 years were 26% and 29%, respectively. Of the patients without a donor, 61% (35 of 57) received autologous stem cell transplantation in first CR. Three patients died due to complications, 19 patients relapsed, and 13 patients are in continuing remission. Preliminary results showed that cytogenetic characteristics had a major impact on treatment outcome. The actuarial 2-year survival of patients with good risk or intermediate risk was 52%, versus 28% in the poor risk group. Thus, the results obtained after autologous stem cell transplantation compare favorably to the long-term results obtained with chemotherapy alone (9,45,49).

A full two-thirds of the patients with MDS who may benefit from allogeneic bone marrow transplantation lack a suitable family donor. However, the development of efficient, worldwide registries of HLA-typed, volunteer, unrelated donors has made allogeneic bone marrow transplantation with fully or partially matched, unrelated donors a realistic alternative. Three recent analyses reported an 18–38% disease-free survival for MDS patients who received bone marrow stem cells from unrelated donors (50–52). Nonrelapse mortality was higher compared with that of HLA-identical related recipients, and increased age was significantly associated with increased risk of death from nonrelapse causes (51,52). A disease-free survival rate of 36% in patients younger than 20 years is very encouraging and is similar to the results obtained with histocompatible sibling transplantation. Conversely, the poor outcome of the 22 patients older than 40 years transplanted with stem cells from unrelated donors indicates that such patients should not be transplanted with unrelated donors unless they are treated in investigational protocols in specialized transplant centers. For the remaining patients, autologous stem cell transplantation is a reasonable alternative.

## VI. CONCLUDING REMARKS

Careful clinical evaluation of the prognostic factors, such as age, probability for achieving CR, and availability of a matched unrelated donor, should guide the treating physician in advising the patient of the available treatment options. Further analysis and prospective studies may identify MDS patients who will benefit from intensive antileukemic therapy followed by autologous stem cell transplantation. A substantial number of patients may not reach the autologous stem cell transplant procedure owing to failure to induce remission or failure to collect sufficient numbers of stem cells. Investigational therapeutic strategies should be developed for these patients.

## REFERENCES

1. Mufti GJ, Stevens JR, Oscier DG, Hamblin TJ, Machin D. Myelodysplastic syndromes: a scoring system with prognostic significance. Br J Haematol 1985; 59: 425–433.
2. Bennett JM, Catovsky D, Daniel MT, Flandrin G, Galton DA, Gralnick HR, Sultan C. Proposals for the classification of the myelodysplastic syndromes. Br J Haematol 1982; 51:189–199.
3. Kantarjian HM, Keating MJ, Walters RS, Smith TL, Cork A, McCredie KB, Freireich EJ. Therapy-related leukemia and myelodysplastic syndrome: clinical, cytogenetic, and prognostic features. J Clin Oncol 1986; 4:1748–1757.
4. de Witte T, Suciu S, Peetermans M, Fenaux P, Strijckmans P, Hayat M, Jaksic B, Selleslag D, Zittoun R, Dardenne M, Solbu G, Zwierzina H, Muus P. Intensive chemotherapy for poor prognosis myelodysplasia (MDS) and secondary acute myeloid leukemia (sAML) following MDS of more than 6 months duration. A pilot study by the Leukemia Cooperative Group of the European Organisation for Research and Treatment in Cancer (EORTC-LCG). Leukemia 1995; 9:1805–1811.
5. Yunis JJ, Rydell RE, Oken MM, Arnesen MA, Mayer MG, Lobell M. Refined chromosome analysis as an independent prognostic indicator in de novo myelodysplastic syndromes. Blood 1986; 67:1721–1730.
6. Geddes AA, Bowen DT, Jacobs A. Clonal karyotype abnormalities and clinical progress in the myelodysplastic syndrome. Br J Haematol 1990; 76:194–202.
7. Greenberg P, Cox C, LeBeau MM, Fenaux P, Morel P, Sanz G, Sanz M, Vallespi T, Hamblin T, Oscier D, Ohyashiki K, Toyama K, Aul C, Mufti G, Bennett J. International scoring system for evaluating prognosis in myelodysplastic syndromes. Blood 1997; 89:2077–2088.
8. Appelbaum FR, Anderson J. Allogeneic bone marrow transplantation for myelodysplastic syndrome: outcomes analysis according to IPSS score. Leukemia 1998; 12(suppl 1):S25–S29.
9. Aul C, Gattermann N, Schneider W. Age-related incidence and other epidemiological aspects of myelodysplastic syndromes. Br J Haematol 1992; 82:358–367.

10. De Witte T, Muus P, De Pauw B, Haanen C. Intensive antileukemic treatment of patients younger than 65 years with myelodysplastic syndromes and secondary acute myelogenous leukemia. Cancer 1990; 66:831–837.

11. De Witte T, Zwaan F, Hermans J, Vernant J, Kolb H, Vossen J, Lönnqvist B, Beelen D, Ferrant A, Gmür J, Liu Yin X, Troussard J, Cahn J, Van Lint M, Gratwohl A. Allogeneic bone marrow transplantation for secondary leukaemia and myelodysplastic syndrome: a survey by the Leukaemia Working Party of the European Bone Marrow Transplantation Group (EBMTG) Br J Haematol 1990; 74:151–155.

12. De Witte T, Gratwohl A. Bone marrow transplantation for myelodysplastic syndrome and secondary leukaemias. Br J Haematol 1993; 84:361–364.

13. Anderson JE, Appelbaum FR, Fisher LD, Schoch G, Shulman H, Anasetti C, Bensinger WI, Bryant E, Buckner CD, Doney K, Martin PJ, Sanders JE, Sullivan KM, Thomas ED, Witherspoon RP, Hansen JA, Storb R. Allogeneic bone marrow transplantation for 93 patients with myelodysplastic syndrome. Blood 1993; 82:677–681.

14. O'Donnell MR, Long GD, Parker PM, Niland J, Nademanee A, Amylon M, Chao N, Negrin RS, Schmidt GM, Slovak ML, Smith EP, Snyder DS, Stein AS, Traweek T, Blume KG, Forman SJ. Busulphan/cyclophosphamide as conditioning regimen for bone marrow transplantation for myelodysplasia. J Clin Oncol 1995; 13:2973–2977.

15. Geller RB, Vogelsang GB, Wingard JR, Yeager AM, Burns WH, Santos GW, Saral R. Successful marrow transplantation for acute myelocytic leukemia following therapy for Hodgkin's disease. J Clin Oncol 1988; 6:1558–1561.

16. Mc Millan AK, Goldstone AH, Linch DC, Gribben JG, Patterson KG, Richards JD, Franklin I, Boughton BJ, Milligan DW, Leyland MM, Hutchison RM, Newland AC. High dose chemotherapy and autologous bone marrow transplantation in acute myeloid leukemia. Blood 1990; 76:480–488.

17. Öberg G, Simonsson B, Smedmyr B, Björkstrand B, Colombat P, Coser P, Ferrant A, Goldstone AH, Helbig W, Löfvenberg E, McCarthy D, Polli E, Reifers J, Sundström C, Tötterman TH, Wahlin A, Wiesneth M. Is haematological reconstitution seen after ABMT in MDS patients? Bone Marrow Transpl 1989; 4(suppl 2):52.

18. Laporte JP, Isnard F, Lesage S, Fenaux P, Douay L, Lopez M, Stacowiak J, Najman A, Gorin NC. Autologous bone marrow transplantation with marrow purged by mafosfamide in seven patients with myelodysplastic syndromes in transformation (AML-MDS): a pilot study. Leukemia 1993; 7:2030–2033.

19. Armitage JO, Dick FR, Needleman SW, Burns CP. Effect of chemotherapy for the dysmyelopoietic syndrome. Cancer Treat Rep 1981; 65:601–605.

20. Mertelsmann R, Tzvithaler H, To L, Gee TS, McKenzie S, Schauer P, Friedman A, Arlin Z, Cirrincione C, Clarkson B. Morphological classification, response to therapy, and survival in 263 adult patients with acute nonlymphoblastic leukemia. Blood 1980; 56:773–781.

21. Michels SD, Saamur J, Arthur DC, Robinson LL, Brunning RD. Refractory anemia with excess of blasts in transformation hematologic and clinical study of 52 patients. Cancer 1989; 64:2340–2346.

22. Invernizzi R, Pecci A, Rossi G, Pelizzari AM, Giusto M, Tinelli C, Ascari E. Idarubicin and cytosine arabinoside in the induction and maintenance therapy of high-risk myelodysplastic syndromes. Haematologica 1997; 82:660–663.

23. Preisler HD, Raza A, Barcos M, Azarnia N, Larson R, Browman G, Walker I, Grunwald H, D'Arrigo P, Stein A, Bloom M, Goldberg J, Gottlieb A, Bennett J, Kirshner J, Priore R. High-dose cytosine arabinoside in the treatment of preleukemic disorders: a leukemia intergroup study. Am J Hematol 1986; 23:131–134.

24. Richard C, Iriondo A, Garijo J, Baro J, Conde E, Recio M, Cuadrado MA, Bello C, Zubizarreta A. Therapy of advanced myelodysplastic syndrome with aggressive chemotherapy. Oncology 1989; 46:6–9.

25. Tricot G, Boogaerts MA. The role of aggressive chemotherapy in the treatment of myelodysplastic syndromes. Br J Haematol 1986; 63:477–483.

26. Aul C, Schneider W. Treatment of advanced myelodysplastic syndrome: trend toward more aggressive chemotherapy. Hamatol Bluttransfus 1990; 33:382–386.

27. Sonneveld P, van Dongen JJ, Hagemeijer A, van Lom K, Nooter K, Schoester M, Adriaansen HJ, Tsuruo T, de Leeuw K. High expression of the multidrug resistance P-glycoprotein in high risk myelodysplasia is associated with immature phenotype. Leukemia 1993; 7:963–969.

28. Fenaux P, Morel P, Rose C, Laï JL, Jouet JP, Bauters F. Prognostic factors in adult de novo myelodysplastic syndromes treated by intensive chemotherapy. Br J Haematol 1991; 77:497–501.

29. Ruutu T, Hanninen A, Jarventie G, Koistinen P, Koivunen E, Katka K, Nousiainen T, Oksanen K, Pelliniemi TT, Remes K, Timonen T, Violin E, Elonen E. Intensive chemotherapy of poor prognosis myelodysplastic syndromes (MDS) and acute myeloid leukemia following MDS with idarubicin and cytarabine. Leuk Res 1997; 21: 133–138.

30. Bernasconi C, Alessandrino EP, Bernasconi P, Bonfichi M, Lazzarino M, Canevori A, Castelli G, Brusamolino E, Pagnucco G, Castagnola C. Randomized clinical study comparing aggressive chemotherapy with or without G-CSF support for high-risk myelodysplastic syndromes and secondary acute myeloid leukemia evolving from MDS. Br J Haematol 1998; 102:678–683.

31. de Witte T, Hermans J, Vossen J, Bacigalupo A, Meloni G, Jacobsen N, Ruutu T, Ljungman P, Gratwohl A, Runde V, Niederwieser D, van Biezen A, Devergie A, Cornelissen J, Jouet JP, Arnold R, Apperley J. Haematopoietic stem cell transplantation for patients with myelodysplastic syndromes and secondary acute myeloid leukaemias: a report on behalf of the Chronic Leukaemia Working Party of the European Group for Blood and Marrow Transplantation (EBMT). Br J Haematol 2000; 110:620–630.

32. Estey E, Pierce S, Kantarjian H, O'Brien S, Beran M, Andreeff M, Escudier S, Koller C, Kornblau S, Robertson L, et al. Treatment of myelodysplastic syndromes with AML-type chemotherapy. Leuk Lymphoma 1993; 11(suppl 2):59–63.

33. Bernstein SH, Brunetto VL, Davey FR, Wurster-Hill D, Mayer RJ, Stone RM, Schiffer CA, Bloomfield CD. Acute myeloid leukemia-type chemotherapy for newly diagnosed patients without antecedent cytopenias having myelodysplastic syndrome as defined by French-American-British criteria: a Cancer and Leukemia Group B Study. J Clin Oncol 1996; 14:2486–2494.

34. Estey E, Thall P, Beran M, Kantarjian H, Pierce S, Keating M. Effect of diagnosis (refractory anemia with excess of blasts, refractory anemia with excess of blasts in transformation, or acute myeloid leukemia [AML]) on outcome of AML-type chemotherapy. Blood 1997; 90:2969–2977.

35. Seymour JF, Estey EH. The prognostic significance of auer rods in myelodysplasia. Br J Haematol 1993; 85:67–76.
36. Gajewski JL, Ho WG, Nimer SD, Hirji KF, Gekelman L, Jacobs AD, Champlin RE. Efficacy of intensive chemotherapy for acute myelogenous leukemia associated with preleukemic syndrome. J Clin Oncol 1989; 7:1637–1645.
37. Fenaux P, Laï JL, Quiquandon I, Preudhomme C, Dupriez B, Facon T, Lorthois C, Lucidarme D, Bauters F. Therapy-related myelodysplastic syndrome and leukemia with no unfauvorable cytogenetic findings have a good response to intensive chemotherapy: a report on 15 cases. Leuk Lymphoma 1991; 5:117–125.
38. Vaughan WP, Karp JE, Burke PJ. Effective chemotherapy of acute myelocytic leukemia occurring after alkylating agent or radiation therapy for prior malignancy. J Clin Oncol 1983; 1:204–207.
39. Estey EH. How I treat older patients with AML. Blood 2000; 96:1670–1673.
40. Aguayo A, Kantarjian H, Manshouri T, Gidel C, Estey E, Thomas D, Koller C, Estrov Z, O'Brien S, Keating M, Freireich E, Albitar M. Angiogenesis in acute and chronic leukemias and myelodysplastic syndromes. Blood 2000; 96:2240–2245.
41. Sievers EL, Appelbaum FR, Spielberger RT, Forman SJ, Flowers D, Smith FO, Shannon-Dorcy K, Berger MS, Bernstein ID. Selective ablation of acute myeloid leukemia using antibody-targetted chemotherapy: a phase I study of an anti-CD33 calicheomicin immunoconjugate. Blood 1999; 93:3678–3684.
42. Aivado M, Rong A, Germing U, Gatterman N, Kobbe G, Rieth C, Haas R, Aul C. Long-term remission after intensive chemotherapy in advanced myelodysplastic syndromes is generally associated with restoration of polyclonal haemopoiesis. Br J Haematol 2000; 110:884–886.
43. Delforge M, Demuynck H, Vandenberghe P, Verhoef G, Zachee P, van Duppen VV, Marijnen P, Van den Berghe H, Boogaerts MA. Polyclonal primitive hematopoietic progenitors can be detected in mobilized peripheral blood from patients with high-risk myelodysplastic syndromes. Blood 1995; 86:3660–3667.
44. De Witte T, Van Biezen A, Hermans J, Labopin M, Runde V, Or R, Meloni G, Mauri SB, Carella A, Apperley J, Gratwohl A, Laporte JP. Autologous bone marrow transplantation for patients with myelodysplastic syndrome (MDS) or acute myeloid leukemia following MDS. Chronic and Acute Leukemia Working Parties of the European Group for Blood and Marrow Transplantation. Blood 1997; 90:3853–3857.
45. Carella AM, Dejana A, Lerma E, Podesta M, Benvenuto F, Chimirri F, Parodi C, Sessarego M, Prencipe E, Frassoni F. In vivo mobilization of karyotypically normal peripheral blood progenitor cells in high-risk MDS, secondary or therapy-related acute myelogenous leukemia. Br J Haematol 1996; 95:127–130.
46. Demuynck H, Delforge M, Verhoef GE, Zachee P, Vandenberghe P, Van den Berghe H, Boogaerts MA. Feasibility of peripheral blood progenitor cell harvest and transplantation in patients with poor-risk myelodysplastic syndromes. Br J Haematol 1996; 92:351–359.
47. Wattel E, Solary E, Leleu X, Dreyfus F, Brion A, Jouet JP, Hoang-Ngoc L, Maloisel F, Guerci A, Rochant H, Gratecos N, Casassus P, Janvier M, Brice P, Lepelley P, Fenaux P. A prospective study of autologous bone marrow or peripheral blood stem cell transplantation after intensive chemotherapy in myelodysplastic syndromes. Francais des Myelodysplasies. Group Ouest-Est d'etude des Leucemies aiguees myeloides. Leukemia 1999; 13:524–529.

48. De Witte T, Suciu S, Boogaerts M, Labar B, Archimbaud E, Aul C, Selleslag D, Ferrant A, Weijermans P, Mandelli F, Amadori S, Jehn U, Muus P, Demuynck H, Dardenne M, Willemze R, Gratwohl A, Apperley J. The influence of cytogenetic abnormalities on treatment outcome after intensive antileukemic therapy for patients with high risk MDS and AML following MDS. A joint study of the EORTC, EBMT, SAKK, GIMEMA Leukemia Groups. Blood 1996; 88(suppl 1):454a.

49. Parker JE, Pagliuca A, Mijovic A, Cullis JO, Czepulkowski B, Rassam SM, Samaratunga IR, Grace R, Gover PA, Mufti GJ. Fludarabine, cytarabine, G-CSF and idarubicin (FLAG-IDA) for the treatment of poor-risk myelodysplastic syndromes and acute myeloid leukemia. Br J Haematol 1997; 99:939–944.

50. Kernan NA, Bartsch G, Ash RC, Beatty PG, Champlin R, Filipovich A, Gajewski J, Hansen JA, Henslee-Downey J, McCullough J, McGlave P, Perkins HA, Phillips GL, Sanders J, Stroncek D, Thomas ED, Blume K. Analysis of 462 transplantations from unrelated donors facilitated by the National marrow Donor Program. N Engl J Med 1993; 328:593–602.

51. Arnold R, de Witte T, van Biezen A, Hermans J, Jacobsen N, Runde V, Gratwohl A, Apperley JF. Unrelated bone marrow transplantation in patients with myelodysplastic syndromes and secondary acute myeloid leukemia: an EBMT survey. European Blood and Marrow Transplantation Group. Bone Marrow Transplant 1998; 21: 1213–1216.

52. Anderson JE, Anasetti E, Appelbaum FR, Schoch G, Gooley TA, Hansen JA, Buckner CD, Sanders JE, Sullivan KM, Storb R. Unrelated donor marrow transplantation for myelodysplasia (MDS) and MDS-related acute myeloid leukemia. Br J Haematol 1996; 93:59–67.

# 17

# Allogeneic Bone Marrow Transplantation in the Myelodysplastic Syndromes*

**Jeanne E. Anderson**
*University of Washington, Seattle, Washington*

## I. SUMMARY

Allogeneic bone marrow transplantation (BMT) is the only treatment modality that has consistently been demonstrated to cure patients with the myelodysplastic syndromes (MDS). Since the early 1980s, numerous publications have reported the results with BMT for over 700 patients with MDS and the lead patients are now disease-free for more than 16 years. Overall, these studies show that approximately 40% of patients are likely to be cured with allogeneic BMT. The best results have been reported for patients with refractory anemia who receive marrow from fully matched related donors, with 75% long-term disease-free survival rates. Factors that are associated with an increased risk of relapse and, thereby, shorter disease-free survival include increased blast percentage and poor-risk karyotype. Factors that are associated with an increased risk of nonrelapse mortality and, in some studies, shorter disease-free survival include longer disease duration, advanced patient age, therapy-related MDS, male patients, and use of mismatched or unrelated donors. However, favorable results have been seen in small studies of patients 55–66 years of age and of patients with refractory anemia undergoing matched unrelated donor BMT. In the opinion of this author, allogeneic BMT is appropriate therapy for patients with high- or intermediate-risk dis-

---

* Reprinted from Anderson JE, ''Bone Marrow Transplantation for Myelodysplasia,'' *Blood Reviews* 2000; 14:63–77, by permission of the publisher, Churchill Livingstone.

ease (risk category based on the International Prognostic Scoring System). The use of allogeneic BMT for patients with low-risk disease is not well defined, but may be appropriate for particularly young individuals or those with a life-threatening single cytopenia. The use of nonmyeloablative preparative regimens for allogeneic BMT is currently undergoing investigation, but results are too preliminary to make definitive recommendation for use outside of clinical trials.

## II. INTRODUCTION

The myelodysplastic syndromes (MDS) include a group of clonal hematopoietic disorders characterized by impaired maturation of hematopoietic cells, progressive peripheral cytopenias, and a tendency to progress into acute myeloid leukemia (AML). The French-American-British (FAB) Cooperative Group recognizes five distinct forms of pathology in MDS: (1) refractory anemia (RA), (2) refractory anemia with ring sideroblasts (RARS), (3) refractory anemia with excess blasts (RAEB), (4) refractory anemia with excess blasts in transformation (RAEB-T), and (5) chronic myelomonocytic leukemia (CMML) (1). Although the World Health Organization has recently proposed an alternative classification system (2), the conventional FAB system is used in this chapter. The median survival after diagnosis of MDS is approximately 2–3 years, and most patients die from complications related to marrow failure or AML (3–6). Survival and likelihood of developing AML can be predicted based on numerous scoring systems, with the International Prognostic Scoring System (IPSS) being the most widely used. (4). Using the number of peripheral cytopenias, marrow blast percentage, and karyotype, this scoring system differentiates patients with primary MDS into four distinct risk groups (low, intermediate-1, intermediate-2, and high risk) with median survival ranging from 0.4 to 5.7 years (4). Patients with therapy-related MDS have generally not been included in prognostic scoring systems, and most experience suggests that patients with secondary MDS will have a worse prognosis than those with primary MDS.

Because of advanced age, the majority of patients with MDS are generally managed solely with supportive care, which includes transfusional support, antimicrobial therapy, and, on occasion, iron chelation (7). Other treatments that have been evaluated in patients with MDS include hormones, differentiating agents, hematopoietic growth factors, immunosuppressive therapy, hypomethylating agents, low-dose chemotherapy, and intensive induction chemotherapy (7–9). Except in the rare individual with RAEB or RAEB-T and normal cytogenetics treated with intensive chemotherapy, these treatments can be considered palliative, at best, and not curative. The observation of clonality in early hematopoietic stem cells likely explains why MDS is incurable with such conventional therapies. Only with complete eradication of the marrow and replacement using stem cells from a normal donor have cures been achieved. Although restrictions based on patient age and donor availability limit the use of allogeneic bone marrow transplantation (BMT) to a small number of patients with MDS, the potential for cure has encouraged extensive investigation of this therapeutic option. This chapter reviews in detail the major findings of allogeneic BMT for MDS. All of the data presented are derived from studies using myeloablative regimens, except for section X, which discusses the use of nonmyeloablative regimens.

## III. OVERVIEW OF ALLOGENEIC BMT FOR MDS

The first report on the use of allogeneic BMT for MDS was published in 1984 (10). In this study of 10 patients, the first three received a preparative regimen of cyclophosphamide only, which is immunosuppressive, but not myeloablative. The procedure was unsuccessful in all three patients because of disease persistence or recurrence. All subsequent patients transplanted for MDS, therefore, have received myeloablative regimens. Since this initial report, over 700 patients with MDS undergoing allogeneic BMT have been described in single-center and registry reports (11–23). A small number of patients with MDS-related AML are included in some of these reports. Although a wide variety of patient characteristics and transplantation procedures was used, the major end points of relapse and death were relatively similar between these studies. The disease-free survival (DFS) rates range from 23 to 63%. At time of publication of these reports, 37% were disease-free survivors, 21% patients relapsed, and 42% died of transplant-related causes. An outline of the 13 largest studies is shown in Table 1.

Representative of these large published series is an analysis of the first 250 consecutive patients with MDS (excluding the first three conditioned with cyclophosphamide only, described above) who underwent allogeneic BMT in Seattle. Table 2 describes the clinical and transplant characteristics of the patients. Patients with MDS that had evolved into AML, defined as any pretreatment marrow examination showing >30% blasts, are not included in this analysis. Patients with an aplastic marrow and a clonal cytogenetic abnormality are considered to have a variant of RA (24). Less advanced MDS is defined as RA or RARS. Advanced MDS is defined as RAEB, RAEB-T, or CMML. There were a wide variety of pretransplant preparative regimens and posttransplant graft-versus-host disease (GVHD) prophylaxis regimens, chosen based on ongoing studies at the time of transplant.

As of September 1998, with a median follow-up of 6.0 (range, 1.8–16.2) years, 95 patients were alive without evidence of disease; 44 patients relapsed; and 111 patients died of nonrelapse causes. The 5-year actuarial DFS is 38.2%, and the cumulative incidences of relapse and nonrelapse mortality are 17.9% and 43.8%, respectively (Fig. 1). With the lead patient alive and disease-free 16 years

**Table 1** Published Reports on Allogeneic BMT for MDS

| Author Year Reference | No. of pts. Median age Median disease duration | Morphology at BMT, number of patients | Preparative Regimen, Number of patients | Donor, number of patients | Median follow-up | Actuarial DFS (actual number of patients) | Actuarial Relapse (actual number of patients) | Actuarial NRM (actual number of patients) |
|---|---|---|---|---|---|---|---|---|
| Runde 1998 11 | 131 33 yrs 7 mos | RA, 46 RAEB, 35 RAEB-T, 28 CMML, 4 sAML, 18 | TBI-based, 70% | HLA-id sib, 131 | 2.3 yrs | 34% (n = 53) | 39% (n = 28) | 44% (n = 50) |
| Arnold 1998 12 | 118 24 yrs 12 mos | RA, 24 RAEB, 26 RAEB-T, 34 CMML, 12 sAML, 22 | TBI-chemo, 69 Chemo only, 30 Unknown, 19 | Unrelated, 118 | Not stated | 28% (n = 32) | 35% (n = 21) | 58% (n = 65) |
| Anderson 1993 13 | 93 30 yrs 10 mos | RA, 40 RAEB, 31 RAEB-T, 14 CMML, 2 Other, 6 | CY-TBI, 88 BU-CY, 5 | HLA-id sib, 64 Syngeneic, 3 Other family, 20 Unrelated, 6 | 4 yrs | 41% (n = 40) | 28% (n = 17) | 43% (n = 36) |
| Sutton 1996 14 | 71 37 yrs 201 days | RA, 11 RAEB, 21 RAEB-T, 21 sAML, 11 CR, 7 | CY-TRBI, 26 BU-CY, 17 Other, 28 | HLA-id sib, 70 Syngeneic, 1 | 6 yrs | 32% (n = 23) | 48% (n = 24) | 39% (n = 24) |
| Nevill 1998 15 | 60 40 yrs 2.9 mos | RA, 14 RAEB, 11[a] RAEB-T, 14[a] sAML, 12[a] | CY-TBI, 12 BU-CY, 35 Other, 13 | HLA-id sib, 37 Other family, 1 Unrelated, 22 | 5.8 yrs | 29% (n = 20) | 52% (n = 13) | 50% (n = 27) |
| Ballen 1998 16 | 43 34 yrs 6-8 mos | RA, 16 RAEB, 9 RAEB-T, 9 | CY-TBI, 1 BU-CY, 7 CY-TBI-AraC, 31 CBV, 4 | HLA-id sib, 33 Syngeneic, 2 Other family, 4 Unrelated, 4 | 3-4 yrs | (n = 14) | (n = 6) | (n = 23) |

| Study | | FAB[a] | Conditioning | Donor | Follow-up | | | |
|---|---|---|---|---|---|---|---|---|
| Locatelli 1997 [17] | 43<br>2 yrs<br>7 mos | CMML, 43 | Chemotherapy +TBI, 22<br>-TBI, 21 | Related, 29<br>Unrelated, 14 | 11 mos | 31%<br>(n = 14) | 58%<br>(n = 22) | 20%<br>(n = 7) |
| O'Donnell 1995 [18] | 38<br>35 yrs<br>7 mos | Blasts <10%, 20<br>Blasts >10%, 18 | BU-CY, 38 | HLA-id sib, 38 | approx 2 yrs | 38%<br>(n = 14) | 24%<br>(n = 5) | not stated<br>(n = 19) |
| Mattijssen 1997 [19] | 35<br>41 yrs<br>9 mos | RAEB-T, 11<br>RAEB, 7<br>RA, 13<br>CMML, 1<br>AML, 3 | CY-TBI, 9<br>CY-Ida-TBI, 22<br>Other, 4 | HLA-id sib, 32<br>Other family, 1<br>Unrelated, 2 | 1.7 yrs | 39%<br>(n = 14) | 34%<br>(n = 7) | not stated<br>(n = 14) |
| Anderson 1996 [20] | 31<br>41 yrs<br>5 mos | RAEB, 15<br>RAEB-T, 8<br>CMML, 8 | BU-CY-TBI, 31 | HLA-id sib, 22<br>Other family, 3<br>Unrelated, 6 | 1.7 yrs | 23%<br>(n = 8) | 28%<br>(n = 6) | 68%<br>(n = 17) |
| Anderson 1996 [21] | 30<br>29 yrs<br>8 mos | RA, 30 | BU-CY, 30 | HLA-id sib, 16<br>Other family, 1<br>Unrelated, 13 | 2.1 yrs | 63%<br>(n = 19) | 0%<br>(n = 0) | 37%<br>(n = 11) |
| Rattanatharathorn 1993 [22] | 27<br>33 yrs<br>5.6 mos | RA, 9<br>RAEB, 8<br>RAEB-T, 3<br>sAML, 6<br>Other, 1 | BU-CY, 1<br>BU-ARAC-CY, 24<br>BU-TLI, 2 | HLA-id sib, 18<br>Other family, 6<br>Unrelated, 3 | 1.7 yrs | 56%<br>(n = 17) | not stated<br>(n = 1) | not stated<br>(n = 9) |
| Demuynck 1996 [23] | 24<br>30 yrs<br>5 mos | RA, 4<br>RAEB, 4<br>RAEB-T, 9<br>CMML, 1<br>sAML, 6 | CY-TBI<br>± chemotherapy, 24 | HLA-id sib, 16<br>Other family, 5<br>Unrelated | 3.3 yrs | 35%<br>(n = 7) | 25%<br>(n = 6) | 50%<br>(n = 11) |

[a] FAB classification based on highest blast count before BMT.

SCT, stem cell transplantation; DFS, disease-free survival; NRM, nonrelapse mortality; RA, refractory anemia; RAEB, RA with excess blasts; RAEB-T, RAEB in transformation; CMML, chronic myelomonocytic leukemia; sAML, secondary AML; CR, complete remission; CY, cyclophosphamide; TBI, total body irradiation; BU, busulfan; Ida, idarubicin; AraC, cytosine arabinoside; CBV, cyclophosphamide, BCNU, VP-16, TLI, total lymphoid irradiation; HLA-id sib, human leuko-yte antigen identical sibling.

**Table 2** Clinical Characteristics of 250 Patients With MDS Treated With Allogeneic BMT in Seattle Between 1981 and 1996

| | |
|---|---|
| Median age, years (range) | 38 (1–66) |
| Gender | 152 M, 98 F |
| Median disease duration, months (range) | 8 (1–192) |
| Therapy-related MDS (number of patients) | 35 |
| Disease morphology (number of patients) | |
|   Less advanced MDS | |
|     RA or RARS | 106 |
|   Advanced MDS | |
|     RAEB | 76 |
|     RAEB-T | 57 |
|     CMML | 11 |
| Peripheral blood counts at time of SCT | |
|   Median neutrophil count, $10^9$ cells/L | 0.8 (0–50) |
|   Median platelet count, $10^9$ cells/L | 46 (2–435) |
|   Median hematocrit, % | 28.6 (10.1–45.6) |
| Cytogenetic risk classification[a] (number of patient) | |
|   Good | 110 |
|   Intermediate | 53 |
|   Poor | 77 |
|   Not performed | 10 |
| Preparative regimen | |
|   Total body irradiation-containing | 172 |
|   Busulfan-cyclophosphamide | 78 |
| Marrow Source[b] | |
|   Syngeneic | 5 |
|   HLA-identical family member | 142 |
|   Partially matched family member | 33 |
|   Unrelated donor | 70 |

[a] Classification as per reference # 4. Good risk included karyotypes that were normal, or a single del (5q), del (20q), or -Y. Poor risk included complex karyotypes (>3 abnormalities) or abnormalities involving chromosome 7. Intermediate risk included all other cytogenetic patterns.

[b] 247 patients received non-T depleted marrow and 3 received peripheral blood stem cell transplants.

after BMT, these data clearly demonstrate the curative potential of allogeneic BMT. The results of the univariable analysis, the actuarial 5-year DFS, and the cumulative incidences of relapse and nonrelapse mortality are shown in Table 3. The results of the multivariable analysis are shown in Table 4. The transplant year groups were chosen based on the opening of new preparative regimen protocols. Details of the analyses are discussed in relevant sections that follow.

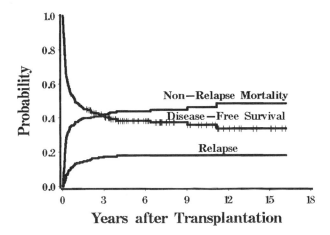

**Fig. 1**  Actuarial DFS and cumulative incidence of relapses and nonrelapse mortality for 250 patients with MDS treated with allogeneic BMT in Seattle between 1981 and 1996. Tick marks represent patients alive in complete continuous remission.

## IV.  DISEASE MORPHOLOGY AND CYTOGENETICS

The two most important independent variables associated with the incidence of relapse and, thereby, DFS are disease morphology and cytogenetic group. Many of the smaller studies and most of the larger studies of allogeneic BMT for MDS have demonstrated that with increasing blast percentage or disease morphology (i.e., RAEB or RAEB-T compared with RA or RARS) there is a higher risk of relapse posttransplant (11–14,18–20,23) and a shorter DFS (11,14). The outcome of the Seattle cohort (Tables 2–4) according to disease morphology is shown graphically in Figure 2.

Approximately 40% of patients with primary MDS have a clonal cytogenetic abnormality (4,6). The IPSS classifies good-risk karyotype as no abnormality or a single abnormality consisting of del(5q), del(20q), or −Y (4). Poor-risk karyotype comprises complex (≥3) or chromosome 7 abnormalities and intermediate-risk karyotype comprises all other abnormalities (4). Several studies have shown that karyotype, classified by either the IPSS or other systems, is predictive of the natural history of MDS (4,6). However, until recently, the prognostic significance of karyotype on outcome following BMT has yielded conflicting results (13–18,20–22). These inconsistent results may have occurred in part because of small sample numbers or the classification system used, as many of these original studies categorized karyotype simply as normal or abnormal. A recent article by

**Table 3**  5-Year Cumulative Incidences of Relapse and Non-Relapse Mortality and Actuarial Disease-free Survival for 250 Patients With MDS Treated With Allogeneic BMT in Seattle Between 1981 and 1996

| Variable | Relapse 5-Yr CI[a] (%) | Univariable p-value | NRM[b] 5-Yr CI[a] (%) | Univariable p-value | DFS 5-Yr CI[a] (%) | Univariable p-value |
|---|---|---|---|---|---|---|
| All patients | 17.9 | — | 43.8 | — | 38.2 | — |
| Age | | | | | | |
| Continuous variable | | 0.0966 | | 0.0038 | | 0.0011 |
| <21 years (n = 48) | 16.7 | | 23.0 | | 60.3 | |
| 21–39 years (n = 85) | 13.1 | | 46.3 | | 40.6 | |
| 40–55 years (n = 96) | 22.7 | | 53.5 | | 23.8 | |
| >55 years (n = 21) | 19.0 | | 38.1 | | 42.9 | |
| Disease Duration | | | | | | |
| Continuous variable | | 0.0152 | | 0.0086 | | 0.2665 |
| <6 months (n = 78) | 23.3 | | 46.3 | | 30.5 | |
| 6–12 months (n = 86) | 22.5 | | 38.0 | | 39.4 | |
| >12 months (n = 86) | 8.3 | | 46.9 | | 44.8 | |
| Morphology | | | | | | |
| Advanced MDS (n = 144) vs. | 27.6 | | 44.9 | | 27.6 | |
| Less advanced MDS (n = 106) | 4.9 | 0.0001 | 42.2 | 0.1209 | 52.7 | 0.0001 |

| | CI[a] | | | | NRM[b] | |
|---|---|---|---|---|---|---|
| Cytogenetics | | | | | | |
| Good risk (n = 110) | 12.1 | | 43.2 | | 44.7 | |
| vs. intermediate risk (n = 53) | 11.4 | 0.3182 | 49.1 | 0.4090 | 39.5 | 0.8226 |
| Good risk vs. poor risk (n = 77) | 31.8 | 0.0001 | 40.6 | 0.4467 | 27.6 | 0.0048 |
| Donor | | | | | | |
| Partially matched related or unrelated (n = 103) | 9.7 | | 51.1 | | 39.1 | |
| vs. matched related (n = 147) | 23.8 | 0.0294 | 38.7 | 0.0261 | 37.6 | 0.5322 |
| Gender | | | | | | |
| Male (n = 152) | 18.2 | | 48.7 | | 33.2 | |
| vs. Female (n = 98) | 17.5 | 0.5322 | 36.3 | 0.0487 | 46.2 | 0.0628 |
| Etiology | | | | | | |
| Therapy-related disease (n = 35) | 22.9 | | 57.1 | | 20.0 | |
| vs. non-therapy-related (n = 215) | 17.2 | 0.0960 | 41.6 | 0.0138 | 41.2 | 0.0026 |
| Transplant Year | | | | | | |
| 1981–1990 (n = 75) vs | 24.0 | | 38.7 | | 37.3 | |
| 1991–1993 (n = 92) | 14.1 | 0.3166 | 46.7 | 0.6746 | 39.1 | 0.9041 |
| 1981–1990 vs. 1994-1996 (n = 83) | 20.6 | 0.5748 | 47.0 | 0.9926 | 32.4 | 0.8146 |

[a] CI = Cumulative incidence.
[b] NRM = Non-relapse mortality.

**Table 4**  Multivariable Analysis of Risk Factors for 250 Patients With MDS Treated With Allogeneic BMT in Seattle Between 1981 and 1996

| Variable | Relative Risk of Relapse | p-value | Relative Risk of of NRM | p-value | Relative Risk of Death or Relapse | p-value |
|---|---|---|---|---|---|---|
| Increasing Age | 1.03 | 0.033 | 1.02 | 0.007 | 1.02 | 0.0006 |
| Increasing Disease Duration | 0.96 | 0.0019 | 1.011 | 0.0002 | NS | |
| Morphology | | | | | | |
| Advanced MDS vs. Less advanced MDS | 6.03 | 0.0002 | NS | | 1.72 | 0.0029 |
| Cytogenetics | | | | | | |
| Good vs. Intermediate risk | NS | | NS | | NS | |
| Good vs. Poor risk | 4.57 | 0.0001 | NS | | 1.62 | 0.015 |
| Donor | | | | | | |
| Partially matched related or unrelated vs. matched related | NS | | 1.76 | 0.0038 | NS | |
| Gender | | | | | | |
| Male vs. female | NS | | 1.94 | 0.0019 | 1.43 | 0.045 |
| Etiology | | | | | | |
| Therapy-related disease vs. Non-therapy related | NS | | 1.99 | 0.0068 | 1.53 | 0.045 |
| Transplant year | | | | | | |
| 1981–1990 vs. 1991–1993 | 0.44 | 0.033 | NS | | NS | |
| 1981–1990 vs. 1994-1996 | 0.24 | 0.0012 | NS | | 0.58 | 0.021 |

NRM, nonrelapse mortality.
NS, not significant.

Nevill et al. was the first study to classify karyotype according to the IPSS (15). In this multivariable analysis, 17 patients with poor-risk cytogenetics had a statistically significantly higher risk of relapse and shorter DFS compared to 40 patients with intermediate or good risk (15). The experience of the Seattle cohort of a larger number of patients with poor-risk cytogenetics ($n = 77$) confirms the findings of Nevill et al. (Tables 3 and 4, Fig. 3). These Seattle data are the first to show that both disease morphology and karyotype are independent predictive factors for relapse and DFS.

These results underscore the importance of monitoring disease morphology and cytogenetics at diagnosis and prior to BMT to provide prognostic information to the patient. These results also suggest that outcome with BMT may be improved if patients are transplanted, if possible, before a poor-risk karyotype or

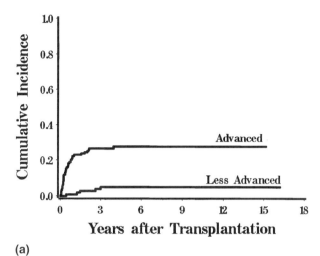

(a)

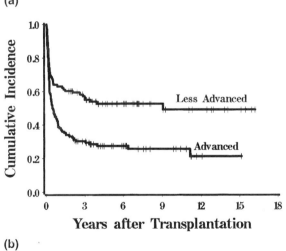

(b)

**Fig. 2** (a) Cumulative incidence of relapse and (b) actuarial DFS for patients with less advanced (RA and RARS, $n = 106$) and advanced (RAEB, RAEB-T, and CMML, $n = 144$) disease morphology for patients with MDS treated with allogeneic BMT in Seattle between 1981 and 1996.

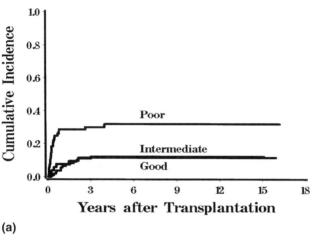

(a)

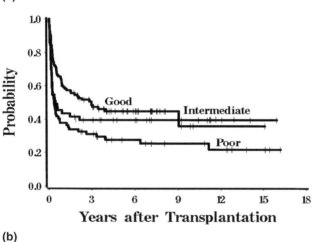

(b)

**Fig. 3**  (a) Cumulative incidence of relapse and (b) actuarial DFS for patients with good ($n = 110$), intermediate ($n = 53$), and poor ($n = 77$) risk cytogenetics for patients with MDS treated with allogeneic BMT in Seattle between 1981 and 1996.

advanced disease morphology develops. It is important to note, however, that the association of poor-risk cytogenetic features and relapse after allogeneic BMT does not appear to extend to patients transplanted with RA or RARS who have never progressed to advanced FAB morphological classification. In a study from Seattle of the first 70 patients with RA (of whom 39 had cytogenetic abnormalities), only one patient relapsed, with a median follow-up of approximately 3.5 years posttransplant (21). Similarly, Nevill et al. and Sutton et al. reported no relapses among 14 and 11 patients transplanted with RA, respectively (14,15). In these studies, the long-term DFS rates among patients receiving human leukocyte antigen (HLA)-identical related-donor BMT were 74 and 73%, respectively (14,21). Other studies have also corroborated the low risk of relapse among patients transplanted for RA, despite the presence of cytogenetic abnormalities (11,12,18,22,23).

## V. TIMING OF BMT

Consideration of disease duration is important in determining the appropriate timing of BMT for MDS, not only because the disease may progress in blast percentage or karyotype during an observation period, but also because longer disease duration may result in greater transplant-related toxicity. Patients with MDS have a particularly high rate of nonrelapse mortality compared to patients with other ''chronic'' diseases, such as chronic myeloid leukemia.

If the pretransplant period of marrow failure among patients with MDS results in complications such as iron overload, HLA alloimmunization, and fungal colonization or infection, then one might expect that prolonged disease duration would result in an inferior outcome after BMT. However, studies that have evaluated the relationship between disease duration and posttransplant outcome have not yielded consistent results (11–15,20,21). This discrepancy may be due to differences in disease duration categories, disease subsets, or pretransplant treatment of patients. The analysis of the 250 patients transplanted in Seattle (Tables 2–4) found that increasing disease duration (entered as a continuous variable) was associated with increased incidence of nonrelapse mortality and, unexpectedly, with decreased incidence of relapse. Consequently, there was no correlation between disease duration and DFS (Fig. 4). It is possible that the effect of disease duration on DFS and nonrelapse mortality among the Seattle cohort is more important among patients with less advanced MDS, since an association was found for both end points in an analysis of 70 patients with less advanced MDS (21), but not in an analysis of 75 patients with advanced MDS (20).

Two studies using disease duration as a dichotomous variable [(<3 vs. ≥3 months (15) or ≤201 vs >201 days (14)] did not find an association between either nonrelapse mortality or DFS among 60 (15) and 71 (14) patients, respectively. On the other hand, two recent studies from the European Group for Blood and Marrow Transplantation (EBMT) did find that shorter disease duration predicted for improved DFS and lower nonrelapse mortality (11,12). The study by Runde et al. evaluated 131 patients with MDS who underwent BMT from HLA-identical siblings, and found the most important time cutoff to be ≤3 versus >3 months (11). In the multivariable analysis, there was a relative risk of 2.41 for greater nonrelapse mortality (95% confidence interval, 1.07–5.45) and a relative

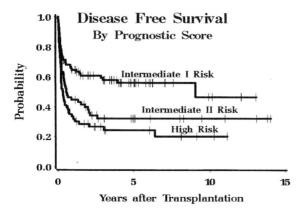

**Fig. 4** Actuarial DFS after allogeneic BMT for patients according to intermediate-1-risk ($n = 94$), intermediate-2-risk ($n = 68$), and high-risk ($n = 77$) International Prognostic Score for patients with MDS treated with allogeneic BMT in Seattle between 1981 and 1996.

risk of 2.01 for shorter DFS (95% confidence interval, 1.09–3.7) among patients with >3 months' compared to ≤3 months' disease duration (11). The study by Arnold et al. evaluated 118 patients who underwent BMT from unrelated donors (12). For a disease duration of <6 months, 6–12 months, and >12 months, the corresponding nonrelapse mortality rates were 29% versus 49% versus 73% ($p = 0.04$) and corresponding DFS rates were 55% versus 34% versus 16% ($p = 0.04$) (12). Although there are discrepancies among studies, given the results of the three large Seattle and EBMT studies, I conclude that the data do support early transplantation in MDS to reduce nonrelapse mortality and improve DFS.

Another approach to determining the appropriate timing for BMT is to compare the outcome with BMT to the outcome without BMT. As described above, the International MDS Risk Analysis Workshop evaluated 816 patients with primary MDS, none of whom received intensive chemotherapy or BMT (4). For patients ≤60 years old, the median survival rates for the low, intermediate-1, intermediate-2, and high-risk groups were 11.8, 5.2, 1.8, and 0.3 years, respectively (4). The IPSS has been applied to 241 patients who underwent allogeneic BMT in Seattle (25). Because of insufficient detail on marrow blast percentage, the score for marrow blasts was modified to be 0 for RA or RARS, 1.0 for RAEB, and 2.0 for RAEB-T. There were 94 patients in the intermediate-1, 68 in the intermediate-2, and 77 in the high-risk groups. Because there were only two patients in the low-risk group, results from this group are not included. There were no differences in nonrelapse mortality rates by IPSS (cumulative incidence of 42% for intermediate-1, 51% for intermediate-2, and 37% for high risk, $p =$

0.5). There were, however, significant differences in relapse rates (cumulative incidence of 2% for intermediate-1, 17% for intermediate-2, and 38% for high risk, $p = 0.0001$) and in 5-year actuarial DFS estimates (56% for intermediate-1, 32% for intermediate-2, and 24% for high risk groups, $p = 0.0003$) (Fig. 4).

The main drawback to comparing these BMT results with the natural history results reported by Greenberg et al. (4) is that the IPSS was not designed to evaluate prognosis at a delayed time after diagnosis, as used in the BMT analysis (25). Nonetheless, the long-term DFS in the intermediate-1, intermediate-2, and high-risk groups appears to be better in the transplanted group than nontransplanted group, thus supporting a decision of immediate BMT for eligible patients within these IPSS risk groups. These data do not address the routine use of allogeneic BMT for patients in the low-risk group. However, it is appropriate to consider early transplantation in select situations of very young patients or those with a life-threatening single cytopenia. Clearly, because of the lack of randomized trials proving a survival benefit of transplantation over less intensive therapy, the decision to proceed to allogeneic transplantation must rest on careful discussion with the patient about his/her individualized risks and benefits.

## VI. IMPACT OF PATIENT AGE

As with many other diseases, there is a clear increase in nonrelapse mortality and decrease in DFS with increasing patient age (Tables 3 and 4) (12,13,18,21). One study also found that older age was associated with shorter DFS because of increased risk of relapse (14). This unexpected finding of increase in relapse rate with older age was also seen in the analysis of the 250 Seattle patients (Table 4), but an explanation is not readily forthcoming. The median age at diagnosis of MDS is approximately 65 years. However, because of the toxicity of allogeneic BMT, most transplant centers have excluded patients above the age of 55 years. In Seattle, there has been cautious exploration of allogeneic BMT for patients up to the age of 66 years (26). In this report, 55 patients with RA ($n = 13$), RAEB ($n = 19$), RAEB-T or AML ($n = 16$), or CMML ($n = 2$) underwent BMT from either a HLA-matched related ($n = 36$), syngeneic ($n = 4$), HLA-mismatched related ($n = 4$), or unrelated ($n = 6$) donor. The median age was 59 (range, 55.3–66.2) years. Using the IPSS, karyotype was classified as low risk in 25, intermediate risk in seven, and high risk in 15 cases. Eight patients had therapy-related MDS. A wide variety of preparative regimens were used, consisting of total-body irradiation (TBI) in 23 and chemotherapy-only in 27 cases. Four patients died before engraftment and the remaining had sustained engraftment. Of 43 survivors beyond day 28, 77% developed acute grades II–IV GVHD (16% grades III–IV). Of 32 patients at risk, 62% have developed chronic GVHD. The actuarial DFS was 42% and the cumulative incidence of relapse was 19%. Among the 22 survivors, at time of last contact, the Karnofsky performance score was 100% for 11, 90–95% for six, and <90% for five patients. Similar to data for younger patients discussed earlier, patients with poor-risk karyotype, increased blasts, high-risk IPSS, and therapy-related MDS had a worse outcome. In addition, patients who received a preparative regimen in which busulfan dosing was adjusted to achieve a steady-state concentration of 600–900 ng/ml had a lower nonrelapse mortality rate and, consequently, higher DFS than patients receiving other preparative regimens. These preliminary results of allogeneic BMT for patients 55–66 years of age are favorable, and suggest that this procedure may be offered to carefully selected individuals in this age range (26).

## VII.  THERAPY-RELATED MDS

Although the etiology of MDS is unknown in the majority of cases, an increasing proportion of patients diagnosed with MDS have developed the disease following treatment with chemotherapy or ionizing radiation or the combination of both. Alkylating agents used for Hodgkin's and non-Hodgkin's lymphoma are the most common drugs associated with the development of therapy-related MDS. Therapy-related MDS typically develops 4–5 years following exposure to the inciting agent, and is associated with chromosome abnormalities in ≥90% of cases, most commonly involving chromosomes 5 and 7 (27). With increasing intensity of chemotherapy for malignancies, such as autologous transplantation for lymphoma, and increasing cure rate for some malignancies there appears to be an increasing incidence of therapy-related MDS (28).

A number of reports on BMT for MDS and secondary AML have included patients with therapy-related MDS and therapy-related AML (11,15,16,18,22, 23,29–34). With complete survival data on 263 of the 275 reported patients with therapy-related MDS or AML, 73 patients (28%) were disease-free survivors, 64 (24%) relapsed, 125 (48%) died of transplant-related causes, and one died of the primary disease. The largest of these studies reported a 6-year actuarial DFS rate of 13%, relapse rate of 47%, and nonrelapse mortality rate of 78% for all 99 patients (29). By FAB subtype, the DFS was 33% for 12 RA/RARS patients, 20% for 18 RAEB patients, and 8% for 67 RAEB-T or AML patients (29).

These data suggest that allogeneic BMT is a feasible treatment option for therapy-related myeloid malignancies, but do not address the question of whether results are different from results for patients with de novo MDS. A study of 18 patients with therapy-related MDS was compared to 25 patients with primary MDS who were transplanted at the same institution (16). The 3-year actuarial DFS rates were 24% for therapy-related and 43% for primary MDS, a difference that did not reach conventional statistical significance (16). As shown in Table 2, 35 of the first 250 patients with MDS who underwent BMT in Seattle had therapy-

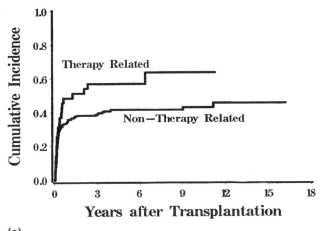

(a)

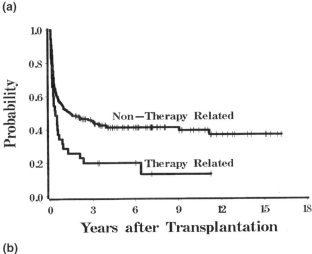

(b)

**Fig. 5**   (a) Cumulative incidence of nonrelapse mortality and (b) actuarial DFS for patients with therapy-related MDS (*n* = 35) and non-therapy-related MDS (*n* = 215) for patients with MDS treated with allogeneic BMT in Seattle between 1981 and 1996.

related MDS. The 5-year DFS for these 35 patients was 20%. In multivariable analysis, there was a significantly shorter DFS owing to a higher incidence of nonrelapse mortality among these 35 patients compared with the remaining patients, and there was no difference in relapse rate (Table 4, Fig. 5). This finding of worse survival due to greater nonrelapse mortality, after adjustment for other factors known to influence outcome, is likely due to the cumulative toxicity associated with treatment for the prior malignancy and toxicity associated with BMT. These results suggest that procedures designed to reduce transplant-related toxicity, such as T-cell depletion, may improve DFS in patients with therapy-related MDS, especially if performed while the patient is at low risk for relapse, i.e., low blast count and without poor-risk cytogenetics.

## VIII.  USE OF UNRELATED DONORS

Most patients transplanted for MDS have received marrow from HLA-matched related individuals, but suitable related donors are only available to a minority of patients who are otherwise eligible for allogeneic BMT. With increasing size of the worldwide registries of HLA-typed volunteer donors, the potential use of unrelated donor transplantation is expanding. The largest published manuscript on the use of unrelated donor BMT for MDS is a review of registry data from the EBMT Group (12). This study included 118 patients transplanted at 49 BMT centers between 1986 and 1996. This group of 118 patients was young (median 24 years). According to FAB classification, 24 had RA or RARS, 26 had RAEB, 34 had RAEB-T, 12 had CMML, and 22 had secondary AML. Eleven of 118 underwent BMT while in first complete remission of RAEB-T or AML. Thirteen of the patients received marrow from a one or two minor HLA-mismatched donor. Preparative regimens and graft-versus-host disease (GVHD) prophylaxis regimens varied, but consisted of T-cell depletion in 36 cases. Primary or secondary graft failure occurred in 18 of 118 patients, but data are not presented to determine whether this high rate of graft failure was due to the use of T-cell depletion. The 2-year actuarial probabilities of DFS, relapse, and transplant-related mortality were 28%, 35%, and 58%, respectively. In the univariable analysis, as outlined in the sections above, there was a lower relapse rate for patients with less advanced MDS, and a greater transplant-related mortality and shorter DFS both for greater patient age and disease duration (12). Relapse rate was lower among patients who developed acute ($p = 0.02$) or chronic ($p = 0.13$) GVHD, but without impact on DFS (12). Another, larger registry report from the National Marrow Donor Program (NMDP) (published in abstract form only) of 320 patients reported a lower rate of engraftment failure (9%) and a similar rate of DFS of 30% (35). In this study, acute GVHD occurred in 53% and chronic GVHD in 38% of patients (35).

Results published from Seattle on the first 52 patients with MDS or MDS-related AML transplanted from unrelated donors using non-T-cell-depleted marrow showed 2-year actuarial probabilities of DFS, relapse, and nonrelapse mortality of 38%, 28%, and 48%, respectively (36), which are relatively similar to the EBMT and NMDP registry analyses (12,35). The risk of relapse was significantly higher among patients with RAEB-T or MDS-related AML compared to RA,

RAEB, or CMML (36). The risk of nonrelapse mortality was significantly higher among older patients and those with longer disease duration (36). At time of publication, 16 of the 19 survivors had a performance status of 90–100% (36). Registry reports on the use of unrelated donor BMT in MDS patients have reported a higher nonrelapse mortality and shorter DFS than the Seattle group (12,33,37,38). In the EBMT study, a total of 49 centers enrolled the total of 118 patients (12), suggesting that probably few patients were transplanted at any individual center. This low volume may contribute to greater transplant-related mortality (39). The most favorable outcome that has been reported for patients with MDS undergoing unrelated donor BMT is among patients with RA who received a busulfan-cyclophosphamide preparative regimen (40). In this analysis, the 3-year actuarial survival was 61% for the 23 patients for whom busulfan was targeted to maintain steady-state concentration of 600–900 mg/ml (40).

The results from the Seattle cohort described in Tables 2–4 included 70 patients transplanted from unrelated donors and 33 from partially matched related donors. In this analysis, when results were compared to those obtained using matched related donors, there was a lower relapse rate, higher nonrelapse mortality rate, and similar DFS for recipients of unrelated or mismatched marrow (Tables 3 and 4). Overall, the use of unrelated donor transplantation for MDS cures at least 30% of eligible patients and may be associated with a higher nonrelapse mortality rate, higher GVHD rate, and lower relapse rate than that obtained with the use of matched related donor transplantation.

## IX. THE CONTROVERSY OF INDUCTION CHEMOTHERAPY BEFORE BMT

Because of the high rate of relapse among patients with RAEB-T and MDS-related AML, many physicians have chosen to administer intensive induction chemotherapy to these patients before allogeneic BMT. This treatment is usually given for one or more of three reasons: (1) life-threatening peripheral cytopenias are present that will improve if remission is obtained; (2) the ability to proceed rapidly to BMT is not readily available; and (3) there is the perception that if a patient achieves remission, the outcome with allogeneic BMT will be improved because of a reduced risk of relapse. Conversely, there are several reasons to suggest that induction chemotherapy before BMT may not improve or may actually worsen long-term survival: (1) if BMT is readily available cytopenias will improve as quickly with BMT as with chemotherapy; (2) complete remission rate with chemotherapy is only 50–60%; (3) the patient may die of toxicity during chemotherapy, thereby preventing BMT altogether; (4) the patient may develop a complication during chemotherapy, such as a fungal infection, that may increase the risk of death with BMT; and (5) the risk of relapse may be equally high for remission patients versus untreated patients, after accounting for karyotype and blast percentage.

Unfortunately, there have been no prospective comparative studies of immediate BMT versus induction chemotherapy followed by BMT. Furthermore, retrospective comparisons of patients transplanted without attempt at remission induction therapy or after such treatment have resulted in contradictory results (14,15,41–45). These contradictory results are likely due to small sample sizes, patient selection, and difficulty in accounting for patients who receive chemotherapy, but do not go to subsequent BMT. In general, patients who fail to obtain a complete remission after induction chemotherapy do poorly with BMT (14,42,44). Patients transplanted after obtaining a complete remission were reported to have a 60% 2-year DFS ($n = 16$) in one study (44) and a 43% 7-year DFS ($n = 7$) in another (14). However, in the latter study, the improved outcome after BMT among complete responders was due to a lower nonrelapse mortality, not a lower relapse rate (14). The study by Nevill et al. included 19 patients who received induction chemotherapy before BMT (15). Four of these 19 were disease-free survivors after BMT, including three of four patients transplanted while in first complete remission. Of the remaining 15 patients who did not achieve remission or relapsed before BMT, only one survived disease-free with the remaining deaths equally divided between relapsed disease and nonrelapse mortality. A study by Copelan et al. consisted of 42 patients with MDS and MDS-related AML who underwent allogeneic BMT, 11 of whom received induction chemotherapy before BMT (41). In addition, the authors report on nine patients with HLA-matched siblings identified, but who died after induction chemotherapy without an attempt at BMT. Among the 19 patients with MDS-related AML who underwent BMT, five of eight who did not versus two of 11 who did receive induction chemotherapy were disease-free survivors (41). Analysis of 46 patients with MDS-related AML and therapy-related AML who underwent BMT without attempt at induction chemotherapy showed a 24% 5-year DFS, which was not significantly different from the 15% 5-year DFS of 20 patients who underwent BMT after induction chemotherapy (while in first or second complete remission or first untreated relapse) (42). Finally, a retrospective review of 51 children with advanced MDS who underwent allogeneic BMT found a trend toward improved event-free survival among the patients who did not receive prior induction chemotherapy compared to those who did (61% vs. 47%, $p = 0.08$) (45).

Assuming a complete remission rate of approximately 50%, and a DFS of approximately 50% after allogeneic BMT for patients transplanted in first complete remission, the overall long-term DFS for patients intended to receive induction chemotherapy followed by BMT would be predicted to be only 25%. This 25% DFS rate is similar to the outcome after BMT for patients with previously untreated RAEB-T and MDS-related AML and patients with de novo AML transplanted in first relapse (46). Therefore, the bias of this author is that induction chemotherapy should not be routinely administered. Only prospective studies or large retrospective studies that account for all patients receiving remission induction chemotherapy (including those who die during such treatment or become ineligible for BMT) will be able to address the use of such pretransplant therapy definitively.

## X. NOVEL APPROACHES TO IMPROVING OUTCOME

### A. Myeloablative Regimens

Innovative approaches to reduce the high risk of relapse after BMT among patients with advanced disease morphology are needed. One approach is the use of novel preparative regimens. One abstract describing the use of busulfan, cyclophosphamide, and cytarabine reported a favorable DFS (52%) and low relapse rate (16%), despite 63% of patients having advanced morphology (47). Several phase II studies in Seattle have evaluated TBI-based regimens (20,48). In the first study, 31 patients with RAEB or RAEB-T received TBI (12 Gy), busulfan (7 mg/kg), and cyclophosphamide (50 mg/kg). In comparison to historical controls receiving cyclophosphamide and TBI, there was a lower relapse rate and higher nonrelapse mortality rate (not statistically significantly different) and similar DFS among the two groups (20). A more recent study evaluated TBI (12 Gy) and busulfan (7 mg/kg) in 26 patients (48). In this study, there was a significantly lower relapse rate, similar nonrelapse mortality rate, and significantly improved DFS compared to the cyclophosphamide-TBI historical controls (48). These favorable data are undergoing formal evaluation in a randomized phase III study within the Southwest Oncology Group. Another ongoing approach to reducing relapse without increasing toxicity is to target radiation specifically to hematopoietic tissues using radiolabeled monoclonal antibodies. Preliminary data among patients with advanced MDS and acute leukemia are promising and studies are ongoing (49).

The reason for the high nonrelapse mortality rate (approximately 40%) seen in patients with MDS treated with allogeneic BMT is not well understood, but may be due to the prolonged period of marrow failure preceding BMT. Studies using T-cell depletion among 22 patients with RA undergoing HLA-matched sibling donor BMT (19,50) have reported DFS rates of 75–80%, which are similar to those reported for similar patients receiving non-T-depleted marrow (14,21). However, there appears to be a much lower incidence of GVHD with the use of T-cell depletion, which may reduce long-term morbidity and mortality. The use of T-cell-depletion techniques among patients with advanced MDS or MDS-related AML resulted in poor results in one study (50) and favorable results in another (51). The use of targeting busulfan to avoid ''toxic'' levels is also an attractive way to reduce toxicity and preliminary results in older patients with

MDS and patients with MDS undergoing unrelated donor transplantation are encouraging (26,40). Finally, administration of busulfan intravenously rather than orally and the use of peripheral blood stem cells rather than bone marrow as a source of allogeneic stem cells may be additional means to improve outcome after transplantation. However, neither of these latter two approaches has been reported in studies comprised solely of MDS patients.

## B. Nonmyeloablative Regimens

Another approach that is designed to reduce toxicity of allogeneic BMT is the use of nonmyeloablative preparative regimens. The concept of nonmyeloablative stem cell transplantation is to minimize the toxicity associated with myeloablative regimens and to allow the graft-versus-malignancy effect of the infused allogeneic cells to provide additional antitumor effect to allow for sustained engraftment and acceptable relapse rates. This approach has been studied in a variety of disease types (52,53), although data specifically on patients with MDS are preliminary and in abstract form only (54–57). One study compared the outcome of 20 MDS patients who received a nonmyeloablative regimen (fludarabine, busulfan, and Campath or fludarabine, idarubicin, and cyarabine) to the outcome of 26 MDS patients who received a myeloablative regimen (busulfan and cyclophosphamide or busulfan, cyclophosphamide, TBI, and Campath) (54). The patients received nonmyeloablative regimens because of advanced age and/or comorbid conditions. The nonmyeloablative regimen was associated with a lower day 100 mortality compared to the myeloablative regimen (5% vs. 23%). At the time of this report three of 20 in the nonablative and one of 26 in the ablative arm had relapsed and the 3-year survival rates were 49% and 54%, respectively (54). Another study detailed the outcome of 18 patients with MDS or MDS-related AML, with a median age of 61 years (55). These patients received a nonmyeloablative preparative regimen of 200 cGy TBI with or without fludarabine (55). At the time this study was presented, three patients had died of nonrelapse causes, five had died of disease progression, and two had either stable disease or a partial remission. Eight of the 18 patients were in continuous complete remission at a median of 246 (range, 120–445) days posttransplant: three of six with RA, one of two with RAEB, none of three with RAEB-T, one of two with CMML, and three of five with MDS-related AML (these five AML patients were in partial or complete remission prior to administration of the preparative regimen). Two other studies presented data on patients with both MDS and acute leukemia and found that results are worse among patients with advanced disease and among patients with chemotherapy-refractory disease (56,57). These preliminary data on nonmyeloablative regimens suggest that, in comparison to standard ablative regimens, this treatment can be safely administered to a greater proportion of patients with MDS (i.e., those with increased age and/or comorbid conditions).

However, the total number of reported patients is small and the follow-up is short, so the rate of durable disease-free survival for any phase of MDS is not yet known.

## XI. CONCLUSIONS

Based on the studies reviewed here, approximately 40% of patients with MDS treated with allogeneic BMT appear to have been cured. The most favorable results are seen among patients with RA who have an HLA-matched related donor, in whom long-term DFS rates of approximately 75% have been achieved. It is possible that with improved transplant techniques (perhaps with use of intravenous busulfan or targeting of drug levels) and with improved patient selection (perhaps with BMT early after diagnosis) cure rates above 75% will be realized for patients with less advanced MDS. Currently, the major limitations in applying allogeneic BMT to the majority of patients are the advanced age of most patients with MDS and the lack of a HLA-compatible related or unrelated donor. In addition, the major limitations to a greater success rate following allogeneic BMT include the increased relapse rate among patients with increased blasts and poor risk cytogenetic features and the increased nonrelapse mortality rate among patients with longer disease duration, patients with therapy-related MDS, male patients, and patients receiving mismatched or unrelated grafts. The use of allogeneic BMT early in the disease course, if possible, before increase in blast percentage, karyotypic evolution, or complications of cytopenias develop may help improve outcome. Although some patients may benefit from the use of remission induction chemotherapy before the start of the preparative regimen, such pretransplant treatment has not been shown to benefit the majority of patients who are at high risk of relapse. In addition, no specific preparative regimen has yet been conclusively shown to be preferable over others, although intriguing pilot data have been reported using a number of novel approaches. The preliminary data on the use of nonmyeloablative preparative regimens suggest this approach may reduce toxicity, but the durability of disease-free survival is not yet known and is likely to be low among patients with advanced MDS.

In the opinion of this author, some general recommendations for the use of allogeneic BMT for patients with MDS can be made given the available data. All patients up to 55 years of age should be evaluated at diagnosis for potential BMT. Patients between 55 and 65 years of age should be considered in select situations, preferably within the context of clinical trials. The use of single HLA-antigen-mismatched related or HLA-matched unrelated donor grafts should be considered at institutions with favorable experience using such alternative donors. Patients with intermediate-1, intermediate-2, or high-risk disease according to the IPSS (which will include patients with either increased blasts or intermediate or poor-risk cytogenetic features) should be considered for transplantation early after diagnosis. The majority of patients with a low-risk score should be observed until evidence of disease progression; however, BMT might be considered in the case of a single life-threatening cytopenia or a particularly young individual with a HLA-matched related donor.

## REFERENCES

1. Bennett JM, Catovsky D, Daniel MT, Flandrin G, Galton DA, Gralnick HR, Sultan C. Proposals for the classification of the myelodysplastic syndromes. Br J Haematol 1982; 51:189–199.
2. Harris NL, Jaffe ES, Diebold J, Flandrin G, Muller-Hermelink HK, Vardiman J, Lister TA, Bloomfield CD. World Health Organization classification of neoplastic diseases of the hematopoietic and lymphoid tissues: report of Clinical Advisory Committee Meeting—Airlie House, Virginia, November 1997. J Clin Oncol 1999; 17:383–389.
3. Aul C, Gattermann N, Heyll A, Germing U, Derigs G, Schneider W. Primary myelo-dysplastic syndromes: analysis of prognostic factors in 235 patients and proposals for an improved scoring system. Leukemia 1992; 6:52–59.
4. Greenberg P, Cox C, LeBeau MM, Fenaux P, Morel P, Sanz G, Sanz M, Vallespi T, Hamblin T, Oscier D, Ohyashiki K, Toyama K, Aul C, Mufti G, Bennett J. International scoring system for evaluating prognosis in myelodysplastic syndromes. Blood 1997; 89:2079–2088.
5. Sanz GF, Sanz MA, Vallespi T, Canizo MC, Torrabadella M, Garcia S, Irriguible D, San Miguel JF. Two regression models and a scoring system for predicting survival and planning treatment in myelodysplastic syndromes: a mutivariate analysis of prognostic factors in 370 patients. Blood 1989; 74:395–408.
6. Morel P, Hebbar M, Lai JL, Duhamel A, Preudhomme C, Wattel E, Bauters F, Fenaux P. Cytogenetic analysis has strong independent prognostic value in de novo myelodysplastic syndromes and can be incorporated in a new scoring system: a report on 408 cases. Leukemia 1993; 7:1315–1323.
7. Cazzola M, Anderson JE, Ganser A, Hellstrom-Lindberg E. A patient-oriented approach to treatment of myelodysplastic syndromes. Haematologica 1998; 83:910–935.
8. Silverman LR, Demakos EP, Peterson B, Odchimar-Reissig R, Nelson D, Kornblith AB, Stone R, Holland JC, Powell BL, DeCastro C, Ellerton J, Larson RA, Schiffer CA, Holland JF. A randomized controlled trial of subcutaneous azacitidine (AZA-C) in patients with the myelodysplastic syndrome (MDS): A study of the Cancer and Leukemia Group B (CALGB). Proceedings of ASCO Meeting. J Clin Oncol 1998; 17(suppl):14a.
9. Gassmann W, Schmitz N, Loffler H, De Witte T. Intensive chemotherapy and bone marrow transplantation for myelodysplastic syndromes. Semin Hematol 1996; 33:196–205.
10. Appelbaum FR, Storb R, Ramberg RE, Shulman HM, Buchner CD, Clift RA, Deeg

HJ, Fefer A, Sanders J, Stewart P. Allogeneic marrow transplantation in the treatment of preleukemia. Ann Intern Med 1984; 100:689–693.

11. Runde V, de Witte T, Arnold R, Gratwohl A, Hermans J, van Biezen A, Niederwieser D, Labopin M, Walter-Noel MP, Bacigalupo A, Jacobsen N, Ljungman P, Carreras E, Kolb HJ, Aul C, Apperley J. Bone marrow transplantation from HLA-identical siblings as first-line treatment in patients with myelodysplastic syndromes: early transplantation is associated with improved outcome. Chronic Leukemia Working Part of the European Group for Blood and Marrow Transplantation. Bone Marrow Transplant 1998; 21:255–261.

12. Arnold R, de Witte T, van Biezen A, Hermans J, Jacobsen N, Runde V, Gratwohl A, Apperley JF. Unrelated bone marrow transplantation in patients with myelodysplastic syndromes and secondary acute myeloid leukemia: an EBMT survey. European Blood and Marrow Transplantation Group. Bone Marrow Transplant 1998; 21: 1213–1216.

13. Anderson JE, Appelbaum FR, Fisher LD, Schoch G, Shulman H, Anasetti C, Bensinger WI, Bryant E, Buckner CD, Doney K, Martin PJ, Sanders JE, Sullivan KM, Thomas ED, Witherspoon RP, Hansen JA, Storb R. Allogeneic bone marrow transplantation for 93 patients with myelodysplastic syndrome. Blood 1993; 82:677–681.

14. Sutton L, Chastang C, Ribaud P, Jouet JP, Kuentz M, Attal M, Reiffers J, Tigaud JM, Rio B, Dauriac C, Legros M, Dreyfus F, Lioure B, Troussard X, Milpied N, Witz F, Oriol P, Cahn JY, Michallet M, Gluckman E, Ifrah N, Pico JL, Vilmer E, Leblond V. Factors influencing outcome in de novo myelodysplastic syndromes treated by allogeneic bone marrow transplantation: a long-term study of 71 patients. Societe Francaise de Greffe de Moelle. Blood 1996; 88:358–365.

15. Nevill TJ, Fung HC, Shepherd JD, Horsman DE, Nantel SH, Klingemann HG, Forrest DL, Toze CL, Sutherland HJ, Hogge DE, Naiman SC, Le A, Brockington DA, Barnett MJ. Cytogenetic abnormalities in primary myelodysplastic syndrome are highly predictive of outcome after allogeneic bone marrow transplantation. Blood 1998; 92:1910–1917.

16. Ballen KK, Gilliland DG, Guinan EC, Hsieh CC, Parsons SK, Rimm IJ, Ferrara JL, Bierer BE, Weinstein HJ, Antin JH. Bone marrow transplantation for therapy-related myelodysplasia: comparison with primary myelodysplasia. Bone Marrow Transplant 1997; 20:737–743.

17. Locatelli F, Niemeyer C, Angelucci E, Bender-Gotze C, Burdach S, Ebell W, Friedrich W, Hasle H, Hermann J, Jacobsen N, Klingebiel T, Kremens B, Mann G, Pession A, Peters C, Schmid HJ, Stary J, Suttorp M, Uderzo C, van't Veer-Korthof ET, Vossen J, Zecca M, Zimmermann M. Allogeneic bone marrow transplantation for chronic myelomonocytic leukemia in childhood: a report from the European Working Group on Myelodysplastic Syndrome in Childhood. J Clin Oncol 1997; 15:566–573.

18. O'Donnell MR, Long GD, Parker PM, Niland J, Nademanee A, Amylon M, Chao N, Negrin RS, Schmidt GM, Slovak ML, Smith EP, Snyder DS, Stein AS, Traweek T, Glume KG, Forman SJ. Busulfan/cyclophosphamide as conditioning regimen for allogeneic bone marrow transplantation for myelodysplasia. J Clin Oncol 1995; 13: 2973–2979.

19. Mattijssen V, Schattenberg A, Schaap N, Preijers F, De Witte T. Outcome of allogeneic bone marrow transplantation with lymphocyte-depleted marrow grafts in adult patients with myelodysplastic syndromes. Bone Marrow Transplant 1997; 19:791–794.

20. Anderson JE, Appelbaum FR, Schoch G, Gooley T, Anasetti C, Bensinger WI, Bryant E, Buckner CD, Chauncey T, Clift RA, Deeg JH, Doney K, Flowers M, Hansen JA, Martin PJ, Matthews DC, Nash RA, Sanders JE, Shulman H, Sullivan KM, Witherspoon RP, Storb R. Allogeneic marrow transplantation for myelodysplastic syndrome with advanced disease morphology: a phase II study of busulfan, cyclophosphamide, and total-body irradiation and analysis of prognostic factors. J Clin Oncol 1996; 14:220–226.

21. Anderson JE, Appelbaum FR, Schoch G, Gooley T, Anasetti C, Bensinger WI, Bryant E, Buckner CD, Chauncey TR, Clift RA, Doney K, Flowers M, Hansen JA, Martin PJ, Matthews DC, Sanders JE, Shulman H, Sullivan KM, Witherspoon RP, Storb R. Allogeneic marrow transplantation for refractory anemia: a comparison of two preparative regimens and analysis of prognostic factors. Blood 1996; 87:51–58.

22. Ratanatharathorn V, Karanes C, Uberti J, Lum LG, de Planque MM, Schultz KR, Cronin S, Dan ME, Mohamed A, Hussein M, Sensenbrenner LL. Busulfan-based regimens and allogeneic bone marrow transplantation in patients with myelodysplastic syndromes. Blood 1993; 81:2194–2199.

23. Demuynck H, Verhoef GE, Zachee P, Emonds MP, van der Schueren E, van den Berghe H, Vandenberghe P, Casteels-Van Daele M, Boogaerts MA. Treatment of patients with myelodysplastic syndromes with allogeneic bone marrow transplantation from genotypically HLA-identical sibling and alternative donors. Bone Marrow Transplant 1996; 17:745–751.

24. Appelbaum FR, Barrall J, Storb R, Ramberg R, Doney K, Sale GE, Thomas ED. Clonal cytogenetic abnormalities in patients with otherwise typical aplastic anemia. Exp Hematol 1987; 15:1134–1139.

25. Appelbaum FR, Anderson J. Allogeneic bone marrow transplantation for myelodysplastic syndrome: outcomes analysis according to IPSS score. Leukemia 1998; 12(suppl 1):S25–S29.

26. Deeg HJ, Shulman HM, Anderson JE, Bryant EM, Gooley TA, Slattery JT, Anasetti C, Fefer A, Storb R, Appelbaum FR. Allogeneic and syngeneic marrow transplantation for myelodysplastic syndrome in patients 55 to 66 years of age. Blood 2000; 95:1188–1194.

27. Pedersen-Bjergaard J, Pedersen M, Roulston D, Philip P. Different genetic pathways in leukemogenesis for patients presenting with therapy-related myelodysplasia and therapy-related acute myeloid leukemia. Blood 1995; 86:3542–3552.

28. Stone RM. Myelodysplastic syndrome after autologous transplantation for lymphoma: the price of progress. Blood 1994; 83:3437–3440.

29. Witherspoon RP, Deeg HJ. Allogeneic bone marrow transplantation for secondary leukemia or myelodysplasia. Haematologica 1999; 84:1085–1087.

30. Le Maignan C, Ribaud P, Maraninchi D, et al. Bone marrow transplantation for mutagen-related leukemia or myelodysplasia. Exper Hematol 1990; 18:660.

31. Bandini G, Rosti G, Calori E, Albertazzi L, Tura S. Allogeneic bone marrow trans-

plantation for secondary leukaemia and myelodysplastic syndrome. Br J Haematol 1990; 75:442–444.

32. De Witte T. Response to "Allogeneic bone marrow transplantation for secondary leukaemia and myelodysplastic syndrome." Br J Haematol 1990; 75:443–444.

33. Bunin NJ, Casper JT, Chitambar C, Hunter J, Truitt R, Menitove J, Camitta BM, Ash R. Partially matched bone marrow transplantation in patients with myelodysplastic syndromes. J Clin Oncol 1988; 6:1851–1855.

34. Yakoub-Agha I, de La Salmoniere P, Ribaud P, Sutton L, Wattel E, Kuentz M, Jouet JP, Marit G, Milpied N, Deconinck E, Gratecos N, Leporrier M, Chabbert I, Caillot D, Damaj G, Dauriac C, Dreyfus F, Francois S, Molina L, Tanguy ML, Chevret S, Gluckman E. Allogeneic bone marrow transplantation for therapy-related myelodysplastic syndrome and acute myeloid leukemia: a long-term study of 70 patients— report of the French society of bone marrow transplantation. J Clin Oncol 2000; 18: 963–971.

35. Castro-Malaspina H, Collins JER, Gajewski J, Harris R, Ramsay N, Deeg HJ Unrelated donor marrow transplantation for myelodysplastic syndromes (MDS). Blood 1997; 90:106a.

36. Anderson JE, Anasetti C, Appelbaum FR, Schoch G, Gooley TA, Hansen JA, Buckner CD, Sanders JE, Sullivan KM, Storb R. Unrelated donor marrow transplanation for myelodysplasia (MDS) and MDS-related acute myeloid leukaemia. Br J Haematol 1996; 93:59–67.

37. Sierra J, Carreras E, Rozman C, Champlin R, Rowlings P, Horowitz M. Bone marrow transplantation for myelodysplasia: the IBMTR data. Leuk Res 1997; 21(suppl): S51.

38. Kernan NA, Bartsch G, Ash RC, Beatty PG, Champlin R, Filipovich A, Gajewski J, Hansen JA, Henslee-Downey J, McCullough J, et al. Analysis of 462 transplantations from unrelated donors facilitated by the National Marrow Donor Program. N Engl J Med 1993; 328:593–602.

39. Dresse MF, Boogaerts M, Vermylen C, Noens L, Ferrant A, Schots R, Doyen C, Bron D, Berneman Z, Ferster A, Benoit Y, Demuynck H, Beguin Y. The belgian experience in unrelated donor bone marrow transplantation: identification of center experience as an important prognostic factor. Haematologica 1999; 84:637–642.

40. Bjerke J, Anasetti C, Gooley T, Appelbaum F, Hansen J, Anderson J, Slattery J, Storb R, Deeg HJ. Unrelated donor (URD) bone marrow transplantation (BMT) for refractory anemia (RA). Blood 1998; 92(suppl):142a.

41. Coplean EA, Penza SL, Elder PJ, Ezzone SA, Scholl MD, Bechtel TP, Belt PS, Avalos BR. Analysis of prognostic factors for allogeneic marrow transplantation following busulfan and cyclophosphamide in myelodysplastic syndrome and after leukemic transformation. Bone Marrow Transplant 2000; 25:1219–1222.

42. Anderson JE, Gooley TA, Schoch G, Anasetti C, Bensinger WI, Clift RA, Hansen JA, Sanders JE, Storb R, Appelbaum FR. Stem cell transplantation for secondary acute myeloid leukemia: evaluation of transplantation as initial therapy or following induction chemotherapy. Blood 1997; 89:2578–2585.

43. Alessandrino EP, Astori C, Van Lint MT, et al. Myelodysplastic syndrome or leukemia developing after MDS treated by allogeneic bone marrow transplantation: outcome of 90 adult patients. Leuk Res 1997; 21(suppl):S52.

44. DeWitte T, Zwaan F, Hermans J, Vernant J, Kolb H, Vossen J, Lonnqvist B, Beelen D, Ferrant A, Gmur J, et al. Allogeneic bone marrow transplantation for secondary leukaemia and myelodysplastic syndrome: a survey by the Leukaemia Working Party of the European Bone Marrow Transplantation Group (EBMTG). Br J Haematol 1990; 74:151–155.

45. Niemeyer C, Duffner U, Bender-Gotze C, Dini G, Ebell W, Egeler M, Hasle H, Heilmann C, Klingebiehl T, Kremens B, Messina C, Nurnberger W, Uderzo C, Zintl F, Zecca M, Nollke P, Locatelli F. AML-type intensive chemotherapy prior to stem cell transplantation (SCT) does not improve survival in children and adolescents with primary myelodysplastic syndromes (MDS). Blood 2000; 96(suppl):521a.

46. Clift RA, Buckner CD, Appelbaum FR, Schoch G, Petersen FB, Bensinger WI, Sanders J, Sullivan KM, Storb R, Singer J, Hansen JA, Thomas D. Allogeneic marrow transplantation during untreated first relapse of acute myeloid leukemia. J Clin Oncol 1992; 10:1723–1729.

47. Karanes C, Abella E, Du W, Klein J, Dansey R, Cassells L, Peters W, Baynes R. Allogeneic bone marrow transplantation (alloBMT) in myelodysplastic syndromes (MDS). Blood 1998; 92:659a.

48. Anderson JE, Appelbaum FR, Deeg HJ, Storb R. Phase II study of busulfan (BU) and total body irradiation (TBI) as a novel preparative regimen in allogeneic marrow transplantation (BMT) for advanced myelodysplastic syndrome. Leuk Res 1999; 23(suppl):S83.

49. Matthews DC, Appelbaum FR, Eary JF, Mitchell D, Press OW, Bernstein ID. Phase I study of [131]I-anti-CD45 antibody plus cyclophosphamide and total body irradiation for advanced acute leukemia and myelodysplastic syndrome. Blood 1997; 90(suppl): 417a.

50. Castro-Malaspina H, Childs B, Papadopoulos E, et al. T-cell depleted (SBA-E-) bone marrow transplantation for myelodysplastic syndromes. Leuk Res 1997; 21(suppl): S51.

51. O'Donnell PV, Noga SJ, Grever M, Vogelsang GB, Jones RJ. Using engineered allografts to improve transplant outcome in myelodysplastic syndrome (MDS). Blood 1997; 90(suppl):229a.

52. Giralt S, Estey E, Albitar M, van Besien K, Rondón G, Anderlini P, O'Brien S, Khouri I, Gajewski J, Mehra R, Claxton D, Andersson B, Beran M, Prezepiorka D, Koller C, Kornblau S, Körbling M, Keating M, Kantarjian H, Champlin R. Engraftment of allogeneic hematopoietic progenitor cells with purine analog-containing chemotherapy: harnessing graft-versus-leukemia without myeloablative therapy. Blood 1997; 89:4531–4536.

53. Slavin S, Nagler A, Naparstek E, Kapelushnik Y, Aker M, Cividalli G, Varadi G, Kirschbaum M, Ackerstein A, Samuel S, Amar A, Brautbar C, Ben-Tal O, Eldor A, Or R. Nonmyeloablative stem cell transplantation and cell therapy as an alternative to conventional bone marrow transplantation with lethal cytoreduction for the treatment of malignant and nonmalignant hematologic diseases. Blood 1998; 91: 756–763.

54. Parker JE, Shafi T, Mijovic A, Pagliuca A, Devereux S, Garg M, Yin JA, Potter M, Prentice HG, Byrne J, Russell NH, Mufti GJ. Allogeneic stem cell transplantation

(SCT) in MDS:interim results of outcome following non-myeloablative conditioning compared to standards preparative regimens Blood 2000; 96(suppl):554a.

55. Cao TM, McSweeney PA, Niederwieser D, Sahebi F, Sandmaier BM, Chauncey TR, Maris MB, Forman SJ, Blume KG, Shizuru JA, Storb RF. Non-myeloablative allogeneic hematopoietic cell transplantation (AHCT) for patients with myelodysplastic syndromes (MDS) and myeloproliferative disorders (MPD). Blood 2000; 96(suppl):170a.

56. Rezvani K, Lalancette M, Szydlo R, Mackinnon S, Blaise D, Slavin S, Alessandrino EP, Michallet M, Niederwieser N, Apperley J, Frassoni F. Non-myeloablative stem cell transplant (NMSCT) in AML, ALL, and MDS: Disappointing outcome for patients with advanced phase disease. Blood 2000; 96(suppl):479a.

57. Shimoni A, Khouri I, Donato M, Anderlini P, Andersson B, Ueno N, Champlin R, Giralt S. Allogeneic transplantation with non-myeloablative or reduced intensity conditioning: the intensity of the conditioning regimen is related to outcome in patients with active disease but not in those in remission at the time of transplantation. Blood 2000; 96(suppl):199a.

# 18

# Therapeutic Strategies in the Care of Patients with Myelodysplastic Syndromes

**Dragana Milojković and Ghulam J. Mufti**
*Guy's, King's, and St Thomas' School of Medicine and King's College Hospital, London, England*

## I. INTRODUCTION

The myelodysplastic syndromes (MDS) comprise a heterogenous group of clonal hematopoietic stem cell disorders characterized by progressive cytopenia and qualitative abnormalities in the erythroid, granulocytic, and megakaryocytic series, and are associated with frequent evolution to acute myeloid leukemia (AML). Augmented apoptosis, leading to ineffective hematopoiesis and peripheral cytopenias, has been observed (1), but the precise nature of the genetic lesions that lead to clonal hematopoiesis and leukemic transformation is unknown. The clonality of MDS has been confirmed by the high number of nonrandom cytogenetic abnormalities (2) and by X-chromosome inactivation analysis (3). Numerous therapeutic modalities have been instituted to eliminate the dysplastic clone or induce clonal differentiation. The identification of risk factors for disease progression and the establishment of prognostic indicators for individual patients has been invaluable in the approach to patient management.

## II. PROGNOSIS

Following the introduction of the French-American-British (FAB) Cooperative Group criteria for the diagnosis and classification of MDS in 1982 (4), some consistency in the prognostic factors related to survival has been noted in a number of large studies using the FAB subgroup morphological criteria (5–7). The disease characteristics, which can predict the natural history in an individual patient, have been documented in an effort to determine indicators for appropriate therapy. Nevertheless, it is evident that no single feature can identify the likely clinical course and outcome in an individual patient owing to the marked heterogeneity of the disease.

Consequently, a number of scoring systems have been developed, all of which provide *general* indicators of outcome, as they do not encompass the multistep nature of MDS. Most systems have involved the prognostic parameters of bone marrow blast percentage, hemoglobin concentration, platelet count, and neutrophil count (5–12). Three main categories of risk have been identified: high, intermediate, and low risk, with predicted median survival times of 4–8 months, 14–18 months, and 34–62 months, respectively. To assess outcome, scores have been based on the presence of abnormal localization of immature precursors (ALIP) (13), marrow fibrosis (12), karyotypic abnormalities (11,14), elevated lactate dehydrogenase (LDH) (10), and age. The most recently described scoring system is the International Prognostic Scoring System (IPSS) (7), which utilizes a multivariate analysis of patient characteristics derived from previous scoring systems. IPSS has improved the prognostic power considerably. Patients are placed into distinctive risk groups for median survival, of which four groups are identified: low (5.7 years), intermediate-1 (INT-1: 3.5 years), intermediate-2 (INT-2: 1.2 years), and high (0.4 years). It is therefore recommended that, where possible, management decisions be based on the patient's IPSS score in the context of the overall clinical picture.

## III. TREATMENT STRATEGIES

Although the natural history of MDS is variable, about 50% of patients die from cytopenic complications and an additional 20–30% transform to AML (15). The main therapeutic objectives are the elimination of the abnormal clone and reestablishment of polyclonal hematopoiesis, which are targeted by a variety of approaches from the induction of differentiation and intensive chemotherapy to bone marrow transplantation. However, owing to the advanced age of the majority of patients with MDS, supportive care has remained the most frequently employed therapeutic modality.

## A. Differentiation Therapy

### 1. Erythropoietin Therapy in Myelodysplastic Syndromes

More than 80% of patients with MDS are anemic at presentation (16), and 40% are transfusion-dependent. Anemia and transfusion dependency can often cause significant morbidity, with long-term blood product transfusion support complicated by a high incidence of reactions to the transfused blood products and secondary hemochromatosis (17). The need for transfusion is a sign of severe, advanced MDS and correlates with the degree of erythroid and trilineage dysplasia. Patients requiring transfusions typically have bone marrow characterized by hyperplasia plus increased apoptosis in bone marrow precursors (18). Erythroid progenitor growth is reduced, with a more marked defect of burst-forming unit-erythroid (BFU-E) compared with colony-forming unit-erythroid (CFU-E).

Erythropoietin (EPO) is a relatively late-acting factor that prevents apoptosis and sustains differentiation of erythroid precursors (19), acting mainly on CFU-E and on a portion of the late BFU-E that causes CFU-E generation (20). In anemic MDS patients, there is a wide variation in endogenous serum EPO levels (4–870 U/L), which has not been found to correlate with FAB subtype or transfusion requirement (21).

Stimulation of erythroid progenitor growth in vitro can be achieved with combinations of hematopoietic growth factors, interleukin-3 (IL-3), and EPO. Clinically, the response to EPO has been poor and continuous maintenance treatment is necessary and costly. Hence, there has been an attempt to establish clinical variables that predict response to treatment. Subcutaneously administered recombinant human erythropoietin (r-HuEPO) induces an overall response in 20–30% of MDS patients. However, a considerable therapeutic range of r-HuEPO has been employed in clinical trials evaluating this treatment modality: 30 U/kg–12,000 U/kg, three times a week (22). If successful, an erythroid response will usually occur within the first 2 months of r-HuEPO treatment.

Responsiveness to EPO therapy is increased in a rather well-defined subset of MDS patients (listed here in the relative order of effectiveness): those with no transfusion requirement, endogenous serum EPO concentrations of less than 200 U/L, normal cytogenetics, and blast count of less than 10% (23). (See Table 1.) This characterization of EPO-responsive MDS patients is supported by a meta-analysis of 205 patients from 17 studies that showed no response to EPO therapy in patients with refractory anemia with ringed sideroblasts (RARS) who had serum EPO concentrations ≥ 200 U/L (20). Interestingly, the meta-analysis also identified a group with a response rate ≥ 50%: those with no transfusion requirement and MDS other than RARS, irrespective of serum EPO concentrations (20). Other studies have shown serum EPO concentration <100 mU/mL to be predictive of response, particularly in refractory anemia (RA) patients (21); however, low endogenous EPO concentrations have not reliably predicted a response (24).

**Table 1**  Predictors of Erythroid
Response with Erythropoeitin
Therapy in Patients with
Myelodysplastic Syndromes

| Predictors of EPO responsiveness |
| --- |
| No transfusion requirement<br>Low serum EPO (<200 U/L)<br>No cytogenetic abnormality<br>Blast count < 10%<br>RA subtype<br>Absence of ringed sideroblasts<br>High bone marrow erythroid index<br>Detectable pretreatment BFU-E<br>Female sex |

RA, refractory anemia; BFU-E, burst-forming unit–erythrocyte.

Subcutaneous administration of r-HuEPO, together with granulocyte colony-stimulating factor (G-CSF), appears to produce the best erythroid response
rate, with a response frequency of 38%, which is greater than that achieved with
any previous study of EPO monotherapy. The EPO/G-CSF combination is particularly effective for patients with RARS (25) when the baseline serum EPO concentration is <500 U/L and transfusion requirements are low (<2 units/month);
the response rate achieved is 60%. It is interesting that a correlation has been
noted between elevated levels of the cytokine, tumor necrosis factor-$\alpha$ (TNF-$\alpha$),
and lack of response to EPO therapy in MDS patients. This observation likely
reflects the evidence that TNF-$\alpha$ inhibits the production of endogenous EPO,
which implicates TNF-$\alpha$ in the pathogenesis of apoptosis in MDS (24). Patients
with RA or refractory anemia with excess blasts (RAEB) may respond well to
EPO alone, but the inclusion of G-CSF provides additional benefit. Response
rates of up to 50% have been achieved, but the response disappears altogether
in some patients when G-CSF is withdrawn, implying synergism between G-CSF
and EPO (26). Pretreatment with G-CSF is not necessary for a response to the
combination treatment (27). A review of 98 MDS patients has shown that those
patients with a low transfusion need (<2 units/month) and serum EPO concentrations <100 U/L achieve a response rate of 78% (16) when treated with EPO/
G-CSF combination therapy for at least 10 weeks. In this retrospective study,
response rates for patients with RA, RARS, RAEB, and refractory anemia with
excess blasts in transformation (RAEB-t) were 27%, 45%, 38%, and 20%, respec-

tively, with a median duration of response of 11–24 months. Higher erythroid response rates have been described with prolonged combination treatment (e.g., erythroid response rate of 80% after 36 weeks) in patients with disease duration of less than 6 months (28).

Although costly, treatment with EPO/G-CSF has few side effects— namely, mild flu-like symptoms, splenomegaly, and thrombocytopenia. Perhaps the most positive outcome of the combination therapy is the observation that some patients have maintained their response for >5 years (16). Although initially of concern, G-CSF has not been found to accelerate disease progression (29); indeed, responding patients have shown a decrease in the percentage of blasts (16). However, it should be emphasized that no randomized clinical trials have been carried out comparing G-CSF and/or EPO therapy versus supportive care with respect to survival, quality of life, and leukemic transformation.

Patients with clonal cytogenetic abnormalities are more likely to have immature myelopoiesis and are therefore EPO-unresponsive. Female patients appear to have a better response than male patients (16), which could be due to a lower resting serum EPO concentration. No dose-response or time-to-response has been established for EPO therapy in MDS patients in studies described to date, which probably reflects the high degree of patient variability.

Although there is no evidence as yet that growth factor therapy prolongs survival or delays disease progression, a sufficient body of data supports these outcomes with EPO/G-CSF therapy in selected patients. It is recommended that RA and RAEB patients with no or low transfusion requirement (<2 units/month) and basal EPO concentrations <200 U/L be considered for a trial treatment period of EPO alone at a dose of 10,000 U/day for 6 weeks. For those patients who do not respond, additional daily G-CSF, with or without doubling the dose of EPO, should be considered. The dose of G-CSF should be increased weekly from 75 μg to 150 μg to 300 μg to establish a white cell count between 6-10 × $10^9$/L. When the maximum response is achieved, the G-CSF can be reduced to three times a week, and EPO reduced from 5 to 4 to 3 days a week at 4-weekly intervals. Patients with RARS and serum EPO concentrations <500 U/L requiring transfusion support should be started on EPO and G-CSF combination therapy from the outset.

Erythroid responses have not been as convincing when EPO is combined with granulocyte-monocyte colony-stimulating factor (GM-CSF). In a review of 66 MDS patients treated with EPO (150 IU/kg 3 times/week) and GM-CSF (0.3– 5.0 μg/kg/day), a hemoglobin response (increase ≥ 2 g/dl) occurred in only 9% of patients (30). Other data support the combination of GM-CSF and EPO in patients with low-risk MDS, with a reported erythroid response rate of 35% (24) to 46% (31). Similarly, Economopoulos et al. noted a good erythroid response in patients with RARS only (32). A limited erythropoietic response has also been attained following EPO combined with recombinant human IL-3, but the response is not much better than that obtained with EPO alone while significant toxicity due to IL-3 is observed (33).

## 2. Immunosuppressive Therapy

It is possible that there is a degree of immune-mediated cytopenia in MDS. Autologous T cells from MDS patients have been found to inhibit erythroid colony-forming cells (34) and granulocyte-macrophage colony formation (35). Antithymocyte globulin (ATG) therapy is known to induce the release of growth factors (36,37), causing an increase in hematopoietic progenitor cells (38). Immunosuppressive ATG therapy may also improve bone marrow function by reducing lymphocyte-mediated marrow suppression, which may occur by eliminating clonally expanded, activated T cells thereby allowing the reexpansion of the normal repertoire (37). The ability of ATG to induce a hematological response in MDS patients has been assessed clinically. Following single-cycle treatment with ATG (40 mg/kg/day $\times$ 4 days), 44% of MDS patients with <20% blasts became transfusion-independent (39). Maximal responses are observed in RA patients and in patients with a coexisting paroxysmal nocturnal hemoglobinuria (PNH) clone (40), but improvement in hematopoiesis has been additionally observed in patients with hypoplastic MDS (41). (See Table 2.)

In a multi-institutional study of 30 ATG-treated MDS patients (RA = 19; RARS = 4; RAEB = 6; childhood MDS = 1), nine (35%) showed a response (complete remission = 1; partial remission = 8). Eight of the responders had RA, and one had RARS. No responses occurred in patients with RAEB. Prior to receiving ATG therapy, 11 patients showed hypocellular bone marrows. The most important predictor of response in this study was the presence of <5% marrow blasts (42). Other studies have shown that normal cytogenetics, presence of PNH clone, and low transfusion requirement predict good responses to ATG.

**Table 2** Predictors of Hematological
Response with Antithymocyte Globulin
Immunosuppressive Therapy in Patients with
Myelodysplastic Syndromes

| Predictors of ATG responsiveness |
| --- |
| Younger age |
| Short interval between diagnosis and treatment |
| Short interval of transfusion dependence |
| RA subtype |

RA, refractory anemia.

Although responses are usually durable, in cases that relapse, further responses can be achieved by repeating the treatment using ATG derived from a species different from that which was used to induce the initial response. Principles of effectiveness of immunosuppression in subgroups of MDS are taken further by ongoing studies that include the use of purine analogs, such as fludarabine, and anti-CD52 CAMPATH-1 monoclonal antibodies.

Cyclosporine A (CSA) exerts a potent immunosuppressive effect by blocking IL-2 production, thereby inhibiting expansion of cytotoxic lymphocytes and possibly suppressing T-cell production of recognized inhibitors of hematopoiesis, such as TNF-$\alpha$ and interferons. A substantial hematological improvement (82% response rate) has been observed in CSA-treated patients with RA (43), regardless of bone marrow cellularity. Smaller studies of hypoplastic RA patients have confirmed a beneficial effect with CSA therapy (41,44).

## 3. Other Therapeutic Agents

There remain a number of treatment modalities of limited therapeutic value (45) that are not routinely recommended to induce a hematological response. (See Table 3.) Some agents, such as corticosteroids (46), may be of possible benefit, but they should be used in defined clinical research protocols only. Amifostine is a cytoprotective prodrug that is metabolized to the pharmacologically active intracellular aminothiol (47), which both protects and stimulates hematopoiesis (48). In a phase I/II study, 18 MDS patients received treatment with intravenous amifostine in escalating doses from 100 to 1,200 mg/m$^2$ (49). Single of multilineage hematological responses were observed in 83% of patients, with 78% of patients having a 50% or greater increase in absolute neutrophil count, 43% show-

**Table 3** Differentiation Therapies Not Recommended for Patients with Myelodysplastic Syndromes Because of Their Limited Therapeutic Value in Inducing Hematological Responses

| Therapeutic agents not recommended for the treatment of anemia |
| --- |
| 13-*cis* retinoic acid |
| Vitamin D3 analogs |
| All-*trans* retinoic acid |
| Interferon-$\alpha$ |
| Pentoxyfilline |
| Pyridoxine |

ing >50% increase from baseline in platelets, and 33% of transfusion-dependent patients having ≥50% reduction in transfusion needs (49). The promising results achieved from this and other studies (50) have prompted further assessment of amifostine in the form of future randomized trials.

## B. Nonintensive Chemotherapy

Patient management strategies based on low-dose chemotherapy generally involve agents for which there is insufficient evidence to support their use. (See Table 4). However, 5-azacytidine, a DNA hypomethylating agent, has produced encouraging results with respect to response rates in specific MDS patient populations. DNA hypermethylation is associated with tumor suppressor gene silencing, and hypermethylation of the cell-cycle regulator $p15^{INK4b}$ has been reported to occur in 8% of low-risk MDS cases (51), 38% of MDS cases with >10% blasts (52), and 78% of high-risk MDS/sAML cases. Reversal of aberrant $p15^{INK4b}$ methylation has been tested as a therapeutic strategy to abrogate the abnormal cell proliferation and differentiation known to occur in MDS (53). Treatment with 5-azacytidine achieves a response in 49% of MDS cases (54), whereas treatment with its deoxy relative, decitabine (5-aza-2'-deoxycytidine), a more potent inhibitor of DNA methylation, has resulted in a slightly greater rate of success (54%) in elderly subjects (55), those with advanced MDS, and those with an IPSS high-risk score (53,56). 5-Azacytidine is deserving of further evaluation for its efficacy in MDS and studies are in progress to assess whether the above-noted responses are indicative of an improved overall survival. Encouraging results have also been obtained with low-dose melphalan, an alkylating agent, in elderly patients with high-risk MDS (57,58).

### 1. Novel Therapeutic Approaches

*a. Farnesyl Transferase Inhibitors.* Most studies have concluded that MDS arises as a result of neoplastic transformation in a single pluripotent hematopoietic stem cell. The transforming ability of activated *RAS* genes has been well

**Table 4**  Nonintensive Chemotherapeutic Agents Not Recommended for Patients with Myelodysplastic Syndromes Owing to Insufficient Evidence Supporting Their Use

| Nonintensive chemotherapeutic agents not recommended for the treatment of MDS |
| --- |
| Low-dose cytosine arabinoside (Ara-C) |
| Idarubicin |
| Thioguanine |

documented (59) and *RAS* mutations are one of the most frequent genetic lesions in MDS patients, being identified in up to 33% of patients (60). In a study of 220 evaluable MDS patients, compared with patients without the *RAS* mutation, those with a mutated *RAS* allele had a significantly shorter survival (19 vs. 39 months) and a higher rate of leukemic progression (70% vs. 20%) (61). Farnesyl transferase inhibitors (FTIs) have been developed as inhibitors of RAS protein signaling. One FTI product in development, R115777, has shown antileukemic activity in a phase I trial in poor-risk acute leukemias (62). Clinical responses occurred in 29% of patients, including two complete remissions (CR), with an absence of detectable N-*RAS* gene mutations in all cases. The use of R115777 and other FTIs in MDS merits further evaluation.

*b. Antiangiogenesis Therapy.* Angiogenesis has been implicated in tumor growth, vascularity, and metastasis. The degree of tumor vascularization is thought to be a negative prognostic factor indicating aggressive disease (63). An increase in the vascularity of bone marrow biopsies and levels of plasma angiogenic factors, such as vascular endothelial growth factor (VEGF), has been found in MDS (64), suggesting a role for angiogenesis in the pathophysiology of MDS. Therapies that target angiogenesis are now emerging. One selective inhibitor of VEGF receptors, SU5416, has potent antiangiogenic activity (65) and is currently being evaluated for the treatment of MDS.

Thalidomide is also an antiangiogenic agent, and has been shown to possess specific immunomodulatory properties such as the inhibition of TNF-$\alpha$ synthesis (66). Significant hematological responses have been noted in 16 of 31 (52%) thalidomide-treated MDS patients, particularly in those with RA and RARS (67). Multicenter, phase I/II studies of thalidomide therapy for patients with low-risk MDS are in progress.

## C.  Intensive Chemotherapy

Intensive chemotherapy in MDS patients is marked by prolonged hypoplasia (postulated to be due to a fewer number of bone marrow stem cells) and subsequent mortality, low remission rates, and a short duration of remission. Indeed, patients are rarely able to tolerate more than two cycles of chemotherapy and a substantial number develop significant drug resistance (68). Therefore, there is a reluctance to treat with intensive-chemotherapy regimens until the disease has progressed to AML, although treatment at this stage results in a less successful outcome. Several studies of intensive chemotherapy for poor-prognosis MDS prior to transformation to AML have been conducted (15).

The results of combination chemotherapy have been disappointing, with short remission duration (5–15 months) (69,70), high relapse rates (44–89%) (71,72), and poor long-term survival (73). In 10 studies of intensive chemotherapy in high-risk MDS patients conducted between 1995 and 1999 (Table 5), the

**Table 5** Clinical Trials of Intensive Chemotherapy in Patients with Myelodysplastic Syndromes Conducted Between 1995 and 1999

| Study | Patient number | Regimen | Complete remission | Outcome |
|---|---|---|---|---|
| Beran et al., 1999 (71) | 59 | HD Ara-C/Topotecan | 61% | Median survival: 60 weeks |
| Estey et al., 1999 (175) | 62 | Flu/Ara-C/Ida ± G-CSF/ATRA | 51% | Median survival: 28 weeks |
| Ossenkoppele et al., 1999 (98) | 64 | Daunomycin/Ara-C ± G-CSF | 63% | 2-year overall survival: up to 29% |
| Bernasconi et al., 1998 (97) | 105 | Ida/VP/Ara-C ± G-CSF | 38% | Median overall survival: 18.7 months |
| Parker et al., 1997 (69) | 19 | Flu/Ara-C/Ida/G-CSF | 78% | 42% relapsed at median of 5 months |
| Ruutu et al., 1997 (72) | 40 | Ida/Ara-C | 58% | Median survival: 12 months |
| Wattel et al., 1997 (70) | 99 | Ara-C/anthracycline | 41% | 4-year survival: 14% |
| Bernstein et al., 1996 (76) | 33 | Ara-C/anthracycline | 79% | Median survival: 13 months |
| Economopoulos et al., 1996 (176) | 22 | Ida/Ara-C/GM-CSF | 55% | Median survival: 24 months |
| de Witte et al., 1995 (99) | 50 | Ida/Ara-C | 54% | Median survival: 14 months |

HD Ara-C, high-dose cytosine arabinoside; Flu, fludarabine; Ida, idarubicin; ATRA, all-*trans*-retinoic acid; VP, etoposide; G-CSF, granulocyte colony-stimulating factor; GM-CSF, granulocyte-macrophage colony-stimulating factor.

percentage of patients achieving CR ranged from 38% to 79%. Although CR rates have been noted to be lower than those achieved in de novo AML patients similarly treated (74) and comparable only in younger patients with RAEB-t (70,75), others have found no discernible difference in patients with RAEB, RAEB-t, or AML (76,77). These latter groups of patients, however, are not comparable as they are not representative of MDS as a whole since most patients were under the age of 65.

Although bone marrow transplantation (BMT) offers a potential cure, this procedure is available to only a small percentage of patients owing to donor availability. Thus, the search for more effective chemotherapeutic regimens for the treatment of these disorders continues. Anthracyclines, which exert their antitumor effect by DNA binding, free radical production, and topoisomerase II inhibition (78), remain the most important component in combination regimens with cytosine arabinoside (Ara-C), etoposide, and/or fludarabine in the majority of effective protocols. To date, there have been no prospective, randomized, controlled trials in MDS patients assessing the outcome following intensive chemotherapy compared with supportive care alone.

## 1. Multidrug Resistance

Overexpression of the multiple drug resistance 1 (*MDR1*) gene, which codes for the transmembrane efflux pump P-glycoprotein (Pgp), has been described in MDS patients (68,79). Indeed, the low response rate of post-MDS AML to chemotherapy has been attributed to drug-resistant disease, strengthened by the findings of increased MDR1 transcripts in this patient population (80) and the detection of Pgp in MDS compared with de novo AML (79). In AML, Pgp expression correlates with an immature blast phenotype, positivity for CD34 antigen, a poor response to chemotherapy, and short survival. Pgp expression in MDS has been studied in relation to treatment and outcome (81), with Pgp positivity rare in "low risk" MDS (RA and RARS: two of 12 cases) as opposed to "high risk" MDS [RAEB, RAEB-t, and chronic myelomonocytic leukemia (CMML): 25 of 60 cases] and MDS/AML (seven of 10 cases). A trend toward more frequent progression to AML and shortened survival was observed for Pgp-positive cases, and only 14% of Pgp-positive cases achieved CR with intensive anthracycline-Ara-C chemotherapy compared with 69% of Pgp-negative cases.

An inverse correlation has been noted between CR rates achieved with daunorubicin-cytarabine combination chemotherapy and an elevated expression of MDR1 mRNA (79). Idarubicin is reputed to be less affected by Pgp, which is associated with anthracycline resistance (82). Leukemic cell lines that express the MDR phenotype take up and retain idarubicin to a greater extent than daunorubicin (83). Idarubicin is more effective in these circumstances and is also more efficient in inhibiting clonogenic growth of these cell lines. The combination of idarubicin and continuous infusion of high-dose cytarabine has resulted in an improved CR rate in patients with AML and RAEB-t compared with historical controls (82).

## 2. Chemotherapeutic Agents and Combination Regimens

In vitro studies have shown that fludarabine is a very effective DNA synthesis terminator (84) and has a potentiating effect on Ara-C by increasing its intracellular concentration (85). The activity of fludarabine on a number of enzymes involved in DNA repair and DNA replication, such as DNA polymerases, ribonucleotide reductase, DNA gyrase, and DNA ligase, implies a role as a biochemical modulator. Pharmacokinetic studies have already shown evidence of an increased remission rate, with higher intracellular levels of the triphosphate Ara-CTP (86). In vitro cytotoxicity of Ara-C is related to Ara-CTP, which can be incorporated into nascent DNA, leading to chain termination. It is proposed that fludarabine triphosphate inhibits ribonucleoside reductase, lowering intracellular deoxyribonucleoside triphosphate pools, with subsequent increases in deoxycytidine kinase activity and accumulation of Ara-CTP. The formation of Ara-CTP after combined fludarabine and Ara-C therapy in vivo is approximately doubled (87).

Using this information, the antileukemic potency of fludarabine/Ara-C combination chemotherapy has been tested in patients with AML and MDS and shown to be effective (88). Additionally, in a study of 57 patients with high-risk MDS, who failed to achieve CR with fludarabine and high-dose Ara-C (89), the induction failure rate was lower than that in a differently treated group of patients (30% vs. 43%). A decrease in fatal infections, with a reduction in bacterial (but not fungal) infections, as a cause of induction death was noted. Interestingly, fungal infections emerged as a leading cause of infectious mortality. Although not supported in this study, fludarabine-based regimens have been associated with unusual opportunistic infections (90).

In vitro results suggest that the addition of G-CSF before, during, and after Ara-C administration can increase the chemosensitivity of AML to Ara-C (91), which has led to the incorporation of G-CSF in this regimen. The combination of G-CSF with fludarabine/Ara-C has shown a higher response rate (64% overall CR rates in AML vs. 52% in those not receiving G-CSF). If G-CSF is given prechemotherapy, the efficacy of fludarabine/Ara-C may be enhanced by the stimulation of leukemic progenitor cells into cycle (92), thereby increasing the fraction of cells in phases of the cell cycle most sensitive to cytarabine (93). G-CSF also augments the rate of active triphosphate synthesis, such as F-Ara-ATP and Ara-CTP, in circulating blasts (94), decreasing the ability of blasts to repair Ara-C-induced DNA damage and altering Ara-C pharmacokinetics.

The delivery of growth factors postchemotherapy has also been initiated to reduce hematological toxicity by stimulating regenerating hematopoiesis (95).

After completion of chemotherapy in patients with previously treated acute leukemia, G-CSF administration has been found to decrease the period of neutropenia by 1 week and consequently reduce the frequency of septicemia (96,97). In patients with poor-risk MDS, the use of G-CSF during and after induction therapy resulted in a significantly reduced neutrophil recovery time (12 days), although no effect on the incidence of CR or infection rates was noted (91,98). Bernasconi et al. have found that although postchemotherapy growth factor support increases the number of responders, it does not modify either the remission duration or overall survival (97). The studies of fludarabine/Ara-C, with or without G-CSF, have revealed that two-thirds of patients achieve CR (85,91).

In a study of 47 patients with de novo MDS treated with an anthracycline protocol, the CR rate achieved was 47% and the mortality from hypoplasia 21% (75). Following fludarabine, cytarabine, and G-CSF (FLAG) chemotherapy, 112 patients with de novo untreated AML and MDS achieved a CR rate of 63% (91). Another group of investigators reported a 78% CR rate in de novo MDS/MDS-AML (69). In an idarubicin-based protocol, a CR rate of 54% was observed in 50 patients with poor-prognosis MDS and sAML/MDS (99). FLAG/Ida is an effective cytotoxic regimen for the treatment of high-risk MDS, with minimal toxicity and rapid hematopoietic recovery.

## 3. Response to Intensive Chemotherapy

A poorer response rate among MDS patients treated with intensive chemotherapy has been observed compared with AML patients, who achieve CR rates in excess of 80%. Patients with MDS are usually older, less able to survive a prolonged period of treatment-induced cytopenia, and often have resistant disease (100). However, the heterogeneity of the MDS patients treated with chemotherapy makes it difficult to interpret most studies and make generalizations. Recently, the FAB distinctions between MDS (particularly, the RAEB and RAEB-t subtypes) and AML have been found to have little therapeutic relevance (76), with similar treatment outcomes observed in all patients (CR rate of 79% and 68%, median CR duration of 11 and 15 months, and median survival of 13 and 16 months for MDS and AML groups, respectively). Estey et al. have suggested a trend for patients with RAEB-t to have an improved event-free survival from the start of treatment compared with RAEB or AML patients (77), but no difference with respect to other outcomes.

In contrast, a higher CR rate has been observed among patients with RAEB-t (70) compared with other FAB subtypes (69% vs. 19%, respectively), and an even greater rate is observed for RAEB-t patients with a normal karyotype: 80% and a median actuarial disease-free survival of 18 months (75). A significantly shorter survival has been described for patients with RAEB (7,101). Other subgroups of MDS that achieve high CR rates and prolonged remissions are those with a large excess of marrow blasts (20–30%), peripheral blasts > 5%, and the presence of Auer rods at diagnosis (75,102). (See Table 6.)

An improved outcome is seen in patients with normal cytogenetics, particularly without the involvement of chromosome 5 or 7 (70,75,100). Karyotype has been described as being the only parameter significantly correlated with disease-free survival: median actuarial disease-free interval was 16.5 months in patients with a normal karyotype versus 4 months in patients with abnormal cytogenetics (75).

It has been shown that a sub-group of patients of younger age, with no prior chemotherapy exposure, has a more favorable response (69,70,76,103) and may achieve prolonged symptom-free survival following intensive-treatment regimens compared with older patients. Although favorable karyotypes are more common in younger patients, this characteristic alone does not account for the full impact of age on outcome. However, following treatment with intensive chemotherapy in patients younger than age 60 with poor-prognosis MDS and a diagnosis of more than 6 months' duration, age has been found to have no significant impact on CR (99).

A short interval from diagnosis to treatment (<3 months) plays an important role in the acquisition of CR and appears to influence the duration of post-chemotherapy-induced hypoplasia (69). Additionally, the rate of disease progression has been identified as the most significant predictive factor in achieving CR (104). MDS patients with rapidly progressive disease achieve CR more easily following intensive chemotherapy, and those patients diagnosed within 3 months of initiation of treatment needed fewer courses of chemotherapy to reach CR (1.1 vs. 2). At 5 years, 33% were alive, whereas those with a longer interval from diagnosis to treatment initiation (>3 months) survived less than 20 months.

MDS-related secondary AML (MDS/sAML) occurs in 20–30% of patients

**Table 6**   Factors Predictive of Responsiveness to Intensive Chemotherapy in Patients with Myelodysplastic Syndromes

| Prognostic factors for intensive chemotherapy |
| --- |
| Normal karyotype |
| RAEB-t > RAEB subtype |
| Presence of Auer rods |
| Absence of antecedent hematological disorder |
| No previous cytotoxic therapy |
| Younger age |

RAEB-t, refractory anemia with excess blasts in transformation; RAEB, refractory anemia with excess blasts.

with MDS and responds unfavorably to chemotherapy (75). In MDS/sAML, the reported CR rate following standard remission-induction therapy was on average 36%. Although a median duration of remission ranging from 7 to 25 months has been described, in most studies the duration was less than 1 year (73).

From all of these studies of intensive chemotherapy, it is apparent that chemotherapy alone is inadequate to achieve prolonged disease-free survival in most patients with MDS. Intensive chemotherapy cannot be recommended in low-risk patients, whose median survival without treatment is 11.8 years (7). In high-risk patients aged <65 years, response to remission-induction therapy can assist in determining patient eligibility for stem cell transplantation, as the outcome for nonresponding patients is very poor (105–107). Patients aged >65 years and those ineligible for stem cell transplantation should be considered for intensive chemotherapy alone. Cohort studies suggest that among high-risk MDS patients, those with RAEB-t lacking an independent adverse risk factor (e.g., karyotype, age performance status, time to diagnosis) achieve the best response to intensive "AML-type" chemotherapy (70). On this basis, intensive chemotherapy is recommended only in such RAEB-t patients. No one chemotherapy combination regimen is considered superior at this time, but most regimens incorporate Ara-C with an anthracycline (etoposide and/or fludarabine). In the remaining high-risk MDS patients, it is recommended that two courses of remission induction be delivered only if hematopoietic progenitor cell transplantation is proposed as consolidation.

## D. Allogeneic Bone Marrow Transplantation

Since MDS is characterized by an expansion of an abnormal clone of pluripotent stem cells, it is logical to attempt to eradicate the abnormal clone using myeloablative therapy and reestablish normal hematopoiesis by allogeneic bone marrow transplantation (allo-BMT) (108). It is evident that allo-BMT alone offers a potential cure for MDS, with early transplantation showing encouraging results by lowering nonrelapse mortality as well as the posttransplant relapse rate (109), leading to long-term, disease-free survival. No other treatment modalities have proven to be of benefit over supportive care, and traditional treatments are not curative as the associated median survival is 15 months after diagnosis (99,110). As MDS is rare in patients under age 50 and many younger patients lack an HLA-identical donor, data for the efficacy of BMT in these patients have been scant until 1990. Roughly 30% of younger patients with MDS/sAML will have an HLA-identical sibling donor and about 5% a one-HLA locus-mismatched, related donor (111). Several studies of allo-BMT have shown disease-free survival rates of 26–63% (Table 7), but nonrelapse mortality rates of 32–55%. Data from the International Bone Marrow Transplant Registry revealed an overall 3-year survival of 53% ± 7% in 272 patients with RA or RARS receiving matched

**Table 7**  Clinical Trials of Allogeneic Transplantation for Myelodysplastic Syndromes

| Study | Patient number | Marrow source | Regimen | Median age (range) (years) | Follow-up (median) (months) | GVHD prophylaxis | DFS (%) | Relapse (%) | TRM (NRM) |
|---|---|---|---|---|---|---|---|---|---|
| Copelan et al., 2000 (121) | 42 | HLA identical $n = 35$ 1 HLA locus mis-match $n = 3$ VUD $n = 4$ | Bu-Cy ± other | 46 (11–62) | From 1984 to 1999 | CSA + MP CSA + MTX | 35 | 21 | 36 |
| Deeg et al., 2000 (129) | 50 | HLA identical $n = 40$ HLA-nonidentical $n = 4$ VUD $n = 6$ | Cy-TBI Cy-TMI Bu-TBI Bu-Cy | 59 (55–66) | 26 | CSA + MTX Other None | OS = 44% | 22 | (40) |
| Appelbaum et al., 1998 (127) | 251 | HLA matched: 59% HLA partial match: 13% VUD: 28% | Bu-Cy Chemo-TBI | 38 | 1981–1996 | MTX/CSP | 40 | 18 | (20%) age < 20 (50%) age > 50 |
| Nevill et al., 1998 (107) | 60 | HLA identical $n = 37$ 1 HLA locus mis-match $n = 1$ VUD $n = 22$ | Bu-Cy Bu-Cy+ other Cy-TBI Cy-TBI+ other | 40 (15–55) | 70 | CSA ± MTX ± other CSA + TCD ± MP MTX ± MP | EFS = 29% | 42 | (50) |
| Runde et al., 1998 (126) | 131 | HLA identical | Chemo ± TBI | 33 (2–55) | 27 | CSA ± MTX MTX TCD: 12% | 41 | 21 | 38 |
| Ballen et al., 1997 (135) | 25 | HLA matched $n = 20$ HLA partial match $n = 3$ VUD $n = 2$ | Ara-C/Cy-TBI Cy-TBI Bu-Cy | 36 (20–54) | 36 | MTX ± CSA MTX/CSA ± other TCD FK506 | 43 | 4 | 60 |
| Mattijssen et al., 1997 (148) | 35 | HLA identical $n = 32$ 2 locus mismatch $n = 1$ VUD $n = 2$ | Cy-TBI ± Ida other | 41 (23–60) | 20 | TCD: 100% CSA | 39 | 20 | 40 |
| Anderson et al., 1996 (125) | a) 31 | (a) HLA matched $n = 23$ HLA partial match $n = 2$ VUD $n = 6$ | (a) Bu-Cy-TBI | (a) 41 (16–54) | (a) 1990–1993 | (a) MTX ± CSA ± FK506 CSA ± MP Other ± Mab | (a) 26 | (a) 19 | (a) (55) |
| | b) 44 | (b) HLA matched $n = 34$ HLA partial match $n = 8$ VUD $n = 2$ | (b) Cy-TBI | (b) 36 (1–55) | (b) 1982–1990 | (b) CSA/MTX ± MP | (b) 27 | (b) 39 | (b) (34) |

| Reference | % | HLA status | Conditioning | Age (range) | Year | GVHD prophylaxis | Survival | | |
|---|---|---|---|---|---|---|---|---|---|
| Anderson et al., 1996 (115) | a) 30<br>b) 38 | (a) HLA matched n = 17, VUD n = 13<br>(b) VUD/HLA mismatched n = 29 | (a) Bu-Cy<br>(b) Cy-TBI | (a) 29 (5–53)<br>(b) 28 | (a) 1990–1993<br>(b) 1981–1990 | (a) CSA + MTX, CSA + steroids, FK506 + MTX<br>(b) — | (a) 63<br>(b) 60 | (a) 0<br>(b) 3 | (a) (37)<br>(b) (39) |
| Sutton et al. 1996 (105) | 71 | HLA identical | Cy-TBI, Bu-Cy, Other ± TBI | 37 (5–55) | 72 | CSA ± MTX, MTX, TCD: 11%, None | EFS = 32% | 34 | 34 |
| Anderson et al., 1995 (109) | 93 | HLA matched n = 82, syngene.c n = 3, VUD n = 6 | Cy-TBI, Bu-Cy | 30 (1–60) | 73 | MTX ± CSA ± steroids | 41 | 19 | 40 |
| O'Donnell et al., 1995 (177) | 38 | HLA identical | Bu-Cy | 35 (5–55) | Up to 60 months | CSA + prednisolone | 37 | 13 | (50) |
| Anderson et al., 1993 (119) | 93 | HLA matched n = 64, Syngeneic n = 3, 1-3 HLA locus mismatch n = 20, VUD n = 6 | Cy-TBI, Bu-Cy | 30 (1–60) | 1981–1990 | MTX ± CSA ± steroids, None | 43 | 18 | 39 |
| Ratanatharathorn et al., 1993 (142) | 27 | HLA matched n = 24, VUD n = 3 | Bu-TLI, Bu-Cy, Bu-Cy-Ara-C | 33 (4–54) | 20 | CSA + MP | 63 | 4 | 33 |
| Nevill et al., 1992 (132) | 23 | HLA matched | Bu-Cy | 35 (18–55) | 27 | CSA ± MTX ± MP | 35 | 22 | 43 |
| Appelbaum et al., 1990 (116) | 59 | HLA identical n = 45, HLA partial match n = 14 | Cy-TBI/other, Bu-Cy | 29 (4–54) | 1981–1988 | MTX ± CSA, CSA/MTX/steroids, None | 47 | 14 | 40 |
| De Witte et al., 1990 (117) | 78 | HLA matched | Chemo ± TBI | 32 (mean) (2–52) | 27 | —, TCD: 28% | 45 | 23 | (32) |
| Longmore et al., 1990 (130) | 23 | HLA matched | Cy-TBI, Bu-Cy, Ara-C-Cy-TBI, BCNU-VP-Cy | 23 (3–46) | 36 | — | 43 | 17 | 39 |
| O'Donnell et al., 1987 (118) | 20 | HLA matched | Cy-TBI, Bu-Cy, Ara-C-Cy-TBI, VP-TBI, Bu-VP-TBI | 36 (4–48) | 35 | — | 35 | 20 | 45 |

GVHD, graft-versus-host disease; HLA, human leukocyte antigens; VUD, volunteer unrelated transplant; Bu, busulfan; Cy, cyclophosphamide; Ara-C, cytosine arabinoside; Ida, idarubicin; VP, etoposide; TBI, total-body irradiation; TMI, TBI (with liver and lung sheilding); TLI, total lymphoid irradiation; MTX, methotrexate; CSA, cyclosporine; MP, methylprednisolone; TCD, T-cell-depleted bone marrow; Mab, monoclonal antibody; DFS, disease-free survival; TRM, transplant-related mortality; NRM, nonrelapse mortality.

sibling allogeneic transplants between 1991 and 1997; by contrast, in 745 patients with RAEB, RAEB-t, or CMML, the 3-year probability of survival was 36% ± 4% (112). (See Fig. 1.) More recently, an analysis of 1378 transplants reported to the European Group for Blood and Marrow transplantation (EBMT) has estimated the disease-free survival and estimated relapse risk at 3 years to be 36% (for both parameters) for 885 patients transplanted with stem cells from matched siblings (113).

The status of the underlying disease is a major factor influencing disease-free survival. An increased incidence of relapse is noted with more advanced disease after allo-BMT (114); other indicators of poor prognosis following allo-BMT include RAEB-t and sAML. The very low relapse rates noted in RA patients (108,115) suggests that the neoplastic stem cell clone has not yet developed mechanisms of resistance to the myeloablative regimen and/or that any remaining clonal cells can be eliminated by the allogeneic graft-versus-MDS effect. Several studies have shown no relapse in patients with RA and RARS (115–117). However, Anderson et al. have shown that patients with RA or hypoplastic MDS have indeed relapsed, but this appears to be a rare occurrence (109). Out of 38 patients with RA, of whom 22 are disease-free survivors, only one relapse has been re-

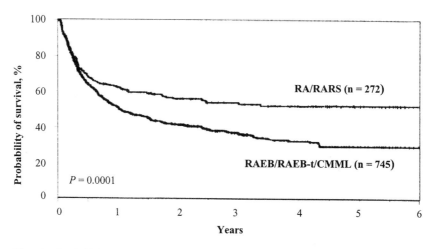

**Fig. 1** Probability of survival after 1,017 HLA-identical sibling bone marrow transplantation for myelodysplastic syndromes by French-American-British (FAB) Cooperative Group classification: 1991–1997. RA, refractory anemia; RARS, refractory anemia with ringed sideroblasts; RAEB, refractory anemia with excess blasts; RAEB-t, refractory anemia with excess blasts in transformation; CMML, chronic myelomonocytic leukemia. [From Bredeson et al., 2000 (112). Reprinted by permission, courtesy of IBMTR/ABMTR.]

ported (115). In untreated, or minimally treated RA, the relapse rate is close to zero (115) and stable RAEB has favorable results. Disease-free survival has been on the order of 60%, with procedure-related deaths approximating 30–40% (116,117). The results are more impressive among patients with RA, RARS, and RAEB (if the blast count is <10%) (116,118,119), whereas a negative correlation exists between >10% blasts and overall survival (117,118). Analysis of the EBMT has shown a 3-year disease-free survival rate of 32% for 18 patients transplanted for RAEB and 27% for 11 patients transplanted for RAEB-t (120). Actuarial relapse rates are higher among patients with excess blasts at the time of transplantation compared with those without excess blasts (49% vs. 4%, respectively), resulting in a lower disease-free survival (31% vs. 54%, respectively) (109). Late relapses occur, particularly in patients with RAEB (120). Appelbaum et al. have described a cumulative probability of relapse of 45% for patients with RAEB and RAEB-t following allo-BMT, with half the relapses occurring more than 1 year after transplantation (116).

Data presented by the EBMT show that the success of allo-BMT for MDS/sAML is closely related to disease stage. The actuarial disease-free survival rate at 2 years posttransplant for MDS patients with untreated RA, untreated RAEB, RAEB-t, and untreated sAML was 58%, 74%, 50%, and 18%, respectively (117). Similar findings have been reported by other investigators; the disease-free survival of RA patients and patients with high-risk MDS transplanted in CR was 50% and 60%, respectively, but no high-risk MDS patient transplanted during persistent disease survived (114). Those transplanted when their disease relapsed following intensive chemotherapy and those with resistant disease who underwent allo-BMT invariably had a poor prognosis, with no patient surviving more than 2 years (117).

The results of allo-BMT in MDS are more favorable in younger patients (age < 40) (109). (See Table 8.) The Seattle report (119) noted the improved overall and disease-free survival at 4 years (48% for age < 40 and 17% for age ≥ 40 at 4 years), due to a significant decrease in nonrelapse mortality at 4 years (38% for age < 40 years and 68% for age ≥ 40 at 4 years). Others have reported a disease-free survival rate of 43% among patients aged < 37, compared with 21% among patients aged 37–55 (105). Transplant-related mortality increases with age (121) owing to a decreased ability to tolerate the toxicity of therapy and to an increased incidence and severity of both acute and chronic graft-versus-host disease (GVHD) (122). In addition, an increased incidence of nonmalignant deaths is observed in the older age group (116).

Other observers have described an overall transplant-related mortality at 5 years of 50% in older patients with more advanced disease (114). A recent study following allogeneic and syngeneic marrow transplantation for MDS in 50 patients aged 55–66 showed that 44% of patients were alive at a median of 2.2 years (range: 0.7–7.1 years), with a Kaplan-Meier survival estimate of 46% and

**Table 8**  Prognostic Factors of Survival in
Allogeneic Bone Marrow Transplantation (Allo-BMT)
for Patients with Myelodysplastic Syndromes

| Factors influencing overall survival in allo-BMT |
| --- |
| Older age |
| Morphology:RAEB/RAEB-t |
| Cytogenetic analysis: high-risk cytogenetics |
| High IPSS prognostic score |
| Marrow fibrosis |
| Use of MTX in posttransplant immunosuppression |

RAEB, refractory anemia with excess blasts; RAEB-t, refractory anemia with excess blasts in transformation; IPSS, International Prognostic Scoring System; MTX, methotrexate.

a relapse-free survival estimate of 42% (123). It has also been noted that the 1- and 2-year survival rates of selected MDS patients aged > 50 who received allo-BMT were not dissimilar to those for younger patients (124). In patients with excess blasts, older age has also predicted for greater relapse (115).

A shorter disease duration is associated with improved overall survival and disease-free survival, primarily due to the decrease in nonrelapse mortality (109,115,119,125–128). (See Table 9.) The effect of disease duration on outcome has been reported to be most pronounced only in those with an interval of ≥5 years from diagnosis to transplantation (116). However, in a multivariate analysis of 70 patients transplanted for RA, where disease duration was found to be an

**Table 9**  Prognostic Factors of
Nonrelapse Mortality in Allogeneic
Bone Marrow Transplantation for
Patients with Myelodysplastic
Syndromes

| Factors increasing nonrelapse mortality in allo-BMT |
| --- |
| Prolonged disease duration |
| Donor source (mismatched donors) |
| Therapy-related MDS |
| Older age |
| Marrow fibrosis |

independent predictive variable, the 3-year actuarial survival was 65% for patients transplanted within the first year after diagnosis ($n = 40$), compared with 50% for patients receiving transplants 1 or more years after diagnosis ($n = 30$) and 30% for patients receiving transplants 5 or more years after diagnosis ($n = 10$) (115). Conversely, in an assessment of outcome following allo-BMT in older patients, superior survival rates were found in patients diagnosed with MDS more than 12 months pretransplant (129).

The degrees of marrow cellularity and marrow fibrosis have not been found to have a statistically significant impact on overall survival, disease-free survival, relapse, or nonrelapse mortality in a study of 59 allo-BMT recipients; however, of six patients with grade 3 or 4 myelofibrosis, none survived (116). Furthermore, marrow fibrosis before BMT appears to be an adverse prognostic factor according to some studies (119,130). Other investigators have shown that greater marrow cellularity pretransplant is associated with a lower risk of dying of nonrelapse causes (125).

Conflicting evidence exists for the influence of marrow cytogenetics on event-free survival post-allo-BMT in MDS. Cytogenetic factors, which strongly influence the spontaneous outcome of MDS, are not always found to influence the outcome following BMT (131). Studies have shown that patients with clonal cytogenetic abnormalities have a significantly better overall and disease-free survival than those without, the difference being due to a significantly increased incidence of nonrelapse mortality in those without cytogenetic abnormalities. However, patients with noncomplex cytogenetic abnormalities have been found to have a lower probability of relapse than those with more complex abnormalities or no abnormalities (0%, 57%, and 67%, respectively; $p < 0.02$) (116). Conversely, in a review of patients with allo-BMT in RA only, the distinction between normal and abnormal karyotype had no effect on survival (54% vs. 63% 3-year actuarial survival; $p = 0.23$) (115), but small patient numbers have limited these findings and others believe this result to be artefactual. With a larger cohort of patients and longer follow-up, cytogenetic abnormalities were no longer significantly associated with an improved outcome (119,132) and in particular those patients with high-risk cytogenetic abnormalities tended to do worse (129). (See Table 10.) In a retrospective multivariate analysis of 60 MDS and sAML patients post-allo-BMT, only the cytogenetic category was predictive of event-free survival, with poor-risk cytogenetics predictive of an unfavorable outcome (107). (See Fig. 2.) It has also been shown that the absence of cytogenetic abnormalities at the time of transplantation is associated with improved overall and disease-free survival rates, and is an independent predictor of lower nonrelapse mortality rates.

Neither patient nor donor cytomegalovirus (CMV) status has been shown to have a statistically significant influence on outcome, although survival has been suggested to be worse in CMV-seropositive patients ($p = 0.11$) (116,133). A higher white cell count at the time of transplant is associated with improved

**Table 10**  Prognostic Factors of
Relapse in Allogeneic Bone Marrow
Transplantation for Patients with
Myelodysplastic Syndromes

| Factors predictive of relapse in allo-BMT |
| --- |
| High-risk cytogenetics |
| High marrow blast % (>10%) |
| Morphology: RAEB/RAEB-t |
| Prolonged disease duration |
| Older age |
| HLA-identical donor |

RAEB, refractory anemia with excess blasts;
RAEB-t, refractory anemia with excess
blasts in transformation; HLA, human leukocyte antigens.

disease-free survival and it would appear that this is an independent predictor of improved survival (125). Interestingly, a higher neutrophil count before transplantation was found to be associated with an increased risk of death by the same group in a study of allo-BMT for RA patients (119).

Intensive chemotherapy pretransplantation has been shown to reduce relapse rates and is the favored approach of European BMT centers, particularly in advanced MDS cases (114,117,120). In contrast, other data have not confirmed these findings (105,107), and most MDS patients in North America have been transplanted without prior induction therapy (116). Indeed, MDS patients with leukemic transformation who undergo early transplantation have been observed to have a significantly better disease-free survival than those treated with prior chemotherapy (121).

To resolve the issue of BMT as first-line therapy, a retrospective analysis was undertaken to study the outcome of HLA-identical sibling BMT in 131 MDS or sAML patients <50 years of age who did not receive conventional induction treatment prior to BMT (126). The cumulative 5-year disease-free survival rate was 34%, similar to the result obtained in patients pretreated with chemotherapy (118,119,130,132). Patients without excess blasts had an excellent prognosis with a 5-year disease-free survival of 52% and relapse risk of 13%, as opposed to RAEB-t patients who achieve a 5-year disease-free survival rate of only 19%. The overall improved outcome was mainly due to a lower risk for treatment-related mortality if the transplant was performed within 3 months of diagnosis. Previously, a 2-year disease-free survival rate of 60% had been obtained for pa-

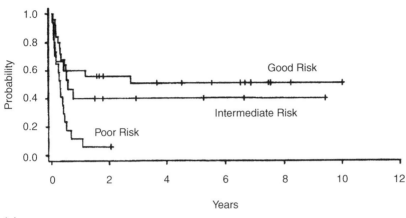

**(a)**

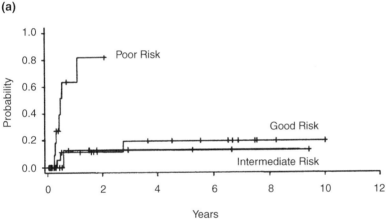

**(b)**

**Fig. 2** (a) Event-free survival after allogeneic bone marrow transplantation for patients with good- ($n$ = 25), intermediate- ($n$ = 15), and poor- ($n$ = 17) risk cytogenetics. (b) Actuarial risk of relapse after allogeneic bone marrow transplantation for patients with good- ($n$ = 25), intermediate- ($n$ =15), and poor- ($n$ = 17) risk cytogenetics. [From Nevill et al., 1998 (107). Reprinted by permission, courtesy of *Blood*.]

tients transplanted in CR after intensive chemotherapy (117). The results are less favorable for patients who have a partial response to chemotherapy (2-year disease-free survival: 18%) or those who relapse or are refractory to aggressive chemotherapy, with few surviving after allo-BMT (117). Demuynck et al. have found that out of 24 MDS patients, none of the nine high-risk patients transplanted with persistent disease survived (114).

In the assessment of disease etiology, therapy-related MDS (tMDS) secondary to chemotherapy or radiotherapy for an initial cancer diagnosis has a worse outcome (129), particularly if CR is not achieved after induction chemotherapy. Patients typically have a rapidly progressive disease with fatal outcome and their neoplastic clones usually have distinct chromosome abnormalities (134). In a univariate analysis of RA patients, survival was lower among patients whose disease was caused by prior cytotoxic therapy, compared with all other patients (20% vs. 63% for 3-year actuarial survival; $p = 0.05$) (115). Although not as successful in this setting as in primary disorders, allo-BMT remains a potential curative treatment. In a review of 70 patients with tMDS ($n = 31$) and therapy-related acute leukemia ($n = 39$), the estimated 2-year overall survival was 30% (133), a rate similar to that seen in earlier studies (106,135). (See Table 11.) Reasons for the failure of achieving long-term survival post-allo-BMT have been shown to be equally divided among relapse, interstitial pneumonia, and GVHD (116,118).

## 1. Preparative Regimens for Allogeneic Bone Marrow Transplantation in MDS

As patients with advanced disease morphology have a higher relapse rate and lower disease-free survival rate, the outcomes obtained with a more ablative preparative regimen were assessed and compared with conventional cyclophosphamide (Cy) and total body irradiation (TBI) (125). Single-agent Cy therapy has been shown to be insufficient to eradicate the malignant clone in MDS (116). A combination preparative regimen consisting of busulfan (Bu) plus Cy and TBI was chosen based on encouraging results with this regimen in patients with advanced hematological malignancies (136). The 23% 3-year actuarial disease-free survival rate for 31 RAEB and RAEB-t patients treated with Bu/Cy/TBI was not statistically significantly different from the 30% 3-year actuarial disease-free survival rate observed in 38 MDS patients treated with Cy/TBI. After correcting for differences in disease and transplant characteristics, there appeared to be a greater antileukemic effect with Bu/Cy/TBI although this benefit was offset by increased toxicity (125). Similarly, in RA patients who underwent allo-BMT, no significant difference in outcome was established for the two preparative regimens evaluated: 3-year actuarial disease-free survival rates were similar for the Cy/TBI and Bu/Cy groups (60% vs. 63%, respectively; $p = 0.9$) (115). Additionally, no difference in the relapse and nonrelapse mortality rates between the two groups was noted (115). However, other prospective, randomized trials comparing Bu/Cy with Cy/TBI have concluded that the latter regimen yields superior results (137,138).

The major distinction between preparative regimes has been the use of TBI-containing and chemotherapy-only protocols. TBI was included in most BMT-

**Table 11** Clinical Trials of Allogeneic Transplantation for Treatment-Related Myelodysplastic Syndromes

| Study | Patient number | Marrow source | Regimen | Median age (range) (years) | Follow-up | GVHD prophylaxis | DFS (%) | Relapse (%) |
|---|---|---|---|---|---|---|---|---|
| Witherspoon et al., 2001 (178) | tMDS $n$ = 55 (tAML $n$ = 56) | HLA matched $n$ = 60 Partial match $n$ = 9 VUD $n$ = 42 | Cy-TBI Bu-Cy Other | — | 1971–1999 | MTX/CSA/FK506 | (at 5 yrs): RAEB-$t$ = 18% RAEB = 17% RA = 42% | (at 5 yrs): RAEB-$t$ = 40% RAEB = 26% RA = 0% |
| Yakoub-Agha et al., 2000 (133) | tMDS $n$ = 31 (tAML) $n$ = 39 | HLA identical $n$ = 59 HLA partial match $n$ = 3 VUD $n$ = 8 | Cy-TBI Bu-Cy Other-TBI | 37 (16–55) | Median; 8 yrs | MTX ± steroids CSA ± steroids CSA/MTX Mab ± other TCD:9% | Estimated 2-yr OS: 18% | Estimated at 2 yrs: 70% |
| Anderson et al., 1997 (106) | sAML/MDS $n$ = 29 (tAML $n$ = 17) | SCT: allogeneic $n$ = 43 syngeneic $n$ = 3 | Cy-TBI Bu/other-TBI Chemotherapy alone | 41.9 (6–61) | 1994–1996 | MTX ± CSA CSA ± steroids CSA ± FK506 | 5-yr actuarial estimate: 35% | 5-yr actuarial estimate: 24% |
| Ballen et al., 1997 (135) | 18 | HLA matched $n$ = 15 HLA partial match $n$ = 1 VUD $n$ = 2 | Ara-C/Cy-TBI Bu-Cy other | 32 (14–52) | Median; 36 mths | MTX ± CSA MTX/CSA ± other TCD None | 24 | 22 |

tMDS, treatment-related MDS; tAML, treatment-related AML; sAML/MDS, secondary AML, MDS related; SCT, stem cell transplantation; Mab, monoclonal antibody; mths, months; DFS, disease-free survival; OS, overall survival; TRM, transplant-related mortality; NRM, nonrelapse mortality; Bu, busulfan; Cy, cyclophosphamide; TBI, total-body irradiation; Ara-C, cytosine arabinoside; MTX, methotrexate; CSA, cyclosporine; TCD, T-cell-depleted bone marrow.

conditioning regimens until a novel combination of oral Bu and parenteral Cy was investigated in advanced AML patients undergoing allo-BMT; the combination showed good antileukemic activity and acceptable toxicity (139). The dose of Cy was subsequently modified, which reduced toxicity (140). The Bu/Cy preparative regimen has also been investigated in MDS patients. In six major clinical studies, there was no apparent difference in the relapse rate or relapse-free survival among patients who received chemotherapy-based or TBI-based regimes (108,117–119,130,132). In some studies, the use of Bu does not appear to improve disease-free survival or the rate of relapse (132). However, in a smaller series of eight MDS patients (141), four received Bu/Cy with no relapses occurring among patients who received a Bu-based regimen, despite RAEB or RAEB-t morphology. A review of published series of transplantation for MDS (109) determined that the most favorable outcome was for those patients receiving Bu-containing regimes, in spite of a high percentage of patients with excess blasts (63% actuarial disease-free survival) (142). When Bu plasma concentrations have been targeted to 600–900 ng/ml in older MDS patients undergoing allo-BMT, greater survival has been noted in all FAB categories (123).

G-CSF has been added to a preparative regimen of Cy/TBI in an attempt to improve the chemosensitivity of leukemic cells and, consequently, transplant outcome (143). In a pilot study involving 13 advanced MDS patients thus treated, at a median follow-up of 39 months, the projected 5-year disease-free and overall survival were 67.7% and 75.5%, respectively, with only one patient showing cytogenetic relapse. A larger trial of G-CSF as a component of an allo-BMT preparative regimen is clearly warranted to evaluate its efficacy.

### 2. Posttransplant Immunosuppressive Regimens

Patients who receive less intensive GVHD prophylaxis without methotrexate (MTX) as part of a posttransplant immunosuppression regimen have a higher nonrelapse mortality rate. In a study of 31 MDS patients, those who had an HLA genotypically or phenotypically-matched donor (53%) were randomized to receive less intensive GVHD prophylaxis consisting of CSA with or without methylprednisolone (MP) (125). These patients were also at a high risk of relapse; consequently their increased incidence of GVHD could have been associated with a higher incidence of graft-versus-leukemia (see below). The remaining patients (47%) had HLA-mismatched or unrelated donors and received MTX-containing regimens. Most of the patients not given MTX (71%) died of GVHD-associated complications. In addition, there was a twofold higher nonrelapse mortality rate despite the more favorable donor type, compared with those who received CSA and MTX. These findings confirm previous reports of increased GVHD incidence associated with allo-BMT among MDS patients not treated with MTX; 40% of patients treated with CSA/MTX prophylaxis developed acute GVHD, compared with 83% of those receiving CSA/MP in a study of 23 patients of whom 22 received an HLA-matched sibling donor transplant (132).

## 3. Character of Marrow Graft

Unsatisfactory results have been reported with volunteer unrelated donor transplants (108,144); however the follow-up period has been too short to determine potential efficacy. (See Table 12.) Up to 50% treatment-related deaths have been described in protocols using volunteer unrelated donors (145). Ratanatharathorn et al. have described an increased disease-free survival rate among MDS patients receiving a genotypically matched marrow graft (142). In a study of 27 patients, those who received a genotypically matched marrow graft had a significantly better disease-free survival than patients receiving a nongenotypic marrow graft ($p = 0.2$). Kaplan-Meier analyses projected an overall disease-free survival of 56% $\pm$ 13% for patients receiving a nongenotypically matched marrow graft compared with 78% $\pm$ 10% for patients who received a genotypically matched marrow graft. Uberti et al. have found that the only feature to have a significant favorable influence on event-free survival was a marrow graft from a genotypically matched donor; the event-free survival of patients receiving a genotypic marrow graft was 76% compared with 23% for those receiving a nongenotypic marrow graft ($p = 0.02$) (108). Anderson et al. have shown that in RA patients, the use of mismatched or unrelated donor marrow was not associated with a statistically significantly worse outcome (3-year actuarial disease-free survival: 50% vs. 64% for the remaining patients) (115). In a different report reviewing MDS patients with either excess blasts or life-threatening cytopenias, Anderson et al. found the 5-year actuarial disease-free survival for recipients of a genotypically matched sibling or twin marrow to be similar to other marrow sources (39% vs. 44%; $p = 0.7$), but a trend toward greater relapse was noted in the matched versus nonmatched group (109).

Other investigators have shown less favorable results. The report from the National Marrow Donor Program of 32 unrelated donor transplants showed actuarial disease-free survival of 18% at 2 years (144). Indeed, when reviewing patients transplanted with advanced disease morphology, Anderson et al. found that transplantation with HLA genotypically identical marrow was associated with a fourfold increase in the relative risk of relapse compared with alternative related and unrelated donors (3-year actuarial risk of relapse: 57% vs. 18%, respectively) (125). The lower relapse rate among recipients of an HLA-mismatched or unrelated marrow has suggested a graft-versus-MDS effect.

The Chronic Leukaemia Working Party of the EBMT has collected data on 118 patients of median age 24 who underwent a volunteer unrelated donor transplant for the treatment of MDS or sAML between 1986 and 1996 (146). In total, the actuarial probability of survival at 2 years was 28%, relapse risk 35%,

**Table 12** Clinical Trials of Volunteer Unrelated Donor Transplantation in Myelodysplastic Syndromes

| Study | Patient number | Marrow source | Regimen | Age range (median) | Follow-up (months) | GVHD prophylaxis | DFS (%) | Relapse (%) |
|---|---|---|---|---|---|---|---|---|
| Arnold et al., 1998 (146) | 118 | Identical $n = 105$ 1/2 HLA locus mismatch $n = 13$ | Chemo ± TBI $n = 69$ Chemo ± serotherapy $n = 30$ Data unavailable $n = 19$ | 0.3–53 (24) | 24 | CSA $n = 8$ MTX $n = 2$ CSA + MTX $n = 25$ Other $n = 44$ TCD $n = 36$ Data unavailable $n = 3$ | 28 | 35 |
| Nevill et al., 1998 (107) | 22 | Identical $n = 16$ 1 HLA locus mismatch $n = 2$ Single allele mismatch $n = 4$ | Bu-Cy Bu-Cy+ other Cy-TBI Cy-TBI+ other | 40 (15–55) | 70 (median) | CSA ± MTX ± Other $n = 42$ CSA ± TCD ± MP $n = 17$ MTX ± MP $n = 1$ | EFS = 32% | 23 |
| Anderson et al., 1996 (111) | 52 | Identical $n = 34$ 1 HLA locus mismatch $n = 17$ 2 HLA locus mismatch $n = 1$ | Bu/Cy $n = 19$ Bu/Cy/TBI $n = 7$ Cy/TBI $n = 26$ | 1–53 (33) | 24 | CSA + MTX $n = 47$ FK506 + MTX $n = 5$ | 38 | 28 |

GVHD, graft-versus-host disease; DFS, disease-free survival; TRM, transplant-related mortality; NRM, nonrelapse mortality; HLA, human leukocyte antigen; TBI, total-body irradiation; Bu, busulfan; Cy, cyclophosphamide; CSA, cyclosporine; MTX, methotrexate; TCD, T-cell-depleted bone marrow; MP, methyl-prednisolone.

and treatment-related mortality 58%, which is similar to previous studies of volunteer unrelated donor transplantation (111). The transplant-related mortality was significantly influenced by the age of the recipient (81% at >35 years), and older age was significantly associated with an increased risk of death from causes other than relapse. Patients with a low blast count (i.e., RA and RAEB patients) had a lower probability of relapse (13% and 15%, respectively) compared with RAEB-t or sAML (29% and 45%, respectively). A total of 47% of evaluable patients had acute GVHD (grade II–IV), while 38% of evaluable patients developed chronic GVHD. Late mortality of patients with chronic GVHD has emphasized that longer follow-up of patients is necessary to determine durability of posttransplant volunteer unrelated donor outcome (111). The 3-year overall survival was demonstrated to be 23% ± 6% by the International Bone Marrow Transplant Registry for 314 patients receiving unrelated transplants between 1991 and 1997. (See Fig. 3.) Despite the procedural toxicity, increased risk of graft failure, and early and late complications of GVHD, volunteer unrelated donor BMT has an established role for selected MDS patients.

## 4. Graft-Versus-Leukemia Effect

The immune reactivity of allogeneic lymphocytes plays a major role in the control of leukemia after BMT. The observation that BMT is associated with an antitumor effect not explained by pretransplant chemotherapy or radiation has led to

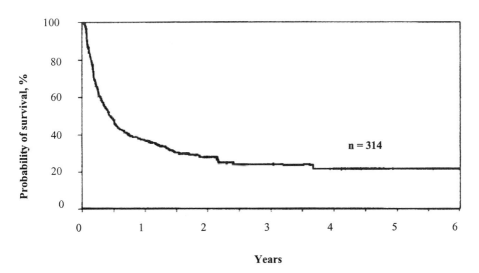

**Fig. 3**  Probability of survival after 314 unrelated bone marrow transplants for myelodysplastic syndromes: 1991–1997. (From International Bone Marrow Transplant Registry.)

the recognition of what is referred to as a graft-versus-leukemia effect. T lympho-cytes are probably responsible for GVHD and the graft-versus-leukemia effect, as depletion of T lymphocytes decreases the incidence and severity of GVHD, but increases the risk of graft failure and disease relapse (147). Following volunteer unrelated donor transplantation, patients with acute GVHD (grade II–IV) had a probability of relapse of 26%, compared with 42% for patients with either no acute GVHD or grade I GVHD (146). In previously reported MDS patient groups, the incidence of fatal GVHD was 20–35% in studies of allo-BMT without T-cell depletion, but in a study of 35 MDS patients, all of whom received lympho-cyte-depleted marrow grafts, the percentage of patients who died of GVHD was only 6% (148). An overall relapse rate of 20% was found to be similar to that in previously reported series (109), which could be explained by the intensive pretreatment the patients received.

The experience with donor leukocyte infusions in MDS is limited to a few case reports (149–152), and the results in acute leukemia have been disappointing (153). The graft-versus-leukemia effect of donor lymphocyte infusions in mar-row-grafted patients has been reviewed in a large group of patients with chronic myeloid leukemia (CML), AML, acute lymphoblastic leukemia (ALL), polycy-themia vera with osteomyelofibrosis, and MDS. Five patients with MDS who had relapsed post-BMT were treated with infusions of donor lymphocytes. CR was induced in one of four evaluable MDS patients who had not responded or who did not receive intensive chemotherapy before donor lymphocyte infusions. Donor lymphocytes were infused for consolidation of chemotherapy-induced re-mission in one patient with MDS; however, this remission was not durable. The study described a total incidence of 41% of grade II or higher GVHD (risk factors included T-cell depletion from the previous marrow graft) and a 34% occurrence of myelosuppression. The median survival for patients with AML/MDS was 248 days (154).

The concept of allogeneic stem cell transplantation with minimally myelo-suppresive conditioning therapy, which reduces the intensity of pretransplant con-ditioning balanced by increasing the level of immunosuppression to harness the graft-versus-leukemia effect, is currently reshaping thinking about transplantation (155,156). Recently, comparison between conventional allo-BMT in 26 patients and nonmyeloablative preparative regimens in 10 patients with MDS has shown that less intensive conditioning allowed for a greater median patient age (48.5 vs. 37.5 years) and did not exclude patients with preexisting organ damage (90% incidence in the nonmyeloablative group) (18). Using the FBC protocol (fludara-bine 30 mg/m$^2$ × 5, busulphan 4 mg/kg × 2, and CAMPATH-1H 20 mg × 5 with CSA/MTX GVHD prophylaxis), full donor engraftment was achieved in 100% of cases transplanted in CR. The duration of neutropenia was diminished, with a consequent reduction in supportive care. Acute GVHD (≥grade II) was observed in 30% and 64% of patients receiving nonablative and ablative protocols, respectively. At follow-up (1–13 months), 80% of patients are in continuing CR. The preliminary nature of these results needs to be addressed with longer follow-up of larger numbers of patients. The long-term consequences of low-intensity conditioning regimens, the overall incidence of GVHD, and the impact of low-dose irradiation are yet to be determined. However, the resultant low-regimen-related toxicity, rapid hematological recovery, and reduced frequency of GVHD makes minimally myelosuppressive conditioning therapy a promising effective therapy.

## 5. Summary Comments on Allogeneic BMT

Because of the variable natural history of MDS, patient selection for such an intensive therapeutic approach as BMT becomes a major issue. Patients with MDS and appropriate donors (HLA-identical sibling), particularly those aged < 40, should undergo marrow transplantation early during the disease course, before the disease progresses or induces life-threatening complications and cytopenia, which may adversely affect or prevent transplantation (119). Allogeneic transplantation with an HLA-matched, unrelated donor may be offered to younger patients (aged < 35 years) with poor-risk MDS. However, allo-BMT with minimally myelosuppressive conditioning therapy has enabled transplantation to become available to a wider group of patients, particularly older patients and those with comorbid medical conditions.

A review of the prognostic factors suggests that allo-BMT should be considered in RAEB or RAEB-t patients, those with marked cytopenia (neutrophil count $< 0.5 \times 10^9/L$ or platelet count $< 20 \times 10^9/L$), poor prognostic cytogenetic abnormalities, or a combination of these factors, as the average survival of such patients is less than 1 year. Induction of CR pretransplant, early transplantation, and blasts < 5% are associated with a lower incidence of leukemia recurrence. Hence, the policy at King's College Hospital in London is to induce remission if the marrow contains > 5% blasts or if complex cytogenetics (e.g., monosomy 7) are detected in the majority of the metaphases.

A recommended length of time from diagnosis to transplantation that would be acceptable for MDS patients is not clearly defined, but owing to the natural history of the disease it would be advisable to pursue the option of transplantation immediately after diagnosis with the knowledge that donor availability is in the order of 35–40%. It has been suggested that transplantation should be considered for patients with RA aged < 56 with an HLA-matched or unrelated donor if the following poor prognostic features are present at diagnosis: platelet count < 100,000, hemoglobin < 9 g/dl, or complex cytogenetic abnormalities; marrow blast percentage is not considered as these patients have a median survival of 3 years or less, regardless of this percentage (115), An overall long-term disease-free survival of greater than 60% is attainable for such patients with RA.

## E. Autologous Bone Marrow Transplantation

For those not eligible for allo-BMT, autologous bone marrow transplantation (ABMT) may provide an alternative therapeutic approach. The rationale behind ABMT is based on the assumption that the impressive antileukemic effect of allo-BMT was due to myeloblative therapy, although it was also recognized that part of the allogeneic effect was immunologically mediated and associated with GVHD (154). In AML, most studies have concluded that although ABMT in first CR increases relapse-free survival compared with chemotherapy alone, no increase in overall survival has been observed, effectively due to the higher mortality associated with BMT (157).

A potential disadvantage with the use of ABMT in hematological malignancies is the possibility of contamination of the harvested bone marrow by residual leukemic cells. Relapse, due to either residual host disease or reinfused malignant cells, remains a major cause of treatment failure post-ABMT. To prolong remission rates, a number of investigators have advocated bone marrow purging techniques (158), but there is only limited data suggesting that purging autografts produces any benefit with respect to relapse rates and disease-free survival. ABMT with marrow purged by mafosfamide has been assessed in seven patients with MDS in transformation after achieving CR (159). Engraftment was delayed and occurred at a median of 41 and 120 days for white cell counts $> 1 \times 10^9/$ L and platelets $> 50 \times 10^9/$L, respectively, although faster engraftment times have been reported (160). Four patients relapsed and one patient died from transplant-related toxicity; however, two patients remained alive and well at 10 and 28 months (159).

There has been limited experience with ABMT in MDS patients (161,162). In the largest study, 79 patients with MDS and MDS/sAML were assessed following ABMT in first CR (161). The 2-year survival, disease-free survival, and relapse rates were 39%, 34%, and 64%, respectively. The relapse risk was $>$ 55% for all stages and all disease categories. Patients younger than 40 years had a significantly better disease-free survival (39%) than patients older than age 40 (25%) ($p = 0.04$), owing to such factors as the duration of disease before treatment and the absence of cytogenetic abnormalities. The disease-free survival at 2 years was 28% for the cohort of 55 patients transplanted for MDS/sAML, but 51% for a matched control group transplanted for de novo AML ($p = 0.025$). Relapse rates were 69% for patients with MDS/sAML and 40% for those with de novo AML ($p = 0.007$). The higher relapse rates in the MDS/sAML group imply a higher burden of residual disease in these patients, resulting in a lower disease-free survival in comparison to similarly treated de novo AML patients. Sufficient numbers of hematopoietic stem cells are present in MDS patients to allow adequate repopulation after ABMT as demonstrated by the low treatment-related mortality rate (10%). Additional prospective studies will contribute to the identification of MDS patients who will benefit from intensive chemotherapy followed by ABMT.

## F. Peripheral Blood Stem Cell Transplantation

A significant number of patients are not eligible for ABMT owing to delayed hematopoietic recovery after intensive chemotherapy and poor marrow harvests. It has been long established that in patients in whom bone marrow harvest is excluded because of extensive bone marrow damage following prior chemotherapy and radiotherapy, peripheral blood progenitor cell harvest remains possible (162,163). Accordingly, in selected patients with high risk MDS, adequate peripheral blood stem cell (PBSC) collection appears feasible. The encouraging data obtained in AML (164) have prompted investigators to explore the role of PBSCT in MDS. This approach in high-risk MDS patients has achieved reduced transplant-related toxicity and has significantly accelerated hematopoietic reconstitution, diminishing the hazards of a prolonged period of cytopenia and the need for supportive care (165,166).

Following high-dose chemotherapy, the mobilization and harvesting of polyclonal immature hematopoietic progenitors in patients with high-risk MDS can be achieved (167,168). Using polymerase chain reaction (PCR) analysis for the human androgen receptor (HUMARA) gene to assess X chromosome inactivation, only polyclonal CD34+ stem cells have been shown in the PBSC harvests of female patients who originally presented with RAEB-t and who were subsequently treated with intensive chemotherapy in combination with growth factors, thereby restoring polyclonal myeloid hematopoiesis after high-dose chemotherapy (167). It is suggested that restoration and harvesting of a normal polyclonal stem cell compartment in MDS should occur early in the disease course, before the normal residual stem cell compartment has become completely replaced by a malignant monoclonal population. This could explain the difficulty of harvesting cells in patients with documented secondary MDS, owing to the initial slow progression of the disease (165).

In a study of 21 patients with high-risk MDS (169), PBSCs were harvested following mobilization with G-CSF alone or during the recovery phase of intensive chemotherapy combined with G-CSF. Fifteen patients achieved an adequate CD34+ progenitor yield of $>1 \times 10^6$/kg. A better yield was obtained after mobilization with growth factors alone and thought to be secondary to the longer delay after intensive chemotherapy before proceeding to the harvest. No leukemic relapse occurred during growth factor treatment. Twelve patients proceeded to PBSCT after a standard Bu/Cy regimen without growth factor support. The median time to absolute neutrophil count $> 0.5$ and $> 1.0 \times 10^9$/L was 14 days (range: 10–18) and 16 days (range: 11–25), respectively. Platelets were self-supporting at a level of $\geq 20 \times 10^9$/L after a median of 41 days (range: 8–144).

Platelet recovery has been observed to be delayed when compared with published data for PBSCT in AML (170). A higher number of progenitor cells could be necessary for platelet engraftment as it has been shown that for rapid platelet engraftment, $2.5 \times 10^6$ CD34+ cells/kg is recommended. Repopulation data after at least 100 days follow-up were compared for 10 patients receiving ABMT versus seven patients receiving PBSCT. The mean number of granulocyte-macrophage colony-forming units (CFU-GM) ($\times 10^4$/kg) reinfused in the ABMT group was 5.2 compared with 68.5 in the PBSCT group. Posttransplant leukocyte regeneration was three times as rapid in the PBSCT group. Of 10 ABMT recipients, five were still transfusion-dependent 100 days posttransplant in contrast to one of seven PBSCT patients (171).

Immune reconstitution (by assessment of the rate and pattern of recovery of total lymphocytes, T-cell subsets, B cells, and NK cells) has been compared following recovery phase PBSCT, ABMT, and allo-BMT (172). The PBSCT group had a significantly faster recovery of total lymphocyte count, total T cells (CD3+ cells), CD8+ cells, and CD4+ cells than the allogeneic group, and reconstitution following ABMT was intermediate, falling between PBSCT and allo-BMT.

In the follow-up of MDS patients post-PBSCT, early relapse (within 21 months) has been noted (166,169). The risk of PBSC tumor contamination remains a concern, particularly since returning a larger quantity of progenitor cells in PBSCT owing to the higher harvesting yield compared with conventional ABMT may increase the probability of reinfusing the malignant clone. One approach to tumor contamination has been to positively select CD34+ cells from stem cells harvested using affinity purification techniques (173). Large numbers of hematopoietic progenitor cells can be harvested, as measured by the CD34+ cells or myeloid progenitors (i.e., CFU-GM). In a study evaluating tumor cell contamination of leukapheresis prior to autologous PBSCT in AML and MDS patients, it was found that PBSC collections were not contaminated by leukemic cells if the bone marrow was disease-free (174), but this was not predictive of long-term disease-free survival. However, leukapheresis prior to autologous PBSCT is often not feasible because of the low levels of circulating CD34+ cells following G-CSF priming in MDS cases, which precludes selection.

PBSCT, therefore, may be an alternative treatment option for patients who lack an allogeneic marrow donor. In those high-risk MDS patients who possess an independent adverse risk factor, it is recommended that intensive remission-induction chemotherapy be offered only if stem cell transplantation is proposed as consolidation. Although encouraging, it is evident that the role of ASCT is yet to be clearly defined and follow-up is currently too short to establish the outcome regarding long-term cure rates. The guidelines followed at King's College in relation to chemotherapy and transplantation are summarized in Figure 4 (low-risk/INT-1 MDS patients ≤65 years of age) and Figure 5 (high-risk/INT-2

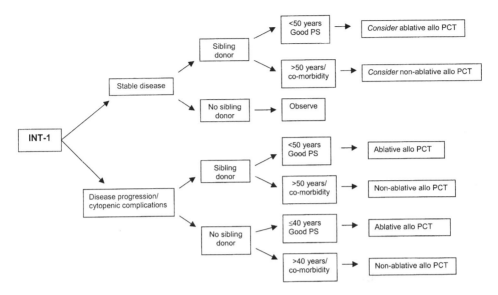

**Fig. 4** King's College Hospital (London) guidelines for the management of low/intermediate-1 (INT-1) risk MDS patients ≤ 65 years. PS, performance score; PCT, peripheral cell transplantation.

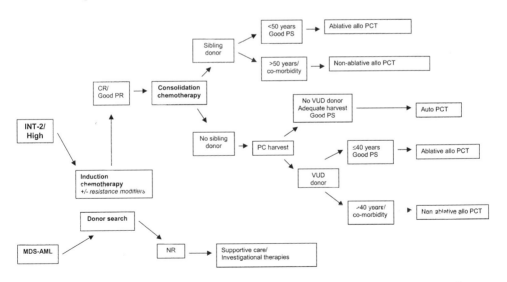

**Fig. 5** King's College Hospital (London) guidelines for the management of intermediate-2 (INT-2)/high-risk MDS and MDS-AML patients ≤ 65 years. PR, prognosis; PS, performance score; PC, peripheral cell; VUD, voluntary unrelated donor; PCT, peripheral cell transplantation; NR, no response.

MDS and MDS-AML patients ≤65 years of age). It is recognized, however, that different units may follow very different policies because of a paucity of available data and the selected patient groups referred to specialist tertiary units.

## IV. CONCLUDING REMARKS

Owing to the heterogenous nature of MDS, the development of precise, effective treatment approaches has been challenging. Refinement of prognostic indicators has proved valuable in establishing risk groups, which should also aid the direction of patient management and individualized therapy.

The mainstay of treatment remains supportive care for the majority of MDS patients. To date, only allo-BMT is effective in eradicating the malignant clone and reconstituting normal hematopoiesis; however, this is available to only a limited number of patients. Advances in PBSCT, including minimally myelosuppressive transplantation (minitransplantation), may increase the number of patients eligible for allo-BMT. Alternatively, treatment with newer cytokines, singly or in combination with growth factors, may be more effective in modifying the course of the disease and providing supportive therapy. The availability of newer differentiating agents that provide a greater trilineage response, either alone or in combination therapy, may improve the outcome, particularly in view of the advanced age of the majority of patients.

With further technological progress in gene therapy and immunotherapy, therapeutic advances at the molecular level become attainable. Appropriate clinical trials evaluating these approaches are invaluable in providing results for improvement in the treatment of patients with these disorders.

## REFERENCES

1.  Parker JE, Fishlock KL, Mijovic A, Czepulkowski B, Pagliuca A, Mufti GJ. 'Low-risk' myelodysplastic syndrome is associated with excessive apoptosis and an increased ratio of pro- versus anti-apoptotic bcl-2-related proteins. Br J Haematol 1998; 103:1075–1082.
2.  Anastasi J, Feng J, Le Beau MM, Larson RA, Rowley JD, Vardiman JW. Cytogenetic clonality in myelodysplastic syndromes studied with fluorescence in situ hybridization: lineage, response to growth factor therapy, and clone expansion. Blood 1993; 81:1580–1585.
3.  Tsukamoto N, Morita K, Maehara T, Okamoto K, Karasawa M, Omine M, Naruse T. Clonality in myelodysplastic syndromes: demonstration of pluripotent stem cell origin using X-linked restriction fragment length polymorphisms. Br J Haematol 1993; 83:589–594.
4.  Bennett JM, Catovsky D, Daniel MT, Flandrin G, Galton DA, Gralnick HR, Sultan

C. Proposals for the classification of the myelodysplastic syndromes. Br J Haematol 1982; 51:189–199.

5.  Mufti GJ, Stevens JR, Oscier DG, Hamblin TJ, Machin D. Myelodysplastic syndromes: a scoring system with prognostic significance. Br J Haematol 1985; 59: 425–433.

6.  Sanz GF, Sanz MA, Vallespi T, Canizo MC, Garcia S, Torrabadella M, San Miguel JF, Irriguible D. [Prediction of survival in myelodysplastic syndrome. Analysis of 2 scoring systems with prognostic value]. Sangre (Barc) 1989; 34:41–46 [Spanish].

7.  Greenberg P, Cox C, LeBeau MM, Fenaux P, Morel P, Sanz G, Sanz M, Vallespi T, Hamblin T, Oscier D, Ohyashiki K, Toyama K, Aul C, Mufti G, Bennett J. International scoring system for evaluating prognosis in myelodysplastic syndromes. Blood 1997; 89:2079–2088.

8.  Goasguen JE, Garand R, Bizet M, Bremond JL, Gardais J, Callat MP, Accard F, Chaperon J. Prognostic factors of myelodysplastic syndromes—a simplified 3-D scoring system. Leuk Res 1990; 14:255–262.

9.  Verhoef G, DeWolf-Peeters C, Kerim S, Van De Broeck J, Mecucci C, Van den Berghe H, Boogaerts M. Update on the prognostic implication of morphology, histology, and karyotype in primary myelodysplastic syndromes. Hematol Pathol 1991; 5:163–175.

10. Aul C, Gattermann N, Heyll A, Germing U, Derigs G, Schneider W. Primary myelodysplastic syndromes: analysis of prognostic factors in 235 patients and proposals for an improved scoring system. Leukemia 1992; 6:52–59.

11. Morel P, Hebbar M, Lai JL, Duhamel A, Preudhomme C, Wattel E, Bauters F, Fenaux P. Cytogenetic analysis has strong independent prognostic value in de novo myelodysplastic syndromes and can be incorporated in a new scoring system: a report on 408 cases. Leukemia 1993; 7:1315–1323.

12. Cunningham I, MacCallum SJ, Nicholls MD, Byth K, Hewson JW Arnold B, Motum PI, Mulligan SP, Crane GG. The myelodysplastic syndromes: an analysis of prognostic factors in 226 cases from a single institution. Br J Haematol 1995; 90: 602–606.

13. Lambertenghi-Deliliers G, Annaloro C, Soligo D, Oriani A. The diagnostic and prognostic value of bone marrow immunostaining in myelodysplastic syndromes. Leuk Lymphoma 1998; 28:231–239.

14  Pfeilstocker M, Reisner R, Nosslinger T, Gruner H, Nowotny H, Tuchler H, Schlogl E, Pittermann E, Heinz R. Cross-validation of prognostic scores in myelodysplastic syndromes on 386 patients from a single institution confirms importance of cytogenetics. Br J Haematol 1999; 106:455–463.

15. Ganser A, Hoelzer D. Clinical course of myelodysplastic syndromes. Hematol Oncol Clin North Am 1992; 6:607–618.

16. Hellstrom-Lindberg E., Negrin R, Stein R, Krantz S, Lindberg G, Vardiman J, Ost A, Greenberg P. Erythroid response to treatment with G-CSF plus erythropoietin for the anaemia of patients with myelodysplastic syndromes: proposal for a predictive model. Br J Haematol. 1997; 99:344–351.

17. Gupta P, LeRoy SC, Luikart SD, Bateman A, Morrison VA. Long-term blood product transfusion support for patients with myelodysplastic syndromes (MDS): cost analysis and complications. Leuk Res 1999; 23:953–959.

18. Parker JE, Mufti GJ, Rasool F, Mijovic A, Devereux S, Pagliuca A. The role of apoptosis, proliferation, and the Bcl-2-related proteins in the myelodysplastic syndromes and acute myeloid leukemia secondary to MDS. Blood 2000; 96:3932–3938.

19. Nijhof W, de Haan G, Pietens J, Dontje B. Mechanistic options of erythropoietin-stimulated erythropoiesis. Exp Hematol 1995; 23:369–375.

20. Hellstrom-Lindberg, E. Efficacy of erythropoietin in the myelodysplastic syndromes: a meta-analysis of 205 patients from 17 studies. Br J Haematol 1995; 89: 67–71.

21. Rose EH, Abels RI, Nelson RA, McCullough DM, Lessin L. The use of r-HuEpo in the treatment of anaemia related to myelodysplasia (MDS). Br J Haematol 1995; 89:831–837.

22. Mittelman M, Lessin LS. Clinical application of recombinant erythropoietin in myelodysplasia. Hematol Oncol Clin North Am 1994; 8:993–1009.

23. Mittelman M, Floru S, Djaldetti M. Subcutaneous erythropoietin for treatment of refractory anemia in hematologic disorders. Blood 1992; 80:841–843.

24. Stasi R, Pagano A, Terzoli E, Amadori S. Recombinant human granulocyte-macrophage colony-stimulating factor plus erythropoietin for the treatment of cytopenias in patients with myelodysplastic syndromes. Br J Haematol 1999; 105:141–148.

25. Hellstrom-Lindberg E, Birgegard G, Carlsson M, Carneskog J, Dahl IM, Dybedal I, Grimfors G, Merk K, Tangen JM, Winqvist I, et al. A combination of granulocyte colony-stimulating factor and erythropoietin may synergistically improve the anaemia in patients with myelodysplastic syndromes. Leuk Lymphoma 1993; 11:221–228.

26. Negrin RS, Stein R, Doherty K, Cornwell J, Vardiman J, Krantz S, Greenberg PL. Maintenance treatment of the anemia of myelodysplastic syndromes with recombinant human granulocyte colony-stimulating factor and erythropoietin: evidence for in vivo synergy. Blood 1996; 87:4076–4081.

27. Hellstrom-Lindberg E, Ahlgren T, Beguin Y, Carlsson M, Carneskog J, Dahl IM, Dybedal I, Grimfors G, Kanter-Lewensohn L, Linder O, Luthman M, Lofvenberg E, Nilsson-Ehle H, Samuelsson J, Tangen JM, Winqvist I, Oberg G, Osterborg A, Ost A. Treatment of anemia in myelodysplastic syndromes with granulocyte colony-stimulating factor plus erythropoietin: results from a randomized phase II study and long-term follow-up of 71 patients. Blood 1998; 92:68–75.

28. Mantovani L, Lentini G, Hentschel B, Wickramanayake PD, Loeffler M, Diehl V, Tesch H. Treatment of anaemia in myelodysplastic syndromes with prolonged administration of recombinant human granulocyte colony-stimulating factor and erythropoietin. Br J Haematol 2000; 109:367–375.

29. Negrin RS, Haeuber DH, Nagler A, Kobayashi Y, Sklar J, Donlon T, Vincent M, Greenberg PL. Maintenance treatment of patients with myelodysplastic syndromes using recombinant human granulocyte colony-stimulating factor. Blood 1990; 76: 36–43.

30. Thompson JA, Gilliland DG, Prchal JT, Bennett JM, Larholt K, Nelson RA, Rose EH, Dugan MH. Effect of recombinant human erythropoietin combined with granulocyte/macrophage colony-stimulating factor in the treatment of patients with

myelodysplastic syndrome. GM/EPO MDS Study Group. Blood 2000; 95:1175–1179.

31. Bernell P, Stenke L, Wallvik J, Hippe E, Hast R. A sequential erythropoietin and GM-CSF schedule offers clinical benefits in the treatment of anaemia in myelodysplastic syndromes. Leuk Res 1996; 20:693–699.

32. Economopoulos T, Mellou S, Papgeorgiou E, Pappa V, Kokkinou V, Stathopoulou B, Pappa M, Raptis S. Treatment of anemia in low risk myelodysplastic syndromes with granulocyte-macrophage colony-stimulating factor plus recombinant human erythropoietin. Leukemia 1999; 13:1009–1012.

33. Miller AM, Noyes WE, Taetle R, List AF. Limited erythropoietic response to combined treatment with recombinant human interleukin 3 and erythropoietin in myelodysplastic syndrome. Leuk Res 1999; 23:77–83.

34. Sugawara T, Endo K, Shishido T, Sato A, Kameoka J, Fukuhara O, Yoshinaga K, Miura A. T cell-mediated inhibition of erythropoiesis in myelodysplastic syndromes. Am J Hematol 1992; 41:304–305.

35. Smith MA, Smith JG. The occurrence subtype and significance of haemopoietic inhibitory T cells (HIT cells) in myelodysplasia: an in vitro study. Leuk Res 1991; 15:597–601.

36. Nimer SD, Golde DW, Kwan K, Lee K, Clark S, Champlin R. In vitro production of granulocyte-macrophage colony-stimulating factor in aplastic anemia: possible mechanisms of action of antithymocyte globulin. Blood 1991; 78:163–168.

37. Molldrem JJ, Jiang YZ, Stetler-Stevenson M, Mavroudis D, Hensel N, Barrett AJ. Haematological response of patients with myelodysplastic syndrome to antithymocyte globulin is associated with a loss of lymphocyte-mediated inhibition of CFU-GM and alterations in T-cell receptor Vbeta profiles. Br J Haematol 1998; 102:1314–1322.

38. Killick SB, Marsh JC, Gordon-Smith EC, Sorlin L, Gibson FM. Effects of antithymocyte globulin on bone marrow CD34+ cells in aplastic anaemia and myelodysplasia. Br J Haematol 2000; 108:582–591.

39. Molldrem JJ, Caples M, Mavroudis D, Plante M, Young NS, Barrett AJ. Antithymocyte globulin for patients with myelodysplastic syndrome. Br J Haematol 1997; 99:699–705.

40. Dunn DE, Tanawattanacharoen P, Boccuni P, Nagakura S, Green SW, Kirby MR, Kumar MS, Rosenfeld S, Young NS. Paroxysmal nocturnal hemoglobinuria cells in patients with bone marrow failure syndromes. Ann Intern Med 1999; 131:401–408.

41. Biesma DH, van den Tweel JG, Verdonck LF. Immunosuppressive therapy for hypoplastic myelodysplastic syndrome. Cancer 1997; 79:1548–1551.

42. Killick SB, Marsh JCW, Cavenagh JD, Mijovic A, Peacock J, Mufti G, Gordon-Smith EC, Bowen DT. A pilot study of antithymocyte globulin (ATG) in the treatment of patients with low risk MDS (submitted).

43. Jonasova A, Neuwirtova R, Cermak J, Vozobulova V, Mocikova K, Siskova M, Hochova I. Cyclosporin A therapy in hypoplastic MDS patients and certain refractory anaemias without hypoplastic bone marrow. Br J Haematol 1998; 100:304–309.

44. Catalano L, Selleri C, Califano C, Luciano L, Volpicelli M, Rocco S, Varriale G,

Ricci P, Rotoli B. Prolonged response to cyclosporin-A in hypoplastic refractory anemia and correlation with in vitro studies. Haematologic 2000; 85:133–138.

45. Santini V, Ferrini PR. Differentiation therapy of myelodysplastic syndromes: fact or fiction? Br J Haematol 1998; 102:1124–1138.

46. Raza A, Qawi H, Lisak L, Andric T, Dar S, Andrews C, Venugopal P, Gezer S, Gregory S, Loew J, Robin E, Rifkin S, Hsu WT, Huang RW. Patients with myelodysplastic syndromes benefit from palliative therapy with amifostine, pentoxifylline, and ciprofloxacin with or without dexamethasone. Blood 2000; 95:1580–1587.

47. List AF. Hematopoietic stimulation by amifostine and sodium phenylbutyrate: what is the potential in MDS? Leuk Res 1998; 22(suppl 1):S7-11.

48. List AF, Heaton R, Glinsmann-Gibson B, Capizzi RL. Amifostine protects primitive hematopoietic progenitors against chemotherapy cytotoxicity. Semin Oncol 1996; 23:58–63.

49. List AF, Brasfield F, Heaton R, Glinsmann-Gibson B, Crook L, Taetle R, Capizzi R. Stimulation of hematopoiesis by amifostine in patients with myelodysplastic syndrome. Blood 1997; 90:3364–3369.

50. Grossi A, Fabbri A, Santini V, Leoni F, Nozzoli C, Longo G, Pagliai G, Ciolli S, Rossi Ferrini P. Amifostine in the treatment of low-risk myelodysplastic syndromes. Haematologica 2000; 85:367–371.

51. Uchida T, Kinoshita T, Nagai H, Nakahara Y, Saito H, Hotta T, Murate T. Hypermethylation of the p15INK4B gene in myelodysplastic syndromes. Blood 1997; 90:1403–1409.

52. Quesnel B, Guillerm G, Vereecque R, Wattel E, Preudhomme C, Bauters F, Vanrumbeke M, Fenaux P. Methylation of the p15(INK4b) gene in myelodysplastic syndromes is frequent and acquired during disease progression. Blood 1998; 91: 2985–2990.

53. Wijermans P, Lubbert M, Verhoef G, Bosly A, Ravoet C, Andre M, Ferrant A. Low-dose 5-aza-2'-deoxycytidine, a DNA hypomethylating agent, for the treatment of high-risk myelodysplastic syndrome: a multicenter phase II study in elderly patients. J Clin Oncol 2000; 18:956–962.

54. Silverman LR, Holland JF, Weinberg RS, Alter BP, Davis RB, Ellison RR, Demakos EP, Cornell CJ, Carey RW, Schiffer C. Effects of treatment with 5-azacytidine on the in vivo and in vitro hematopoiesis in patients with myelodysplastic syndromes. Leukemia 1993; 7(suppl 1):21–29.

55. Wijermans PW, Krulder JW, Huijgens PC, Neve P. Continuous infusion of low-dose 5-Aza-2'-deoxycytidine in elderly patients with high-risk myelodysplastic syndrome. Leukemia 1997; 11(suppl 1):S19–S23.

56. Zagonel V, Lo Re G, Marotta G, Babare R, Sardeo G, Gattei V, De Angelis V, Monfardini S, Pinto A. 5-Aza-2'-deoxycytidine (Decitabine) induces trilineage response in unfavourable myelodysplastic syndromes. Leukemia 1993; 7(suppl 1): 30–35.

57. Omoto E, Deguchi S, Takaba S, Kojima K, Yano T, Katayama Y, Sunami K, Takeuchi M, Kimura F, Harada M, Kimura I. Low-dose melphalan for treatment of high-risk myelodysplastic syndromes. Leukemia 1996; 10:609–614.

58. Denzlinger C, Bowen D, Benz D, Gelly K, Brugger W, Kanz L. Low-dose melphalan induces favourable responses in elderly patients with high-risk myelodysplastic

syndromes or secondary acute myeloid leukaemia. Br J Haematol 2000; 108:93–95.

59. Reuter CW, Morgan MA, Bergmann L. Targeting the Ras signaling pathway: a rational, mechanism-based treatment for hematologic malignancies? Blood 2000; 96:1655–1669.

60. Yunis JJ, Boot AJ, Mayer MG, Bos JL. Mechanisms of ras mutation in myelodysplastic syndrome. Oncogene 1989; 4:609–614.

61. Paquette RL, Landaw EM, Pierre RV, Kahan J, Lubbert M, Lazcano O, Isaac G, McCormick F, Koeffler HP. N-ras mutations are associated with poor prognosis and increased risk of leukemia in myelodysplastic syndrome. Blood 1993; 82:590–599.

62. Karp JE, Lancet JE, Kaufmann SH, End DW, Wright JJ, Bol K, Horak I, Tidwell ML, Liesveld J, Kottke TJ, Ange D, Buddharaju L, Gojo I, Highsmith WE, Belly RT, Hohl RJ, Rybak ME, Thibault A, Rosenblatt J. Clinical and biologic activity of the farnesyltransferase inhibitor R115777 in adults with refractory and relapsed acute leukemias: a phase 1 clinical-laboratory correlative trial. Blood 2001; 97: 3361–3369.

63. Mendel DB, Laird AD, Smolich BD, Blake RA, Liang C, Hannah AL, Shaheen RM, Ellis LM, Weitman S, Shawver LK, Cherrington JM. Development of SU5416, a selective small molecule inhibitor of VEGF receptor tyrosine kinase activity, as an anti-angiogenesis agent. Anticancer Drug Des 2000; 15:29–41.

64. Aguayo A, Kantarjian H, Manshouri T, Gidel C, Estey E, Thomas D, Koller C, Estrov Z, O'Brien S, Keating M, Freireich E, Albitar M. Angiogenesis in acute and chronic leukemias and myelodysplastic syndromes. Blood 2000; 96:2240–2245.

65. Vajkoczy P, Menger MD, Vollmar B, Schilling L, Schmiedek P, Hirth KP, Ullrich A, Fong TA. Inhibition of tumor growth, angiogenesis, and microcirculation by the novel Flk-1 inhibitor SU5416 as assessed by intravital multi-fluorescence video-microscopy. Neoplasia 1999; 1:31–41.

66. Marriott JB, Muller G, Dalgleish AG. Thalidomide as an emerging immunotherapeutic agent. Immunol Today 1999; 20:538–540.

67. Raza A, Meyer P, Dutt D, Zorat F, Lisak L, Nascimben F, duRandt M, Kaspar C, Goldberg C, Loew J, Dar S, Gezer S, Venugopal P, Zeldis J. Thalidomide produces transfusion independence in long-standing refractory anemias of patients with myelodysplastic syndromes. Blood 2001; 98:958–965.

68. Holmes J, Jacobs A, Carter G, Janowska-Wieczorek A, Padua RA. Multidrug resistance in haemopoietic cell lines, myelodysplastic syndromes and acute myeloblastic leukaemia. Br J Haematol 1989; 72:40–44.

69. Parker JE, Pagliuca A, Mijovic A, Cullis JO, Czepulkowski B, Rassam SM, Samaratunga IR, Grace R, Gover PA, Mufti GJ. Fludarabine, cytarabine, G-CSF and idarubicin (FLAG-IDA) for the treatment of poor-risk myelodysplastic syndromes and acute myeloid leukaemia. Br J Haematol 1997; 99:939–944.

70. Wattel E, De Botton S, Luc Lai J, Preudhomme C, Lepelley P, Bauters F, Fenaux P. Long-term follow-up of de novo myelodysplastic syndromes treated with intensive chemotherapy: incidence of long-term survivors and outcome of partial responders. Br J Haematol 1997; 98:983–991.

71. Beran M, Estey E, O'Brien S, Cortes J, Koller CA, Giles FJ, Kornblau S, Andreeff M, Vey N, Pierce SR, Hayes K, Wong GC, Keating M, Kantarjian H. Topotecan and cytarabine is an active combination regimen in myelodysplastic syndromes and chronic myelomonocytic leukemia. J Clin Oncol 1999; 17:2819–2830.

72. Ruutu T, Hanninen A, Jarventie G, Koistinen P, Koivunen E, Katka K, Nousiainen T, Oksanen K, Pelliniemi TT, Remes K, Timonen T, Volin L, Elonen E. Intensive chemotherapy of poor prognosis myelodysplastic syndromes (MDS) and acute myeloid leukemia following MDS with idarubicin and cytarabine. Leuk Res 1997; 21: 133–138.

73. Hamblin TJ. Intensive chemotherapy in myelodysplastic syndromes. Blood Rev 1992; 6:215–219.

74. Hiddemann W, Jahns-Streubel G, Verbeek W, Wormann B, Haase D, Schoch C. Intensive therapy for high-risk myelodysplastic syndromes and the biological significance of karyotype abnormalities. Leuk Res 1998; 22(suppl 1):S23–S26.

75. Fenaux P, Morel P, Rose C, Lai JL, Jouet JP, Bauters F. Prognostic factors in adult de novo myelodysplastic syndromes treated by intensive chemotherapy. Br J Haematol 1991; 77:497–501.

76. Bernstein SH, Brunetto VL, Davey FR, Wurster-Hill D, Mayer RJ, Stone RM, Schiffer CA, Bloomfield CD. Acute myeloid leukemia-type chemotherapy for newly diagnosed patients without antecedent cytopenias having myelodysplastic syndrome as defined by French-American-British criteria: a Cancer and Leukemia Group B Study. J Clin Oncol 1996; 14:2486–2494.

77. Estey E, Thall P, Beran M, Kantarjian H, Pierce S, Keating M. Effect of diagnosis (refractory anemia with excess blasts, refractory anemia with excess blasts in transformation, or acute myeloid leukemia [AML]) on outcome of AML-type chemotherapy. Blood 1997; 90:2969–2977.

78. Andrivon W, Saucier JM, Auclair C, Monneret C, Florent JC, Guillosson JJ, Nafziger J. Enhanced topoisomerase II-induced DNA breaks and free radical production by a new anthracycline with potent antileukemic activity. Leuk Res 1996; 20: 119–126.

79. Marie JP, Zittoun R, Sikic BI. Multidrug resistance (mdr1) gene expression in adult acute leukemias: correlations with treatment outcome and in vitro drug sensitivity. Blood 1991; 78:586–592.

80. Sato H, Gottesman MM, Goldstein LJ, Pastan I, Block AM, Sandberg AA, Preisler HD. Expression of the multidrug resistance gene in myeloid leukemias. Leuk Res 1990; 14:11–21.

81. Lepelley P, Soenen V, Preudhomme C, Lai JL, Cosson A, Fenaux P. Expression of the multidrug resistance P-glycoprotein and its relationship to hematological characteristics and response to treatment in myelodysplastic syndromes. Leukemia 1994; 8:998–1004.

82. Estey EH, Kantarjian H, Keating M. Idarubicin plus continuous-infusion high-dose cytarabine as treatment for patients with acute myelogenous leukemia or myelodysplastic syndrome. Semin Oncol 1993; 20:1–5.

83. Berman E, McBride M. Comparative cellular pharmacology of daunorubicin and idarubicin in human multidrug-resistant leukemia cells. Blood 1992; 79:3267–3273.

84. Plunkett W, Huang P, Gandhi V. Metabolism and action of fludarabine phosphate. Semin Oncol 1990; 17:3–17.
85. Gandhi V, Estey E, Keating MJ, Plunkett W. Fludarabine potentiates metabolism of cytarabine in patients with acute myelogenous leukemia during therapy. J Clin Oncol 1993; 11:116–124.
86. Estey EH, Keating MJ, McCredie KB, Freireich EJ, Plunkett W. Cellular ara-CTP pharmacokinetics, response, and karyotype in newly diagnosed acute myelogenous leukemia. Leukemia 1990; 4:95–99.
87. Keating MJ, O'Brien S, Robertson LE, Kantarjian H, Dimopoulos M, McLaughlin P, Cabanillas F, Gregoire V, Li YY, Gandhi V, et al. The expanding role of fludarabine in hematologic malignancies. Leuk Lymphoma 1994; 14(suppl 2):11–16.
88. Estey E, Plunkett W, Gandhi V, Rios MB, Kantarjian H, Keating MJ. Fludarabine and arabinosylcytosine therapy of refractory and relapsed acute myelogenous leukemia. Leuk Lymphoma 1993; 9:343–350.
89. Anderlini P, Luna M, Kantarjian HM, O'Brien S, Pierce S, Keating MJ, Estey EH. Causes of initial remission induction failure in patients with acute myeloid leukemia and myelodysplastic syndromes. Leukemia 1996; 10:600–608.
90. Cheson BD. Infectious and immunosuppressive complications of purine analog therapy. J Clin Oncol 1995; 13:2431–2448.
91. Estey E, Thall P, Andreeff M, Beran M, Kantarjian H, O'Brien S, Escudier S, Robertson LE, Koller C, Kornblau S, et al. Use of granulocyte colony-stimulating factor before, during, and after fludarabine plus cytarabine induction therapy of newly diagnosed acute myelogenous leukemia or myelodysplastic syndromes: comparison with fludarabine plus cytarabine without granulocyte colony-stimulating factor. J Clin Oncol 1994; 12:671–678.
92. Bernell P, Kimby E, Hast R. Recombinant human granulocyte-macrophage colony-stimulating factor in combination with standard induction chemotherapy in acute myeloid leukemia evolving from myelodysplastic syndromes: a pilot study. Leukemia 1994; 8:1631–1639.
93. Tafuri A, Andreeff M. Kinetic rationale for cytokine-induced recruitment of myeloblastic leukemia followed by cycle-specific chemotherapy in vitro. Leukemia 1990; 4:826–834.
94. Gandhi V, Estey E, Du M, Nowak B, Keating MJ, Plunkett W. Modulation of the cellular metabolism of cytarabine and fludarabine by granulocyte-colony-stimulating factor during therapy of acute myelogenous leukemia. Clin Cancer Res 1995; 1:169–178.
95. Ganser A, Heil G, Kolbe K, Maschmeyer G, Fischer JT, Bergmann L, Mitrou PS, Heit W, Heimpel H, Huber C, et al. Aggressive chemotherapy combined with G-CSF and maintenance therapy with interleukin-2 for patients with advanced myelodysplastic syndrome, subacute or secondary acute myeloid leukemia—initial results. Ann. Hematol 1993; 66:123–125.
96. Ohno R, Tomonaga M, Kobayashi T, Kanamaru A, Shirakawa S, Masaoka T, Omine M, Oh H, Nomura T, Sakai Y, et al. Effect of granulocyte colony-stimulating factor after intensive induction therapy in relapsed or refractory acute leukemia. N Engl J Med 1990; 323:871–877.
97. Bernasconi C, Alessandrino EP, Bernasconi P, Bonfichi M, Lazzarino M, Canevari

A, Castelli G, Brusamolino E, Pagnucco G, Castagnola C. Randomized clinical study comparing aggressive chemotherapy with or without G-CSF support for high-risk myelodysplastic syndromes or secondary acute myeloid leukaemia evolving from MDS. Br J Haematol 1998; 102:678–683.

98. Ossenkoppele GJ, van der Holt B, Verhoef GE, Daenen SM, Verdonck LF, Sonneveld P, Wijermans PW, van der Lelie J, van Putten WL, Lowenberg B. A randomized study of granulocyte colony-stimulating factor applied during and after chemotherapy in patients with poor risk myelodysplastic syndromes: a report from the HOVON Cooperative Group. Dutch-Belgian Hemato-Oncology Cooperative Group. Leukemia 1999; 13:1207–1213.

99. de Witte T, Suciu S, Peetermans M, Fenaux P, Strijckmans P, Hayat M, Jaksic B, Selleslag D, Zittoun R, Dardenne M, et al. Intensive chemotherapy for poor prognosis myelodysplasia (MDS) and secondary acute myeloid leukemia (sAML) following MDS of more than 6 months duration. A pilot study by the Leukemia Cooperative Group of the European Organisation for Research and Treatment in Cancer (EORTC-LCG). Leukemia 1995; 9:1805–1811.

100. Fenaux P, Preudhomme C, Hebbar M. The role of intensive chemotherapy in myelodysplastic syndromes. Leuk Lymphoma 1992; 8:43–49.

101. Fenaux P, Preudhomme C, Helene Estienne M, Morel P, Lai JL, Gardin C, Jouet JP, Bauters F. de novo myelodysplastic syndromes in adults aged 50 or less. A report on 37 cases. Leuk Res 1990; 14:1053–1059.

102. Mertelsmann R, Tzvi Thaler H, To L, Gee TS, McKenzie S, Schauer P, Friedman A, Arlin Z, Cirrincione C, Clarkson B. Morphological classification, response to therapy, and survival in 263 adult patients with acute nonlymphoblastic leukemia. Blood 1980; 56:773–781.

103. Tricot G. Boogaerts MA. The role of aggressive chemotherapy in the treatment of the myelodysplastic syndromes. Br J Haematol 1986; 63:477–483.

104. Hirst WJ, Mufti GJ. The rate of disease progression predicts the quality of remissions following intensive chemotherapy for myelodysplastic syndromes. Leuk Res 1994; 18:797–804.

105. Sutton L, Chastang C, Ribaud P, Jouet JP, Kuentz M, Attal M, Reiffers J, Tigaud JM, Rio B, Dauriac C, Legros M, Dreyfus F, Lioure B, Troussard X, Milpied N, Witz F, Oriol P, Cahn JY, Michallet M, Gluckman E, Ifrah N, Pico JL, Vilmer E, Leblond V. Factors influencing outcome in de novo myelodysplastic syndromes treated by allogeneic bone marrow transplantation: a long-term study of 71 patients Societe Francaise de Greffe de Moelle. Blood 1996; 88:358–365.

106. Anderson JE, Gooley TA, Schoch G, Anasetti C, Bensinger WI, Clift RA, Hansen JA, Sanders JE, Storb R, Appelbaum FR. Stem cell transplantation for secondary acute myeloid leukemia: evaluation of transplantation as initial therapy or following induction chemotherapy. Blood 1997; 89:2578–2585.

107. Nevill TJ, Fung HC, Shepherd JD, Horsman DE, Nantel SH, Klingemann HG, Forrest DL, Toze CL, Sutherland HJ, Hogge DE, Naiman SC, Le A, Brockington DA, Barnett MJ. Cytogenetic abnormalities in primary myelodysplastic syndrome are highly predictive of outcome after allogeneic bone marrow transplantation. Blood 1998; 92:1910–1917.

108. Uberti JP, Ratanatharathorn V, Karanes C, Sensenbrenner LL. Allogeneic bone

marrow transplantation in patients with myelodysplastic syndromes. Leuk Lymphoma 1994; 14:379–385.

109. Anderson JE, Appelbaum FR, Storb R. An update on allogeneic marrow transplantation for myelodysplastic syndrome. Leuk Lymphoma 1995; 17:95–99.

110. Cheson BD. The myelodysplastic syndromes: current approaches to therapy. Ann Intern Med 1990; 112:932–941.

111. Anderson JE, Anasetti C, Appelbaum FR, Schoch G, Gooley TA, Hansen JA, Buckner CD, Sanders JE, Sullivan KM, Storb R. Unrelated donor marrow transplantation for myelodysplasia (MDS) and MDS-related acute myeloid leukaemia. Br J Haematol 1996; 93:59–67.

112. Bredeson C. Report on state of the art in blood and marrow transplantation—the IBMTR/ABMTR Summary Slides with guide. IBMTR/ABMTR newsletter (supported by an unrestricted educational grant from Sangstat Medical Corporation) 2000; 7:3–10.

113. de Witte T, Hermans J, Vossen J, Bacigalupo A, Meloni G, Jacobsen N, Ruutu T, Ljungman P, Gratwohl A, Runde V, Niederwieser D, van Biezen A, Devergie A, Cornelissen J, Jouet JP, Arnold R, Apperley J. Haematopoietic stem cell transplantation for patients with myelo-dysplastic syndromes and secondary acute myeloid leukaemias: a report on behalf of the Chronic Leukaemia Working Party of the European Group for Blood and Marrow Transplantation (EBMT). Br J Haematol 2000; 110:620–630.

114. Demuynck H, Verhoef GE, Zachee P, Emonds MP, van der Schueren E, Van den Berghe H, Vandenberghe P, Casteels-Van Daele M, Boogaerts MA. Treatment of patients with myelodysplastic syndromes with allogeneic bone marrow transplantation from genotypically HLA-identical sibling and alternative donors. Bone Marrow Transplant 1996; 17:745–751.

115. Anderson JE, Appelbaum FR, Schoch G, Gooley T, Anasetti C, Bensinger WI, Bryant E, Buckner CD, Chauncey TR, Clift RA, Doney K, Flowers M, Hansen JA, Martin PJ, Matthews DC, Sanders JE, Shulman H, Sullivan KM, Witherspoon RP, Storb R. Allogeneic marrow transplantation for refractory anemia: a comparison of two preparative regimens and analysis of prognostic factors. Blood 1996; 87:51–58.

116. Appelbaum FR, Barrall J, Storb R, Fisher LD, Schoch G, Ramberg RE, Shulman H, Anasetti C, Bearman SI, Beatty P. Bone marrow transplantation for patients with myelodysplasia. Pretreatment variables and outcome. Ann Intern Med 1990; 112:590–597.

117. De Witte T, Zwaan F, Hermans J, Vernant J, Kolb H, Vossen J, Lonnqvist B, Beelen D, Ferrant A, Gmur J, et al. Allogeneic bone marrow transplantation for secondary leukaemia and myelodysplastic syndrome: a survey by the Leukaemia Working Party of the European Bone Marrow Transplantation Group (EBMTG). Br J Haematol 1990; 74:151–155.

118. O'Donnell MR, Nademanee AP, Snyder DS, Schmidt GM, Parker PM, Bierman PJ, Fahey JL, Stein AS, Krance RA, Stock AD, et al. Bone marrow transplantation for myelodysplastic and myeloproliferative syndromes. J Clin Oncol 1987; 5:1822–1826.

119. Anderson JE, Appelbaum FR, Fisher LD, Schoch G, Shulman H, Anasetti C, Ben-

singer WI, Bryant E, Buckner CD, Doney K. Allogeneic bone marrow transplantation for 93 patients with myelodysplastic syndrome. Blood 1993; 82:677–681.

120. De Witte T, Gratwohl A. Bone marrow transplantation for myelodysplastic syndrome and secondary leukaemias. Br J Haematol 1993; 84:361–364.

121. Copelan EA, Penza SL, Elder PJ, Ezzone SA, Scholl MD, Bechtel TP, Belt PS, Avalos BR. Analysis of prognostic factors for allogeneic marrow transplantation following busulfan and cyclophosphamide in myelodysplastic syndrome and after leukemic transformation. Bone Marrow Transplant 2000; 25:1219–1222.

122. Carlens S, Ringden O, Remberger M, Lonnqvist B, Hagglund H, Klaesson S, Mattsson J, Svahn BM, Winiarski J, Ljungman P, Aschan J. Risk factors for chronic graft-versus-host disease after bone marrow transplantation: a retrospective single centre analysis. Bone Marrow Transplant 1998; 22:755–761.

123. Deeg HJ, Shulman HM, Anderson JE, Bryant EM, Gooley TA, Slattery JT, Anasetti C, Fefer A, Storb R, Appelbaum FR. Allogeneic and syngeneic marrow transplantation for myelodysplastic syndrome in patients 55 to 66 years of age. Blood 2000; 95:1188–1194.

124. Du W, Dansey R, Abella EM, Baynes R, Peters WP, Klein J, Akhtar L, Cherednikova L, Karanes C. Successful allogeneic bone marrow transplantation in selected patients over 50 years of age—a single institution's experience. Bone Marrow Transplant 1998; 21:1043–1047.

125. Anderson JE, Appelbaum FR, Schoch G, Gooley T, Anasetti C, Bensinger WI, Bryant E, Buckner CD, Chauncey T, Clift RA, et al. Allogeneic marrow transplantation for myelodysplastic syndrome with advanced disease morphology: a phase II study of busulfan, cyclophosphamide, and total-body irradiation and analysis of prognostic factors. J Clin Oncol 1996; 14:220–226.

126. Runde V, de Witte T, Arnold R, Gratwohl A, Hermans J, van Biezen A, Niederwieser D, Labopin M, Walter-Noel MP, Bacigalupo A, Jacobsen N, Ljungman P, Carreras E, Kolb HJ, Aul C, Apperley J. Bone marrow transplantation from HLA-identical siblings as first-line treatment in patients with myelodysplastic syndromes: early transplantation is associated with improved outcome. Chronic Leukemia Working Party of the European Group for Blood and Marrow Transplantation. Bone Marrow Transplant 1998; 21:255–261.

127. Appelbaum FR, Anderson J. Bone marrow transplantation for myelodysplasia in adults and children: when and who? Leuk Res 1998; 22(suppl 1):S35–S39.

128. Witherspoon RP, Deeg HJ. Allogeneic bone marrow transplantation for secondary leukemia or myelodysplasia. Haematologica 1999; 84:1085–1087.

129. Deeg HJ, Appelbaum FR. Hematopoietic stem cell transplantation in patients with myelodysplastic syndrome. Leuk Res 2000; 24:653–663.

130. Longmore G, Guinan EC, Weinstein HJ, Gelber RD, Rappeport JM, Antin JH. Bone marrow transplantation for myelodysplasia and secondary acute nonlymphoblastic leukemia. J Clin Oncol 1990; 8:1707–1714.

131. Sutton L, Leblond V, Ribaud P, Jouet JP. Indications and timing of allogeneic bone marrow transplantation in myelodysplastic syndromes. Leuk Lymphoma 1997; 27: 475–485.

132. Nevill TJ, Shepherd JD, Reece DE, Barnett MJ, Nantel SH, Klingemann HG, Phillips GL. Treatment of myelodysplastic syndrome with busulfancyclophosphamide

conditioning followed by allogeneic BMT. Bone Marrow Transplant 1992; 10:445–450.

133. Yakoub-Agha I, de La Salmoniere P, Ribaud P, Sutton L, Wattel E, Kuentz M, Jouet JP, Marit G, Milpied N, Deconinck E, Gratecos N, Leporrier M, Chabbert I, Caillot D, Damaj G, Dauriac C, Dreyfus F, Francois S, Molina L, Tanguy ML, Chevret S, Gluckman E. Allogeneic bone marrow transplantation for therapy-related myelodysplastic syndrome and acute myeloid leukemia: a long-term study of 70 patients-report of the French society of bone marrow transplantation. J Clin Oncol 2000; 18:963–971.

134. Pedersen-Bjergaard J, Philip P, Larsen SO, Jensen G, Byrsting K. Chromosome aberrations and prognostic factors in therapy-related myelodysplasia and acute non-lymphocytic leukemia. Blood 1990; 76:1083–1091.

135. Ballen KK, Gilliland DG, Guinan EC, Hsieh CC, Parsons SK, Rimm IJ, Ferrara JL, Bierer BE, Weinstein HJ, Antin JH. Bone marrow transplantation for therapy-related myelodysplasia: comparison with primary myelodysplasia. Bone Marrow Transplant 1997; 20:737–743.

136. Petersen FB, Buckner CD, Appelbaum FR, Clift RA, Sanders JE, Bensinger WI, Storb R, Witherspoon RP, Sullivan KM, Bearman SI, et al. Busulfan, cyclophosphamide and fractionated total body irradiation as a preparatory regimen for marrow transplantation in patients with advanced hematological malignancies: a phase I study. Bone Marrow Transplant 1989; 4:617–623.

137. Ringden O, Ruutu T, Remberger M, Nikoskelainen J, Volin L, Vindelov L, Parkkali T, Lenhoff S, Sallerfors B, Ljungman P. A randomized trial comparing busulfan with total body irradiation as conditioning in allogeneic marrow transplant recipients with leukemia: a report from the Nordic Bone Marrow Transplantation Group. Blood 1994; 83:2723–2730.

138. Blaise D, Maraninchi D, Archimbaud E, Reiffers J, Devergie A, Jouet JP, Milpied N, Attal M, Michallet M, Ifrah N. Allogeneic bone marrow transplantation for acute myeloid leukemia in first remission: a randomized trial of a busulfan-Cytoxan versus Cytoxan-total body irradiation as preparative regimen: a report from the Group d'Etudes de la Greffe de Moelle Osseuse. Blood 1992; 79:2578–2582.

139. Santos GW, Tutschka PJ, Brookmeyer R, Saral R, Beschorner WE, Bias WB, Braine HG, Burns WH, Elfenbein GJ, Kaizer H, et al. Marrow transplantation for acute nonlymphocytic leukemia after treatment with busulfan and cyclophosphamide. N Engl J Med 1983; 309:1347–1353.

140. Tutschka PJ, Copelan EA, Klein JP. Bone marrow transplantation for leukemia following a new busulfan and cyclophosphamide regimen. Blood 1987; 70:1382–1388.

141. Belanger R, Gyger M, Perreault C, Bonny Y, St-Louis J. Bone marrow transplantation for myelodysplastic syndromes. Br J Haematol 1988; 69:29–33.

142. Ratanatharathorn V, Karanes C, Uberti J, Lum LG, de Planque MM, Schultz KR, Cronin S, Dan ME, Mohamed A, Hussein M. Busulfan-based regimens and allogeneic bone marrow transplantation in patients with myelodysplastic syndromes. Blood 1993; 81:2194–2199.

143. Okamoto S, Takahashi S, Wakui M, Ishida A, Tanosaki R, Ikeda Y, Asano S. Treatment of advanced myelodysplastic syndrome with a regimen including recom-

binant human granulocyte colony-stimulating factor preceding allogeneic bone marrow transplantation. Br J Haematol 1999; 104:569–573.

144. Kernan NA, Bartsch G, Ash RC, Beatty PG, Champlin R, Filipovich A, Gajewski J, Hansen JA, Henslee-Downey J, McCullough J, et al. Analysis of 462 transplantations from unrelated donors facilitated by the National Marrow Donor Program. N Engl J Med 1993; 328:593–602.

145. Gajewski JL, Ho WG, Feig SA, Hunt L, Kaufman N, Champlin RE. Bone marrow transplantation using unrelated donors for patients with advanced leukemia or bone marrow failure. Transplantation 1990; 50:244–249.

146. Arnold R, De Witte T, van Biezen A, Hermans J, Jacobsen N, Runde V, Gratwohl A, Apperley JF. Unrelated bone marrow transplantation in patients with myelodysplastic syndromes and secondary acute myeloid leukemia: an EBMT survey. European Blood and Marrow Transplantation Group. Bone Marrow Transplant 1998; 21:1213–1216.

147. Horowitz MM, Gale RP, Sondel PM, Goldman JM, Kersey J, Kolb HJ, Rimm AA, Ringden O, Rozman C, Speck B, et al. Graft-versus-leukemia reactions after bone marrow transplantation. Blood 1990; 75:555–562.

148. Mattijssen V, Schattenberg A, Schaap N, Preijers F, De Witte T. Outcome of allogeneic bone marrow transplantation with lymphocyte-depleted marrow grafts in adult patients with myelodysplastic syndromes. Bone Marrow Transplant 1997; 19:791–794.

149. Tsuzuki M, Maruyama F, Kojima H, Ezaki K, Hirano M. Donor buffy coat infusions for a patient with myelodysplastic syndrome who relapsed following allogeneic bone marrow transplantation. Bone Marrow Transplant 1995; 16:487–489.

150. Bressoud A, Chapuis B, Roux E, Cabrol C, Jeannet M, Roosnek E, Helg C. Donor lymphocyte infusion for a patient with relapsing myelodysplastic syndrome after allogeneic bone marrow transplantation. Blood 1996; 88:1902–1903.

151. Okumura H, Takamatsu H, Yoshida T. Donor leucocyte transfusions for relapse in myelodyplastic syndrome after allogeneic bone marrow transplantation. Br J Haematol 1996; 93:386–388.

152. Castagna L, El Weshi A, Bourhis JH, Ribrag V, Naccache P, Vantelon JM, Brault P, Pico JL. Successful donor lymphocyte infusion (DLI) in a patient with myelodysplastic syndrome (MDS) after failure of T-cell-depleted bone marrow transplantation (TD-BMT). Br J Haematol 1998; 103:284–285.

153. MacKinnon S. Who may benefit from donor leucocyte infusions after allogeneic stem cell transplantation? (review). Br J Haematol 2000; 110:12–17.

154. Kolb HJ, Schattenberg A, Goldman JM, Hertenstein B, Jacobsen N, Arcese W, Ljungman P, Ferrant A, Verdonck L, Niederwieser D, et al. Graft-versus-leukemia effect of donor lymphocyte transfusions in marrow grafted patients. European Group for Blood and Marrow Transplantation Working Party Chronic Leukemia. Blood 1995; 86:2041–2050.

155. Slavin S, Nagler A, Naparstek E, Kapelushnik Y, Aker M, Cividalli G, Varadi G, Kirschbaum M, Ackerstein A, Samuel S, Amar A, Brautbar C, Ben-Tal O, Eldor A, Or R. Nonmyeloablative stem cell transplantation and cell therapy as an alternative to conventional bone marrow transplantation with lethal cytoreduction for the

treatment of malignant and nonmalignant hematologic diseases. Blood 1998; 91: 756–763.

156. Milojkovic D, Mufti GJ. Extending the role of allogeneic stem-cell transplantation. Lancet 2001; 357:652–654.

157. Zittoun RA, Mandelli F, Willemze R, de Witte T, Labar B, Resegotti L, Leoni F, Damasio E, Visani G, Papa G, et al. Autologous or allogeneic bone marrow transplantation compared with intensive chemotherapy in acute myelogenous leukemia. European Organization for Research and Treatment of Cancer (EORTC) and the Gruppo Italiano Malattie Ematologiche Maligne dell'Adulto (GIMEMA) Leukemia Cooperative Groups. N Engl J Med 1995; 332:217–223.

158. Bensinger WI. Should we purge? Bone Marrow Transplant 1998; 21:113–115.

159. Laporte JP, Isnard F, Lesage S, Fenaux P, Douay L, Lopez M, Stachowiak J, Najman A, Gorin NC. Autologous bone marrow transplantation with marrow purged by mafosfamide in seven patients with myelodysplastic syndromes in transformation (AML-MDS): a pilot study. Leukemia 1993; 7:2030–2033.

160. Bishop MR, Jackson JD, Tarantolo SR, O'Kane-Murphy B, Iversen PL, Bayever E, Joshi SM, Sharp JG, Pierson JL, Warkentin PI, Armitage JO, Kessinger A. Ex vivo treatment of bone marrow with phosphorothioate oligonucleotide OL(1)p53 for autologous transplantation in acute myelogenous leukemia and myelodysplastic syndrome. J.Hematother 1997; 6:441–446.

161. De Witte T, Van Biezen A, Hermans J, Labopin M, Runde V, Or R, Meloni G, Mauri SB, Carella A, Apperley J, Gratwohl A, Laporte JP. Autologous bone marrow transplantation for patients with myelodysplastic syndrome (MDS) or acute myeloid leukemia following MDS. Chronic and Acute Leukemia Working Parties of the European Group for Blood and Marrow Transplantation. Blood 1997; 90: 3853–3857.

162. Wattel E, Solary E, Leleu X, Dreyfus F, Brion A, Jouet JP, Hoang-Ngoc L, Maloisel F, Guerci A, Rochant H, Gratecos N, Casassus P, Janvier M, Brice P, Lepelley P, Fenaux P. A prospective study of autologous bone marrow or peripheral blood stem cell transplantation after intensive chemotherapy in myelodysplastic syndromes. Groupe Francais des Myelodysplasies. Group Ouest-Est d'etude des Leucemies aigues myeloides. Leukemia 1999; 13:524–529.

163. Kessinger A, Armitage JO, Landmark JD, Smith DM, Weisenburger DD. Autologous peripheral hematopoietic stem cell transplantation restores hematopoietic function following marrow ablative therapy. Blood 1988; 71:723–727.

164. Vellenga E, van Putten WL, Boogaerts MA, Daenen SM, Verhoef GE, Hagenbeek A, Jonkhoff AR, Huijgens PC, Verdonck LF, van der Lelie J, Schouten HC, Gmur J, Wijermans P, Gratwohl A, Hess U, Fey MF, Lowenberg B. Peripheral blood stem cell transplantation as an alternative to autologous marrow transplantation in the treatment of acute myeloid leukemia? Bone Marrow Transplant 1999; 23:1279–1282.

165. Demuynck H, Delforge M, Verhoef GE, Zachee P, Vandenberghe P, Van den Berghe H, Boogaerts MA. Feasibility of peripheral blood progenitor cell harvest and transplantation in patients with poor-risk myelodysplastic syndromes. Br J Haematol 1996; 92:351–359.

166.  Russell JA, Larratt L, Brown C, Turner AR, Chaudhry A, Booth K, Woodman RC, Wolff J, Valentine K, Stewart D, Ruether JD, Ruether BA, Klassen J, Jones AR, Gyonyor E, Egeler M, Dunsmore J, Desai S, Coppes MJ, Bowen T, Anderson R, Poon MC. Allogeneic blood stem cell and bone marrow transplantation for acute myelogenous leukemia and myelodysplasia: influence of stem cell source on outcome. Bone Marrow Transplant 1999; 24:1177–1183.

167.  Delforge M, Demuynck H, Vandenberghe P, Verhoef G, Zachee P, van Dupper V, Marijnen P, Van den Berghe H, Boogaerts MA. Polyclonal primitive hematopoietic progenitors can be detected in mobilized peripheral blood from patients with high-risk myelodysplastic syndromes. Blood 1995; 86:3660–3667.

168.  Carella AM, Dejana A, Lerma E, Podesta M, Benvenuto F, Chimirri F, Parodi C, Sessarego M, Eprencipe F, Frassoni F. In vivo mobilization of karyotypically normal peripheral blood progenitor cells in high-risk MDS, secondary or therapy-related acute myelogenous leukaemia. Br J Haematol 1996; 95:127–130.

169.  Boogaerts MA. Stem cell transplantation and intensified cytotoxic treatment for myelodysplasia. Curr Opin Hematol 1998; 5:465–471.

170.  Sanz MA, de la Rubia J, Sanz GF, Martin G, Martinez J, Jarque I, Sempere A, Gomis F, Senent L, Soler MA et al. Busulfan plus cyclophosphamide followed by autologous blood stem-cell transplantation for patients with acute myeloblastic leukemia in first complete remission: a report from a single institution. J Clin Oncol 1993; 11:1661–1667.

171.  Boogaerts MA, Verhoef GE, Demuynck H. Treatment and prognostic factors in myelodysplastic syndromes. Baillieres Clin Haematol 1996; 9:161–183.

172.  Roberts MM, To LB, Gillis D, Mundy J, Rawling C, Ng K, Juttner CA. Immune reconstitution following peripheral blood stem cell transplantation, autologous bone marrow transplantation and allogeneic bone marrow transplantation. Bone Marrow Transplant 1993; 12:469–475.

173.  Henschler R, Brugger W, Luft T, Frey T, Mertelsmann R, Kanz L. Maintenance of transplantation potential in ex vivo expanded CD34(+)-selected human peripheral blood progenitor cells. Blood 1994; 84:2898–2903.

174.  Testoni N, Lemoli RM, Martinelli G, Carboni C, Pelliconi S, Ottaviani E, Ruggeri D, Rizzi S, Motta MR, Visani G, Tura S. Autologous peripheral blood stem cell transplantation in acute myeloblastic leukaemia and myelodysplastic syndrome patients: evaluation of tumour cell contamination of leukaphereses by cytogenetic and molecular methods. Bone Marrow Transplant 1998; 22:1065–1070.

175.  Estey EH, Thall PF, Pierce S, Cortes J, Beran M, Kantarjian H, Keating MJ, Andreef M, Freireich E. Randomized phase II study of fludarabine + cytosinde arabinoside + indarubicin +/− all-trans retinoic acid +/− granulocyte colony-stimulating factor in poor prognosis newly diagnosed acute myeloid leukemia and myelodysplastic syndrome. Blood 1999; 93:2478–2484.

176.  Economopoulos T, Papageorgiou E, Stathakis N, Constantinidou M, Parharidou A, Kostourou A, Dervenoulas J, Raptis S. Treatment of high risk myelodysplastic syndromes with idarubicin and cytosine arabinoside supported by granulocyte-macrophage colony-stimulating factor (GM-CSF). Leuk Res 1996; 20:385–390.

177.  O'Donnell MR, Long GD, Parker PM, Niland J, Nademanee A, Amylon M, Chao N, Negrin RS, Schmidt GM, Slovak ML, et al. Busulfan/cyclophosphamide as con-

ditioning regimen for allogeneic bone marrow transplantation for myelodysplasia. J Clin Oncol 1995; 13:2973–2979.

178.  Witherspoon RP, Deeg HJ, Storer B, Anasetti C, Storb R, Appelbaum FR. Hematopoietic stem-cell transplantation for treatment-related leukemia or myelodysplasia. J Clin Oncol 2001; 19:2134–2141.

# Index

ABC transporters, 266–272
acantholysis, 68
S-adenosyl-methionine, 315
African Americans, 32
age
  and anemia, in MDS, 350–351
  and chemotherapy, 362, 422, 424,
    478
  and dysplasia, 16
  hypocellular marrow, 126–127,
    131–132
  and immunosuppressive therapy,
    384
  as incidence factor, 17, 20, 32,
    203, 299
  and marrow transplant, 422, 450–
    451, 453, 457, 483–484,
    493
  and P-glycoprotein, 276
  prognostic value, 7, 8–9, 209,
    233, 424

[age]
  and stem cell transplant, 426,
    427–428
  trends, 203
  *See also* children
alcohol, 23, 35, 47
ALIPs (blast clusters), 216
alkaloids, indole, 277
alkylating agents
  AML marrow, 141
  case report, 148
  in children, 317
  dose response, 145
  mechanism, 144
  for primary cancers, 153, 155
  and *RAS,* 144
  specific agents, 40, 145
  summary, 142
allergic granulomatosis, 67
*ALL1* gene, 106–107
alloimmunization, 352